ESSENTIAL CLINICAL ANATOMY

Second Edition

ESSENTIAL CLINICAL ANATOMY

Second Edition

Keith L. Moore, MSC, PhD, FIAC, FRSM

Professor Emeritus, Division of Anatomy, Department of Surgery
Faculty of Medicine, University of Toronto
Toronto, Ontario, Canada
and former Professor and Head of Anatomy, University of Manitoba
and Professor and Chair of Anatomy, University of Toronto

Anne M.R. Agur, BSC(OT), MSC, PhD

Associate Professor, Divisions of Anatomy and Biomedical
    Communications
Department of Surgery, and Departments of Physical and Occupational
    Therapy
Faculty of Medicine, University of Toronto
Toronto, Ontario, Canada

With the assistance and dedication of
Valerie Oxorn, BA, MA, MSC, BMC
Marion Moore, BA

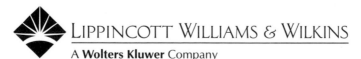

LIPPINCOTT WILLIAMS & WILKINS
A **Wolters Kluwer** Company
Philadelphia • Baltimore • New York • London
Buenos Aires • Hong Kong • Sydney • Tokyo

Editor: Betty Sun
Managing Editor: Dana Battaglia
Marketing Manager: Aimee Sirmon
Senior Production Editor: Karen M. Ruppert
Designer: Armen Kojoyian
Compositor: Graphic World
Printer: Quebecor

The publisher is not responsible (as a matter of product liability, negligence, or otherwise) for any injury resulting from any material contained herein. This publication contains information relating to general principles of medical care that should not be construed as specific instructions for individual patients. Manufacturers' product information and package inserts should be reviewed for current information, including contraindications, dosages, and precautions.

Printed in the United States of America
First Edition, 1995

Library of Congress Cataloging-in-Publication Data

Moore, Keith L.
    Essential clinical anatomy / Keith L. Moore, Anne M.R. Agur ; with the assistance and dedication of Valerie Oxorn, Marion Moore.— 2nd ed.
       p. ; cm.
    Compilation of material extracted from: Clinically oriented anatomy / Keith L. Moore. 4th ed. and Grant's atlas of anatomy / Anne M.R. Agur. 10th ed.
    Includes bibliographical references and index.
    ISBN 0-7817-2830-4
    1. Human anatomy. 2. Human anatomy—Atlases. I. Agur, A. M. R. II. Moore, Keith L. Clinically oriented anatomy. III. Agur, A. M. R. Grant's atlas of anatomy. IV. Title.
    [DNLM: 1. Anatomy—Handbooks. QS 39 M822e 2002]
    QM23.2 .M673 2002
    611—dc21

               2001050697

The publishers have made every effort to trace the copyright holders for borrowed material. If they have inadvertently overlooked any, they will be pleased to make the necessary arrangements at the first opportunity.

To purchase additional copies of this book, call our customer service department at **(800) 638-3030** or fax orders to **(301) 824-7390.** International customers should call **(301) 714-2324.**

Visit Lippincott Williams & Wilkins on the Internet: http://www.LWW.com. Lippincott Williams & Wilkins customer service representatives are available from 8:30 am to 6:00 pm, EST.

02 03 04 05 06
1 2 3 4 5 6 7 8 9 10

Preface to Second Edition

The first edition of *Essential Clinical Anatomy* (1995) evolved from a perceived need for a concise yet thorough textbook of clinical anatomy that would give students approaching anatomy for the first time—especially medical students and those in the allied health sciences—some guidance concerning the amount of anatomy they are expected to know. The growing endorsement of *Essential Clinical Anatomy* indicates that the book is filling a need for many students. Some use the book as their primary source of clinical anatomy and use its parent, *Clinically Oriented Anatomy*, by the same senior author and Dr. Arthur Dalley, as a reference.

The text of this edition has been completely revised, keeping in mind comments received from students, colleagues, and reviewers. *A main aim of the book is to provide a well-illustrated text with an appropriate amount of anatomical material in a readable and interesting form.* We received strong suggestions from most users for slightly more information—descriptive and illustrative material. Chapter 1, *Introduction to Clinical Anatomy,* has been expanded by adding more explanatory material and several new illustrations. Similar changes have been made to other chapters; more diagnostic images have been added. The "blue boxes" containing clinical material have been expanded somewhat to illustrate the practical importance of correlating preclinical and clinical subjects.

The terminology conforms with the International Anatomical Terminology—*Terminologia Anatomica* (TA)—approved in 1998 by the International Federation of Anatomists. Commonly used other terms appear in parenthesis—e.g., sternal angle (angle of Louis)—so that all users will understand what structures are being described.

We welcome your comments and suggestions for improvements in the next edition of this book.

Keith L. Moore
Anne M.R. Agur

Preface to First Edition

It is clear that many students and practitioners in the health care professions and related disciplines require a compact yet thorough textbook of clinical anatomy. The parent of this book, *Clinically Oriented Anatomy* (COA), by the senior author, is recommended as a resource for more complete and detailed descriptions of human anatomy and its relationship and importance to medicine and surgery.

Essential Clinical Anatomy is an overview of the important aspects of anatomy described in COA. The number of structures described is limited to those deemed likely to be important to the practitioner. Furthermore, the structures receive an amount of attention that is roughly proportionate to their importance. Presentations are brief and

- Provide a basic text of human anatomy for use in current health sciences curricula
- Present an appropriate amount of anatomical material in a readable and interesting form
- Provide a concise clinically oriented anatomical reference for clinical courses in subsequent years
- Serve as a rapid review when preparing for examinations, particularly the national boards
- Offer enough information for those wishing to refresh their knowledge of anatomy

Essential Clinical Anatomy is a concise text with a strong clinical orientation and many descriptive figures and tables. Most illustrations are in full color and are designed to highlight important facts and show their relationship to clinical medicine and surgery. Some illustrations are from *Grant's Atlas,* by the junior author; others are from COA. Current diagnostic imaging techniques (radiographs, CTs, and MRIs) are also included to demonstrate anatomy as it is often viewed clinically. Interspersed in blue boxes and white boxes with blue borders are clinical comments that relate anatomy to clinical practice. They are introduced with the intention of illustrating the importance of correlating preclinical and clinical subjects.

Surface anatomy is emphasized because the examination of every patient involves applied knowledge of this approach to the study of anatomy. Bony and other anatomical landmarks are used as points of reference during physical examinations and for surgical approaches to internal organs. The fundamental aim of surface anatomy is visualization of the structures that lie beneath the skin. Surface anatomy information is presented in white boxes headed with a pink bar.

The terminology conforms with the sixth edition of *Nomina Anatomica* (1989). To facilitate communication, unofficial widely used alternative terms appear in parentheses [e.g., uterine tube (Fallopian tube), omental bursa (lesser sac), and rectouterine pouch (pouch of Douglas)]. Many terms are anglicized for those who prefer not to use Latin terms [e.g., deep brachial artery (profundus brachii artery) and hip bone (os coxae)].

We welcome your comments and suggestions for improvements in the next edition.

Keith L. Moore
Anne M.R. Agur

Acknowledgments

We again thank the medical artist, *Kam Yu,* who prepared the superb new color illustrations for the first edition of *Essential Clinical Anatomy.* Similar excellent artistic skills are displayed in this edition by *Valerie Oxorn.* She prepared all new illustrations for this edition. Other illustrations from the fourth edition of *Clinically Oriented Anatomy* and the tenth edition of *Grant's Atlas* were prepared by Angela Cluer, Nina Kilpatrick, Stephen Mader, David Mazierski, Sari O'Sullivan, Bart Vallecoccia, and J/B Woolsey Associates.

The publisher gratefully acknowledges the expert contribution of Dr. Ming Jee Lee, Senior Tutor in Clinical Anatomy and Cell Biology, Biomedical Communications, Faculty of Medicine, University of Toronto, in the preparation of many of the drawings in this work.

The authors are also indebted to all those who made constructive criticisms, especially Dr. Arthur Dalley, Professor, Department of Cell Biology at Vanderbilt University School of Anatomy in Nashville, TN; Dr. Thomas H. Quinn, Professor of Anatomy and Surgery, Creighton University School of Medicine in Omaha, NE; and Dr. Lois Newman, Honorary Associate Professor of Anatomy, Department of Anatomy, Pathology, and Cell Biology, Jefferson Medical College in Philadelphia, PA.

Many people—some unknowingly—helped us by perusing parts of the manuscript and/or providing constructive criticisms of the text and illustrations in the first edition:

- *Dr. Peter Abrahams,* Clinical Anatomist, Girton College, Cambridge, England
- *Dr. Robert D. Acland,* Professor of Surgery/Microsurgery, Division of Plastic and Reconstructive Surgery, Department of Surgery, University of Louisville, Louisville, KY
- *Dr. Helen L. Block,* Attending Physician, Emergency Department, Long Island Jewish Medical Center, Forest Hills, NY
- *Dr. Stephen W. Carmichael,* Professor and Chair, Department of Anatomy, Mayo Clinic/Mayo Foundation/Mayo Medical School, Rochester, MN
- *Dr. James D. Collins,* Professor of Radiological Sciences, University of California, Los Angeles School of Medicine/Center for Health Sciences, Los Angeles, CA
- *Dr. Ralph Ger,* Professor of Anatomy and Structural Biology, Albert Einstein College of Medicine; Professor of Surgery, State University of New York at Stony Brook; Associate Chairman, Department of Surgery, Nassau County Medical Centre, Great Neck, NY
- *Dr. Duane E. Haines,* Professor and Chairman, Department of Anatomy, University of Mississippi Medical Center, Jackson, MS
- *Dr. Todd R. Olson,* Professor of Anatomy and Structural Biology, Albert Einstein College of Medicine, Bronx, NY
- *Dr. Tamiko Sato,* Associate Professor of Cell Biology and Anatomy, New York Medical College, Valhalla, NY
- *Professor Phillip V. Tobias,* Department of Anatomy and Human Biology, University of Witwatersrand, Johannesburg, Republic of South Africa
- *Professor Colin P. Wendell-Smith,* Department of Anatomy and Physiology, University of Tasmania, Tasmania, Australia

We wish to thank the editorial and production team at Lippincott Williams & Wilkins, especially Susan Katz, Vice President, Medical Education and Health Professions; Nancy Evans, Editorial Director; Dana Battaglia, Managing Editor; Kathleen Scogna, Senior Developmental Editor; Jonathan Dimes, Art Director; Lisa Donohoe, Developmental Editor; and Loftin Paul Montgomery, Jr., Editorial Assistant, who made our work on this edition a pleasurable experience.

Keith L. Moore
Anne M.R. Agur

Contents

1 Introduction to Clinical Anatomy

*E*ssential Clinical Anatomy relates the structure and function of the body to what is commonly required in the general practice of medicine, dentistry, and the allied health sciences. Because the number of details in anatomy overwhelms many beginning stu- dents, *Essential Clinical Anatomy* simplifies, correlates, and integrates the information so that understanding may be achieved. The *clinical correlation boxes* (blue boxes) illustrate clinical applications of anatomy.

1

APPROACHES TO STUDYING ANATOMY

There are three main approaches to studying anatomy: systemic, regional, and surface anatomy.

- **Systemic anatomy** is an approach to anatomical study organized by *organ systems,* such as the cardiovascular system, emphasizing an overview of the system throughout the body.
- **Regional anatomy** is an approach to anatomical study based on regions, parts, or divisions of the body, such as the abdomen, emphasizing the relationships of various systemic structures (e.g., muscles, nerves, and arteries) within the region, part, or division of the body (Fig. 1.1).
- **Clinical anatomy** is an approach to anatomical study based on regions and/or systems, emphasizing the practical application of anatomical knowledge to the solution of clinical problems, and/or

the application of clinical observations to expand anatomical knowledge.

Surface anatomy—the study of the living body at rest and in action—is used in the three main approaches to studying anatomy. Surface anatomy describes the configuration of the surface of the body, especially its relationship to deeper parts such as bones and muscles. *The physical examination of patients is a clinical extension of surface anatomy.* A main aim of surface anatomy is the visualization of structures that lie under the skin. In people with stab wounds, for example, the physician has to visualize deep structures that might be injured.

SYSTEMS OF BODY

In this introductory chapter, the systemic approach to the study of anatomy is used. In subsequent chapters, the clinical and regional approaches to the study of anatomy are used

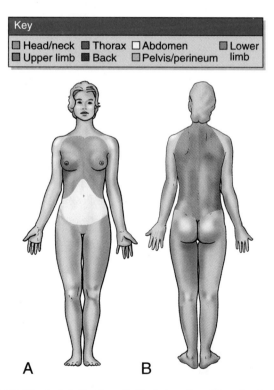

Key

☐ Head/neck ■ Thorax ☐ Abdomen   ■ Lower
■ Upper limb ■ Back   ☐ Pelvis/perineum   limb

A   B

FIGURE 1.1   Regions of body. A. Anterior view. **B.** Posterior view. All anatomical descriptions are based on the assumption that the person is standing in the anatomical position illustrated here.

because dissections and surgical procedures are performed region by region and not system by system. Brief descriptions of the systems of the body and their branches of study (in parentheses) follow:

- The **integumentary system** (dermatology) consists of the skin (integument) and its appendages such as the hair and nails. The skin, an extensive sensory organ, forms a protective covering for the body.
- The **skeletal system** (osteology) consists of bones and cartilage. It provides support for the body and protects vital organs; the ribs and sternum protect the heart and lungs for example. The muscular system acts on the skeletal system to produce movement.
- The **articular system** (arthrology) consists of joints and their associated ligaments. It connects the bony parts of the skeletal system and provides the sites at which movements occur. Thus, much of the skeletal, articular, and muscular systems constitute the *locomotor system*. They work together to produce *locomotion* — changes in posture or position as well as movement from place to place. The structures involved in locomotion are the muscles, bones, joints, and ligaments, as well as the arteries, veins, and nerves that supply oxygen and nutrients to them, remove waste from them, and stimulate them to act.
- The **muscular system** (myology) is composed of muscles that contract to move parts of the body, especially the bones that articulate at joints.
- The **nervous system** (neurology) consists of the *central nervous system* (brain and spinal cord) and the *peripheral nervous system* (cranial and spinal nerves, together with their motor and sensory endings). *The nervous system responds to the environment and internal conditions and* stimulates the appropriate response. It also controls and coordinates the functions of the various systems.
- The **circulatory system** (angiology) consists of the cardiovascular and lymphatic systems, which function in parallel to distribute fluids within the body. The **cardiovascular system** consists

of the heart and blood vessels that propel and conduct blood through the body. The **lymphatic system** is a network of lymphatic vessels that withdraws excess extracellular fluid (lymph) from the body's interstitial (intercellular) fluid compartment, filters it through lymph nodes, and returns it to the bloodstream.

- The **alimentary system** or digestive system (gastroenterology) is composed of the organs associated with the ingestion, mastication (chewing), deglutition (swallowing), digestion, absorption of nutrients, and the elimination of solid wastes in the form of feces (stool).
- The **respiratory system** (pulmonology) consists of the air passages and lungs that supply oxygen and eliminate carbon dioxide.
- The **urinary system** (urology) consists of the kidneys, ureters, urinary bladder, and urethra, which, respectively, produce, transport, store, and intermittently excrete liquid waste (urine). The kidneys also regulate fluid and acid-base balance.
- The **reproductive system** (gynecology and andrology) consists of the genital organs, such as the ovaries and testes, which are concerned with reproduction.
- The **endocrine system** (endocrinology) consists of ductless glands, such as the thyroid gland, that produce hormones that are distributed by the circulatory system to all parts of the body to reach the receptor organs. Endocrine glands influence metabolism and coordinate and regulate other body processes, including those associated with the menstrual cycle or the events of pregnancy.

ANATOMICAL VARIATIONS

Although anatomy books describe the structure of the body observed in most people, the structure of different people varies considerably in its details. Students are often frustrated because the bodies they are examining or dissecting do not conform to the atlas or textbook they are using. Students should expect anatomical variations when dissecting or studying prosected specimens. *There is a normal range of ethnic and racial variations; they* are not birth defects. Bones of the skeleton vary among themselves, not only in their basic shape, but also in lesser details of surface structure. There is also a wide variation in the size, shape, and form of the attachment of muscles. Similarly, there is variation in the method of division of vessels and nerves with the greatest variation occurring in veins, followed by arteries and nerves. The frequency of variations often differs among various human groups. *Congenital anomalies* (birth defects) are caused by genetic factors such as chromosomal abnormalities or environmental factors such as drugs and viruses (Moore and Persaud, 1998; Moore et al., 2000).

ANATOMICAL AND MEDICAL TERMINOLOGY

Anatomy has an international vocabulary that is the foundation of medical terminology. It is important that physicians, dentists, and other health professionals throughout the world use the same terms. Although *eponyms* (names of structures derived from the names of persons) are not used in official anatomical terminology, those commonly used by clinicians appear in parentheses throughout this book to help reduce ambiguity and misunderstanding. Similarly, formerly used terms appear in parentheses on first mention; for example, internal thoracic artery (internal mammary artery). The terminology in this book conforms with the *Terminologia Anatomica: International Anatomical Terminology* (1998).

ANATOMICAL POSITION

All anatomical descriptions are expressed in relation to the anatomical position (Fig. 1.1) to ensure that the descriptions are not ambiguous. The anatomical position refers to persons—regardless of the actual position they may be in—as if they were standing erect, with their:

- Head, eyes, and toes directed anteriorly (forward)
- Upper limbs by the sides with the palms facing anteriorly

- Lower limbs together with the feet directed anteriorly.

ANATOMICAL PLANES

Anatomical descriptions are based on four anatomical planes that pass through the body in the anatomical position (Fig. 1.2). There are many sagittal, frontal, and transverse planes but there is only one median plane.

The main use of anatomical planes is to describe sections and images of the body.

- **Median plane** (median sagittal plane) is the vertical plane passing longitudinally through the center of the body—dividing it into right and left halves.

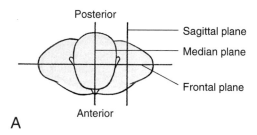

A

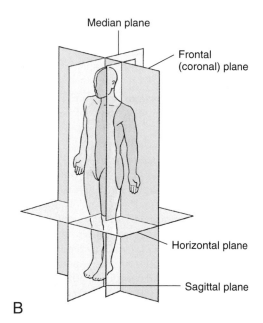

B

FIGURE 1.2   Planes of body. A. Superior view. **B.** Anterolateral view. Anatomical descriptions are based on four planes that pass through the body in the anatomical position.

- **Sagittal planes** are vertical planes passing through the body parallel to the median plane. It is helpful to give a point of reference indicating its position, such as a sagittal plane through the midpoint of the clavicle.
- **Frontal planes** (coronal planes) are vertical planes passing through the body *at* right angles to the median plane, dividing it into anterior (front) and posterior (back) portions.
- **Horizontal planes** (transverse planes) are planes passing through the body at right angles to the median and frontal planes. A horizontal plane divides the body into superior (upper) and inferior (lower) parts. It is helpful to give a reference point indicating its level, such as a horizontal plane through the umbilicus. Radiologists refer to horizontal planes as *transaxial planes* or simply axial planes that are perpendicular to the long axis of the body and limbs.

TERMS OF RELATIONSHIP AND COMPARISON

Various adjectives, explained and illustrated in Table 1.1 and arranged as pairs of opposites (such as superior and inferior), describe the relationship of parts of the body in the anatomical position by comparing the relative position of two structures with each other, a single structure relative to the surface or the midline, or a structure to the "ends" of the body and its extensions (nose or forehead, and tips of fingers and toes). For example, the eyes are superior to the nose, whereas the nose is inferior to the eyes.

Combined terms describe intermediate positional arrangements. For example:

- *Inferomedial* means nearer to the feet and closer to the median plane; for example, the anterior parts of the ribs run inferomedially.
- *Superolateral* means nearer to the head and farther from the median plane.

Proximal and **distal** are directional terms that are used when describing positions, for example, whether structures are nearer to the trunk or point of origin (i.e., proximal). **Dorsum** refers to the superior or dorsal surface (back) of any part that protrudes anteriorly from the body, such as the *dorsum of the foot or hand*. It is easier to understand why these surfaces are considered dorsal if one thinks of a plantigrade animal that walks on its soles, such as a dog. The **sole** indicates the inferior aspect or bottom of the foot, much of which is in contact with the ground when standing barefooted. The **palm** refers to the flat of the hand, exclusive of the thumb and fingers, and is the opposite of the dorsum of the hand.

TERMS OF LATERALITY

Paired structures having right and left members such as the kidneys are **bilateral,** whereas those occurring on one side only are **unilateral** (e.g., the spleen). **Ipsilateral** means occurring on the same side of the body; the right thumb and right great toe are ipsilateral, for example. **Contralateral** means occurring on the opposite side of the body; the right hand is contralateral to the left hand.

TERMS OF MOVEMENT

Various terms (such as *flexion and extension*) describe movements of the limbs and other parts of the body (Table 1.2). Movements take place at joints where two or more bones or cartilages articulate with one another. They are described as pairs of opposites (e.g., abduction and adduction).

INTEGUMENTARY SYSTEM

The skin, the largest organ of the body, consists of a superficial cellular layer, the **epidermis,** and a deep connective tissue layer, the **dermis** (Fig. 1.3). *The skin provides:*

- *Protection for the body* from injury, fluid loss (e.g., in minor burns), and invading organisms
- *Heat regulation* through sweat glands and blood vessels
- *Sensation* (e.g., pain) by way of superficial nerves and their sensory endings.

TABLE 1.1.   COMMONLY USED TERMS OF RELATIONSHIP AND COMPARISON

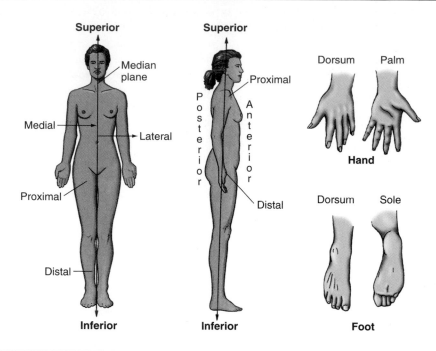

Term	Meaning	Usage
Superior (cranial)	Nearer to head	Heart is superior to stomach
Inferior (caudal)	Nearer to feet	Stomach is inferior to heart
Anterior (ventral)	Nearer to front	Sternum is anterior to heart
Posterior (dorsal)	Nearer to back	Kidneys are posterior to intestine
Medial	Nearer to median plane	Fifth digit (little finger) is on medial side of hand
Lateral	Farther from median plane	First digit (thumb) is on lateral side of hand
Proximal	Nearer to trunk or point of origin (e.g., of a limb)	Elbow is proximal to wrist, and the proximal part of an artery is its beginning
Distal	Farther from trunk or point of origin (e.g., of a limb)	Wrist is distal to elbow and distal part of lower limb is the foot
Superficial	Nearer to or on surface	Muscles of arm are superficial to its bone (humerus)
Deep	Farther from surface	Humerus is deep to arm muscles
Dorsum	Dorsal surface of hand or foot	Veins are visible in dorsum of hand
Palm	Palmar surface of hand	Skin creases are visible on palm
Sole	Plantar surface of foot	Skin is thick on sole of foot

TABLE 1.2.   TERMS OF MOVEMENT

Flexion means bending of a part or decreasing the angle between body parts. **Extension** means straightening a part or increasing the angle between body parts.

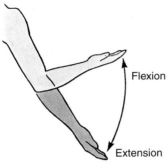

Flexion and extension of forearm at elbow joint

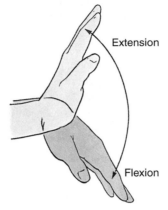

Flexion and extension of hand at wrist joint

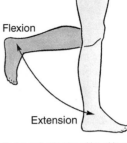

Flexion and extension of leg at knee joint

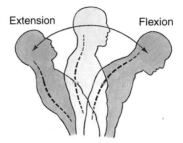

Flexion and extension of vertebral column at intervertebral joints

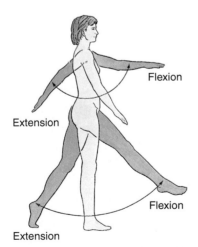

Flexion and extension of upper limb at shoulder joint and lower limb at hip joint

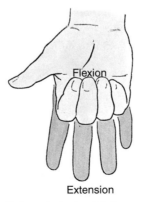

Flexion and extension of digits (fingers) at interphalangeal joints

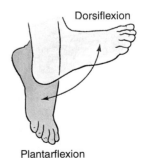

Dorsiflexion and plantarflexion of foot at ankle joint

continued

TABLE 1.2. *CONTINUED*

Abduction means moving away from the median plane of the body in the frontal plane. **Adduction** means moving toward the median plane of the body in the coronal plane. In the digits (fingers and toes), abduction means spreading them, and adduction refers to drawing them together. **Rotation** means moving a part of the body around its long axis. *Medial rotation* turns the anterior surface medially and *lateral rotation* turns this surface laterally. **Circumduction** is the circular movement of the limbs, or parts of them, combining in sequence the movements of flexion, extension, abduction, and adduction. **Pronation** is a medial rotation of the forearm and hand so that the palm faces posteriorly. **Supination** is a lateral rotation of the forearm and hand so that the palm faces anteriorly, as in the anatomical position. Eversion means turning sole of foot outward. Inversion means turning sole of foot inward. **Protrusion** (protraction) means to move the jaw anteriorly. **Retrusion** (retraction) means to move the jaw posteriorly. **Elevation** raises or moves a part superiorly. **Depression** lowers or moves a part inferiorly.

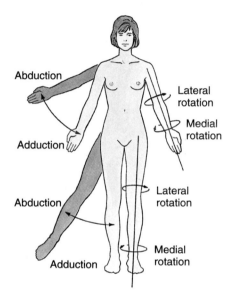

Abduction and adduction of right limbs and rotation of left limbs at glenohumeral and hip joints, respectively

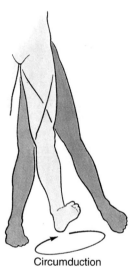

Circumduction (circular movement) of lower limb at hip joint

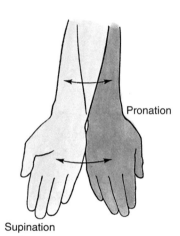

Pronation and supination of forearm at radioulnar joints

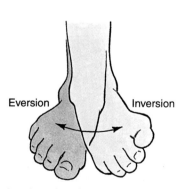

Inversion and eversion of foot at subtalar and transverse tarsal joints

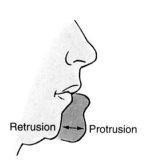

Protrusion and retrusion of jaw at temporomandibular joints

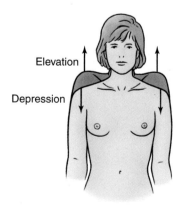

Elevation and depression of shoulders

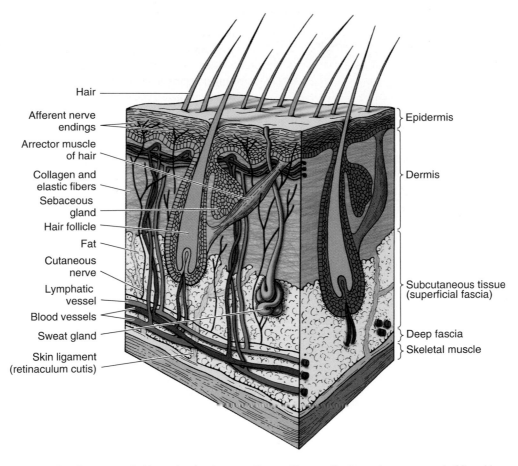

Hair

Afferent nerve
endings

Arrector muscle
of hair

Collagen and
elastic fibers

Sebaceous
gland

Hair follicle

Fat

Cutaneous
nerve

Lymphatic
vessel

Blood vessels

Sweat gland

Skin ligament
(retinaculum cutis)

Epidermis

Dermis

Subcutaneous tissue
(superficial fascia)

Deep fascia

Skeletal muscle

FIGURE 1.3   Structure of skin and subcutaneous tissue. Observe the layered arrangement of the skin and the hairs and glands embedded in the skin and subcutaneous tissue.

The **deep layer of the dermis** is formed by a dense layer of interlacing *collagen* and *elastic fibers*. These fibers provide skin tone and account for the strength and toughness of the skin. The deep layer of the dermis also contains hair follicles, with their associated smooth arrector (arrector pili) muscles and sebaceous glands. Contraction of the *arrector muscles* erects the hairs, causing "goose bumps."

The **subcutaneous tissue** (superficial fascia, hypodermis) is composed of loose connective tissue and fat. Located between the dermis and underlying deep fascia, the subcutaneous tissue contains the deepest parts of sweat glands, the blood and lymphatic vessels, and cutaneous nerves that are distributed to the skin. The **deep fascia** is a dense, organized connective tissue layer that invests deep structures such as the muscles and neurovascular bundles. **Skin ligaments** (L. retinacula cutis)—numerous small fibrous bands—extend through the subcutaneous tissue and attach the deep surface of the dermis to the underlying deep fascia. These ligaments determine the mobility of the skin over deep structures.

SKIN INCISIONS AND WOUNDS
Tension lines (cleavage or Langer's lines) in the skin keep the skin under tension. When the collagen fibers in the dermis are interrupted by an incision, the wound gapes. Surgeons make their incisions parallel with the tension lines when possible. Skin incisions along these lines usually heal well with minimal scarring because the lines of force pull the cut surfaces together. An incision across a tension line disrupts and disturbs the collagen fibers and

Continued

may produce excessive scarring. Stab wounds in the skin by an ice pick, for example, are usually slitlike rather than rounded because the pick splits the collagen fibers in the dermis and allows the wound to gape.

Stretch Marks in Skin
The collagen and elastic fibers in the dermis form a tough, flexible meshwork of tissue. The skin can distend considerably when the abdomen enlarges during pregnancy, for example. However, if stretched too far, it can result in damage to the collagen fibers in the dermis. Bands of thin wrinkled skin, initially red, become purple and later white. Stretch marks appear on the abdomen, buttocks, thighs, and breasts. These marks also form in obese individuals and generally fade after pregnancy and weight loss.

Burns
Burns are tissue injuries caused by thermal, electrical, radioactive, or chemical agents.
- In *first degree burns* the damage is limited to the superficial part of the epidermis.
- In *second degree burns* the damage extends through the epidermis into the superficial part of the dermis. However, the sweat glands and hair follicles are not damaged.
- In *third degree burns* the entire epidermis and dermis are destroyed. Loss of blood plasma by exudation from the burn site occurs. In these cases a skin autograph is required for skin healing.

SKELETAL SYSTEM

The skeleton of the body is composed of bones and cartilages (Fig. 1.4). **Bone**—*a living tissue*—is a highly specialized, hard form of connective tissue that forms most of the skeleton and is the chief supporting tissue of the body. *Bones provide:*

- Protection for vital structures
- Support for the body
- The mechanical basis for movement
- Storage for salts (e.g., calcium)
- A continuous supply of new blood cells.

Cartilage—a resilient, semirigid form of connective tissue—forms parts of the skeleton where more flexibility is necessary (e.g., the *costal cartilages* that attach the ribs to the sternum). The articulating surfaces of bones participating in a synovial joint are capped with **articular cartilage** that provides gliding sur-

faces for free movement of the articulating bones (see blue ends of humerus [Fig. 1.4*A*]). The proportion of bone and cartilage in the skeleton changes as the body grows; the younger a person is, the greater the contribution of cartilage. The bones of a newborn are soft and flexible because they are mostly composed of cartilage.

The skeletal system has two main parts (Fig. 1.4):

- The **axial skeleton** consists of the bones of the head (cranium), neck (hyoid bone and cervical vertebrae), and trunk (ribs, sternum, vertebrae, and sacrum).
- The **appendicular skeleton** consists of the bones of the limbs, including those forming the pectoral (shoulder) and pelvic girdles (bony rings to which the upper and lower limbs are attached).

BONES

There are two types of bone: **compact** and **spongy.** The differences between these types of bone (Fig. 1.5) depend on the relative amount of solid matter and the number and size of the spaces they contain. All bones have a superficial thin layer of compact bone around a central mass of spongy bone, except where the latter is replaced by a **medullary (marrow) cavity.** Within this cavity of adult bones, and between the spicules of spongy bone, blood cells and platelets are formed. The architecture of spongy and compact bone varies according to function. Compact bone provides strength for weightbearing. In long bones, designed for rigidity and attachment of muscles and ligaments, the amount of compact bone is greatest near the middle of the **shaft** (body) of the bone where it may buckle. The superficial thin layer of compact bone is called *cortical bone.*

Classification of Bones
Bones are classified according to their shape (Fig. 1.4).

- **Long bones** are tubular structures, such as the humerus in the arm; the actual length

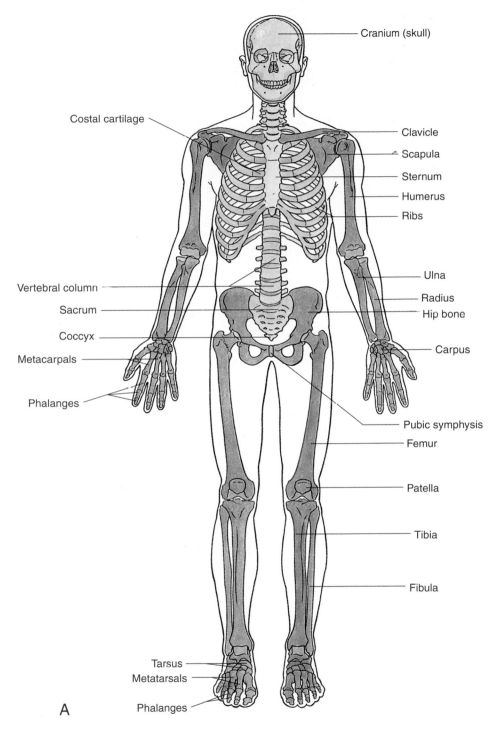

Cranium (skull)

Costal cartilage

Clavicle

Scapula

Sternum

Humerus

Ribs

Ulna

Vertebral column

Radius

Sacrum

Hip bone

Coccyx

Metacarpals

Carpus

Phalanges

Pubic symphysis

Femur

Patella

Tibia

Fibula

Tarsus

Metatarsals

Phalanges

A

FIGURE 1.4   Skeletal system. A. Anterior view. **B.** Posterior view. The appendicular skeleton is shown in *purple* to distinguish it from the axial skeleton (*yellow*). Cartilages are colored *blue.* Bone markings and formations are shown on the right side.

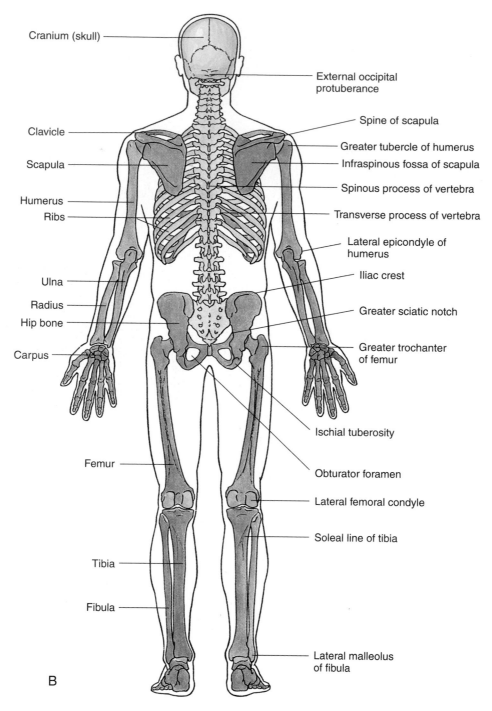

Cranium (skull)

External occipital protuberance

Spine of scapula

Clavicle

Greater tubercle of humerus

Scapula

Infraspinous fossa of scapula

Humerus

Spinous process of vertebra

Ribs

Transverse process of vertebra

Lateral epicondyle of humerus

Ulna

Iliac crest

Radius

Greater sciatic notch

Hip bone

Greater trochanter of femur

Carpus

Ischial tuberosity

Femur

Obturator foramen

Lateral femoral condyle

Soleal line of tibia

Tibia

Fibula

Lateral malleolus of fibula

B

FIGURE 1.4   *Continued.*

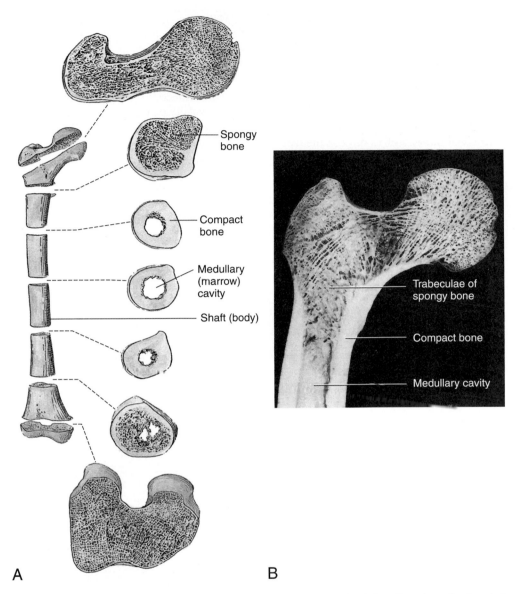

FIGURE 1.5 **Sections of bones.** **A.** Transverse sections of femur. **B.** Frontal section of proximal end of femur. The shaft (body) of a living bone is a tube of compact bone, the medullary (marrow) cavity of which contains marrow. Observe the tension and pressure lines (trabeculae) related to the weight-bearing function of this bone.

of the bones has little to do with this classification (e.g., the phalanges [finger bones] are also classified as long bones).

- **Short bones** are cuboidal and are found only in the ankle (tarsus) and wrist (carpus).
- **Flat bones** usually serve protective functions; the flat bones of the cranium, for example, protect the brain.
- **Irregular bones,** such as those in the face, have various shapes other than long, short, or flat.
- **Sesamoid bones,** such as the patella (knee cap), develop in certain tendons and are found where tendons cross the ends of long bones in the limbs. These bones protect the tendons from excessive wear and often change the angle from which the tendons pass to their attachments.

- **Malleolus:** rounded prominence (e.g., lateral malleolus of fibula)
- **Notch:** indentation at the edge of a bone (e.g., greater sciatic notch in posterior border of hip bone)
- **Protuberance:** projection of bone (e.g., external occipital protuberance of cranium)
- **Spine:** thornlike process (e.g., spine of scapula)
- **Process:** projecting spinelike part (e.g., spinous and transverse processes of a vertebra)
- **Trochanter:** large blunt elevation (e.g., greater trochanter of femur)
- **Tubercle:** small raised eminence (e.g., greater tubercle of humerus)
- **Tuberosity:** large rounded elevation (e.g., ischial tuberosity).

HETEROTOPIC BONES

Bones sometimes form in soft tissues where they are not normally present. Horse riders often develop heterotopic bones in their thighs or buttocks (*rider's bones*), probably because of repeatedly bruised (hemorrhagic or bloody) areas that undergo calcification and eventual ossification.

Bone Markings

Bone markings appear wherever tendons, ligaments, and fascia are attached, or where arteries lie adjacent to or enter bones. Other formations occur in relation to the passage of a tendon (often to direct the tendon or improve its leverage) or to control the type of movement occurring at a joint. *Some markings and features of bones are* (Fig. 1.4*B*):

- **Condyle:** rounded articular area (e.g., condyles of femur)
- **Crest:** ridge of bone (e.g., the iliac crest)
- **Epicondyle:** eminence superior to a condyle (e.g., epicondyles of humerus)
- **Facet:** smooth flat area, usually covered with cartilage, where a bone, such as a rib, articulates with another bone (e.g., a vertebra)
- **Foramen:** passage through a bone (e.g., obturator foramen)
- **Fossa:** hollow or depressed area (e.g., infraspinous fossa of scapula)
- **Line:** linear elevation (e.g., soleal line of tibia)

TRAUMA TO BONE AND BONE CHANGES

Bones are living organs that hurt when injured, bleed when fractured, remodel in relationship to stress placed on them, and change with age. Like other organs, bones have blood vessels, lymphatic vessels, and nerves, and they may become diseased. Unused bones, such as in a paralyzed or cast limb, *atrophy* (decrease in size). Bone may be absorbed, which occurs in the mandible after teeth are extracted. Bones *hypertrophy* (enlarge) when they have increased weight to support for a long period.

Trauma to a bone may fracture it. For the fracture to heal properly, the broken ends must be brought together approximating their normal position (*reduction of fracture*). During bone healing, the surrounding fibroblasts (connective tissue cells) proliferate and secrete collagen that forms a *collar of callus* to hold the bones together. Remodelling of bone occurs in the fracture area and the callus calcifies. Eventually, the callus is resorbed and replaced by bone.

Osteoporosis

During old age both the organic and inorganic components of bone decrease, producing *osteoporosis*—a reduction in the quantity of bone (atrophy of skeletal tissue). The bones become brittle, lose their elasticity, and fracture easily.

Bone Development

All bones are derived from mesenchyme (embryonic connective tissue) but by two different processes: *intramembranous ossification* (directly from mesenchyme) and *endochondral ossification* (from cartilage derived from mesenchyme). The histology of a bone is the same either way.

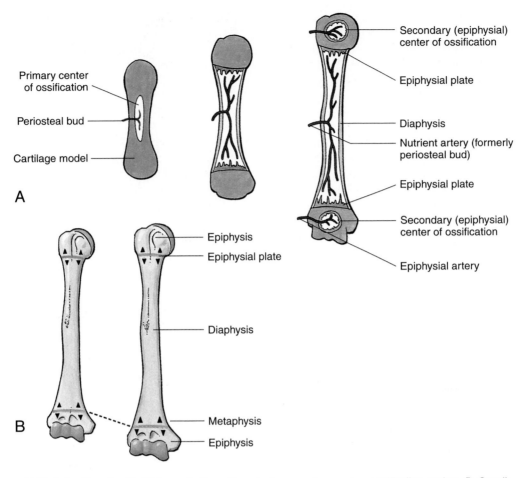

Primary center of ossification

Periosteal bud

Cartilage model

A

Secondary (epiphysial) center of ossification

Epiphysial plate

Diaphysis

Nutrient artery (formerly periosteal bud)

Epiphysial plate

Secondary (epiphysial) center of ossification

Epiphysial artery

Epiphysis

Epiphysial plate

Diaphysis

B

Metaphysis

Epiphysis

FIGURE 1.6   Growth of long bone. A. Formation of primary and secondary ossification centers. **B.** Growth in length of bone occurs on both sides of the epiphysial plates (*arrowheads*).

- In **intramembranous ossification** mesenchymal models of bone form during the embryonic period; direct ossification of the mesenchyme begins in the fetal period.
- In **endochondral ossification** cartilage models of bones form from mesenchyme during the fetal period and subsequently (after birth in large part) bone replaces most of the cartilage.

A brief description of endochondral ossification explains how long bones grow. The mesenchymal cells condense and differentiate into *chondroblasts*—dividing cells in growing cartilage tissue—that form a *cartilage model* (Fig. 1.6). In the midregion of the bone model, the cartilage calcifies (becomes impregnated with calcium salts), and periosteal capillaries

(capillaries from the fibrous sheath surrounding the model) grow into the calcified cartilage of the bone model and supply its interior. These blood vessels, together with associated osteogenic (bone-forming) cells, form a **periosteal bud.** The capillaries initiate the **primary ossification center,** so named because the bone tissue it forms replaces most of the cartilage in the main body of the bone model. The shaft or body of a bone ossified from a primary ossification center is the **diaphysis.**

Most **secondary ossification centers** appear in other parts of the developing bone after birth; the parts of a bone ossified from these centers are **epiphyses.** The flared part of the diaphysis nearest the epiphysis is the **metaphysis** (Fig. 1.6B). For growth to continue, the bone formed from the primary center in the diaphysis does not fuse with that formed from the secondary centers in the epiphyses until the bone reaches its adult size. Thus, during growth of a long bone, cartilaginous **epiphysial plates** intervene between the diaphysis and epiphyses. These growth plates are eventually replaced by bone at each of its two sides, diaphysial and epiphysial. When this occurs, bone growth ceases and the diaphysis fuses with the epiphyses (*synostosis*). The seam formed during this process is particularly dense and is recognizable in radiographs as an **epiphysial line** (Fig. 1.7). The epiphysial fusion of bones occurs progressively from the age of puberty to maturity.

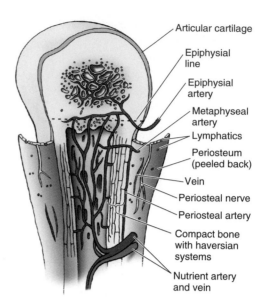

FIGURE 1.7   Vasculature and innervation of a long bone. The bulk of compact bone is composed of haversian canal systems (osteons). The haversian canal in the system houses one or two small blood vessels for nourishing the osteocytes (bone cells).

ACCESSORY BONES

Accessory (supernumerary) bones develop when additional ossification centers appear and form extra bones. Many bones develop from several centers of ossification (sites of earliest bone formation), and the separate parts normally fuse. Sometimes one of these centers fails to fuse with the main bone, giving the appearance of an extra bone; however, careful study shows that the apparent extra bone is a missing part of the main bone. It is important to know that *accessory bones are common in the foot* so as not to mistake them for bone chips in radiographs and other medical images. Circumscribed areas of bone are often seen along the sutures of the skull where the flat bones come together. These small wormlike bones are *sutural bones* (wormian bones).

Assessment of Bone Age

Knowledge of the sites where ossification centers occur, the times of their appearance, the rate at which they grow, and the times of fusion of the sites (times when synostosis occurs) is used to determine the age of a person. The main criteria to determine bone age are:

- Appearance of calcified material in the diaphysis and/or epiphyses
- Disappearance of the dark line representing the epiphysial plate (absence of this line indicates epiphysial fusion has occurred); fusion occurs at specific times for each epiphysis. Fusion of epiphyses with the diaphysis occurs 1 to 2 years earlier in girls than in boys.

Determination of bone age can be helpful in predicting adult height in early- or late-maturing adolescents and in establishing the approximate age of human skeletal remains in medicolegal cases.

Vasculature and Innervation of Bones

Arteries enter bones from the **periosteum**—the fibrous connective tissue membrane investing bones (Fig. 1.7). **Periosteal arteries** enter at numerous points and supply the bone; these arteries nourish the compact bone. Consequently, a bone from which the periosteum has been removed dies. Near the center of the shaft of the bone, a **nutrient artery** passes obliquely through the compact bone and supplies the spongy bone and bone marrow. **Metaphysial** and **epiphysial arteries** supply the ends of the bones.

Veins accompany arteries through the *nutrient foramina*. Many large veins leave through foramina near the articular ends of the bones. Bones containing marrow have numerous large veins. **Lymphatics** (lymphatic vessels) are abundant in the periosteum. **Nerves** accompany the blood vessels supplying bones. The **periosteum** is richly supplied with sensory nerves—**periosteal nerves**—that carry pain fibers. The periosteum is especially sensitive to tearing or tension, which explains the acute pain from bone fractures. Bone itself is relatively sparsely supplied with sensory endings. Within bones, *vasomotor nerves* cause constriction or dilation of blood vessels, regulating blood flow through the bone marrow.

AVASCULAR NECROSIS

Loss of blood supply to an epiphysis or other parts of a bone results in death of bone tissue—*avascular necrosis* (G. nekrosis, deadness). After every fracture, small areas of adjacent bone undergo necrosis. In some fractures, avascular necrosis of a large fragment of bone may occur.

JOINTS

A joint is an articulation—the place of union or junction between two or more rigid components (bones, cartilages, or even parts of the same bone). Joints exhibit a variety of form and function. Some joints have no movement; others allow only slight movement, and some are freely movable, such as the glenohumeral (shoulder) joint.

Classification of Joints

The **three types of joint** are classified according to the manner or type of material by which the articulating bones are united (Table 1.3):

- **Fibrous joints are united by fibrous tissue;** the amount of movement occurring at a fibrous joint depends in most cases on the length of the fibers uniting the articular bones. A **syndesmosis** type of fibrous joint unites the bones with a sheet of fibrous tissue, either a ligament or fibrous membrane. Consequently, this type of joint is partially movable. The dense **interosseous membrane** in the forearm is a sheet of fibrous tissue that joins the radius and ulna in a syndesmosis. A *gomphosis* or *dentoalveolar syndesmosis* is a type of fibrous joint in which a peglike process fits into a socket articulation between the root of the tooth and the alveolar process (socket).
- **Cartilaginous joints are united by cartilage or fibrocartilage** (a combination of cartilage and fibrous tissue).

- **Articulating surfaces of synovial joints are covered with cartilage and united by a fibrous capsule.** A synovial membrane encloses the articulating surfaces within a joint cavity. **Synovial joints**—the most common type of joint—provide free movement between the bones they join and are typical of nearly all limb joints. Synovial joints contain *synovial fluid* and are lined with a **synovial membrane** consisting of vascular connective tissue that produces synovial fluid. Synovial fluid serves the dual function of nourishing the articular cartilage and lubricating the joint surfaces. *Distinguishing features of a synovial joint are:*

- A **joint cavity**
- **Articular cartilage** covers the bone ends
- Articulating surfaces and joint cavity are enclosed by an **articular** or **joint capsule** (fibrous capsule lined with synovial membrane).

Synovial joints are usually reinforced by accessory ligaments that are either separate (extrinsic) or are a thickening of a part of the fibrous capsule (intrinsic). Some synovial joints have other distinguishing features such as fibrocartilaginous *articular discs,* which are present when the articulating surfaces of the bones are incongruous. The **six major types of synovial joint** are classified according to the shape of the articulating surfaces and/or the type of movement they permit (Table 1.4).

Vasculature and Innervation of Joints

Joints receive blood from articular arteries that arise from vessels around the joint. The arteries often anastomose (communicate) to form networks (anastomoses), allowing continuous blood supply in the various positions of the joint. *Articular veins*—communicating veins (see Fig. 1.12C)—accompany the arteries and, like them, are located in the articular capsule, mostly in the synovial membrane.

Joints have a rich nerve supply; the nerve endings are numerous in the articular capsule. In the distal parts of limbs, the *articular nerves* are branches of the cutaneous nerve supplying the overlying skin. Otherwise, most articular

TABLE 1.3. TYPES OF JOINT

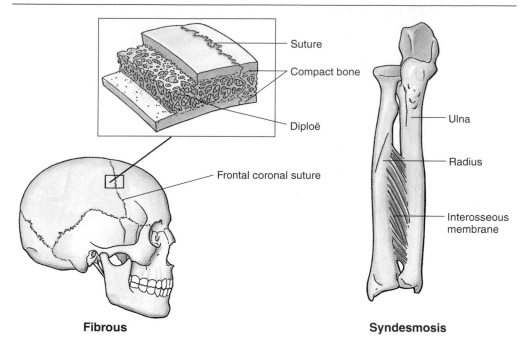

Fibrous

Syndesmosis

In fibrous joints, articulating bones are joined by fibrous tissue. Sutures of the cranium are examples of a type of fibrous joint where bones are close together and united by fibrous tissue, often interlocking along a wavy line. Flat bones consist of two plates of compact bone separated by spongy bone and marrow (diploë). In a syndesmosis, the bones are joined by a sheet of fibrous tissue (e.g., interosseous membrane joining forearm bones).

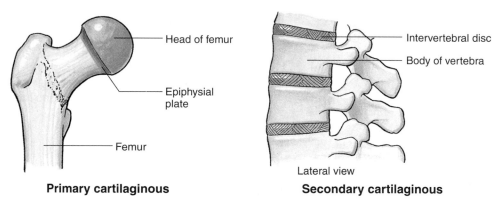

Primary cartilaginous

Secondary cartilaginous

In cartilaginous joints, articulating bones are united by fibrocartilage or hyaline cartilage. Common type of synchrondrosis is that in a developing long bone where bony epiphysis and body are joined by an epiphysial plate. In a symphysis the binding tissue is a fibrocartilaginous disc (e.g., between two vertebrae).

A synovial joint (articulation) is characterized by a joint cavity; the two bones are separated by a joint cavity containing synovial fluid but are joined by an articular capsule (fibrous capsule lined with synovial membrane). The bearing surfaces of the bones are covered with articular cartilage. Synovial joints are the most common and important type of joint functionally. They provide free movement between the bones they join and are typical of nearly all joints of the limbs.

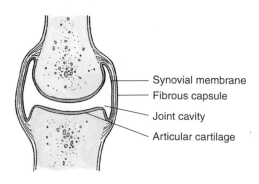

Synovial joint

TABLE 1.4.   TYPES OF SYNOVIAL JOINT

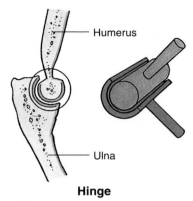

Hinge

Hinge joints (uniaxial) permit flexion and extension only (e.g., elbow joint).

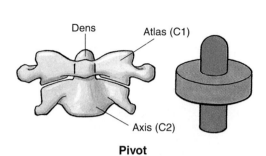

Pivot

Pivot joints (uniaxial) allow rotation. A round process of bone fits into a bony ligamentous socket; e.g., atlantoaxial joint between the atlas (C1) and axis (C2).

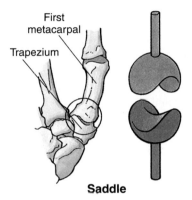

Saddle

Saddle joints (biaxial) are shaped like a saddle; i.e., they are concave and convex where bones articulate.

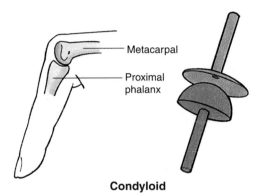

Condyloid

Condyloid joints (biaxial) permit flexion and extension, abduction and adduction, and circumduction [e.g., metacarpophalangeal (knuckle) joints of digits].

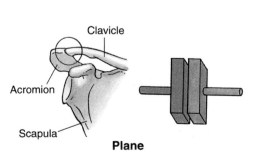

Plane

Plane joints permit gliding or sliding movements (e.g., acromioclavicular joint).

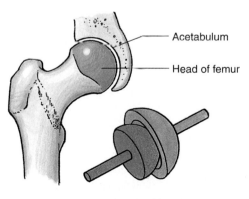

Ball and socket

Ball and socket joints (multiaxial) permit movement in several axes (e.g., flexion-extension, abduction-adduction, medial and lateral rotation, and circumduction). A rounded head fits into a concavity.

nerves are branches of nerves that supply the muscles that cross and therefore move the joint. *Hilton's law states that the nerves supplying a joint also supply the muscles moving the joint and the skin covering their attachments.* Joints transmit a sensation called *proprioception*—information that provides an awareness of movement and position of the parts of the body.

DEGENERATIVE JOINT DISEASE

Synovial joints are well designed to withstand wear but heavy use over several years can cause degenerative changes. Beginning early in adult life and progressing slowly thereafter, aging of articular cartilage occurs on the ends of the articulating bones, particularly those of the hip, knee, vertebral column, and hands. *These irreversible degenerative changes in joints result in the articular cartilage becoming less effective as a shock absorber and a lubricated surface.* As a result, the articulation becomes vulnerable to the repeated friction that occurs during joint movements. In some people these changes cause considerable pain. *Degenerative joint disease*—osteoarthritis or osteoarthrosis—is often accompanied by stiffness, discomfort, and pain. *Osteoarthritis* is common in older people and usually affects joints that support the weight of their bodies (e.g., hips and knees).

MUSCULAR SYSTEM

Muscle cells—often called *muscle fibers* because they are long and narrow when relaxed—produce contractions that move body parts, including internal organs. The associated connective tissue conveys nerve fibers and capillaries to the muscle fibers as it binds them into bundles or fascicles. Muscles also give form to the body and provide heat. *There are three types of muscle* (Table 1.5):

- **Skeletal muscle,** which moves bones and other structures (e.g., the eyes)
- **Cardiac muscle,** which forms most of the walls of the heart and adjacent parts of the great vessels, such as the aorta
- **Smooth muscle,** which forms part of the walls of most vessels and hollow organs, moves substances through viscera such as the intestine, and controls movement through blood vessels.

SKELETAL MUSCLE

Most skeletal muscles are attached directly or indirectly through tendons to bones, cartilages, ligaments, or fascia, or to some combination of these structures. Some skeletal muscles are attached to organs (the eyeball, for example), to skin (such as the facial muscles), and to mucous membrane (intrinsic tongue muscles that alter its shape). When a muscle contracts and shortens, one of its attachments usually remains fixed and the other one moves. Attachments of muscles are commonly described as the origin and insertion; the *origin* is usually the proximal end of the muscle that remains fixed during muscular contraction, and the *insertion* is usually the distal end of the muscle that is movable. However, some muscles can act in both directions under different circumstances. Therefore, the terms *proximal* and *distal* or *medial* and *lateral* are used in this book when describing most muscle attachments. Skeletal muscles produce movements of the skeleton and other parts. Figure 1.8 shows major skeletal muscles; they are often called *voluntary muscles* because individuals control many of them at will. However, some of their actions are automatic (e.g., the diaphragm contracts automatically); a person controls it voluntarily when taking a deep breath. Skeletal muscles are also referred to as "striated" or "striped" muscle because of the striped appearance of their cells (fibers) under microscopy (Table 1.5). *Skeletal muscles produce movement by shortening; they pull and never push;* however, certain phenomena—such as "popping the ears" to equalize air pressure, and the *musculovenous pump* —take advantage of the expansion of muscle bellies during contraction (see Fig. 1.12*B*).

The architecture and shape of skeletal muscles vary. The fleshy part is the **muscle belly** (Fig. 1.9*A*). Some muscles are fleshy throughout but most have **tendons** that attach to bones. When referring to the length of a muscle, both the belly and tendons are included— i.e., *a muscle's length is the distance between its bony attachments.* Some tendons form flat sheets or **aponeuroses** that anchor one muscle

TABLE 1.5. TYPES OF MUSCLE

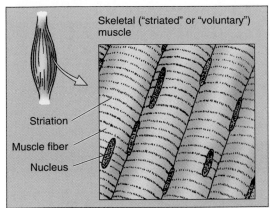

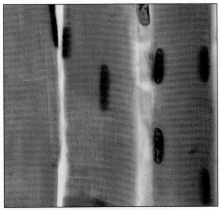

Location	Appearance	Type of Activity	Stimulation
Named muscle (e.g., the biceps of the arm) attached to the skeleton and fascia of limbs, body wall, and head/neck	Large, long, unbranched, cylindrical fibers with transverse striations (stripes) arranged in parallel bundles; multiple, peripherally located nuclei	Strong, quick intermittent (phasic) contraction above a baseline tonus; acts primarily to produce movement or resist gravity	Voluntary (or reflexive) by the somatic nervous system (SNS, p. 38)

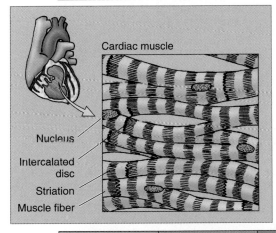

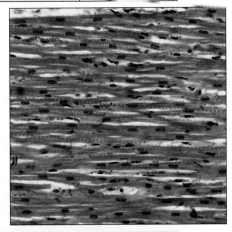

Location	Appearance	Type of Activity	Stimulation
Muscle of heart (myocardium) and adjacent portions of the great vessels (aorta, vena cava)	Branching and anastomosing shorter fibers with transverse striations (stripes) running parallel and connected end-to-end by complex junctions (intercalated discs); single, central nucleus	Strong, quick, continuous rhythmic contraction; acts to pump blood from heart	Involuntary; intrinsically (myogenically) stimulated and propagated; rate and strength of contraction modified by autonomic nervous system (ANS, p. 38)

continued

TABLE 1.5. *CONTINUED*

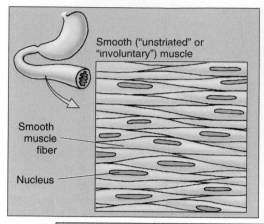
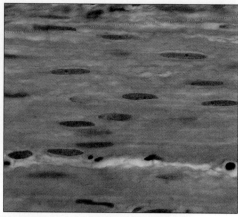

Location	Appearance	Type of Activity	Stimulation
Walls of hollow viscera and blood vessels, iris, and ciliary body of eye; attached to hair follicles of skin (arrector muscle of hair)	Single or agglomerated small, spindle-shaped fibers without striations; single, central nucleus	Weak, slow, rhythmic, or sustained tonic contraction; acts mainly to propel substances (peristalsis) and to restrict flow (vasoconstriction and sphincteric activity)	Involuntary by autonomic nervous system

to another, such as the external oblique muscles of the anterolateral abdominal wall (Fig. 1.9*B*). *Most muscles are named on the basis of their function or the bones to which they are attached.* The abductor digiti minimi, for example, abducts the little finger (L. digiti minimi). The sternocleidomastoid (cleido—clavicle) attaches inferiorly to the sternum and clavicle and superiorly to the mastoid process of the temporal bone of the cranium. Other muscles are named on the basis of their position (medial, lateral, anterior, or posterior) or length (brevis, short; longus, long). *Muscles may be described* or classified according to their shape (Figs. 1.8 and 1.9). For example:

- **Pennate muscles,** which are featherlike (L. pennatus, feather) in the arrangement of their fascicles, and may be uni-, bi-, or multipennate—like the deltoid

- A **fusiform muscle,** which is spindle-shaped (round, thick belly, and tapered ends)—e.g., the biceps brachii
- A **quadrate muscle,** which has four sides (L. quadratus, square)—e.g., the pronator quadratus pronates the forearm (Table 1.2)
- **Circular** or **sphincteral muscle,** which surrounds a body opening or orifice constricting it when contracted—e.g., the orbicularis oculi closes the eye
- **Flat muscles** with parallel fibers often having an aponeurosis—e.g., the external oblique.

The structural unit of a muscle is a **muscle fiber** (Fig. 1.10). A delicate network of collagenous and elastic fibers, the **endomysium,** invests the entire muscle fiber. Parallel muscle fibers are organized into bundles that are covered by a heavier connective tissue covering the **perimysium.** A coarser connective tissue investment, the **epimysium** surrounds the muscle itself. The functional unit of a muscle, consisting of a motor neuron and the muscle fibers it controls, is a **motor unit.** When a nerve impulse reaches a motor neuron in the spinal cord, another impulse is initiated that causes all the muscle fibers supplied by that motor unit to contract simultaneously. The number of muscle fibers in a motor unit varies from one to several hundred according to the size and function of the muscle. Large motor units, where one neuron supplies several hundred muscle fibers, are found in the large trunk and thigh muscles. In the small eye and hand muscles, where precision movements are required, the motor units contain only a few muscle fibers.

Movements result from activation of an increasing number of motor units:

- *Prime movers* or *agonists are the main muscles activated* during a specific movement of the body; they contract actively to produce the desired movement.
- *Antagonists are muscles that oppose the action of prime movers;* as a prime mover contracts, the antagonist progressively relaxes, producing a smooth movement.
- *Synergists complement the action of prime movers,* for example, by preventing movement of the intervening joint when a prime mover passes over more than one joint.
- *Fixators steady the proximal parts of a limb* while movements are occurring in distal parts.

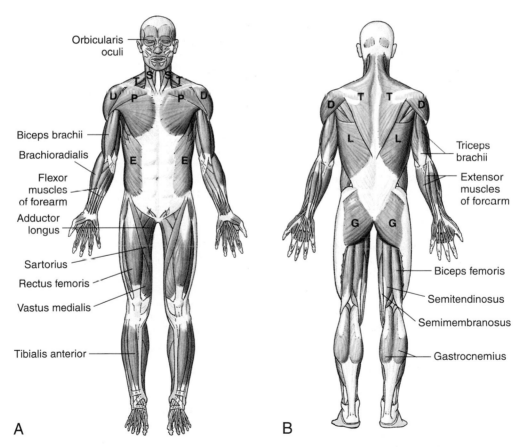

FIGURE 1.8   Skeletal muscles. A. Anterior view. **B.** Posterior view. Some larger muscles are labeled. *S,* sternocleidomastoid; *T,* trapezius; *D,* deltoid; *P,* pectoralis major; *E,* external oblique; *L,* latissimus dorsi; *G,* gluteus maximus.

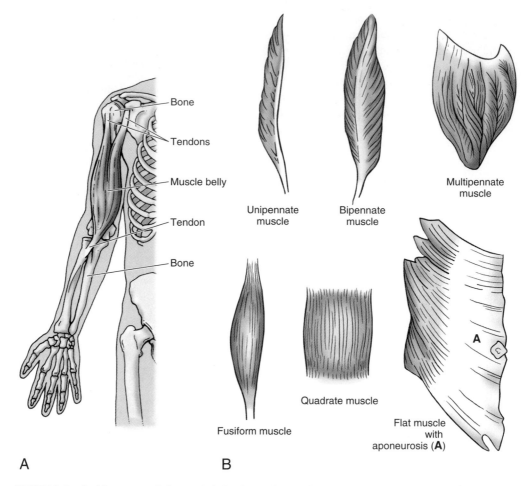

FIGURE 1.9 **Architecture and shape of skeletal muscles. A.** Skeletal muscle in situ. **B.** Fiber arrangement.

The same muscle may act as a prime mover, antagonist, synergist, or fixator under different conditions.

MUSCLE TESTING

Muscle testing helps an examiner diagnose nerve injuries. *There are two common testing methods:*

- The person performs movements that resist those produced by the examiner.
- The examiner performs movements against resistance produced by the person.

When testing flexion of the forearm, for example the examiner asks the person to flex his or her forearm (Table 1.2), while the examiner resists the effort. This technique enables the examiner to gauge the power of the person's movement. Usually muscles are tested in bilateral pairs for comparison.

Electromyography (EMG)

The electrical stimulation of muscles or EMG is another method for testing muscle action. The examiner places surface electrodes over a muscle and asks the person to perform certain movements. The examiner then amplifies and records the differences in electrical action potentials of the muscles. A normal resting muscle shows only a baseline activity (tonus), which disappears only during sleep, paralysis, and when under anesthesia. Contracting muscles demonstrate variable peaks of phasic activity. EMG makes it possible to analyze the activity of an individual muscle during different movements. EMG may also be part of the treatment program for restoring the action of muscles.

Muscular Atrophy

Wasting of muscular tissue of a limb, for example, may result from a primary disorder of muscle or from a lesion of a motor unit. Muscle atrophy may also be caused by immobilization of a limb with a cast.

CARDIAC MUSCLE

Cardiac muscle forms the muscular wall of the heart (Table 1.5)—the *myocardium.* Some cardiac muscle is also present in the walls of the aorta, pulmonary vein, and superior vena cava (SVC). Cardiac muscle contractions are not under voluntary control. Heart rate is regulated intrinsically by a *pacemaker,* composed of special cardiac muscle fibers that are influenced by the autonomic nervous system.

SMOOTH MUSCLE

Smooth muscle—so-called because of the absence of microscopic striations (Table 1.5)—forms a large part of the tunica media (middle

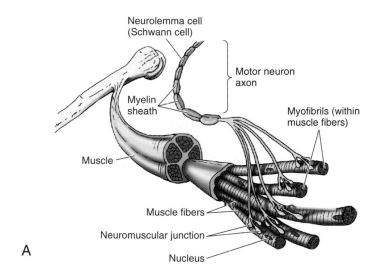

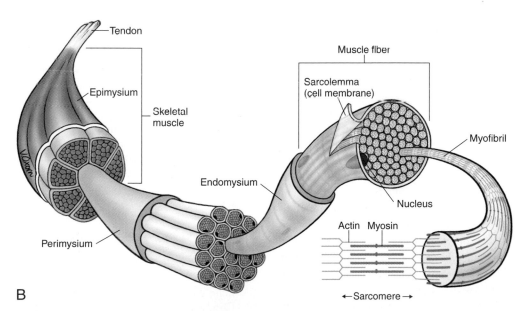

FIGURE 1.10 **Structure of a skeletal muscle and a motor unit. A.** Motor unit. The aggregate of a motor neuron axon and all muscle fibers innervated by it constitute a motor unit. **B.** Epimysium, perimysium, and endomysium. Actin (thin) and myosin (thick) filaments are contractile elements in muscular fibers.

coat) of the walls of most blood vessels (see Fig. 1.12*A*) and the muscular part of the wall of the digestive tract. Smooth muscle is also found in skin—*arrector muscles* associated with hair follicles (Fig. 1.3)—and in the eyeball, where smooth muscle controls lens thickness and pupil size. Like cardiac muscle, smooth muscle is innervated by the ANS (Table 1.5); hence, it is *involuntary muscle* that can undergo partial contraction for long periods. This is important in regulating the size of the lumen of tubular structures; in the walls of the digestive tract, uterine tubes, and ureters, the smooth muscle cells undergo rhythmic contractions (peristaltic waves). This process—*peristalsis*—propels the contents along these tubular structures.

HYPERTROPHY

The *myocardium* responds to increased demands—*compensatory hypertrophy*—by increasing the size of its fibers (cells). When cardiac muscle fibers are damaged during a heart attack, fibrous scar tissue is formed that produces a *myocardial infarct* (MI)—an area of myocardial necrosis (death of myocardial tissue).

   Smooth muscle cells also undergo compensatory hypertrophy in response to increased demands. During pregnancy, the smooth muscle cells in the wall of the uterus increase not only in size (*hypertrophy*) but also in number (*hyperplasia*).

CARDIOVASCULAR SYSTEM

The heart and blood vessels form a *blood transportation network*—the *cardiovascular system* (Fig. 1.11). Through this system, the heart pumps blood through the body's vast system of vessels. The blood carries nutrients, oxygen, and waste products to and from cells. Blood under high pressure leaves the heart and is distributed to the body by a branching system of thick-walled **arteries.** The final distributing vessels—**arterioles**—deliver oxygenated blood to **capillaries,** which form a **capillary bed** where the interchange of oxygen, nutrients, waste products, and other substances with the extracellular fluid occurs (Fig. 1.12*A*). Blood from the capillary bed passes into thin-walled **venules,** which resemble wide capillaries. Venules drain into small **veins** that

open into larger veins. The largest veins, the superior and inferior vena cavae (SVC and IVC), return poorly oxygenated blood to the heart. *The walls of blood vessels have three tunics or coats. Moving from external to internal the separate layers of tissue, tunics, are:*

- Tunica externa
- Tunica media
- Tunica intima

ARTERIES

Arteries carry blood away from the heart and distribute it to the body (Fig. 1.11*A*). Blood passes from the heart through arteries of ever decreasing caliber. The different types of artery are distinguished from each other on the basis of the thickness and differences in the makeup of the coats, especially the tunica media (Figs. 1.12*A* and 1.13). *Artery size is a continuum;* that is, there is a gradual change in morphological characteristics from one type to another. *There are three types of artery:*

- **Elastic arteries** (conducting arteries) are the largest type; the *aorta* and its branches from the *arch of the aorta* are good examples. The maintenance of blood pressure in the arterial system between contractions of the heart results from the elasticity of these arteries. This quality allows them to expand when the heart contracts and to return to normal between cardiac contractions.
- **Muscular arteries** (distributing arteries) such as the femoral artery distribute blood to various parts of the body. Their walls consist chiefly of circularly disposed smooth muscle fibers, which constrict their lumina—interior spaces of the arteries—when they contract. *Muscular arteries regulate the flow of blood to different parts as required by the body.*
- **Arterioles** are the smallest type; they have relatively narrow lumina and thick muscular walls. The degree of arterial pressure within the vascular system is mainly regulated by the degree of tonus (firmness) in the smooth muscle in the arterial walls. If the tonus is above normal, *hypertension* (high blood pressure) results.

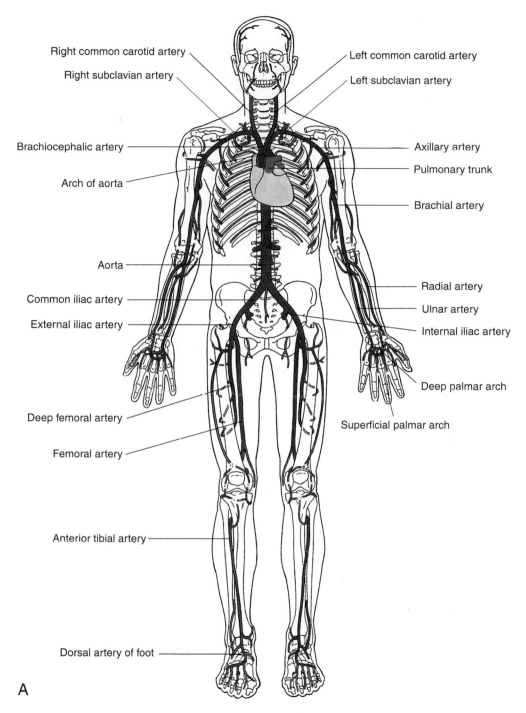

Right common carotid artery

Right subclavian artery

Brachiocephalic artery

Arch of aorta

Aorta

Common iliac artery

External iliac artery

Deep femoral artery

Femoral artery

Anterior tibial artery

Dorsal artery of foot

Left common carotid artery

Left subclavian artery

Axillary artery

Pulmonary trunk

Brachial artery

Radial artery

Ulnar artery

Internal iliac artery

Deep palmar arch

Superficial palmar arch

A

FIGURE 1.11 **Cardiovascular system. A.** Arterial system. **B.** Venous system. Superficial veins are shown in left limbs and deep veins in right limbs. Most arteries carry oxygenated blood away from the heart and most veins carry deoxygenated blood to the heart; however, the pulmonary arteries arising from the pulmonary trunk carry deoxygenated blood (colored blue) to the lungs, and the pulmonary veins carry oxygenated blood (colored red) from the lungs to the heart.

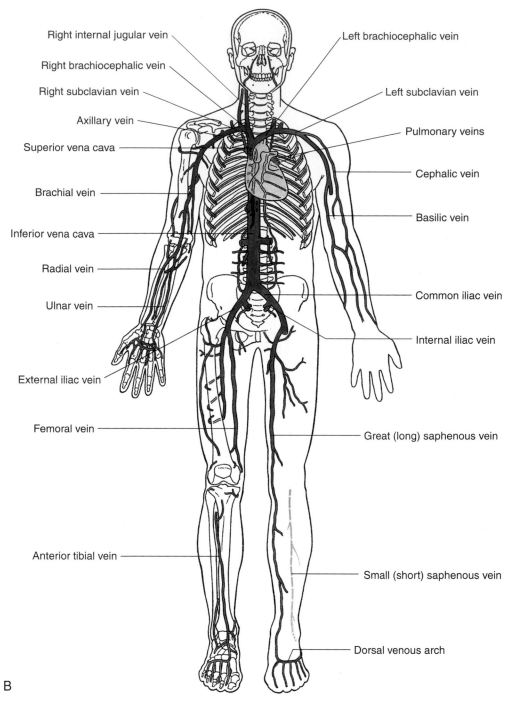

Right internal jugular vein

Right brachiocephalic vein

Right subclavian vein

Axillary vein

Superior vena cava

Brachial vein

Inferior vena cava

Radial vein

Ulnar vein

External iliac vein

Femoral vein

Anterior tibial vein

Left brachiocephalic vein

Left subclavian vein

Pulmonary veins

Cephalic vein

Basilic vein

Common iliac vein

Internal iliac vein

Great (long) saphenous vein

Small (short) saphenous vein

Dorsal venous arch

B

FIGURE 1.11 *Continued.*

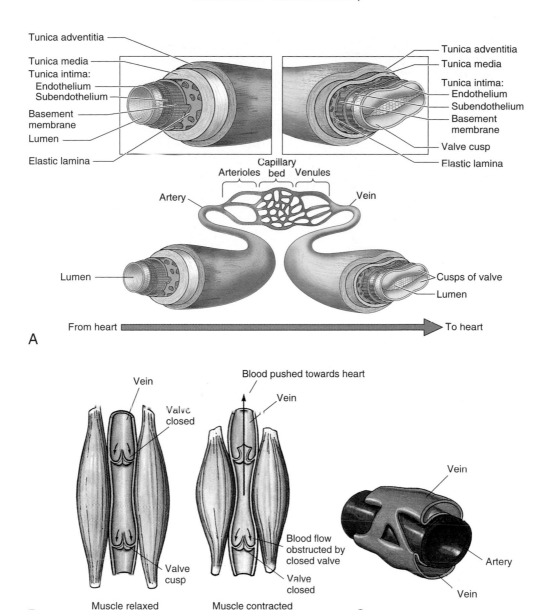

FIGURE 1.12   Blood vessels. A. Structure of blood vessels. Note that the diameter of the vein is greater than that of the artery it accompanies. **B.** The musculovenous pump. Muscular contractions in limbs function with venous valves to move blood toward the heart. The outward expansion of the bellies of contracting muscles becomes a compressive force, propelling blood against gravity. The *arrows* indicate the direction of blood flow. **C.** Muscular artery embraced by its accompanying or companion veins (L. venae communicantes).

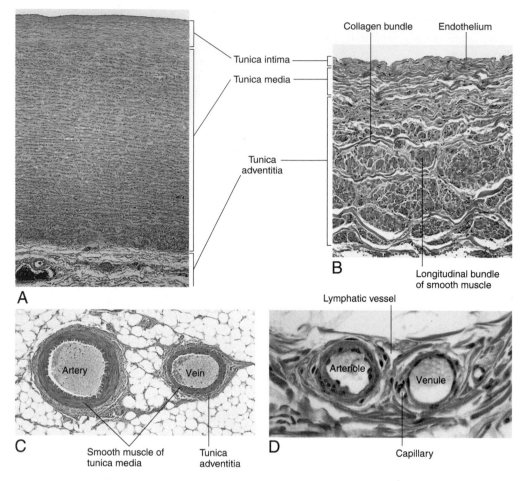

FIGURE 1.13 **Structures of arteries and veins. A.** Elastic artery (aorta, low power). **B.** IVC (low power). **C.** Muscular artery and vein (low power). **D.** Arteriole and venule (high power).

ARTERIOSCLEROSIS AND ISCHEMIC HEART DISEASE

The most common acquired disease of arteries is *arteriosclerosis* (hardening of arteries), a group of diseases characterized by thickening and loss of elasticity of arterial walls. *Atherosclerosis*—a common form of arteriosclerosis—is associated with the buildup of fat (mainly cholesterol) in the arterial walls. Calcium deposits then form *atheromatous plaques* or *atheromas*. The complications of atherosclerosis are *ischemic heart disease* (resulting from inadequate blood supply), *myocardial infarction* (necrosis of heart muscle and heart attack), stroke, and gangrene (e.g., necrosis in parts of the limbs).

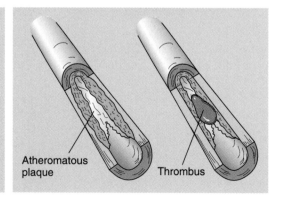

VEINS

Veins return poorly oxygenated blood to the heart from the capillary beds. *The large pulmonary veins are atypical in that they carry well-oxygenated blood from the lungs to the heart.* To make this clear, the pulmonary veins are colored red in Fig. 1.11*A*. Because of the lower blood pressure in the venous system, the walls of veins are thinner than those of their companion arteries (Figs. 1.12*A* and 1.13). The smallest veins—**venules**—unite to form larger veins that usually form *venous plexuses,* such as the **dorsal venous arch** of the foot. *Medium-sized veins* in the limbs and in other locations—where the flow of blood is opposed by the pull of gravity—have **valves** that permit blood to flow toward the heart but not in the reverse direction (Fig. 1.12*B*). **Large veins,** such as the SVC and IVC, are characterized by wide bundles of longitudinal smooth muscle and a well-developed tunica adventitia.

Veins tend to be double or multiple. Systemic veins are more variable than arteries and anastomoses occur more often between them. Those that accompany deep arteries (accompanying or companion veins) occupy a relatively unyielding *vascular sheath* with the artery they accompany (Fig. 1.12*C*). As a result they are stretched and flattened as the artery expands during contraction of the heart, which assists in driving the venous blood toward the heart. The outward expansion of the bellies of contracting skeletal muscles in the legs, for example, compresses the veins, "milking" the blood superiorly toward the heart—the *musculovenous pump* (Fig. 1.12*B*).

CAPILLARIES

Capillaries are simple endothelial tubes connecting the arterial and venous sides of the circulation. They are generally arranged in networks—**capillary beds**—between the arterioles and venules (Figs. 1.12*A* and 1.13*D*). The blood flowing through the capillaries is brought to them by **arterioles** and carried away from them by **venules.** As the hydrostatic pressure in the arterioles forces blood through the capillary bed, oxygen, nutrients, and other cellular materials are exchanged with the surrounding tissue. In some regions, such as in the fingers, there are direct connections between the small arteries and veins proximal to the capillary beds they supply and drain. The sites of such communications—*arteriovenous anastomoses (AV shunts)*—permit blood to pass directly from the arterial to the venous side of the circulation without passing through capillaries. *AV shunts are numerous in the skin,* where they have an important role in conserving body heat.

VARICOSE VEINS

When the walls of veins lose their elasticity, they are weak. A weakened vein dilates under the pressure of supporting a column of blood against gravity. This results in *varicose veins*—abnormally swollen, twisted veins —most often seen in the legs. Varicose veins have a caliber greater than normal and their valve cusps do not meet or have been destroyed by inflammation. These veins have *incompetent valves;* thus, the column of blood ascending toward the heart is unbroken, placing increased pressure on the weakened walls of the veins and exacerbating their varicosities.

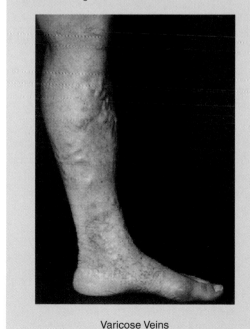

Varicose Veins

LYMPHATIC SYSTEM

The lymphatic system is part of the circulatory system; the other part is the cardiovascular system. The lymphatic system is a vast network of lymphatic vessels—**lymphatics**—that are connected with **lymph nodes**—small masses of lymphatic tissue (Fig. 1.14). The lymphatic system collects surplus extracellular tissue fluid as **lymph.** Lymph is usually clear and watery and has the same constituents as blood plasma. *The lymphatic system consists of:*

- **Lymphatic plexuses,** networks of very small lymphatic vessels—*lymphatic capillaries*—that originate in the intercellular spaces of most tissues
- **Lymphatics,** a bodywide network of lymphatic vessels, originating from lymphatic plexuses, along which lymph nodes are located
- **Lymph nodes,** small masses of lymphatic tissue through which lymph passes on its way to the venous system
- **Aggregations of lymphoid tissue** in the walls of the alimentary canal or digestive tract and in the spleen and thymus
- **Circulating lymphocytes** formed in *lymphoid tissue,* such as lymph nodes and the spleen, and in *myeloid tissue* in red bone marrow.

After traversing one or more lymph nodes, lymph enters larger lymphatic vessels—*lymphatic trunks*—that unite to form either the thoracic duct or the right lymphatic duct (Fig. 1.14).

- The **right lymphatic duct** drains lymph from the body's right upper quadrant—right side of head and neck, the right upper limb, and the right half of the thoracic cavity. The right lymphatic duct ends in the right subclavian vein at its angle of junction with the right internal jugular vein—*the right venous angle.*
- The **thoracic duct** drains lymph from the remainder of the body. This duct begins in the abdomen as a sac—**chyle cistern** (L. cistern chyli)—and ascends through the thorax and enters the junction of the left internal jugular and left subclavian veins—*the left venous angle.*

Superficial lymphatic vessels in the skin and subcutaneous tissue eventually drain into *deep lymphatic vessels* in the deep fascia between the muscles and subcutaneous tissue; the deep vessels accompany the major blood vessels.

The functions of lymphatics include:

- *Drainage of tissue fluid, collection of lymph plasma from the tissue spaces,* and *transport of lymph to the venous system*
- *Absorption and transport of fat,* in which special lymphatic capillaries (*lacteals*) receive all absorbed fat (*chyle*) from the intestine and convey it through the thoracic duct to the venous system
- *Formation of a defense mechanism for the body;* when foreign protein drains from an infected area, antibodies specific to the protein are produced by immunologically competent cells and/or lymphocytes and dispatched to the infected area.

LYMPHANGITIS, LYMPHADENITIS, AND LYMPHEDEMA
The terms *lymphangitis* and *lymphadenitis* refer to inflammation of lymphatic vessels and lymph nodes, respectively. These pathological processes may occur when the lymphatic system is involved in the *metastasis* (spread) of cancer—lymphogenous dissemination of cancer cells. *Lymphedema*—the accumulation of interstitial fluid—occurs when lymph is not drained from an area of the body. For instance, if *cancerous lymph nodes* are surgically removed from the axilla (armpit), lymphedema of the limb may result.

NERVOUS SYSTEM

The nervous system enables the body to react to continuous changes in its external and internal environments. It controls and integrates various activities of the body, such as circulation and respiration. *For descriptive purposes, the human nervous system is divided*

- Structurally into the *central nervous system* (CNS)—brain and spinal cord—and *peripheral nervous system* (PNS)—nerve fibers and cell bodies outside of CNS; because of their locations in the cranium and vertebral column, respectively, the brain and spinal cord are the most protected in the body (Haines, 2001)

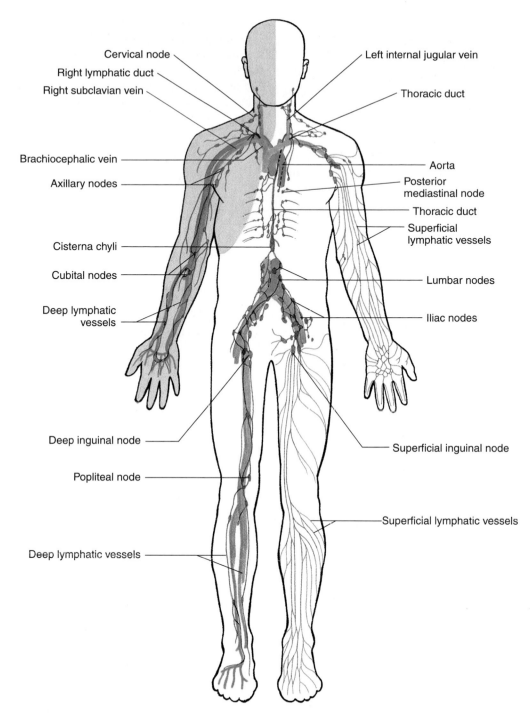

FIGURE 1.14 **Lymphatic system.** Anterior view. Right lymphatic duct drains lymph from right side of head and neck and right upper limb (*shaded*). Thoracic duct drains remainder of the body. Deep lymphatic vessels are shown on the right and superficial lymphatic vessels are shown on the left.

- Functionally into the *somatic nervous system* (SNS)—voluntary nervous system—and *autonomic nervous system* (ANS)—involuntary nervous system.

Nervous tissue consists of two main types of cell: **neurons** (nerve cells) and **neuroglia** (non-neuronal, nonexcitable glia cells). *The neuron is the structural and functional unit of the nervous system that is specialized for rapid communication* (Fig. 1.15). The neuron consists of a **cell body** and processes—**dendrites** and an **axon**—that carry impulses to and away from the cell body, respectively. *Myelin*—layers of lipid and protein substances—form a **myelin sheath** around some axons, greatly increasing the velocity of impulse conduction. Neurons communicate with each other at **synapses**—points of contact between neurons. The communication occurs by means of *neurotransmitters*—chemical agents released or secreted by one neuron, which may excite or inhibit another neuron, continuing or terminating the relay of impulses or the response to them. *Neuroglia* are approximately five times as abundant as neurons and form a major component (scaffolding) of ner-vous tissue. *Neuroglia support, insulate, and nourish the neurons.*

CENTRAL NERVOUS SYSTEM

The CNS consists of the **brain** and **spinal cord** (Fig, 1.16). *The principal roles of the CNS are to:*

- Integrate and coordinate incoming and outgoing neural signals
- Carry out higher mental functions such as thinking and learning.

A collection of nerve cell bodies in the CNS is a **nucleus** (Fig. 1.16*B*). A bundle of

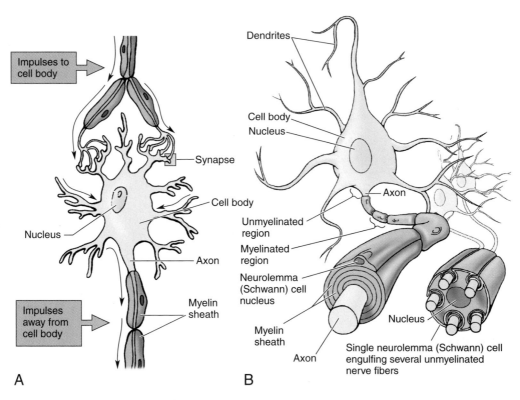

FIGURE 1.15   Structure of a motor neuron. A. Parts of a motor neuron. **B.** Myelinated and unmyelinated nerves.

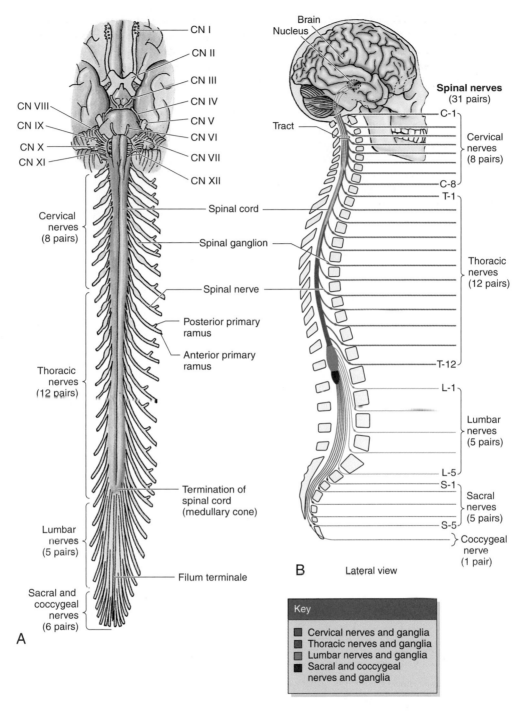

CN I

CN II

CN III

CN IV

CN V

CN VI

CN VII

CN XII

CN VIII

CN IX

CN X

CN XI

Brain

Nucleus

Spinal nerves
(31 pairs)

C-1

Tract

Cervical
nerves
(8 pairs)

C-8

T-1

Cervical
nerves
(8 pairs)

Spinal cord

Spinal ganglion

Spinal nerve

Posterior primary
ramus

Anterior primary
ramus

Thoracic
nerves
(12 pairs)

T-12

Thoracic
nerves
(12 pairs)

L-1

Lumbar
nerves
(5 pairs)

L-5

S-1

Termination of
spinal cord
(medullary cone)

Sacral
nerves
(5 pairs)

S-5

Coccygeal
nerve
(1 pair)

Lumbar
nerves
(5 pairs)

B   Lateral view

Filum terminale

Sacral and
coccygeal
nerves
(6 pairs)

A

Key

■ Cervical nerves and ganglia
■ Thoracic nerves and ganglia
■ Lumbar nerves and ganglia
■ Sacral and coccygeal
  nerves and ganglia

FIGURE 1.16   Basic organization of nervous system. A. Anterior view. *CN,* cranial nerve. **B.** Lateral view.

nerve fibers (axons) connecting neighboring or distant nuclei of the CNS is a **tract.** The nerve cell bodies lie within and constitute the **gray substance** (gray matter); the interconnecting fiber tract systems form the **white substance** (white matter). In transverse sections of the spinal cord, the gray substance appears roughly as an H-shaped area embedded in a matrix of white substance (Fig. 1.17). The struts (supports) of the H are **horns;** therefore, there are *posterior (dorsal)* and *anterior (ventral) gray horns.* Three membranous layers—pia mater, arachnoid mater, and dura mater, collectively constituting the **meninges**—and the cerebrospinal fluid (**CSF**) surround and protect the CNS. The brain and spinal cord are intimately covered on their outer surface by the innermost layer, a delicate, transparent covering—the **pia mater** (pia). CSF is located between the pia and **arachnoid mater** (arachnoid); fine weblike strands—**arachnoid trabeculae**—extend through the CSF, joining the pia and arachnoid. External to the pia and arachnoid is the thick, tough **dura mater** (dura), which is adherent to the internal surface of the cranium but separated from the vertebral column by the *extradural (epidural) space.*

DAMAGE TO CNS

When the CNS is damaged, the injured axons do not recover in most circumstances. Their proximal stumps begin to regenerate, sending sprouts into the area of the lesion; however, growth stops in approximately 2 weeks. As a result, permanent disability follows destruction of a tract in the brain or spinal cord.

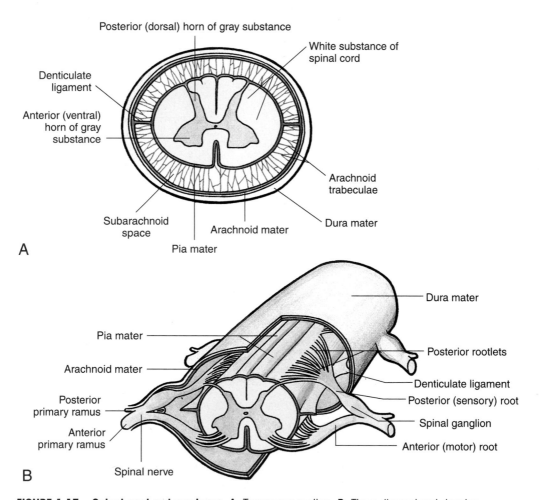

FIGURE 1.17 **Spinal cord and meninges. A.** Transverse section. **B.** Three-dimensional drawing.

PERIPHERAL NERVOUS SYSTEM

The PNS consists of nerve fibers and cell bodies outside the CNS that conduct impulses to or away from the CNS (Fig. 1.16). The PNS is made up of nerves that connect the CNS with peripheral structures. A bundle of nerve fibers (axons) in the PNS, held together by a connective tissue sheath, is a **peripheral nerve,** a strong, whitish cord in living persons. A collection of nerve cell bodies outside the CNS is a ganglion—a **spinal ganglion,** for example. *Peripheral nerves are either cranial or spinal nerves.* Eleven of the twelve pairs of **cranial nerves** arise from the brain; the 12th pair (CN XII) arises mostly from the superior part of the spinal cord. All cranial nerves exit the cranial cavity through foramina (openings) in the cranium (G. kranion, skull). The 31 pairs of **spinal nerves** (8 cervical, 12 thoracic, 5 lumbar, 5 sacral, and 1 coccygeal) arise from the spinal cord and exit through intervertebral foramina in the vertebral column. A **peripheral nerve fiber** (Fig. 1.18) consists of:

- An *axon*—the single process of a neuron
- A *neurolemmal sheath* surrounding a peripheral nerve fiber
- The *endoneurium*—an endoneural connective tissue sheath.

The **axon** under normal conditions conducts nervous impulses away from the cell body. The **neurolemmal sheath** may take two forms, creating two classes of nerve fiber (Fig. 1.15*B*).

- *Myelinated nerve fibers* have a neurolemmal (myelin) sheath consisting of a continuous series of *neurolemma (Schwann) cells* that surround an individual axon and form myelin.
- *Unmyelinated nerve fibers* are engulfed in groups by a single neurolemma cell that does not produce myelin; most fibers in cutaneous nerves are unmyelinated.

Peripheral nerves are fairly strong and resilient because the nerve fibers are supported and protected by **three connective tissue coverings** (Fig. 1.18):

- *Endoneurium,* a delicate connective tissue sheath that surrounds the neurolemma cells and axons

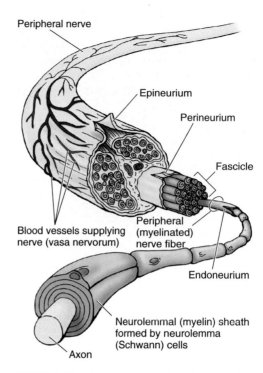

FIGURE 1.18 Arrangement and ensheathment of peripheral nerve fibers.

- *Perineurium,* which encloses a bundle (fascicle) of peripheral nerve fibers, providing an effective barrier against penetration of the nerve fibers by foreign substances
- *Epineurium,* a thick sheath of loose connective tissue that surrounds and encloses the nerve bundles, forming the outermost covering of the nerve; it includes fatty tissues, blood vessels, and lymphatics.

A peripheral nerve is much like a telephone cable, the axons being the individual wires insulated by the neurolemmal sheath and endoneurium, the insulated wires bundled by the perineurium, and the bundles surrounded in turn by the epineurium forming the outer wrapping of the "cable."

PERIPHERAL NERVE DEGENERATION
When peripheral nerves are crushed or severed, their axons degenerate distal to the lesion because they are dependent on their cell bodies for survival. A *crushing nerve injury* damages or kills the axons distal to the injury site; however, the nerve cell bodies usually survive

Continued
and the connective tissue coverings of the nerve are intact. No surgical repair is needed for this type of nerve injury because the intact connective tissue sheaths guide the growing axons to their destinations. *Surgical intervention is necessary if the nerve is cut* because the regeneration of axons requires apposition of the cut ends by sutures through the epineurium. The individual bundles of nerve fibers are realigned as accurately as possible. Compromising a nerve's blood supply for a long period, producing *ischemia* by compression of the vasa nervorum (Fig. 1.18), can also cause nerve degeneration. Prolonged ischemia of a nerve may result in damage no less severe than that produced by crushing or even cutting the nerve.

Somatic Nervous System

The SNS, or voluntary nervous system, composed of somatic parts of the CNS and PNS, provides general sensory and motor innervation to all parts of the body (G. soma), except the viscera in the body cavities, smooth mus-cle, and glands (Fig. 1.19). The *somatic sensory system* transmits sensations of touch, pain, temperature, and position from sensory receptors. The *somatic motor system* permits voluntary and reflexive movement by causing contraction of skeletal muscles, such as occurs when one touches a candle flame.

Autonomic Nervous System

The ANS, classically described as the *visceral motor system,* consists of fibers that innervate involuntary (smooth) muscle, modified cardiac muscle (the intrinsic stimulating and conducting tissue of the heart [Chapter 3]), and glands. However, the visceral efferent (motor) fibers of the ANS are accompanied by visceral afferent (sensory) fibers. In their role as the afferent component of autonomic reflexes and in conducting visceral pain impulses, sensory fibers also regulate visceral function.

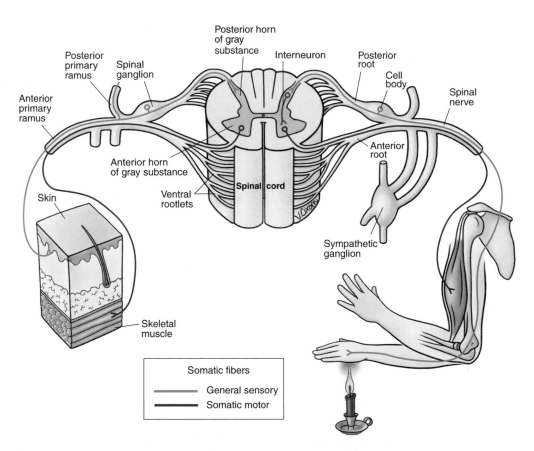

FIGURE 1.19   Components of somatic (spinal) nerves. The somatic motor system permits voluntary and reflexive movement by causing contraction of skeletal muscles, such as occurs when one touches a hot iron.

Visceral Afferent Sensation. Visceral afferent fibers have important relationships to the ANS, both anatomically and functionally. We are usually unaware of the sensory input of these fibers, which provides information about the condition of the body's internal environment. This information is integrated in the CNS, often triggering visceral or somatic reflexes or both. *Visceral reflexes regulate blood pressure and chemistry by altering such functions as heart and respiratory rates and vascular resistance.* Visceral sensation, which reaches a conscious level, is generally categorized as pain that is usually poorly localized and may be perceived as hunger or nausea. Surgeons operating on patients who are under local anesthesia may handle, cut, clamp, or even burn (cauterize) visceral organs without evoking conscious sensation. However, adequate stimulation such as the following may elicit true pain:

- Sudden distention
- Spasms or strong contractions
- Chemical irritants
- Mechanical stimulation, especially when the organ is active
- Pathological conditions (especially *ischemia*—inadequate blood supply) that lower the normal thresholds of stimulation.

Normal activity usually produces no sensation but may do so when there is ischemia. Most visceral reflex (subconscious) sensation and some pain travel in visceral afferent fibers that accompany the parasympathetic fibers retrograde (moving backward). Most visceral pain impulses (from the heart and most organs of the peritoneal cavity) travel centrally along visceral afferent fibers accompanying sympathetic fibers.

Visceral Motor Innervation. The efferent nerve fibers and ganglia of the ANS are organized into two systems or divisions:

- **Sympathetic (thoracolumbar) division.** In general, the effects of sympathetic stimulation are *catabolic*—preparing the body to "flee or fight."
- **Parasympathetic (craniosacral) division.** In general, the effects of parasympathetic stimulation are *anabolic*—promoting normal function and conserving energy.

Although both sympathetic and parasympathetic systems innervate the same structures, they have different (usually contrasting) but coordinated effects (Table 1.6).

Conduction of impulses from the CNS to the effector organ involves a series of two neurons in sympathetic and parasympathetic systems. The cell body of the *1st presynaptic, or preganglionic, neuron* is located in the gray substance of the CNS. Its fiber (axon) synapses only on the cell bodies of *postsynaptic, or postganglionic neurons,* the 2nd neurons in the series. The cell bodies of the *2nd neurons are located in autonomic ganglia* outside the CNS, with fibers terminating on the effector organ (smooth muscle, modified cardiac muscle, or glands). *The anatomical distinction between the two divisions of the ANS is based primarily on the location of the presynaptic cell bodies.* A functional distinction of pharmacological importance in medical practice is that the postsynaptic neurons of the two systems generally liberate different neurotransmitter substances: *norepinephrine by the sympathetic division* (except in the case of sweat glands) and *acetylcholine by the parasympathetic division.*

COMPONENTS OF A TYPICAL SPINAL NERVE. A typical spinal nerve arises from the spinal cord by **nerve rootlets,** which converge to form two **nerve roots** (Fig. 1.19): the *anterior (ventral) root* and the *posterior (dorsal) root.* The anterior and posterior roots unite to form a **mixed spinal nerve** that immediately divides into two rami (branches): a **posterior primary ramus** and an **anterior primary ramus.** As branches of the mixed spinal nerve, the posterior and anterior rami carry both motor and sensory nerves, as do all their subsequent branches.

- The **posterior primary rami** supply nerve fibers to synovial joints of the vertebral column, deep muscles of the back, and the overlying skin.
- The **anterior primary rami** supply nerve fibers to the much larger remaining area, consisting of anterior and lateral regions of the trunk and the upper and lower limbs arising from them.

The *afferent, or sensory, fibers* convey neural impulses to the CNS from sense organs

TABLE 1.6. FUNCTIONS OF AUTONOMIC NERVOUS SYSTEM (ANS)

Organ, Tract, or System		Effect of Sympathetic Stimulation[a]	Effect of Parasympathetic Stimulation[b]
Eyes	Pupil	Dilates pupil (admits more light for increased acuity at a distance)	Constricts pupil (protects pupil from excessively bright light)
	Ciliary body		Contracts ciliary muscle, allowing lens to thicken for near vision (accommodation)
Skin	Arrector muscle of hair	Causes hairs to stand on end ("gooseflesh" or "goose bumps")	No effect (does not reach)[c]
	Peripheral blood vessels	Vasoconstricts (blanching of skin, lips, and turning fingertips blue)	No effect (does not reach)[c]
	Sweat glands	Promotes sweating[d]	No effect (does not reach)[c]
Other glands	Lacrimal glands	Slightly decreases secretion[e]	Promotes secretion
	Salivary glands	Secretion decreases, becomes thicker, more viscous[e]	Promotes abundant, watery secretion
Heart		Increases the rate and strength of contraction; inhibits the effect of parasympathetic system on coronary vessels, allowing them to dilate[e]	Decreases the rate and strength of contraction (conserving energy); constricts coronary vessels in relation to reduced demand
Lungs		Inhibits effect of parasympathetic system, resulting in bronchodilation and reduced secretion, allowing for maximum air exchange	Constricts bronchi (conserving energy) and promotes bronchial secretion
Digestive tract		Inhibits peristalsis, and constricts blood vessels to digestive tract so that blood is available to skeletal muscle; contracts internal anal sphincter to aid fecal continence	Stimulates peristalsis and secretion of digestive juices
			Contracts rectum, inhibits internal anal sphincter to cause defecation
Liver and gallbladder		Promotes breakdown of glycogen to glucose (for increased energy)	Promotes building/conservation of glycogen; increases secretion of bile
Urinary tract		Vasoconstriction of renal vessels slows urine formation; internal sphincter of bladder contracted to maintain urinary continence	Inhibits contraction of internal sphincter of bladder, contracts detrusor muscle of the bladder wall causing urination
Genital system		Causes ejaculation and vasoconstriction resulting in remission of erection	Produces engorgement (erection) of erectile tissues of the external genitals
Suprarenal medulla		Release of adrenaline into blood	No effect (does not innervate)

Underlying general principles:
[a]In general, the effects of sympathetic stimulation are catabolic—preparing body to flee or fight.
[b]In general, the effects of parasympathetic stimulation are anabolic—promoting normal function and conserving energy.
[c]The parasympathetic system is restricted in its distribution to the head, neck, and body cavities (except for erectile tissues of genitalia); otherwise, parasympathetic fibers are never found in the body wall and limbs. Sympathetic fibers, by comparison, are distributed to all vascularized portions of the body.
[d]With the exception of the sweat glands, glandular secretion is parasympathetically stimulated.
[e]With the exception of the coronary arteries, vasoconstriction is sympathetically stimulated; the effects of sympathetic stimulation on glands (other than sweat glands) are the indirect effects of vasoconstriction.

(e.g., the eyes) and from sensory receptors in various parts of the body (e.g., in the skin). Its *efferent, or motor, fibers* convey neural impulses from the CNS to the effector organs (muscles and glands).

The anterior root contains somatic motor fibers from the nerve cell bodies in the anterior horn of the spinal cord. The dorsal root carries general sensory fibers to the posterior horn of the spinal cord. As branches of a *mixed spinal nerve,* the anterior and posterior primary rami carry both motor and sensory nerves, as do all their branches. *The components of a typical spinal nerve include:*

- **Somatic sensory fibers and motor fibers**
  —*General sensory (general somatic afferent)* fibers transmit sensations from the body to the spinal cord; they may be *exteroceptive sensations* (pain, temperature, touch, and pressure) from the skin, or pain and proprioceptive sensations from muscles, tendons, and joints. *Proprioceptive sensations* are unconscious sensations that convey information on joint position and the tension of tendons and muscles, providing information on how the body and limbs are oriented in space.
  —*Somatic motor (general somatic efferent)* fibers transmit impulses to skeletal (voluntary) muscles (Fig. 1.19).

- **Visceral sensory fibers and motor fibers** of the sympathetic and parasympathetic nervous systems
  —*Visceral sensory (general visceral afferent)* fibers transmit reflex or pain sensations from mucous membranes, glands, and blood vessels back to the CNS. Both types of sensory fibers—visceral sensory and general sensory—have their cell bodies within spinal ganglia or sensory ganglia of cranial nerves.
  —*Visceral motor (general visceral efferent)* fibers transmit impulses to involuntary (smooth and cardiac) muscle and glandular tissues. The two varieties of fibers—*presynaptic* and *postsynaptic*—team together to conduct impulses from the CNS to smooth muscle or glands (Fig. 1.20).

- **Connective tissue coverings** (Fig. 1.18).
- **Vasa nervorum,** the blood vessels supplying the nerves.

SYMPATHETIC VISCERAL MOTOR INNERVATION. The cell bodies of presynaptic neurons of the sympathetic division of the ANS are located in the **intermediolateral cell columns** or nucleus (IMLs) of the spinal cord (Fig. 1.21). The paired (right and left) IMLs are a part of the gray substance extending between the 1st thoracic (T1) and the 2nd or 3rd lumbar (L2 or L3) segments of the spinal cord. In horizontal sections of this part of the spinal cord, the IMLs appear as small **lateral horns** of the H-shaped gray substance, looking somewhat like an extension of the cross-bar of the H between the posterior and anterior horns of gray substance. The cell bodies of postsynaptic neurons of the sympathetic nervous system occur in two locations, the paravertebral and prevertebral ganglia (Fig. 1.22):

- **Paravertebral ganglia** are linked to form right and left *sympathetic trunks (chains)* on each side of the vertebral column that extend essentially the length of this column. The superior paravertebral ganglion—the **superior cervical ganglion** of each sympathetic trunk—lies at the base of the cranium. The **ganglion impar** forms inferiorly where the two trunks unite at the level of the coccyx.
- **Prevertebral ganglia** are in the plexuses that surround the origins of the main branches of the abdominal aorta, such as the large **celiac ganglia,** which surround the origin of the *celiac trunk* (artery) arising from the aorta.

Because they are motor fibers, the axons of presynaptic neurons leave the spinal cord through anterior roots and enter the anterior rami of spinal nerves T1 through L2 or L3 (Fig. 1.23). Almost immediately after entering the rami, all the presynaptic sympathetic fibers leave the anterior primary rami of these spinal nerves and pass to the **sympathetic trunks** through white communicating branches or **white rami communicantes.** Within the sympa-

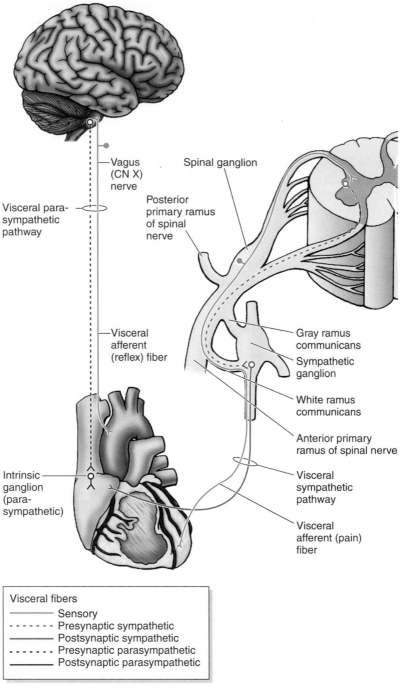

FIGURE 1.20 **Sympathetic and parasympathetic innervation of the heart.**

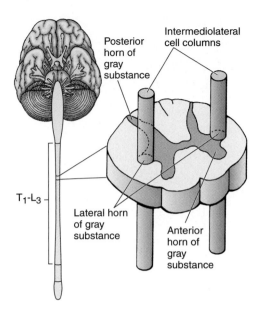

FIGURE 1.21 **Intermediolateral cell columns (IMLs).** The paired IML columns or nuclei constitute the lateral horn of gray substance, seen on section of spinal cord segments T1 through L2 or L3, and consist of the cell bodies of presynaptic neurons of the sympathetic nervous system.

thetic trunks, presynaptic fibers follow one of three possible courses:

- Enter and synapse immediately with a postsynaptic neuron of the paravertebral ganglion at that level
- Ascend or descend in the sympathetic trunk to synapse with a postsynaptic neuron of a higher or lower paravertebral ganglion
- Pass through the sympathetic trunk without synapsing, continuing on through an abdominopelvic splanchnic nerve to reach the prevertebral ganglia.

Presynaptic sympathetic fibers providing autonomic innervation within the head, neck, body wall, limbs, and thoracic cavity follow one of the first two courses, synapsing within the paravertebral ganglia. Presynaptic sympathetic fibers innervating viscera within the abdominopelvic cavity follow the 3rd course.

Postsynaptic sympathetic fibers destined for distribution within the neck, body wall,

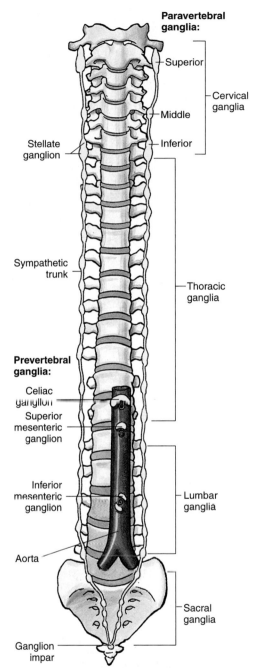

FIGURE 1.22 **Sympathetic ganglia.** *Paravertebral ganglia* are associated with all spinal nerves although at cervical levels eight spinal nerves share three ganglia. *Prevertebral (preaortic) ganglia* occur in the plexuses that surround the origins of the main branches of the abdominal aorta, such as the celiac artery.

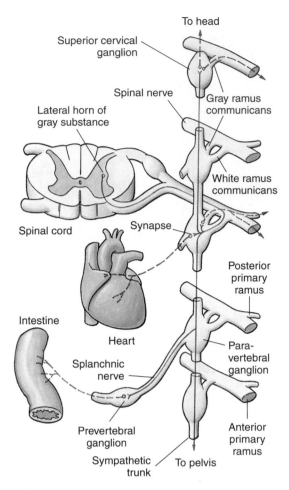

FIGURE 1.23 **Origin and distribution of sympathetic motor fibers.** *Solid lines,* presynaptic fibers; *broken lines,* postsynaptic fibers.

and limbs pass from the paravertebral ganglia of the sympathetic trunks to adjacent anterior rami of spinal nerves (Fig. 1.24) through gray communicating branches or **gray rami communicantes.** They enter all branches of the spinal nerve, including the posterior primary rami, to stimulate contraction of blood vessels (*vasomotion*) and arrector pili muscles associated with hairs (*pilomotion* resulting in "goose bumps"), and to cause sweating (*sudomotion*). Postsynaptic sympathetic fibers that perform these functions in the head (plus innervation of the dilator muscle of the iris) all have their cell bodies in the **superior cervical ganglion** at the superior end of the sympathetic trunk. They pass by means of a *cephalic arterial ra-*

mus to form a **carotid periarterial plexus** (Fig. 1.24), which follow branches of the carotid arteries to their destination.

Splanchnic nerves (Figs. 1.23 and 1.24) convey visceral efferent (autonomic) and afferent fibers to viscera of the body cavities. Postsynaptic sympathetic fibers destined for viscera of the thoracic cavity (e.g., heart, lungs, and esophagus) pass through **cardiopulmonary splanchnic nerves** to enter the cardiac, pulmonary and esophageal plexuses. The presyn-aptic sympathetic fibers involved in innervation of viscera of the abdominopelvic cavity (e.g., the stomach and intestines) pass to the prevertebral ganglia through **abdominopelvic splanchnic nerves** (comprising the greater, lesser, least, and lumbar splanchnic nerves). All presynaptic sympathetic fibers of the abdominopelvic splanchnic nerves, except those involved in innervating the suprarenal (adrenal) glands, synapse in the prevertebral ganglia. The postsynaptic fibers from these ganglia form *periarterial plexuses,* which

follow branches of the abdominal aorta to reach their destination.

Presynaptic sympathetic fibers passing through the prevertebral (celiac) ganglia terminate on cells in the medulla of the suprarenal gland (Fig. 1.25). The suprarenal medullary cells

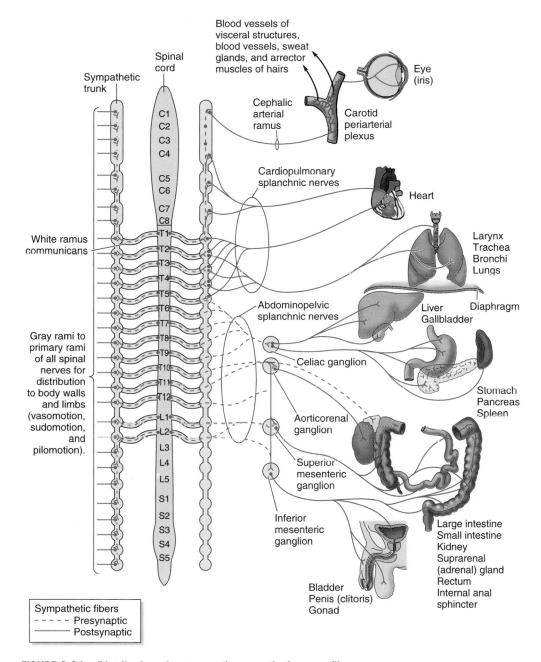

FIGURE 1.24 **Distribution of postsynaptic sympathetic nerve fibers.**

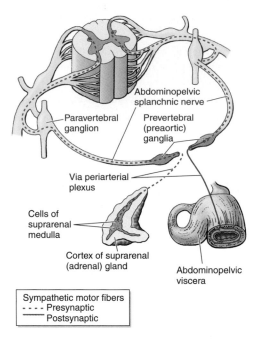

Sympathetic motor fibers
- - - - Presynaptic
———— Postsynaptic

FIGURE 1.25 **Sympathetic supply to medulla of suprarenal gland.** The sympathetic supply to this gland is exceptional. The secretory cells of the medulla are postsynaptic neurons that lack axons or dendrites. Consequently, the suprarenal medulla is supplied directly by presynaptic sympathetic neurons. The neurotransmitters produced by medullary cells are released into the bloodstream to produce a widespread sympathetic response.

function as a special type of postsynaptic neuron that, instead of releasing their neurotransmitter substance onto the cells of a specific effector organ, release it into the blood stream to circulate throughout the body, producing a widespread sympathetic response. As described earlier, postsynaptic sympathetic fibers are components of virtually all branches of all spinal nerves. By this and other means, they extend to and innervate all the body's blood vessels, sweat glands, and many other structures. Thus, the sympathetic nervous system reaches virtually all parts of the body with the rare exception of avascular tissues such as cartilage and nails.

PARASYMPATHETIC VISCERAL MOTOR INNERVATION. Presynaptic parasympathetic neuron cell bodies are located in two sites within the CNS, their fibers exiting by two routes (Fig. 1.26):

- In the gray substance of the brainstem (medulla, pons, and midbrain), the fibers exit the CNS within cranial nerves III, VII, IX, and X; these fibers constitute the **cranial parasympathetic outflow.**
- In the gray substance of the sacral segments of the spinal cord (S2 through S4), the fibers exit the CNS through the ventral roots of spinal nerves S2 through S4 and the pelvic splanchnic nerves that arise from their ventral rami; these fibers constitute the **sacral parasympathetic outflow.**

Not surprisingly, the cranial outflow provides parasympathetic innervation of the head and the sacral outflow provides the parasympathetic innervation of the pelvic viscera. However, in terms of the innervation of thoracic and abdominal viscera, the cranial outflow through the vagus nerve (CN X) is dominant. It provides innervation to all the thoracic viscera and most of the gastrointestinal (GI) tract from the esophagus through most of the large bowel (to its left colic flexure). With regard to the GI tract, the sacral outflow supplies only the descending and sigmoid colon and rectum.

Regardless of the extensive influence of its cranial outflow, the parasympathetic system is much more restricted than is the sympathetic system in its distribution. The parasympathetic system distributes only to the head, visceral cavities of the trunk, and erectile tissues of the external genitalia. With the exception of the latter, it does not reach the body wall or limbs, and except for initial parts of the anterior primary rami of spinal nerves S2 through S4, its fibers are not components of spinal nerves or their branches.

Four discrete pairs of parasympathetic ganglia occur in the head (see Chapters 8 and 10). Elsewhere, presynaptic parasympathetic fibers synapse with postsynaptic cell bodies that occur singly in or on the wall of the target organ (*intrinsic or enteric ganglia*).

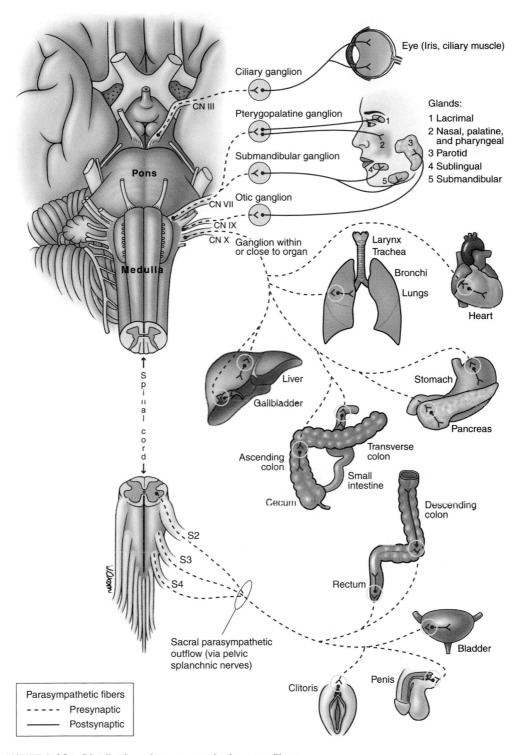

FIGURE 1.26   **Distribution of parasympathetic nerve fibers.**

MEDICAL IMAGING TECHNIQUES

Familiarity with imaging techniques commonly used in clinical settings enables one to recognize abnormalities such as congenital anomalies, tumors, and fractures. The most commonly used diagnostic imaging techniques follow:

- Conventional radiography (plain films)
- Computerized tomography (CT)
- Magnetic resonance imaging (MRI)
- Ultrasonography (sonography).

CONVENTIONAL RADIOGRAPHY

The essence of a radiological examination is that a highly penetrating beam of X-rays transilluminates the patient, showing tissues of differing densities of mass within the body as images of differing densities of light and dark on the X-ray film (Fig. 1.27). A tissue or organ

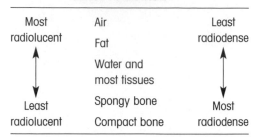

TABLE 1.7.   BASIC PRINCIPLES OF X-RAY IMAGE FORMATION

Most radiolucent ↕ Least radiolucent	Air Fat Water and most tissues Spongy bone Compact bone	Least radiodense ↕ Most radiodense

that is relatively dense in mass (e.g., compact bone in rib) absorbs more X-rays than does a less dense tissue such as spongy bone (Table 1.7). Consequently, a dense tissue or organ produces a relatively transparent area on the X-ray film because relatively fewer X-rays reach the silver slat/gelatin emulsion in the film. Therefore, relatively fewer grains of silver are developed at this area when the film is processed. A very dense substance is *radiopaque,* whereas a substance of less density is *radiolucent.*

COMPUTERIZED TOMOGRAPHY

Computerized tomography (CT) shows images of sections of the body such as the abdomen (Fig. 1.28). A beam of X-rays is passed through the body as the X-ray tube moves in a circle around the body. The amount of radiation absorbed by each different type of tissue of the chosen body plane varies with the amount of fat, cancellous and compact bone, and water density of the tissue in each element. A multitude of linear energy absorptions is measured and stored in a computer that compiles and generates images. CT is excellent for examining bony tissues.

ULTRASONOGRAPHY

Ultrasonography (sonography) gives images of deep structures in the body by recording reflections of pulses of ultrasonic waves directed into the tissues (Fig. 1.29). A common use of diagnostic ultrasound imaging is to examine abdominal organs, such as the kidneys,

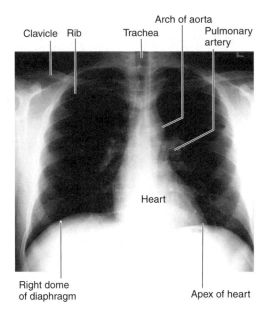

Clavicle   Rib   Trachea   Arch of aorta   Pulmonary artery

Heart

Right dome of diaphragm   Apex of heart

FIGURE 1.27   Radiograph of the thorax (chest). Posteroanterior (PA) projection. (Courtesy of Dr. E.L. Lansdown, Professor of Medical Imaging, University of Toronto, Toronto, Ontario, Canada.)

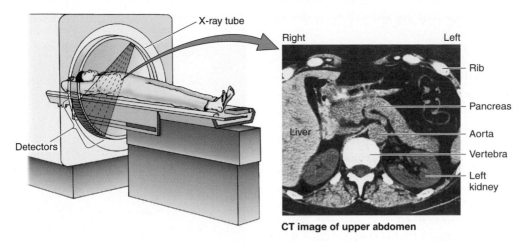

CT image of upper abdomen

FIGURE 1.28   CT scan of upper abdomen. The X-ray tube rotates around the person in the CT scanner and sends a fan-shaped beam of X-rays through the person's upper abdomen from a variety of angles. X-ray detectors on the opposite side of the person's body measure the amount of radiation that passes through a transverse section of the person. A computer reconstructs the CT images from several scans and an abdominal CT scan is produced. The scan is oriented so it appears the way an examiner would view it when standing at the foot of the bed and looking toward a supine person's head.

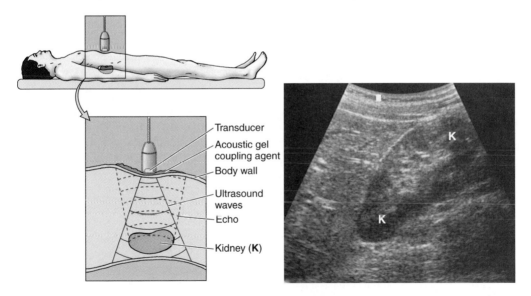

FIGURE 1.29   Ultrasound scan of upper abdomen. The image results from the echo of ultrasound waves from structures of different densities. The image of the right kidney is displayed on a monitor.

and to assess fetal age and well-being during pregnancy.

MAGNETIC RESONANCE IMAGING

Magnetic resonance imaging (MRI) shows images of the body (Fig. 1.30) similar to those produced by CT in that they are planar, but they are better for tissue differentiation. MRI has the great advantage of requiring no radiation. The MRI technique uses the magnetic properties of the hydrogen nucleus excited by radiofrequency transmitted by a coil surrounding the body (see Moore and Dalley [1999] for more details). MRI is better than CT for showing details in soft tissues (e.g., heart and muscles surrounding the thorax), but provides little information about bones.

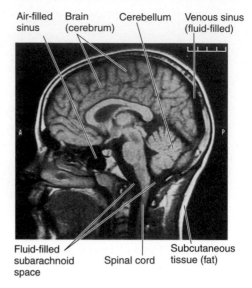

Air-filled sinus Brain (cerebrum) Cerebellum Venous sinus (fluid-filled)

Fluid-filled subarachnoid space Spinal cord Subcutaneous tissue (fat)

FIGURE 1.30   Median MRI of head. Many details of the CNS are visible. Structures in the nasal and oral cavities and upper neck are also shown. The patient is placed in a strong magnetic field that aligns the body's free protons. The aligned protons are "flipped" by radiowaves and emit radiowaves as they flip back. The latter radiowaves are detected by an MRI system and processed by a computer, which produces the MRI scan.

*T*he thorax (chest) is the superior part of the trunk between the neck and abdomen. *The* **thoracic cavity,** surrounded by the **thoracic wall,** contains the heart, lungs, thymus, distal part of the trachea, and most of the esophagus. *Because these structures (includ-*ing the thoracic wall) are constantly moving, *the thorax is one of the most dynamic regions of the body.* To perform a physical examination of the thorax, a working knowledge of its structure and vital organs is required.

THORACIC WALL

The thoracic wall consists of skin, fascia, nerves, vessels, muscles, and bones. The function of the thoracic wall is not only to protect the contents of the thoracic cavity but also to provide the mechanical function of breathing. The *mammary glands* of the breasts are in the subcutaneous tissue overlying the pectoral muscles covering the anterolateral thoracic wall. These muscles usually act on the upper limbs. The thoracic wall is covered internally by *parietal thoracic (endothoracic) fascia.* This deep fascia invests the underlying internal intercostal, subcostal, and transverse thoracic (L. transversus thoracis) muscles forming the *epimysium,* a connective tissue covering. The deep fascia also blends with the periosteum of the ribs and sternum and with the perichondrium of the costal cartilages.

SKELETON OF THORACIC WALL

The skeleton of the thoracic wall (Fig. 2.1) forms an **osteocartilaginous thoracic cage** that protects the heart, lungs, and some upper abdominal organs such as the liver. **The thoracic skeleton (bony thorax) includes:**

- 12 pairs of ribs and costal cartilages
- 12 thoracic vertebrae and intervertebral (IV) discs
- The sternum.

Ribs and Costal Cartilages
The ribs are curved, flat bones that form most of the thoracic cage (Fig. 2.1, *A* and *B*). They are remarkably light in weight yet highly resilient. *There are three types of ribs:*

- **True (vertebrocostal) ribs** (the first seven of the twelve ribs)—so-called because they attach directly to the sternum through their own costal cartilages.
- **False (vertebrochondral) ribs** (the 8th to 10th ribs). Their cartilages are joined to the cartilage of the rib just superior to them; thus, their connection with the sternum is indirect.

- **Floating (free) ribs** (the 11th and 12th ribs). Their cartilages do not connect even indirectly with the sternum; instead, they end in the posterior abdominal musculature.

Costal cartilages form the anterior continuation of the ribs, providing the means by which they reach and articulate with the sternum (Fig. 2.1*A*). Ribs and their cartilages are separated by **intercostal spaces,** which are occupied by intercostal muscles, vessels, and nerves.

Typical ribs (*3rd to 9th*) *have a:*

- **Head** that is wedge-shaped and has two facets, separated by the **crest of the head** (Fig. 2.2*A*); one facet is for articulation with the numerically corresponding vertebra and one facet is for the vertebra superior to it.
- **Neck** that connects the head with the body (shaft) at the level of the tubercle.
- **Tubercle** occurring at the junction of the neck and shaft. The tubercle has a smooth *articular part* for articulating with the corresponding transverse process of the vertebra, and a rough *nonarticular part* for the attachment of the costotransverse ligament.
- **Body** (shaft) that is thin, flat, and curved—most markedly at the **angle** where the rib turns anterolaterally; the concave internal surface has a **costal groove** that protects the intercostal nerve and vessels.

Atypical ribs (*1st, 2nd, and 10th to 12th*) *are dissimilar* (Figs. 2.1 and 2.3):

- The **lst rib** is the broadest (i.e., its body is widest and is nearly horizontal), shortest, and most sharply curved of the seven true ribs; it has two **grooves for the subclavian vessels** on its superior surface, which are separated by a **scalene tubercle** and ridge.
- The **2nd rib** is thinner, less curved, and much longer than the 1st rib; it has two facets on its head for articulation with the bodies of T1 and T2 vertebrae, and a **tubercle** for muscle attachment.
- The **10th to 12th ribs,** like the lst rib, have only one facet on their heads.
- The **11th and 12th ribs** are short and have no necks or tubercles.

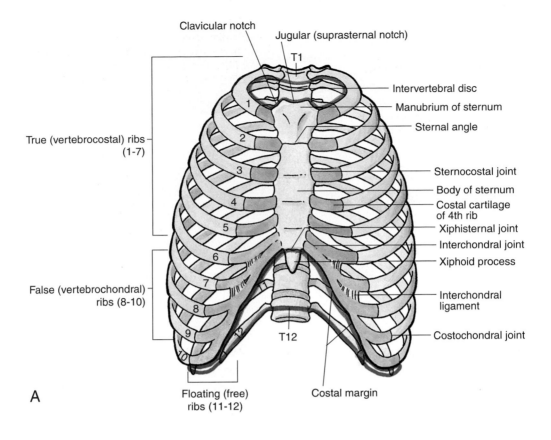

A

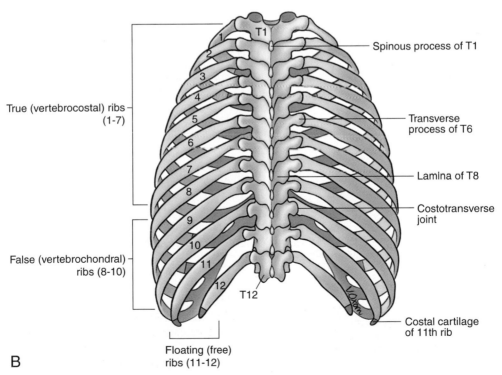

B

FIGURE 2.1 **Thoracic skeleton. A.** Anterior view. Superior and inferior thoracic apertures are outlined in pink. Ribs are numbered 1 to 12. *T1,* body of 1st thoracic vertebrae; *T12,* body of 12th thoracic vertebrae. **B.** Posterior view.

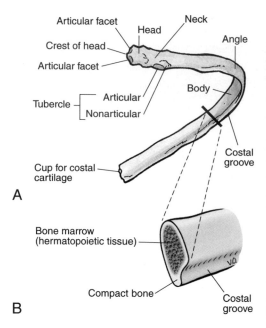

A

B

FIGURE 2.2 Typical rib. A. Posterior view. **B.** Cross section.

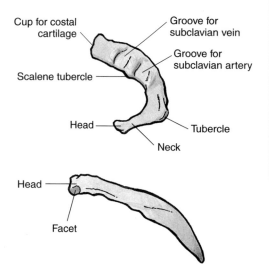

Head

Facet

FIGURE 2.3 Atypical ribs. *Upper,* Superior view of 1st rib. *Lower,* Posterior view of 12th rib.

ROLE OF COSTAL CARTILAGES

Costal cartilages prolong the ribs anteriorly and contribute to the elasticity of the thoracic wall, preventing many blows from fracturing the sternum and/or ribs. In elderly people the costal cartilages undergo calcification, making them radiopaque.

Rib Excision

Rib excision is performed by surgeons who need access to the thoracic cavity. An incision is made through the periosteum along the curve of the rib and a piece of rib is removed. After the operation the rib regenerates from the osteogenic layer of the preserved periosteum.

Rib Fractures

The weakest part of a rib is just anterior to its angle. Rib fractures commonly result from direct blows or indirectly from crushing injuries. The middle ribs are most commonly fractured. Direct violence may fracture a rib anywhere, and its broken end may injure internal organs such as a lung and/or the spleen.

Flail Chest

Flail chest occurs when a sizeable segment of the anterior and/or lateral thoracic wall moves freely because of *multiple rib fractures.* This condition allows the loose segment of the wall to move paradoxically (inward on inspiration and outward on expiration). Flail chest is an extremely painful injury and impairs ventilation, thereby affecting oxygenation of the blood. During treatment, the loose segment is often fixed by hooks and/or wires so that it cannot move.

Supernumerary Ribs

People usually have 12 ribs on each side, but the number may be increased by the presence of cervical and/or lumbar ribs, or decreased by failure of the 12th pair to form. **Cervical ribs** (present in up to 1% of people) articulate with C7 vertebra and are clinically significant because they may compress C8 and T1 nerves, or the inferior trunk of the brachial plexus supplying the upper limb, causing tingling and numbness along the medial border of the forearm. They may also compress the subclavian artery, resulting in *ischemic muscle pain* (caused by poor blood supply) in the upper limb. **Lumbar ribs** are less common than cervical ribs but have clinical significance in that they may confuse the identification of vertebral levels in diagnostic images.

Thoracic Vertebrae

Thoracic vertebrae are typical in that they have *vertebral arches* and *seven processes* for muscular and articular connections (see Chapter 5). *Special features of thoracic vertebrae include:*

- Costal demifacets or facets on their bodies for articulation with the heads of ribs (Fig. 2.4)
- Costal facets on their transverse processes for articulation with the tubercles of ribs, except for the inferior two or three
- Long spinous processes.

Sternum

The sternum is the flat, vertically elongated bone that forms the middle of the anterior part of the thoracic cage. *The sternum consists of three parts: manubrium, body, and xiphoid process* (Figs. 2.1A and 2.5).

The **manubrium,** the superior part of the sternum, is a roughly triangular bone that lies at the level of the bodies of T3 and T4 vertebrae. Its thick superior border is indented by the **jugular notch** (suprasternal notch). On each side of this notch is a **clavicular notch** that ar-

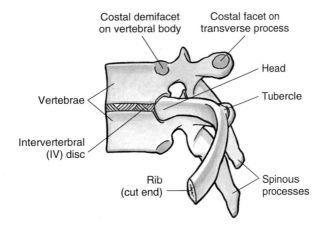

FIGURE 2.4 **Costovertebral articulations of typical rib.** Lateral view.

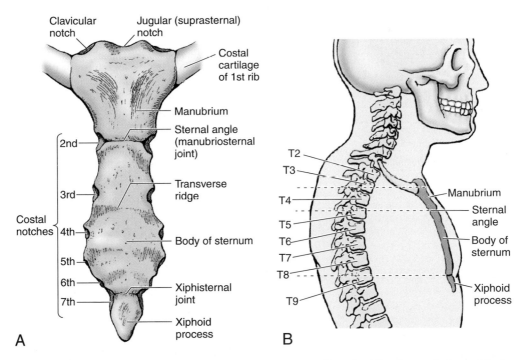

A   B

FIGURE 2.5 **Sternum. A.** Anterior view. **B.** Lateral view. The relationship of the sternum to the vertebral column is shown.

ticulates with the sternal (medial) end of the clavicle. Just inferior to this notch, the costal cartilage of the 1st rib fuses with the lateral border of the manubrium. At the **manubriosternal joint,** the manubrium and body of the sternum lie in slightly different planes; hence, their junction forms a projecting **sternal angle** (angle of Louis). This readily palpable *clinical landmark* is located opposite the second pair of costal cartilages at the level of the intervertebral (IV) disc between T4 and T5 vertebrae (Fig. 2.5*B*).

The **body** of the sternum—longer, narrower, and thinner than the manubrium—is located at the level of T5 through T9 vertebrae. Its width varies because of the scalloping of its lateral borders by the **costal notches** for articulation with the costal cartilages.

The **xiphoid process**—the lower, smallest and most variable part of the sternum—is relatively thin and elongated but varies considerably in form. It lies at the level of T10 vertebra. The process is cartilaginous in young people but more or less ossified in adults older than 40 years.

STERNAL FRACTURES

Sternal fractures are not common but crush injuries can occur during traumatic compression of the thoracic wall (e.g., in automobile accidents when the driver's chest is driven into the steering column). When the body of the sternum is fractured, it is usually a *comminuted fracture* (broken into several pieces). The most common fracture occurs at the sternal angle, resulting in dislocation of the manubriosternal joint. The installation of air bags in vehicles has reduced the number of sternal fractures.

Median Sternotomy

To gain access to the thoracic cavity for surgical operations—on the heart and great vessels, for example—the sternum is divided ("split") in the median plane and retracted (spread apart). After surgery, the halves of the sternum are reunited and held together with wire sutures.

Sternal Biopsies

The sternal body is often used for a *bone marrow needle biopsy* because of its breadth and subcutaneous position. The needle pierces the thin compact bone and enters the spongy bone. Sternal biopsy is commonly used to obtain samples of bone marrow for transplantation.

THORACIC APERTURES

The thoracic cavity communicates with the neck through the kidney-shaped **superior tho-**

racic aperture (Fig. 2.1*A*). Structures entering and leaving the thoracic cavity through this aperture include the trachea, esophagus, vessels, and nerves. The adult superior thoracic aperture measures approximately 6.5 cm anteroposteriorly and 12.5 cm transversely. Because of the obliquity of the first pair of ribs, the superior thoracic aperture slopes anteroinferiorly. *The superior thoracic aperture is bounded by the:*

- First thoracic (T1) vertebra (posterior landmark)
- First pair of ribs and their costal cartilages
- Superior border of manubrium (anterior landmark).

The thoracic cavity communicates with the abdomen through the **inferior thoracic aperture** (Fig. 2.1*A*)—the anatomical thoracic outlet—which is closed by the diaphragm separating the thoracic and abdominal cavities. The inferior thoracic aperture is more spacious than the superior thoracic aperture. Structures passing to or from the thorax to the abdomen pass through openings in the diaphragm, such as the inferior vena cava (IVC) and esophagus, or posterior to it (e.g., aorta). *The inferior thoracic aperture is bounded by the:*

- 12th thoracic vertebra (posterior landmark)
- 11th and 12th pairs of ribs
- Costal cartilages of ribs 7 through 10
- Xiphisternal joint (anterior landmark).

THORACIC OUTLET SYNDROME

When clinicians refer to the superior thoracic aperture as the thoracic "outlet," they are emphasizing the important nerves and arteries that pass through this aperture into the lower neck and upper limb. Hence, various types of thoracic outlet syndrome exist, such as the *costoclavicular syndrome*—pallor and coldness of the skin of the upper limb and diminished radial pulse—resulting from compression of the subclavian artery between the clavicle and the 1st rib, particularly when the angle between the neck and shoulder is increased.

JOINTS OF THORACIC WALL

Movements of the joints of the thoracic wall are frequent during respiration; however, the range of movement at the individual joints is small. Any disturbance that reduces the mobility of these joints interferes with respiration. During deep breathing, the excursions of the thoracic cage (anteriorly, superiorly, or laterally) are considerable. Straightening the back further increases the anteroposterior (AP) diameter of the thorax. *Joints of the thoracic wall* (Table 2.1) occur between the:

- Vertebrae (intervertebral joints)
- Ribs and vertebrae (costovertebral joints: joints of the heads of ribs and costotransverse joints)
- Sternum and costal cartilages (sternocostal joints)
- Sternum and clavicle (sternoclavicular joints)
- Ribs and costal cartilages (costochondral joints)
- Costal cartilages (interchondral joints)
- Parts of the sternum (manubriosternal and xiphisternal joints) in young people—the former and sometimes the latter usually fuses in very old people.

The *intervertebral (IV) joints* between the bodies of adjacent vertebrae are joined together by longitudinal ligaments and IV discs. These joints are discussed with the back (see Chapter 5).

DISLOCATION OF RIBS

A rib dislocation (*slipping rib syndrome*) is the displacement of a costal cartilage from the sternum—*dislocation of a sternocostal joint*. This causes severe pain, particularly during deep respiratory movements. The injury produces a lumplike deformity at the dislocation site. Rib dislocations are common in body contact sports, and possible complications are pressure on or damage to nearby nerves, vessels, and muscles.

Separation of Ribs

A rib separation *refers to dislocation of a costochondral junction*—between the rib and its costal cartilage. In separations of the 3rd to 10th ribs, tearing of the perichondrium and periosteum usually occurs. As a result, the rib may move superiorly, overriding the rib above and causing pain.

MOVEMENTS OF THORACIC WALL

Movements of the thoracic wall and diaphragm during inspiration produce increases in the intrathoracic volume and diameters of the thorax. Consequent pressure changes result in air being drawn into the lungs (inspiration) through the nose, mouth, larynx, and trachea. During passive expiration, the diaphragm, intercostal muscles, and other muscles relax, decreasing *intrathoracic volume* and increasing *intrathoracic pressure,* expelling air from the lungs (expiration) through the same passages. The stretched elastic tissue of the lungs recoils, expelling most of the air. Concurrently, *intra-abdominal pressure decreases.*

The *vertical diameter (height) of the central part of the diaphragm* (Fig. 2.6A) increases during inspiration as the central diaphragm descends (is pulled inferiorly), compressing the abdominal viscera below it. During expiration the vertical diameter returns to normal as the elastic recoil of the lungs produces subatmospheric pressure in the pleural cavities between the lungs and the thoracic wall. As a result of this and the absence of resistance to the previously compressed viscera, the domes of the diaphragm ascend, diminishing the vertical diameter. The *transverse diameter of the thorax* increases slightly when the intercostal muscles contract, raising the middle (lateral-most parts) of the ribs—the *bucket-handle movement* (Fig. 2.6, *A* and *C*). The downwardly curved ribs ascend pivoting at both ends. They move superolaterally like a bucket handle being raised, as it moves away from the side of the bucket. The *anteroposterior (AP) diameter of the thorax* also increases when the intercostal muscles contract (Fig. 2.6, *B* and *C*). Movement of the ribs (primarily 2nd through 6th) at the costovertebral joints about an axis passing through the neck of the ribs causes the ends of the ribs to rise like pump handles—the *pump handle movement* (Fig. 2.6B). Because the ribs slope inferiorly, their elevation also results in anterior-posterior movement of the sternum, especially its inferior end, with slight movement occurring at the manubriosternal joint in young people.

TABLE 2.1. JOINTS OF THORACIC WALL

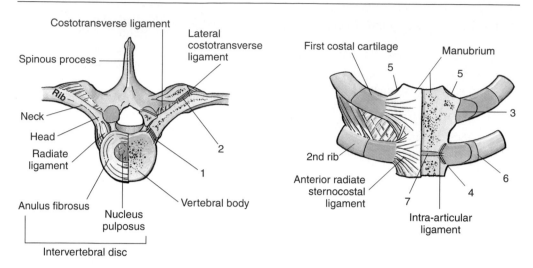

Joint	Type	Articulations	Ligaments	Comments
Intervertebral	Symphysis (secondary cartilaginous joint)	Adjacent vertebral bodies bound together by intervertebral disc	Anterior and posterior longitudinal	
Costovertebral Joints of heads of ribs (1)	Synovial plane joint	Head of each rib with superior demifacet or costal facet of corresponding vertebral body and inferior demifacet or costal facet of vertebral body superior to it	Radiate and intra-articular ligaments of head of rib	Heads of 1st, 11th, and 12th ribs (sometimes 10th) articulate only with corresponding vertebral body
Costotransverse (2)		Articulation of tubercle of rib with transverse process of corresponding vertebra	Lateral and superior costotransverse	11th and 12th ribs do not articulate with transverse process of corresponding vertebrae
Sternocostal (3 and 4)	1st: primary cartilaginous joint	Articulation of 1st costal cartilages with manubrium of sternum		
	2nd to 7th: synovial plane joints	Articulation of 2nd to 7th pairs of costal cartilages with sternum	Anterior and posterior radiate sternocostal	
Sternoclavicular (5)	Saddle type of synovial joint	Sternal end of clavicle with manubrium and 1st costal cartilage	Anterior and posterior sternoclavicular ligaments; costoclavicular ligament	This joint is divided into two compartments by an articular disc
Costochondral (6)	Primary cartilaginous joint	Articulation of lateral end of costal cartilage with sternal end of rib	Cartilage and bone are bound together by periosteum	No movement normally occurs at this joint

continued

TABLE 2.1. *CONTINUED*

Joint	Type	Articulations	Ligaments	Comments
Interchondral (Fig. 2.1*A*)	Synovial plane joint	Articulation between costal cartilages of 6th–7th, 7th–8th, and 8th–9th ribs	Interchondral ligaments	Articulation between costal cartilages of 9th and 10th ribs is fibrous
Manubriosternal (7)	Secondary cartilaginous joint (symphysis)	Articulation between manubrium and body of sternum	These joints often fuse and become a synostosis in older persons	
Xiphisternal (Fig. 2.1*A*)	Primary cartilaginous joint (synchondrosis)	Articulation between xiphoid process and body of sternum		

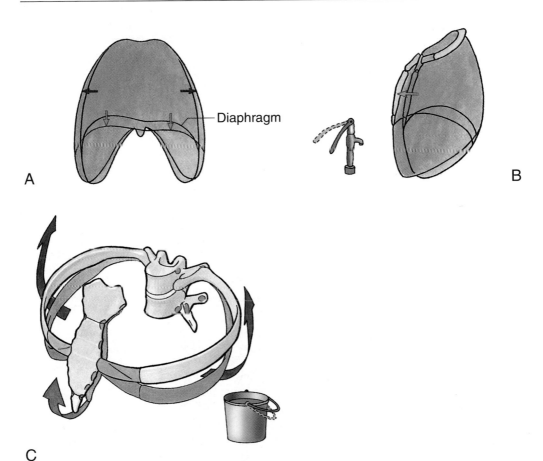

FIGURE 2.6 **Movements of the thoracic wall during inspiration. A.** Increased vertical (*green arrows*) and transverse (*red arrows*) diameters. Anterior view. **B.** Increased anteroposterior (AP) diameter. Lateral view. The AP diameter of the thorax is increased ("pump-handle" movement) with a greater excursion (increase) occurring inferiorly. **C.** Increased anteroposterior (*blue arrow*) and transverse diameters (*red arrows*). Anterolateral view. The middle parts of the lower ribs move laterally when they are elevated ("bucket-handle" movement).

PARALYSIS OF DIAPHRAGM

One can detect paralysis of the diaphragm radiographically by noting its paradoxical movement. Paralysis of half of the diaphragm because of *injury to its motor supply from the phrenic nerve* does not affect the other half because each dome has a separate nerve supply. Instead of descending on inspiration, the paralyzed dome is pushed superiorly by the abdominal viscera that are being compressed by the active side. It falls during expiration in response to the positive pressure in the lungs.

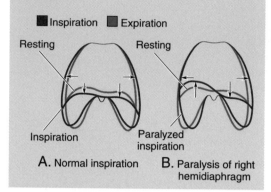

■ Inspiration   ■ Expiration

Resting   Resting

Inspiration   Paralyzed
                   inspiration

A. Normal inspiration   B. Paralysis of right
                          hemidiaphragm

BREASTS

Both men and women have breasts; normally the mammary glands are well developed only in women. **Mammary glands** are located in the subcutaneous tissue of the anterior thoracic wall (Fig. 2.7). At the greatest prominence of the breast is the **nipple,** surrounded by a circular pigmented area—the **areola.** The breast contains up to 20 masses of glandular tissue, each of which is drained by a **lactiferous duct** that opens on the nipple. Just deep to the areola each duct has a dilated portion, a **lactiferous sinus.** The roughly circular **base of the female breast** extends (Fig. 2.8*A*):

- Transversely from the lateral border of the sternum to the midaxillary line—a vertical line intersecting a point midway between the anterior and posterior axillary folds (p. 63)
- Vertically from the 2nd through 6th ribs.

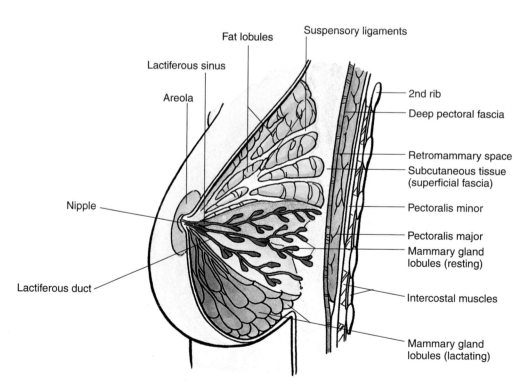

Fat lobules

Suspensory ligaments

Lactiferous sinus

Areola

Nipple

Lactiferous duct

2nd rib

Deep pectoral fascia

Retromammary space

Subcutaneous tissue (superficial fascia)

Pectoralis minor

Pectoralis major

Mammary gland lobules (resting)

Intercostal muscles

Mammary gland lobules (lactating)

FIGURE 2.7   Sagittal section of the female breast. *Upper part,* fat lobules and suspensory ligaments; *middle part,* appearance of glandular tissue in nonlactating (resting) breast; *lower part,* appearance of glandular tissue in lactating breast.

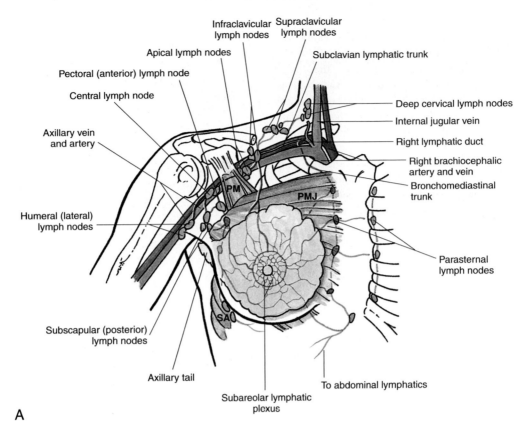

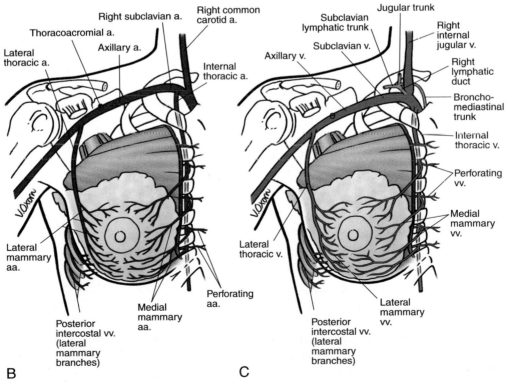

FIGURE 2.8 **Lymphatic drainage and vasculature of the breast. A.** Axillary lymph nodes. **B.** Arteries.
C. Veins. Anterior views of right breast. *PM,* pectoralis minor; *PMJ,* pectoralis major; *SA,* serratus anterior.

A small part of the mammary gland may extend along the inferolateral edge of the pectoralis major muscle toward the axilla (armpit), forming an **axillary tail** (tail of Spence). Two-thirds of the breast rests on the **deep pectoral fascia** covering the pectoralis major; the other third rests on the fascia covering the serratus anterior muscle (Figs. 2.7 and 2.8A). Between the breast and the deep pectoral fascia is a loose connective tissue plane or potential space—the **retromammary space** (bursa). This plane, containing a small amount of fat, allows the breast some degree of movement on the deep pectoral fascia. The mammary gland is firmly attached to the dermis of the overlying skin by skin ligaments (retinacula cutis)—the **suspensory ligaments** (ligaments of Cooper). These ligaments, particularly well developed in the superior part of the gland (Fig. 2.7), help to support the mammary gland lobules. During puberty (8 to 15 years of age), the female breasts normally grow because of glandular development and increased fat deposition. The areolae and nipples also enlarge. Breast size and shape result from genetic, racial, and dietary factors. Further development of the breasts occurs in association with pregnancy.

Vasculature of Breast

The **arterial supply of the breast** (Fig. 2.8B) is derived from:

- Medial mammary branches of perforating branches and anterior intercostal branches of the **internal thoracic artery,** originating from the subclavian artery
- **Lateral thoracic** and **thoracoacromial arteries,** branches of axillary artery
- **Posterior intercostal arteries,** branches of the thoracic aorta in intercostal spaces.

The **venous drainage of the breast** (Fig. 2.8C) is mainly to the **axillary vein,** but there is some drainage to the *internal thoracic vein.*

The **lymphatic drainage of the breast** is important because of its role in the metastasis (spread) of cancer cells. Lymph passes from the nipple, areola, and lobules of the gland to the **subareolar lymphatic plexus** (Fig. 2.8A), and from it:

- Most lymph (more than 75%), especially from the lateral quadrants of the breasts (p. 63), drains to the **axillary lymph nodes** (apical, humeral, central, pectoral, and subscapular) but mainly to the *pectoral (anterior) group.* However, some lymph may drain directly to other axillary nodes, or even to interpectoral, deltopectoral, and supraclavicular, or inferior deep cervical nodes.
- Most of the remaining lymph, particularly from the medial breast quadrants, drains to the **parasternal lymph nodes** or to the opposite breast, while lymph from the lower breast quadrants passes deeply to the inferior phrenic (abdominal) nodes.

Lymph from the axillary nodes drains to infraclavicular and supraclavicular nodes and from them to the **subclavian lymphatic trunk.** Lymph from the parasternal nodes enters the **bronchomediastinal trunks,** which ultimately drain into the respective lymphatic duct.

Nerves of Breast

The nerves of the breasts derive from the anterior and lateral cutaneous branches of the **4th through 6th intercostal nerves** (Fig. 2.9). The branches of the intercostal nerves pass through the deep fascia covering the pectoralis major to reach the skin. The branches thus convey sensory fibers to the skin of the breast and sympathetic fibers to the blood vessels in the breast and smooth muscle in the overlying skin and nipple.

BREAST QUADRANTS
For the anatomical location and description of pathology (e.g., cysts and tumors), the breast is divided into four quadrants. The *axillary tail* is an extension of the upper outer quadrant.

Breast Cancer
Understanding the lymphatic drainage of the breasts is of practical importance in predicting the *metastasis* (spread) of breast cancer. Interference with the lymphatic drainage by cancer produces a leathery thickened appearance of the breast skin. Often the skin is dimpled because of cancerous invasion of the suspensory ligaments. Prominent pores may develop that give the skin an orange peel

appearance (*peau d'orange sign*) because of edema (excess fluid in subcutaneous tissue) resulting from the blocked lymphatic drainage. *Although breast cancer is uncommon in men, the consequences are serious* because the tumor is often undetected until extensive metastases have occurred, as in bones, for example.

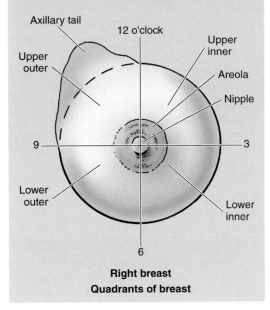

Right breast
Quadrants of breast

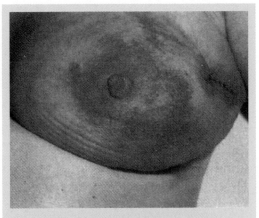

Inflamed carcinoma (cancer) of breast

Supernumerary Breasts and Nipples
Supernumerary breasts (exceeding two)—*polymastia*—or nipples (*polythelia*) may occur superior or inferior to the normal breasts. Usually supernumerary breasts consist only of a rudimentary nipple and areola. A supernumerary breast may appear anywhere along a line extending from the axilla to the groin, the location of the embryonic mammary ridge ("milk line") from which the breasts develop (Moore and Persaud, 1998). In either sex, there may be no breast development (amastia).

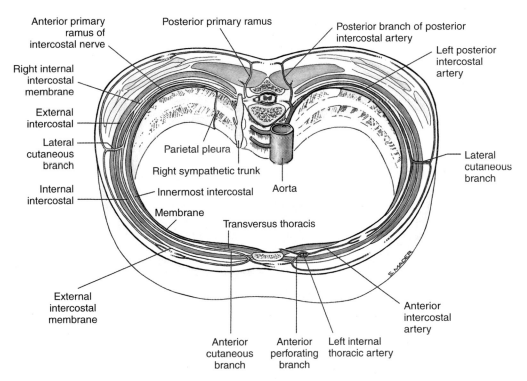

FIGURE 2.9   Transverse section of thorax. Observe the contents of an intercostal space. The diagram is simplified by showing nerves on the right and arteries on the left.

MUSCLES OF THORACIC WALL

Several upper limb muscles attach to the ribs—such as the pectoralis major and serratus anterior (Fig. 2.8A)—as do the anterolateral abdominal muscles and some neck and back muscles. The **pectoral muscles** covering the anterior thoracic wall usually act on the upper limbs; however, the **pectoralis major** and other muscles may also function as accessory muscles of respiration, helping to expand the thoracic cavity when inspiration is deep and forceful (e.g., after a 100-meter dash). The *scalene muscles,* passing from the neck to the lst and 2nd ribs (Chapter 9), also function as accessory respiratory muscles by elevating these ribs during forced inspiration. The intercostal, transverse thoracic (L. transversus thoracis), subcostal, levator costarum, and serratus posterior are muscles of the thorax proper (Table 2.2).

DYSPNEA–DIFFICULT BREATHING

When people with respiratory problems such as *asthma,* emphysema, or with *heart failure* struggle to breathe, they use their accessory respiratory muscles to assist the expansion of their thoracic cavities. They typically lean on a table or their thighs to fix their pectoral girdles (clavicles and scapulae) so the muscles are able to act on their rib attachments and expand the thorax.

Typical intercostal spaces contain fleshy or membranous parts of the three layers of intercostal muscles (Figs. 2.9 and 2.10). The superficial layer is formed by the **external intercostal muscles,** the middle layer is formed by the **internal intercostal muscles,** and the deepest layer is formed by the **innermost intercostal muscles.** Anteriorly, the fleshy external intercostal muscles are replaced by **external intercostal membranes,** and posteriorly the fleshy internal intercostal muscles are replaced by **internal intercostal membranes.**

NERVES OF THORACIC WALL

The thoracic wall has 12 pairs of thoracic spinal nerves. As soon as they pass through the IV foramina, they divide into anterior (ventral) and posterior (dorsal) primary rami (Fig. 2.9). *The anterior rami of T1 to T11 form the inter-*

costal nerves that run along the extent of the intercostal spaces. The anterior primary rami of T12 nerves, inferior to the 12th ribs, form the **subcostal nerves** (see Chapter 3). The posterior primary rami of thoracic spinal nerves pass posteriorly, immediately lateral to the articular processes of the vertebrae, to supply the bones, joints, deep back muscles, and skin of the back in the thoracic region.

Typical intercostal nerves (3rd through 6th) run initially along the posterior aspects of the intercostal spaces, between the parietal pleura (serous lining of thoracic cavity) and the internal intercostal membrane. At first they run across the internal surface of the internal intercostal membrane and muscle near the middle of the intercostal space. Near the angles of the ribs, the nerves pass between the internal intercostal and innermost intercostal muscles. Here the nerves take a course adjacent to their respective rib entering and sheltered by the **costal grooves,** lying just inferior to the intercostal arteries (Figs. 2.10 and 2.11). Collateral branches of these nerves arise near the angles of the ribs and supply the intercostal muscles. The nerves continue anteriorly between the internal and innermost intercostal muscles, giving branches to these and other muscles and giving rise to **lateral cutaneous branches** approximately at the midaxillary line (Fig. 2.9). Anteriorly, the nerves appear on the internal surface of the internal intercostal muscle. Near the sternum the nerves turn anteriorly, passing between the costal cartilages and entering the subcutaneous tissue as **anterior**

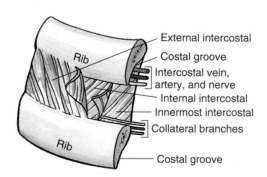

FIGURE 2.10   Contents of typical intercostal space. Note order of structures in the costal groove from superior to inferior: *VAN* (**V**ein, **A**rtery, and **N**erve).

TABLE 2.2. MUSCLES OF THORACIC WALL

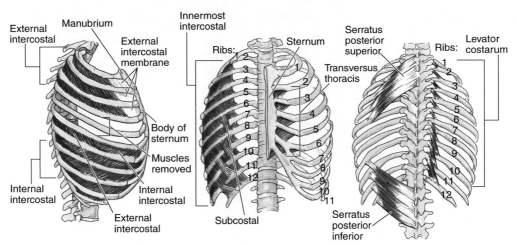

Lateral view   **Anterior view**   **Posterior view**

Muscles	Superior Attachment	Inferior Attachment	Innervation	Main Action[a]
External intercostal	Inferior border of ribs	Superior border of ribs below	Intercostal nerve	Elevate ribs
Internal intercostal				Depress ribs
Innermost intercostal				Probably elevate ribs
Transverse thoracic	Posterior surface of lower sternum	Internal surface of costal cartilages 2–6		Depress ribs
Subcostal	Internal surface of lower ribs near their angles	Superior borders of 2nd or 3rd ribs below		Elevate ribs
Levator costarum	Transverse processes of T7–T11	Subjacent ribs between tubercle and angle	Posterior primary rami of C8–T11 nerves	Elevate ribs
Serratus posterior superior	Ligamentum nuchae, spinous processes of C7 to T3 vertebrae	Superior borders of 2nd to 4th ribs	2nd to 5th intercostal nerves	Elevate ribs
Serratus posterior inferior	Spinous processes of T11 to L2 vertebrae	Inferior borders of 8th to 12th ribs near their angles	Anterior primary rami of 9th to 12th thoracic spinal nerves	Depress ribs

[a]All intercostal muscles keep intercostal spaces rigid, thereby preventing them from bulging out during expiration and from being drawn in during inspiration. Role of individual intercostal muscles and accessory muscles of respiration in moving the ribs is difficult to interpret despite many electromyographic studies.

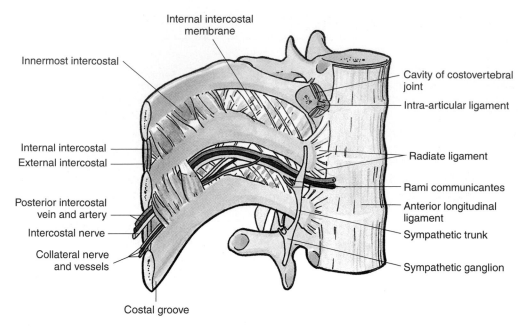

FIGURE 2.11   Dissection of vertebral end of intercostal space. Note attachment of the intercostal nerve to the sympathetic trunk by communicating branches (L. rami communicantes).

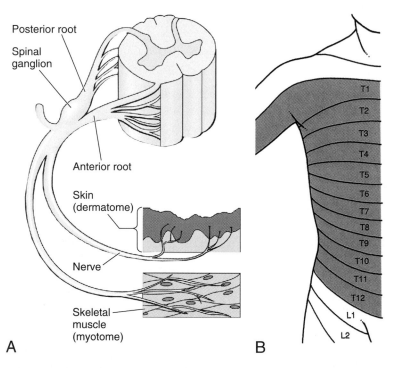

FIGURE 2.12   Dermatomes and myotomes. A. Schematic illustration of the area of skin (dermatome) and skeletal muscle (myotome) innervated by a spinal nerve or segment of spinal cord. **B.** Dermatomes of the thorax (T1 to T12). Anterior view.

cutaneous branches. *Muscular branches* also arise all along the course of the intercostal nerves to supply the subcostal, transverse thoracic, levator costarum, and serratus posterior muscles (Table 2.2). *The 1st and 2nd intercostal nerves are atypical.* In the first part of their course, they pass on the internal surfaces of the 1st and 2nd ribs. Through the posterior ramus and the lateral and anterior cutaneous branches of the anterior ramus, each spinal nerve supplies a striplike area of skin extending from the posterior median line to the anterior median line. These bandlike skin areas—**dermatomes**—are each supplied by the sensory fibers of a single posterior root through the posterior and anterior primary rami of its spinal nerve (Fig. 2.12*A*).

The dermatomes are arranged in a segmental fashion because the thoracoabdominal nerves arise from segments of the spinal cord (Fig. 2.12*B*). Closely related dermatomes such as T4, T5, and T6 overlap considerably. In fact, *a lesion of a single spinal nerve may not produce a noticeable sensory deficit because of the* overlap in the distribution of adjacent spinal nerves. Physicians need a working knowledge of the segmental, or dermatomal, innervation of the skin so they can determine (e.g., with a pin) whether or not a particular segment of the spinal cord is functioning normally. The group of muscles supplied by one pair of intercostal nerves is a **myotome** (Fig. 2.12*A*).

Communicating branches—**rami communicantes**—connect each intercostal nerve, the subcostal nerve, and upper lumbar nerves to the ipsilateral **sympathetic trunk** (Fig. 2.11). Presynaptic fibers leave each nerve as a *white ramus* and pass to a **sympathetic ganglion.** Postsynaptic fibers, destined for the body and limbs, leave all the ganglia of the trunks by means of *gray rami* to join the anterior ramus of the nearest spinal nerve, including all the intercostal nerves. *Sympathetic nerve fibers are thus distributed through the branches of all spinal nerves* to blood vessels, sweat glands, smooth muscle, and muscles of the body wall and limbs.

HERPES ZOSTER INFECTION
Herpes zoster (shingles)—a viral disease of spinal ganglia—is a *dermatomally distributed skin lesion*. The *herpes virus* invades a spinal ganglion and is transported along the axon to the skin where it produces an infection, which causes a sharp burning pain in the dermatome supplied by the involved nerve. A few days later, the skin of the dermatome becomes red and vesicular eruptions appear.

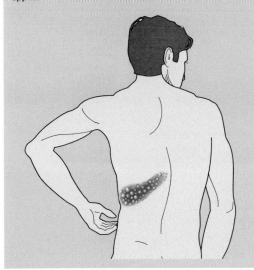

Thoracocentesis
Sometimes it is necessary to insert a hypodermic needle through an intercostal space into the pleural cavity—the potential space between the parietal pleura lining the pulmonary cavity and the visceral pleura covering the lung—to obtain a sample of pleural fluid, or to remove blood or pus. To avoid damage to the intercostal nerve and vessels, the needle is inserted superior to the rib, high enough to avoid the collateral branches.

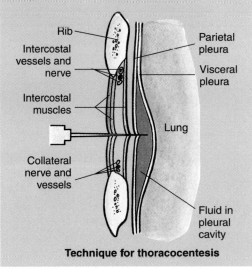
Technique for thoracocentesis

Surface Anatomy of Thoracic Wall

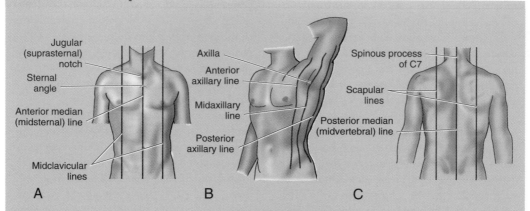

Several bony landmarks and imaginary lines facilitate anatomical descriptions, identification of thoracic areas, and the location of lesions such as a bullet wound:

- **Anterior median (midsternal) line** indicates the intersection of the median plane with the anterior chest wall (**A**).
- **Midclavicular lines** pass through the midpoints of the clavicles, parallel to the anterior median line.
- **Anterior axillary line** runs vertically along the anterior axillary fold (**B**) that is formed by the border of the pectoralis major as it spans from the thorax to the humerus (arm bone).
- **Midaxillary line** runs from the apex (deepest part) of the axilla, parallel to the anterior axillary line.
- **Posterior axillary line,** also parallel to the anterior axillary line, is drawn vertically along the posterior axillary fold formed by the latissimus dorsi and teres major muscles as they span from the back to the humerus.
- **Posterior median (midvertebral) line** is a vertical line described by the tips of the spinous processes of the vertebrae (**C**).
- **Scapular lines** are parallel to the posterior median line and cross the inferior angles of the scapulae.

The **clavicles** lie subcutaneously, forming bony ridges at the junction of the thorax and neck. They can be palpated easily throughout their length, especially where their medial ends articulate with the **manubrium**. The **sternum** also lies subcutaneously in the anterior median line and is palpable throughout its length. *The manubrium of the sternum:*

- Lies at the level of the bodies of **T3 and T4 vertebrae**
- Is anterior to the **arch of the aorta**
- Has a **jugular notch** than can be palpated between the prominent sternal ends of the clavicles
- Has a **sternal angle** where it articulates with sternal body at the level of the **T4/T5 IV disc** and the space between the 3rd and 4th spinous processes.

The **sternal angle** is a palpable landmark that lies at the level of the 2nd pair of costal cartilages. The main bronchi pass inferolaterally from the bifurcation of the trachea at the level of the sternal angle. The **SVC** passes inferiorly deep to the manubrium, projecting as much as a fingerbreadth to the right of this bone. Because the first rib cannot be palpated as it lies deep to the clavicle, **count the ribs and**

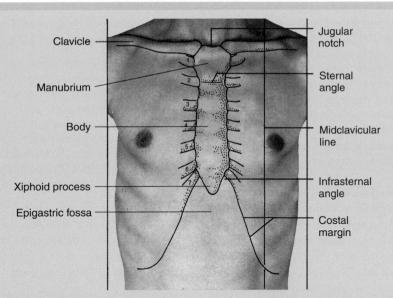

Clavicle

Manubrium

Body

Xiphoid process

Epigastric fossa

Jugular notch

Sternal angle

Midclavicular line

Infrasternal angle

Costal margin

intercostal spaces anteriorly by sliding the fingers laterally from the sternal angle onto the 2nd costal cartilage. Start counting with rib 2 and count the ribs and spaces by moving the fingers inferolaterally. The 1st intercostal space is inferior to the first rib; likewise, the other spaces lie inferior to the similarly numbered ribs.

The **body of the sternum,** lies anterior to the right border of the heart and vertebrae T5 through T9. The **xiphoid process** lies in a slight depression—the **epigastric fossa**— where the converging costal margins form the **infrasternal angle.** This angle is used in *cardiopul-*

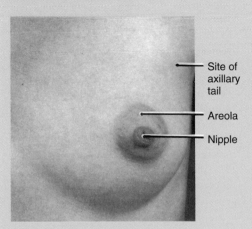

Site of axillary tail

Areola

Nipple

monary resuscitation (CPR) for locating the proper hand position on the inferior part of the body of the sternum. The **costal margins**— formed by the medial borders of the 7th through 10th costal cartilages—are palpable with ease, as they extend inferolaterally from the **xiphisternal joint.** This articulation, often seen as a ridge, is at the level of the inferior border of T9 vertebra.

Breasts are the most prominent surface features of the anterior thoracic wall, especially in women. Their flattened superior surfaces show no sharp demarcation from the anterior surface of the thoracic wall; however, laterally and inferiorly their borders are well defined. The area (cleavage) in the anterior median line—the **intermammary cleft**—is between the breasts. The **nipple** in the midclavicular line is surrounded by a slightly raised and circular pigmented area—the **areola**. Its color varies with the woman's complexion; it darkens during pregnancy and retains its color thereafter. The nipple in men lies anterior to the 4th intercostal space, about 10 cm from the anterior median line. The position of the nipple in women is so inconstant that it is not reliable as a surface landmark for the 4th intercostal space.

VASCULATURE OF THORACIC WALL

The **arterial supply to the thoracic wall** (Fig. 2.13*A*, Table 2.3) derives from the:

- **Thoracic aorta** through posterior intercostal and subcostal arteries
- **Subclavian artery** through the internal thoracic and supreme (superior) intercostal arteries
- **Axillary artery** through superior and lateral thoracic arteries.

The **veins of the thoracic wall** accompany the intercostal arteries and nerves and lie most superiorly in the costal grooves (Figs. 2.10 and 2.13*B*). There are eleven posterior intercostal veins and one subcostal vein on each side. While the posterior intercostal veins anastomose with the anterior intercostal veins—tributaries of the internal thoracic veins—most posterior intercostal veins end in the *azygos venous system* (p. 115) that conveys venous blood to the superior vena cava (SVC).

THORACIC CAVITY AND VISCERA

The thoracic cavity—the space within the thoracic walls—has three compartments (Fig. 2.14*A*):

- Two lateral compartments—the **pulmonary cavities**—that contain the lungs and pleurae (lining membranes)
- A central compartment—the **mediastinum**—that contains all other thoracic structures: the heart, thoracic parts of the great vessels, thoracic part of the trachea, esophagus, thymus, and other structures such as lymph nodes.

The pulmonary cavities are completely separate from each other and, with the lungs and pleurae, occupy the majority of the thoracic cavity. The mediastinum extends from the superior thoracic aperture to the diaphragm.

PLEURAE AND LUNGS

To visualize the relationship of the pleurae and lungs, push your fist into an underinflated

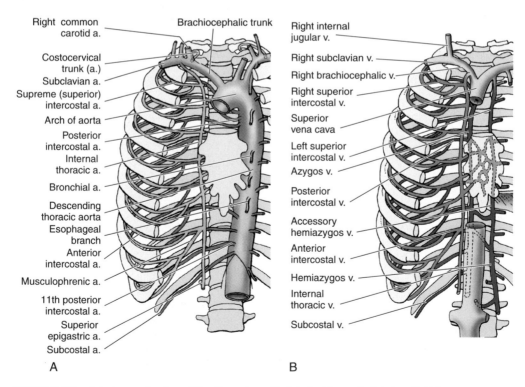

FIGURE 2.13 **Arteries and veins of the thoracic wall.** Anterior views. **A.** Arteries. **B.** Veins.

TABLE 2.3. ARTERIAL SUPPLY TO THORACIC WALL

Artery	Origin	Course	Distribution
Posterior intercostals	Superior intercostal artery (intercostal spaces 1 and 2) and thoracic aorta (remaining intercostal spaces)	Pass between internal and innermost intercostal muscles	Intercostal muscles and overlying skin, parietal pleura
Anterior intercostals	Internal thoracic (intercostal spaces 1–6) and musculophrenic arteries (intercostal spaces 7–9)		
Internal thoracic	Subclavian artery	Passes inferiorly and lateral to sternum between costal cartilages and internal intercostal muscles to divide into superior epigastric and musculophrenic arteries	By way of anterior intercostal arteries to intercostal spaces 1–6
Subcostal	Thoracic aorta	Courses along inferior border of 12th rib	Muscles of anterolateral abdominal wall

balloon (Fig. 2.14*A*). The part of the balloon wall adjacent to the skin of your fist (which represents the lung) is comparable to the *visceral pleura;* the remainder of the balloon represents the *parietal pleura.* The cavity between the layers of the balloon is analogous to the *pleural cavity.* At your wrist (*root of lung*), the inner and outer walls of the balloon are continuous, as are the visceral and parietal layers of pleura, together forming a *pleural sac.* Note that the lung is outside of but surrounded by the pleural sac, just as your fist was surrounded by but outside of the balloon.

Pleurae
Each lung is invested by and enclosed in a serous pleural sac that consists of two continuous membranes—the pleurae (Fig. 2.14):

- The **visceral pleura** (pulmonary pleura) invests the lungs, including the surfaces within the horizontal and oblique fissures; it cannot be dissected from the lungs.
- The **parietal pleura** lines the pulmonary cavities—the bilateral subdivisions of the thoracic cavity lying on either side of the mediastinum and occupied by the lungs.

The **pleural cavity**—the potential space between the visceral and parietal layers of pleura—contains a capillary layer of serous *pleural fluid,* which lubricates the pleural surfaces and allows the layers of pleura to slide smoothly over each other during respiration. Its surface tension also provides the cohesion that keeps the lung surface in contact with the thoracic wall; consequently, the lung expands and fills with air when the thorax expands while still allowing sliding to occur, much like a layer of water between two glass plates.

The **parietal pleura** lines the pulmonary cavities and adheres to the thoracic wall, mediastinum, and diaphragm. *The parietal pleura consists of four parts:*

- **Costal pleura** covers internal surface of thoracic wall
- **Mediastinal pleura** covers lateral aspects of mediastinum—the mass of tissues and organs separating the pulmonary cavities and their pleural sacs
- **Diaphragmatic pleura** covers superior (thoracic) surface of diaphragm on each side of the mediastinum
- **Cervical pleura** (pleural cupula) extends through the superior thoracic aperture into the root of the neck, forming a cup-shaped dome over the apex of the lung. *The summit of the cervical pleura extends 2 to 3 cm superior to the level of the medial third of the clavicle at the level of the neck of the 1st rib.*

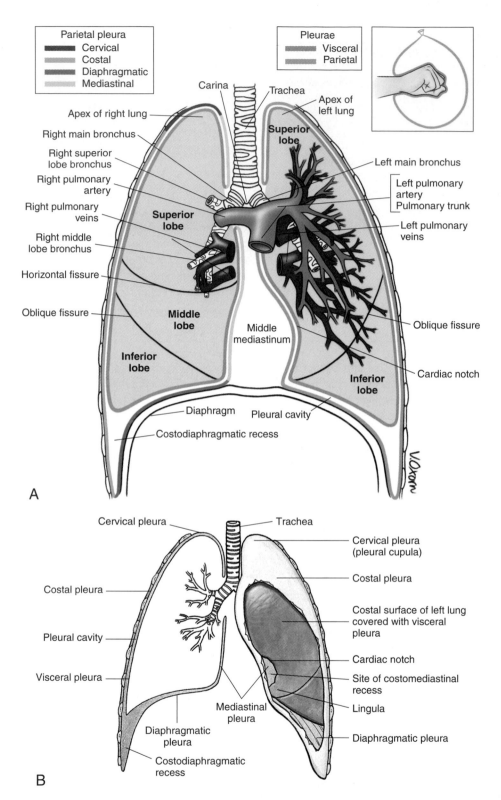

FIGURE 2.14   Lungs and pleurae. A. Overview of respiratory system. Anterior view. The *inset drawing* showing a fist invaginating an underinflated balloon demonstrates the relationship of the lung (represented by fist) to the walls of the pleural sac (parietal and visceral layers of pleura). The cavity of the pleural sac (pleural cavity) is comparable to the cavity of the balloon. **B.** Parts of the parietal pleura and pleural cavities. Anterior view.

The **costal pleura** is separated from the internal surface of the thoracic wall (sternum, ribs, and costal cartilages, intercostal muscles and membranes, and side of thoracic vertebrae) by **endothoracic fascia.** This thin, extrapleural layer of loose connective tissue forms a natural cleavage plane for the surgical separation of the costal pleura from the thoracic wall, allowing the thoracic surgeon to move and place instruments inside the thoracic wall yet remain outside—thereby preventing potential infection from entering the pleural cavities. The endothoracic fascia also forms a thin layer of connective tissue between the diaphragm and the diaphragmatic pleura. The relatively abrupt lines along which the parietal pleura changes direction from one wall of the pleural cavity to another are the **lines of pleural reflection.**

- The **sternal line of pleural reflection** is sharp or abrupt and occurs where the costal pleura becomes continuous with the mediastinal pleura anteriorly.
- The **costal line of pleural reflection** is also sharp and occurs where the costal pleura becomes continuous with the diaphragmatic pleura inferiorly.
- The **vertebral line of pleural reflection** is a much rounder, gradual reflection where the costal pleura becomes continuous with the mediastinal pleura posteriorly.

At the root of the lung the visceral and parietal layers of pleura are continuous; a double layer of parietal pleura—the **pulmonary ligament**—hangs inferiorly from this region (Fig. 2.15). The lungs do not completely occupy the pleural cavities during expiration; thus, the peripheral diaphragmatic pleura is in contact with the lowermost part of the costal pleura. The potential pleural spaces here are the **costodiaphragmatic recesses** (Fig. 2.14)—the pleural-lined "gutters"—that surround the upward convexity of the diaphragm inside the thoracic wall. Similar but smaller pleural recesses are located posterior to the sternum where the costal pleura is in contact with the mediastinal pleura. The potential spaces here are the **costomediastinal recesses** (Fig. 2.14*B*); the left recess is potentially larger (less occupied) because of the cardiac notch in the left lung. The inferior borders of the lungs move further into the pleural recesses during deep inspiration and retreat from them during expiration.

PULMONARY COLLAPSE

If a sufficient amount of air enters the pleural cavity, the surface tension adhering visceral to parietal pleura (lung to thoracic wall) is broken and the lung collapses because of its inherent elasticity (elastic recoil). When a lung collapses, the pleural cavity—normally a potential space (purple)—becomes a real space. The pleural cavity is located between the parietal pleura (blue) and the visceral pleura (red). One lung may be collapsed after surgery, for example, without collapsing the other because the pleural sacs are separate.

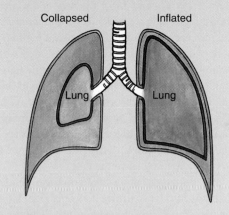

Collapsed   Inflated

Lung   Lung

Pneumothorax, Hydrothorax, Hemothorax, and Chylothorax

Entry of air into the pleural cavity—**pneumothorax**—resulting from a penetrating wound of the parietal pleura or rupture of a lung from a bullet, for example, results in partial collapse of the lung. Fractured ribs may also tear the parietal pleura and produce pneumothorax. The accumulation of a significant amount of fluid in the pleural cavity—**hydrothorax**—may result from *pleural effusion* (escape of fluid into the pleural cavity). This may also occur from leakage from the lung through an opening in the visceral pleura. With a chest wound, blood may also enter the pleural cavity (**hemothorax**); this condition results more often from injury to a major intercostal vessel than from laceration of a lung. Lymph from a torn thoracic duct may also enter the pleural cavity (**chylothorax**). Chyle, a pale white or yellow lymph fluid in the thoracic duct is taken up by the lacteals of the intestines (Chapter 2).

Pleuritis

During inspiration and expiration the normally moist, smooth pleurae make no detectable sound during *auscultation* (listening to breath sounds); however, inflammation of the pleurae—*pleuritis* (pleurisy)—makes the lung surfaces rough. The resulting friction (*pleural rub*) may be heard with a stethoscope. Acute pleuritis is marked by sharp, stabbing pain, especially on exertion, such as climbing stairs, when the rate and depth of respiration may be increased even slightly.

Lungs

The lungs are vital organs of respiration. Their main function is to oxygenate the blood by bringing inspired air into close relation with the venous blood in the pulmonary capillaries. Although cadaveric lungs may be shrunken, hard to the touch, and discolored in appearance, healthy lungs in living people are normally light, soft, and spongy. They are also elastic and recoil to about one-third their size when the thoracic cavity is opened.

The **root of the lung** is formed by the structures entering and emerging from the lung at its hilum (Figs. 2.14 and 2.15). *The root of the lung connects the lung with the heart and trachea.* The root is enclosed within the area of continuity between the parietal and visceral layers of pleura—the **pleural sleeve** or mesopneumonium (mesentery of the lung). The **hilum of the lung** is the area on the medial surface of each lung, the point at which the structures forming the root—the main bronchus, pulmonary vessels, bronchial vessels, lymphatic vessels, and nerves—enter and leave the lung.

The **horizontal and oblique fissures** divide the lungs into lobes (Table 2.4). *The right lung has three lobes, the left lung has two.* The right lung is larger and heavier than the left, but it is shorter and wider because the right dome of the diaphragm is higher and the heart and pericardium bulge more to the left. The anterior margin of the right lung is relatively straight, whereas this margin of the left lung has a deep *cardiac notch.* The cardiac notch primarily indents the anteroinferior aspect of the superior lobe of the left lung. This often creates a thin, tonguelike process of the superior lobe—the **lingula** (Fig. 2.14*B*)—which extends below the cardiac notch and slides in and out of the costomediastinal recess during inspiration and expiration. **Each lung has:**

- An **apex,** the blunt superior end of the lung ascending above the level of the lst rib into the root of the neck that is covered by cervical pleura

- **Three surfaces:** *costal surface*—adjacent to the sternum, costal cartilages, and ribs*; mediastinal surface*—including the hilum of the lung and related medially to the mediastinum and posteriorly to sides of the vertebrae; *diaphragmatic surface*—resting on the convex dome of diaphragm.

- **Three borders:** *anterior border,* where the costal and mediastinal surfaces meet anteriorly and overlap the heart; the *cardiac notch* indents this border of the left lung; *inferior border,* which circumscribes the diaphragmatic surface of lung and separates the diaphragmatic surface from the costal and mediastinal surfaces; *posterior border,* where the costal and mediastinal surfaces meet posteriorly; it is broad and rounded and lies adjacent to the thoracic region of the vertebral column.

TABLE 2.4. LOBES AND FISSURES OF LUNGS

Right lung (three lobes)	Left lung (two lobes)
Superior (upper) lobe separated by horizontal fissure from the middle lobe separated by oblique fissure from the inferior (lower) lobe	Superior (upper) lobe separated by oblique fissure from the inferior (lower) lobe

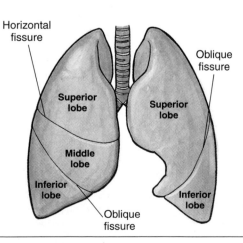

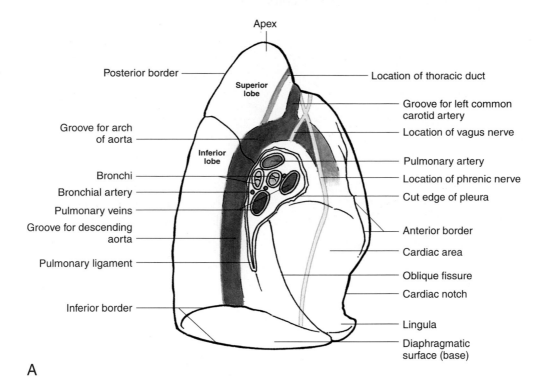

A

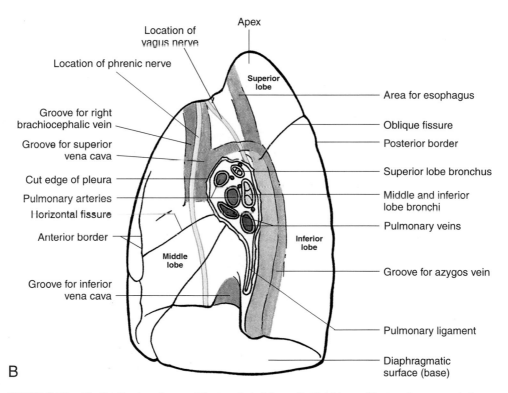

B

FIGURE 2.15 **Mediastinal surfaces of lungs. A.** Left lung. **B.** Right lung. Observe the somewhat pear-shaped depression, the hilum (doorway) of the lung near the center of this surface. The hilum (together with its contents, the pulmonary vessels and bronchi) constitute the root of the lung. The root is where the visceral and parietal pleura are continuous (cut here) and through which the pulmonary vessels and bronchi enter the lung at the hilum. The embalmed lungs have impressions of structures in contact with them (e.g., aorta and superior vena cava).

Surface Anatomy of Pleurae and Lungs

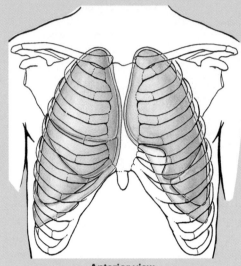

Anterior view

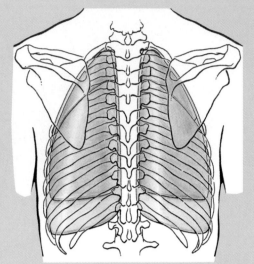

Posterior view

The cervical pleurae and apices of the lungs pass through the superior thoracic aperture into the root of the neck superior and posterior to the clavicles. The anterior borders of the lungs lie adjacent to the anterior line of reflection of the parietal pleura as far inferiorly as the 4th costal cartilages. Here the margin of the left pleural reflection moves laterally and then inferiorly at the cardiac notch to reach the level of the 6th costal cartilage. The anterior border of the left lung is more deeply indented by its cardiac notch. On the right side, the pleural reflection continues inferiorly from the 4th to the 6th costal cartilage, paralleled closely by the anterior border of the right lung. Both pleural reflections pass laterally and reach the midclavicular line at the level of the 8th costal cartilage, the 10th rib at the midaxillary line, and the 12th rib at the scapular line, proceeding toward the spinous process of T10 vertebra. They then proceed toward the spinous process of T12 vertebra. Thus, the parietal pleura extends approximately two ribs inferior to the lung. The *oblique fissure of the lungs* extends from the level of the spinous process of T2 vertebra posteriorly to the 6th costal cartilage anteriorly, which coincides approximately with the vertebral border of the scapula when the upper limb is elevated above the head (causing the inferior angle to be rotated laterally). The *horizontal fissure of the right lung* extends from the oblique fissure along the 4th rib and costal cartilage anteriorly.

Trachea and Bronchi

The **main bronchi** (primary bronchi), one to each lung, pass inferolaterally from the **bifurcation of the trachea** to the lungs at the level of the sternal angle to the hila (plural of hilum) of the lungs (Figs. 2.16 and 2.17*A*). The walls of the trachea and bronchi are supported by C-shaped rings of hyaline cartilage.

- The **right main bronchus** is wider, shorter, and runs more vertically than the left main bronchus as it passes directly to the hilum of the lung
- The **left main bronchus** passes inferolaterally, inferior to the arch of the aorta and anterior to the esophagus and thoracic aorta, to reach the hilum of the lung.

The main bronchi enter the hila of the lungs and branch in a constant fashion within the lungs to form the **bronchial tree.** Each main bronchus divides into **lobar bronchi** (secondary bronchi), two on the left and three on the right, each of which supplies a lobe of the lung. Each lobar bronchus divides into **segmental**

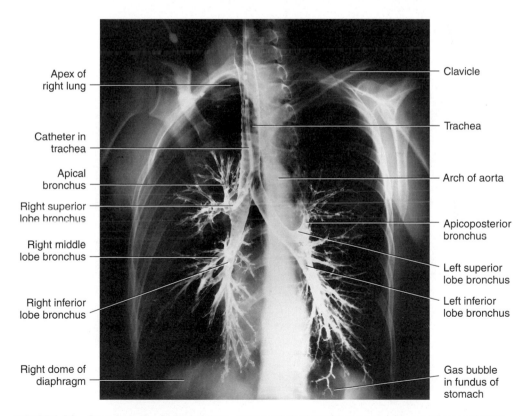

FIGURE 2.16   Bronchogram. Slightly oblique, posteroanterior bronchogram of right and left bronchial tree.

Apex of right lung
Catheter in trachea
Apical bronchus
Right superior lobe bronchus
Right middle lobe bronchus
Right inferior lobe bronchus
Right dome of diaphragm

Clavicle
Trachea
Arch of aorta
Apicoposterior bronchus
Left superior lobe bronchus
Left inferior lobe bronchus
Gas bubble in fundus of stomach

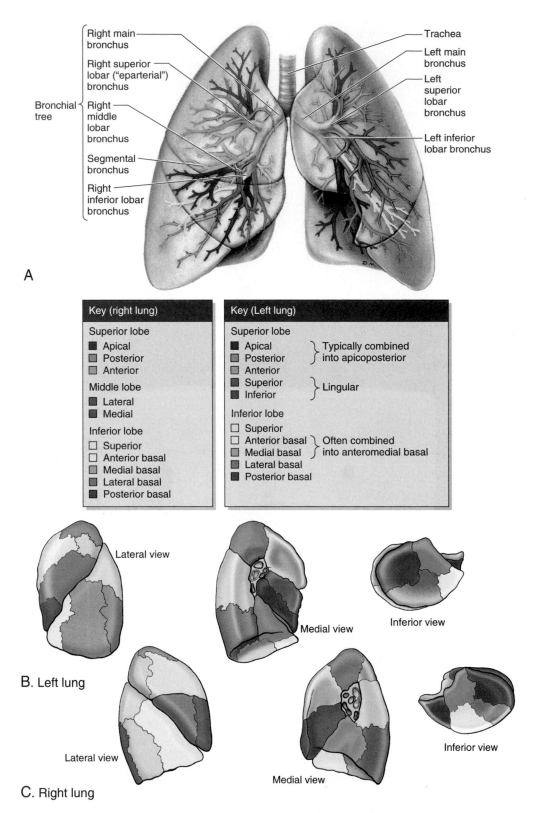

Key (right lung)

Superior lobe
■ Apical
■ Posterior
□ Anterior

Middle lobe
■ Lateral
■ Medial

Inferior lobe
□ Superior
□ Anterior basal
■ Medial basal
■ Lateral basal
■ Posterior basal

Key (Left lung)

Superior lobe
■ Apical   } Typically combined
■ Posterior   into apicoposterior
□ Anterior
■ Superior } Lingular
■ Inferior

Inferior lobe
□ Superior
□ Anterior basal } Often combined
■ Medial basal   into anteromedial basal
■ Lateral basal
■ Posterior basal

A

B. Left lung

Lateral view

Medial view

Inferior view

C. Right lung

Lateral view

Medial view

Inferior view

FIGURE 2.17   Bronchi and bronchopulmonary segments. A. Segmental bronchi. Segmental (tertiary) bronchi are indicated by *colors* (see key). **B.** Bronchopulmonary segments of right lung. **C.** Bronchopulmonary segments of left lung.

bronchi (tertiary bronchi) that supply the bronchopulmonary segments (Fig. 2.17, *B* and *C*). Each **bronchopulmonary segment** is pyramidal, with its apex directed toward the root of the lung and its base at the pleural surface. Each segment is named according to the segmental bronchus that supplies it.

ASPIRATION OF FOREIGN BODIES
Because the right bronchus is wider and shorter and runs more vertically than the left bronchus, aspirated foreign bodies are more likely to enter and lodge in it or one of its branches. A potential hazard encountered by dentists is an aspirated foreign body, such as a piece of tooth, filling material, or a small instrument. Such objects are also most likely to enter the right main bronchus.

Lung Resections
Knowledge of the anatomy of the bronchopulmonary segments is essential for precise interpretations of diagnostic images of the lungs and for surgical resection (removal) of diseased segments. When resecting a bronchopulmonary segment, surgeons follow the interlobar veins to pass between the segments. Bronchial and pulmonary disorders such as tumors or abscesses (collections of pus) often localize in a bronchopulmonary segment, which may be surgically resected. During the treatment of lung cancer, the surgeon may remove a whole lung (*pneumonectomy*), a lobe (*lobectomy*), or one or more bronchopulmonary segments (*segmentectomy*). Knowledge and understanding of the bronchopulmonary segments and their relationship to the bronchial tree is also essential for planning drainage and clearance techniques utilized in physical therapy in enhancing drainage from specific areas (e.g., in pneumonia and cystic fibrosis patients).

Bronchoscopy
When examining the bronchi with a *bronchoscope*—an endoscope for inspecting the interior of the tracheobronchial tree for diagnostic purposes—one can observe

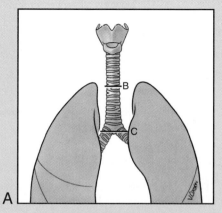
Levels of views B and C

a keel-like ridge—the **carina**—between the orifices of the main bronchi. The carina is a cartilaginous projection of the last tracheal ring. If the tracheobronchial lymph nodes in the angle between the main bronchi are enlarged because cancer cells have metastasized from a bronchogenic carcinoma, for example, the carina is distorted, widened posteriorly, and immobile.

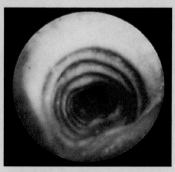
B
Bronchoscopic view of trachea

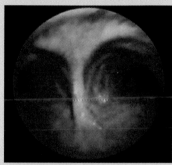
C
Bronchoscopic view of carina

Vasculature and Nerves of Lungs and Pleurae
Each lung has a large **pulmonary artery** supplying blood to it and two **pulmonary veins** draining blood from it (Fig. 2.18). The right and left pulmonary arteries arise from the **pulmonary trunk** at the level of the sternal angle and *carry poorly oxygenated ("venous") blood to the lungs for oxygenation.* The pulmonary arteries pass to the corresponding root of the lung and give off a branch to the superior lobe before entering the hilum. Within the lung each artery descends posterolateral to the main bronchus and divides into **lobar** and **segmental arteries.** Consequently, an arterial branch goes to each lobe and bronchopulmonary segment of the lung, usually on the anterior aspect of

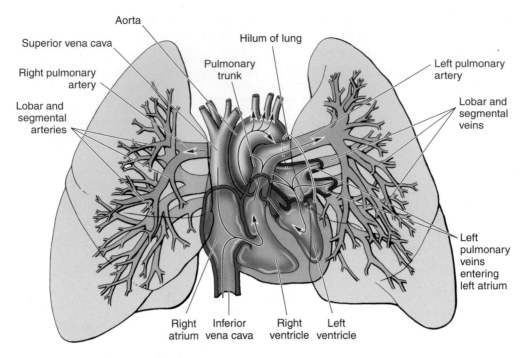

FIGURE 2.18 Pulmonary circulation. Anterior view.

the corresponding bronchus. The **pulmonary veins,** two on each side, *carry well-oxygenated ("arterial") blood from the lungs to the left atrium of the heart.* Beginning in the pulmonary capillaries, the veins unite into larger and larger vessels. Intrasegmental veins drain blood from adjacent bronchopulmonary segments into the intersegmental veins in the septa, which separate the segments. A main vein drains each bronchopulmonary segment, usually on the anterior surface of the corresponding bronchus. The *veins from the parietal pleura* join the systemic veins in adjacent parts of the thoracic wall. The *veins from the visceral pleura* drain into the pulmonary veins.

The **bronchial arteries** supply blood for the nutrition of the structures comprising the root of the lungs, the supporting tissues of the lung, and the visceral pleura (Figs. 2.15 and 2.19*A*). *The left bronchial arteries arise from the thoracic aorta; however, the right bronchial artery may arise from:*

- A superior posterior intercostal artery

PULMONARY THROMBOEMBOLISM

Obstruction of a pulmonary artery by a *thrombus* (immobile blood clot)—*pulmonary thromboembolism*—is a common cause of morbidity (sickness) and mortality (death). A detached thrombus, fat globule, or air bubble travels in the blood to the lungs from a leg or pelvic vein. The embolus (mobile clot) passes through the right side of the heart to a lung through a pulmonary artery. The embolus may lodge in a pulmonary artery—*pulmonary thromboembolism*—or one of its branches. The immediate result is partial or complete obstruction of bloodflow to the lung. The obstruction results in a sector of lung that is ventilated but not perfused with blood. When a large embolus occludes a pulmonary artery, the person suffers *acute respiratory distress* because of a major decrease in the oxygenation of blood and may die in a few minutes. A medium-sized embolus may block an artery supplying a bronchopulmonary segment, producing a *thrombotic infarct*—an area of necrotic (dead) tissue.

- A common trunk from the thoracic aorta with the right 3rd posterior intercostal artery
- A left superior bronchial artery.

The small bronchial arteries provide branches to the upper esophagus and then pass along the posterior aspects of the main bronchi, supplying them and their branches as far distally as the respiratory bronchioles. The distalmost branches of the bronchial arteries anastomose with branches of the pulmonary arteries in the walls of the small bronchi and in the visceral pleura.

The **bronchial veins** (Fig. 2.19B) drain only part of the blood supplied to the lungs by the bronchial arteries; some blood is drained by the pulmonary veins, especially from the more peripheral parts of the distal root of the lung. The right bronchial vein drains into the **azygos**

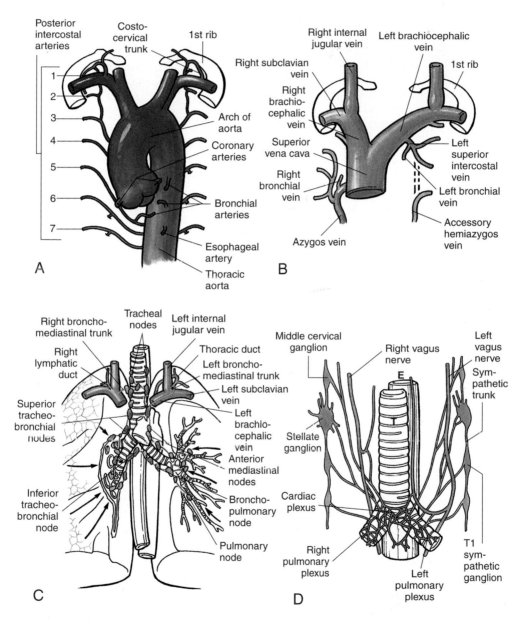

FIGURE 2.19   Vasculature and nerves of lungs and pleurae. A. Arteries. **B.** Veins. **C.** Lymphatics. *Arrows* indicate direction of lymph flow; those on the right indicate flow from the superficial pulmonary lymphatic plexuses; those on the left indicate flow from the deep pulmonary plexuses. **D.** Nerves. *E,* esophagus; *T,* trachea. *Orange,* sympathetic; *green,* parasympathetic; *blue,* plexus.

vein and the left bronchial vein drains into the **accessory hemiazygos vein** or the left superior intercostal vein.

The **lymphatic plexuses in the lungs** communicate freely (Fig. 2.19C).

- *The superficial lymphatic plexus* lies deep to the visceral pleura and drains the lung parenchyma (tissue) and visceral pleura. Lymphatic vessels from the plexus drain into the **bronchopulmonary lymph nodes** (hilar lymph nodes) in the hilum of the lung.
- The *deep lymphatic plexus* is located in the submucosa of the bronchi and in the peribronchial connective tissue. It is largely concerned with draining structures that form the root of the lung. Lymphatic vessels from this plexus drain into the **pulmonary lymph nodes** located along the lobar bronchi. At the hilum of the lung they drain into bronchopulmonary lymph nodes.

Lymph from the superficial and deep plexuses drains from the bronchopulmonary lymph nodes to the superior and inferior **tracheobronchial lymph nodes,** superior and inferior to the bifurcation of the trachea, respectively. Lymph from the tracheobronchial lymph nodes passes to the right and left **bronchomediastinal lymph trunks.** These trunks usually terminate on each side at the junction of the subclavian and internal jugular veins; however, the right bronchomediastinal trunk may first merge with other lymphatic trunks converging here to form the very short **right lymphatic duct.** The left bronchomediastinal trunk commonly terminates in or is replaced by the **thoracic duct.** The superficial (subpleural) lymphatic plexus drains lymph from the *visceral pleura.* Lymph from the *parietal pleura* drains into the lymph nodes of the thoracic wall (intercostal, parasternal, mediastinal, and phrenic). A few vessels from the cervical pleura drain into the axillary lymph nodes.

The **nerves of the lungs and visceral pleura** derive from the pulmonary plexuses located anterior and (mainly) posterior to the roots of the lungs (Fig. 2.19D). These nerve networks contain parasympathetic fibers from the **vagus nerves** (CN X) and sympathetic fibers from the sympathetic trunks. *Parasympathetic ganglion cells*—cell bodies of postsynaptic parasympathetic neurons—are in the **pulmonary plexuses** and along the branches of the bronchial tree. The parasympathetic fibers from the vagus nerves (CN X) are motor to the smooth muscle of the bronchial tree (*bronchoconstrictor*); inhibitor to the pulmonary vessels (*vasodilator*), and secretor to the glands of the bronchial tree (*secretomotor*). *The visceral afferent fibers of CN X are distributed to the:*

- Bronchial mucosa and are probably concerned with cough reflexes
- Bronchial muscles and are involved in stretch reception
- Interalveolar connective tissue and are involved in Herring-Breuer reflexes, the mechanism that tends to limit respiratory excursions
- Pulmonary arteries as pressor receptors and pulmonary veins as chemoreceptors.

Sympathetic ganglion cells—cell bodies of postsynaptic sympathetic neurons—are in the **paravertebral sympathetic ganglia** of the sympathetic trunks. The sympathetic fibers are inhibitor to the bronchial muscle (bronchodilator); motor to the pulmonary vessels (vasoconstrictor), and inhibitor to the alveolar glands of the bronchial tree.

INJURY TO PLEURAE

The visceral pleura is insensitive to pain because its innervation is autonomic (motor and visceral afferent). The autonomic nerves reach the visceral pleura in company with the bronchial vessels. The visceral pleura receives no nerves of general sensation. *The parietal pleura is very sensitive to pain,* particularly the costal pleura, because it is richly supplied by branches of the somatic intercostal and phrenic nerves (see Fig. 2.22A). Irritation of the parietal pleura produces local pain and referred pain to the areas sharing innervation by the same segments of the spinal cord. Irritation of the costal and peripheral parts of the diaphragmatic pleura results in local pain and referred pain along the intercostal nerves to the thoracic and abdominal walls. Irritation of the mediastinal and central diaphragmatic areas of the parietal pleura results in pain that is referred to the root of the neck and over the shoulder (C3 through C5 dermatomes).

Inhalation of Carbon Particles

Lymph from the lungs carries *phagocytes*—cells possessing the property of ingesting carbon particles from inspired air. In many people, especially cigarette smokers, these particles color the surface of the lungs and associated lymph nodes a mottled gray to black. *Smokers' cough* results from inhalation of irritants in tobacco.

Bronchiolar Carcinoma

Bronchiolar carcinoma (CA) is a common type of lung cancer that arises from the epithelium of the bronchial tree. **Lung cancer** is mainly caused by cigarette smoking. Bronchiolar CA usually metastasizes widely because of the arrangement of the lymphatics. The tumor cells probably enter the systemic circulation by invading the wall of a sinusoid or venule in the lung and are transported through the pulmonary veins, left heart, and aorta to all parts of the body, especially the cranium and brain.

MEDIASTINUM

The mediastinum—occupied by the mass of tissue between the pulmonary cavities—is the central compartment of the thoracic cavity (Fig. 2.20). *It does not contain the lungs.* It is covered on each side by mediastinal pleura and contains all the thoracic viscera and structures except the lungs. The mediastinum extends from the *superior thoracic aperture* to the diaphragm inferiorly and from the sternum and costal cartilages anteriorly to the bodies of the thoracic vertebrae posteriorly. The mediastinum in living persons is a highly mobile region because it consists primarily of hollow (liquid or air-filled) visceral structures united only by loose connective tissue, often infiltrated with fat. The major structures in the mediastinum are also surrounded by blood and lymphatic vessels, lymph nodes, nerves, and fat. The looseness of the connective tissue and the elasticity of the lungs and parietal pleura on each side of the mediastinum enable it to accommodate movement, volume, and pressure changes in the thoracic cavity, such as those resulting from movements of the diaphragm, thoracic wall, and tracheobronchial tree during respiration, pulsations of the great arteries, esophagus during swallowing, and movement of the lungs and heart. This connective tissue becomes more fibrous and rigid with age; hence, the mediastinal structures become less mobile. The mediastinum is artificially divided into superior and inferior parts for purposes of description.

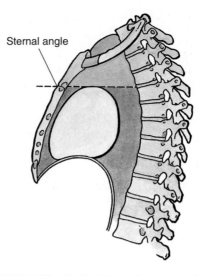

FIGURE 2.20 Mediastinum. *Green*—superior mediastinum. *Purple*—anterior mediastinum. *Yellow*—middle mediastinum. *Blue*—posterior mediastinum.

- *The superior mediastinum* extends inferiorly from the superior thoracic aperture to the horizontal plane—often called the *transverse thoracic plane*—passing through the sternal angle and the IV disc of T4 and T5 vertebra (Fig. 2.20). *The superior mediastinum contains* the SVC, brachiocephalic veins, arch of aorta, thoracic duct, trachea, esophagus, thymus, vagus nerve, left recurrent laryngeal nerve, and phrenic nerve.
- *The inferior mediastinum* between the transverse thoracic plane and the diaphragm is further subdivided by the pericardium into anterior, middle, and posterior parts. *The anterior mediastinum* contains remnants of the thymus, lymph nodes, fat, and connective tissue. *The middle mediastinum* contains the pericardium, heart, roots of the great vessels, arch of azygos vein, and main bronchi. *The posterior mediastinum* contains the esophagus, thoracic aorta, azygos and hemiazygos veins, thoracic duct, vagus nerves, sympathetic trunks, and splanchnic nerves.

Some structures—the esophagus, for example—pass vertically through the mediastinum and therefore lie in more than one mediastinal compartment.

LEVELS OF VISCERA IN MEDIASTINUM

The level of the viscera relative to the mediastinal subdivisions depends on the position of the person. When a person is lying supine, the level of the viscera relative to the subdivisions of the mediastinum are as shown. Anatomical descriptions traditionally describe the level of the viscera as if the person were in this position, that is, lying in bed or on the operating or dissection table. In this position, the abdominal viscera push the mediastinal structures superiorly. However, in the standing position, the levels of the viscera are as shown below. This occurs because the soft structures in the mediastinum (especially the pericardium and its contents), the heart and great vessels, and the abdominal viscera supporting them sag inferiorly under the influence of gravity. This movement of mediastinal structures must be considered during physical and radiological examinations.

Mediastinoscopy

Using a *mediastinoscope,* surgeons can see much of the mediastinum and conduct minor surgical procedures. They insert this tubular, lighted instrument through a small incision in the root of the neck, just superior to the manubrium near the jugular notch. During mediastinoscopy, surgeons may view or biopsy mediastinal lymph nodes to determine if cancer cells have metastasized to them from a bronchogenic carcinoma, for example. The mediastinum can also be explored and biopsies taken by removing part of a costal cartilage.

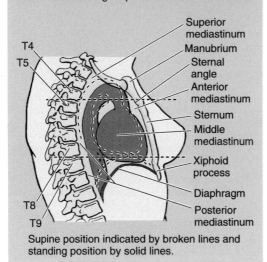

Supine position indicated by broken lines and standing position by solid lines.

HEART AND GREAT VESSELS

The middle mediastinum contains the pericardium, heart, roots of the great vessels, ascending aorta, pulmonary trunk and SVC—passing to and from the heart—arch of azygos vein, and main bronchi.

Pericardium

The pericardium is a *double-walled fibroserous sac* that encloses the heart and the roots of its great vessels (Table 2.5). This conical sac lies posterior to the body of the sternum and the second to sixth costal cartilages at the level of T5 to T8 vertebrae. The tough external fibrous layer of the sac—the **fibrous pericardium**—is

---

TABLE 2.5. LAYERS OF PERICARDIUM AND HEART

Pericardium

External sac called fibrous pericardium
Internal sac called serous pericardium

   Parietal layer—lines fibrous pericardium
   Visceral layer becomes outermost layer
   of wall of heart, the epicardium

Thin film of fluid in pericardial cavity between visceral and parietal layers of serous pericardium allows heart to move freely within pericadrial sac

Heart

Wall of heart is composed of three layers; from superficial to deep,

   Epicardium
   Myocardium
   Endocardium

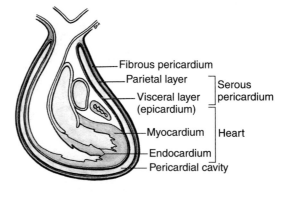

bound to the central tendon of the diaphragm (Fig. 2.21, *A* and *B*). The **serous pericardium** is composed of a single layer of flattened cells forming an epithelium that lines both the internal surface of the fibrous pericardium and the external surface of the heart. The **pericardial sac** is influenced by movements of the heart and great vessels, sternum, and diaphragm because the fibrous pericardium is

- Fused with the tunica adventitia of the great vessels entering and leaving the heart
- Attached to the posterior surface of the sternum by *sternopericardial ligaments*
- Fused with the central tendon of the diaphragm.

The fibrous pericardium protects the heart against sudden overfilling because it is so unyielding and closely related to the great vessels that pierce it superiorly (Fig. 2.21, *A* and *B*). The ascending aorta carries the pericardium superiorly beyond the heart to the level of the sternal angle.

The **pericardial cavity** is the potential space between the opposing layers of the parietal and visceral layers of serous pericardium (Table 2.5). It normally contains a thin film of serous fluid that enables the heart to move and beat in a frictionless environment. The *parietal layer of serous pericardium* fuses to the internal surface of the fibrous pericardium. *The visceral layer of serous pericardium forms the epicardium*—the external layer of the heart wall—and reflects from the heart and great vessels to become continuous with the parietal layer of serous pericardium, where

- The aorta and pulmonary trunk leave the heart; a finger can be inserted into the **transverse pericardial sinus** located posterior to these large vessels and anterior to the SVC (see drawing)
- The SVC, IVC and pulmonary veins enter the heart; these vessels are partly covered by serous pericardium, which forms the **oblique pericardial sinus,** a wide, slitlike recess posterior to the heart. The oblique sinus can be entered inferiorly and will admit several fingers; however, they cannot pass around any of these vessels because the sinus is a blind recess (cul-de-sac).

These pericardial sinuses form during development of the heart as a consequence of folding of the primordial heart tube (Fig. 2.22). As the heart tube folds, its venous end moves posterosuperiorly so that the venous end of the tube lies adjacent to the arterial end, separated by the transverse pericardial sinus. As these vessels expand and move apart, the pericardium is reflected around them to form the boundaries of the oblique pericardial sinus.

SURGICAL SIGNIFICANCE OF TRANSVERSE PERICARDIAL SINUS

The transverse pericardial sinus is especially important to cardiac surgeons. After the pericardial sac has been opened anteriorly, a finger can be passed through the transverse pericardial sinus posterior to the aorta and pulmonary trunk. By passing a surgical clamp or placing a ligature around these vessels, inserting the tubes of a coronary bypass machine, and then tightening the ligature, surgeons can stop or divert the circulation of blood in these large arteries while performing cardiac surgery, such as coronary artery bypass grafting. Cardiac surgery is performed while the patient is on cardiopulmonary bypass.

Pericarditis, Pericardial Effusion, and Cardiac Tamponade

Inflammation of the pericardium—*pericarditis*—usually causes chest pain. Usually the layers of serous pericardium make no detectable sound during auscultation. However, pericarditis makes the surfaces rough and the resulting friction—*pericardial friction rub*—sounds like the rustle of silk when listening with a stethoscope. Certain inflammatory diseases may also produce *pericardial effusion* (passage of fluid from the pericardial capillaries into the pericardial cavity). If there is extensive pericardial effusion, the excess fluid does not allow the heart to expand fully, thereby limiting the inflow of blood to the ventricles. This phenomenon—*cardiac tamponade* (heart compression)—is a potentially lethal condition because the fibrous pericardium is tough and inelastic. Consequently, heart volume is increasingly compromised by the fluid outside

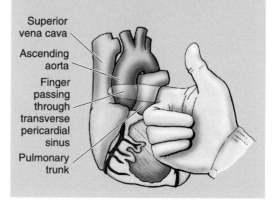

Superior vena cava

Ascending aorta

Finger passing through transverse pericardial sinus

Pulmonary trunk

Continued
the heart but inside the pericardial cavity. When there is a slow increase in the size of the heart—*cardiomegaly*—the pericardium allows the enlargement of heart to occur without compression.

Stab wounds that pierce the heart causing blood to enter the pericardial cavity—*hemopericardium*—also risk producing cardiac tamponade. Hemopericardium may also result from perforation of a weakened area of heart muscle following a heart attack. As blood accumulates, the heart is compressed and circulation fails. The veins of the face and neck become engorged because of compression of the SVC where it enters the pericardium. *Pericardiocentesis* (drainage of serous fluid from pericardial cavity) is usually necessary to relieve the cardiac tamponade. To remove the excess fluid, a wide-bore needle may be inserted through the left 5th or 6th intercostal space near the sternum.

The **arterial supply of the pericardium** is mainly from the **pericardiacophrenic artery** (Fig. 2.21*A*), a slender branch of the **internal thoracic artery** that may accompany or parallel the phrenic nerve to the diaphragm. Smaller contributions of blood to the pericardium come from the

- *Musculophrenic artery,* a terminal branch of the internal thoracic artery
- *Bronchial, esophageal, and superior phrenic arteries* from the thoracic aorta (Fig. 2.19*A*)
- *Coronary arteries* (visceral layer of serous pericardium only).

The **venous drainage of the pericardium** is from the

- *Pericardiophrenic veins,* tributaries of the brachiocephalic (or internal thoracic) veins
- Variable tributaries of azygos venous system (Fig. 2.19*B*).

The **nerve supply of the pericardium** (Figs. 2.19*D* and 2.221*A*) is from the

- *Phrenic nerves* (C3 through C5)—a primary source of sensory fibers
- *Vagus nerves* (CN X)—function uncertain
- *Sympathetic trunks*—vasomotor.

Pain sensations conveyed by the phrenic nerves are commonly referred to the skin of the ipsilateral supraclavicular region (top of shoulder on same side).

Heart and Great Vessels

The heart, slightly larger than a clenched fist (Fig. 2.21*A*), is a double self-adjusting muscular pump, the parts of which work in unison to propel blood to the body. The right side of the heart receives poorly oxygenated blood from the body through the superior vena cava (SVC) and inferior vena cava (IVC) and pumps it through the pulmonary trunk to the lungs for oxygenation. The left side of the heart receives well-oxygenated blood from the lungs through the pulmonary veins and pumps it into the aorta for distribution to the body.

The heart has four chambers: **right** and **left atria** and **right** and **left ventricles.** The atria are receiving chambers that pump blood into the ventricles—the discharging chambers. The synchronous pumping actions of the heart's two atrioventricular (AV) pumps (right and left chambers) constitute the **cardiac cycle**) (Fig. 2.23). The cycle begins with a period of ventricular relaxation (**diastole**) and ends with a period of ventricular contraction (**systole).** Two *heart sounds*—resulting from valve closures—can be heard with a stethoscope: a "lub" sound as the atria transfer blood to the ventricles and a "dub" sound as the ventricles contract and propel blood from the heart. The heart sounds are produced by the snapping shut of the one-way valves that normally keep blood from flowing backward during contractions of the heart. *The wall of each chamber of the heart consists of three layers from superficial to deep* (Table 2.5):

- **Epicardium,** a thin external layer (mesothelium) formed by the visceral layer of serous pericardium
- **Myocardium,** a thick middle layer composed of cardiac muscle
- **Endocardium,** a thin internal layer (endothelium and subendothelial connective tissue) or lining membrane of the heart that also covers its valves.

When the ventricles contract, they produce a wringing motion because of the spiral orientation of the cardiac muscle fibers in the myocardium. This motion propels the blood from the heart. The muscle fibers are anchored to the **fibrous skeleton of the heart** (Fig. 2.24).

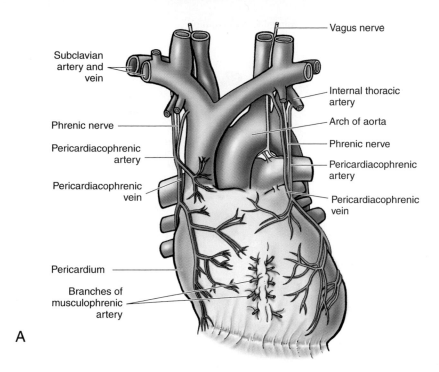

A

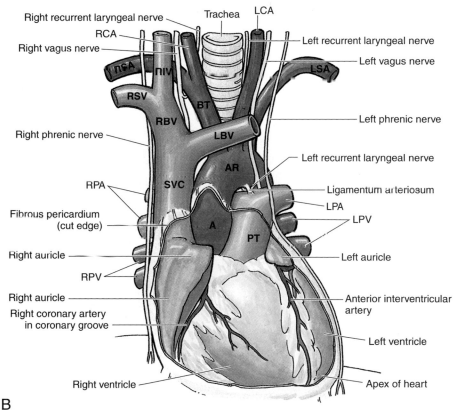

B

FIGURE 2.21 **Pericardium and parts, surfaces, and borders of the heart. A.** Arterial supply and venous drainage of the pericardium. Anterior view. **B.** Sternocostal surface of the heart. Anterior view. **C,** Interior of pericardial sac after removal of the heart. **D.** Base and diaphragmatic surface of the heart. Posteroinferior view. *A,* aorta; *AR,* arch of aorta; *BT,* brachiocephalic trunk; *LBV,* left brachiocephalic vein; *LCA,* left common carotid artery; *LPA,* left pulmonary artery; *LPV,* left pulmonary vein; *LSA,* left subclavian artery; *PT,* pulmonary trunk; *RBV,* right brachiocephalic vein; *RCA,* right common carotid artery; *RIV,* right internal jugular vein; *RPA,* right pulmonary artery; *RPV,* right pulmonary vein; *RSA,* right subclavian artery.

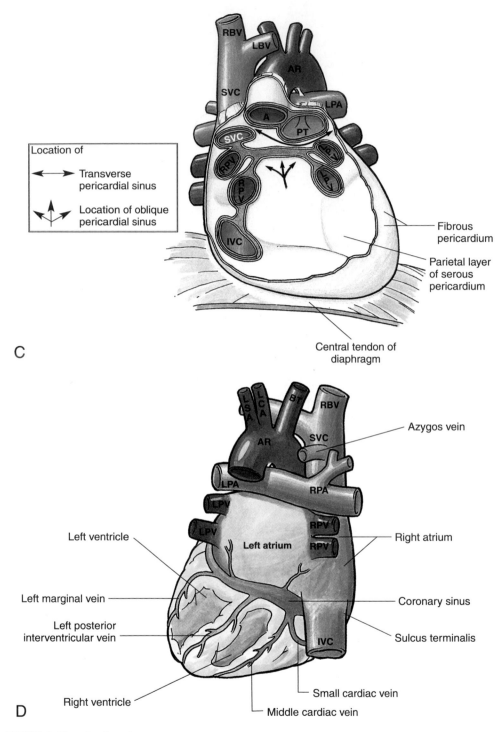

C

FIGURE 2.21 *Continued.*

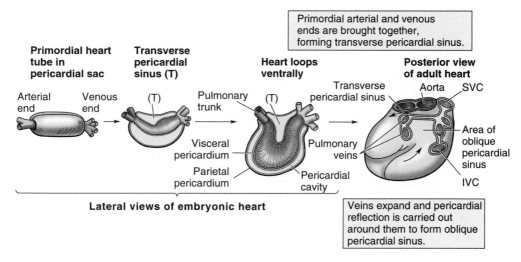

Primordial arterial and venous ends are brought together, forming transverse pericardial sinus.

Primordial heart tube in pericardial sac

Transverse pericardial sinus (T)

Heart loops ventrally

Posterior view of adult heart

Arterial end   Venous end   (T)   Pulmonary trunk   (T)   Transverse pericardial sinus   Aorta   SVC

Visceral pericardium   Pulmonary veins   Area of oblique pericardial sinus

Parietal pericardium   Pericardial cavity   IVC

Lateral views of embryonic heart

Veins expand and pericardial reflection is carried out around them to form oblique pericardial sinus.

FIGURE 2.22   Development of the heart and pericardium. The primordial heart tube invaginates the double-layered pericardial sac (somewhat like placing a hotdog in a bun). The primordial heart then loops ventrally, bringing the primordial arterial and venous ends of the heart together and creating the transverse pericardial sinus between them. The veins expand and move apart. The pericardium is reflected around them to form the boundaries of the oblique pericardial sinus.

The fibrous framework of dense collagen forms four **fibrous rings,** which surround the orifices of the valves, right and left **fibrous trigones,** formed by connecting the rings, and the membranous parts of the interatrial and interventricular septa. **The fibrous skeleton of the heart:**

- Keeps the orifices of the atrioventricular (AV) and semilunar valves patent and from being overly distended by the volume of blood pumping through them
- Provides attachments (origin and insertion) for the leaflets and cusps of the valves
- Provides attachment (origin and insertion) for the myocardium
- Forms an electrical "insulator" by separating the myenterically conducted impulses of the atria and ventricles so that they contract independently, and by surrounding and providing passage for the initial part of the AV bundle.

The heart and roots of the great vessels within the pericardial sac are related anteriorly to the sternum, costal cartilages, and the medial ends of the 3rd through 5th ribs on the left side. The heart and pericardial sac are situated obliquely, about two-thirds to the left and one-third to the right of the median plane. *The heart has an apex, base, three surfaces, and four borders.*

The **apex of the heart** (Fig. 2.21*A*):

- Is formed by the left inferolateral part of the left ventricle
- Is located posterior to the left 5th intercostal space in adults, usually 9 cm from the median plane
- Is where maximal pulsation of the heart (**apex beat**) occurs and underlies the site where the "heartbeat" may be observed or palpated on the thoracic wall.

The **base of the heart** (Fig. 2.21*C*):

- Is the heart's posterior aspect (opposite the apex) as it lies in the thorax
- Is formed mainly by the left atrium, with a lesser contribution by the right atrium
- *Faces posteriorly toward the bodies of vertebrae T6 through T9,* and is separated from them by the pericardium, oblique pericardial sinus, esophagus, and aorta
- Extends superiorly to the bifurcation of the pulmonary trunk and inferiorly to the coronary groove (sulcus)

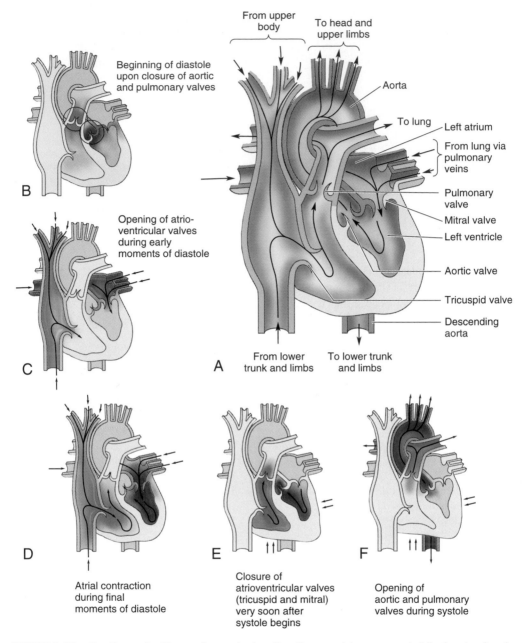

From upper body

To head and upper limbs

Aorta

To lung

Left atrium

From lung via pulmonary veins

Pulmonary valve

Mitral valve

Left ventricle

Aortic valve

Tricuspid valve

Descending aorta

From lower trunk and limbs

To lower trunk and limbs

A

B   Beginning of diastole upon closure of aortic and pulmonary valves

C   Opening of atrio-ventricular valves during early moments of diastole

D   Atrial contraction during final moments of diastole

E   Closure of atrioventricular valves (tricuspid and mitral) very soon after systole begins

F   Opening of aortic and pulmonary valves during systole

FIGURE 2.23   Cardiac cycle. The cardiac cycle describes the complete movement of the heart or heartbeat and includes the period from the beginning of one heartbeat to the beginning of the next one. The cycle consists of *diastole* (ventricular filling) and *systole* (ventricular emptying).

- Receives the pulmonary veins on the right and left sides of its left atrial portion and the superior and inferior venae cavae at the upper and lower ends of its right atrial portion.

The **three surfaces of the heart** (Fig. 2.21, *A* and *C*) are the:

- *Anterior (sternocostal) surface,* formed mainly by the right ventricle
- *Diaphragmatic (inferior) surface,* formed mainly by the left ventricle and partly by the right ventricle; the diaphragmatic surface is related to the central tendon of the diaphragm
- *Pulmonary (left) surface,* formed mainly by the left ventricle; it occupies the cardiac area of the left lung (Fig. 2.15*A*).

The **four borders of the heart** (Fig. 2.25) are the:

- *Right border* (vertical, slightly convex), formed by the right atrium and extending between the 3VC and IVC

- *Inferior border* (nearly horizontal), formed mainly by the right ventricle and only slightly by the left ventricle
- *Left border* (oblique, nearly vertical), formed mainly by the left ventricle and slightly by the left auricle
- *Superior border,* formed by the right and left atria and auricles in an anterior view; the ascending aorta and pulmonary trunk emerge from the superior border, and the SVC enters its right side. Posterior to the aorta and pulmonary trunk and anterior to the SVC, the superior border forms the inferior boundary of the transverse pericardial sinus.

PERCUSSION OF HEART

Percussion defines the density and size of the heart. The classical percussion technique is to create vibration by tapping the chest with a finger while listening and feeling for differences in sound wave conduction. Percussion is performed at the 3rd, 4th, and 5th intercostal spaces from the left anterior axillary line to the right anterior axillary line. Normally the percussion note changes from resonance to dullness (because of the presence of the heart) approximately 6 cm lateral to the left border of the sternum. The

---

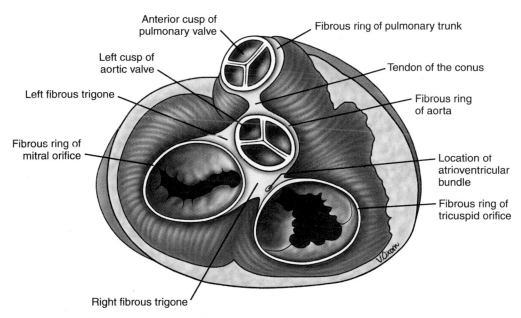

FIGURE 2.24 Fibrous skeleton of the heart. Superior view. The atria have been removed at the coronary groove, leaving the ventricles and valves. The fibrous skeleton is composed of four fibrous rings—each encircling a valve, two trigones, and the membranous parts of the interatrial (not shown) and interventricular septa.

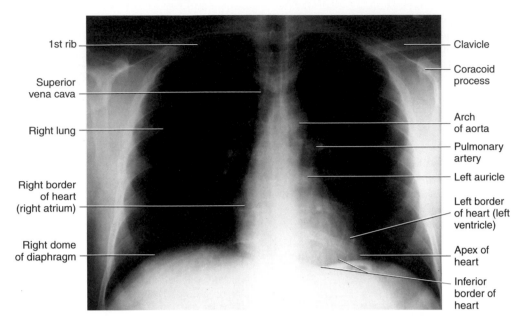

1st rib

Clavicle

Coracoid process

Superior vena cava

Arch of aorta

Pulmonary artery

Right lung

Left auricle

Right border of heart (right atrium)

Left border of heart (left ventricle)

Right dome of diaphragm

Apex of heart

Inferior border of heart

FIGURE 2.25　Posteroanterior radiograph of thorax. Observe the lungs and heart.

Continued
character of the sound changes as different areas of the chest are tapped.

Radiographs of Thorax
Anteroposterior chest films show the contour of the heart and great vessels—the *cardiovascular silhouette* or cardiac shadow (Fig. 2.25). The silhouette contrasts with the clearer areas occupied by the air-filled lungs because the heart and great vessels are full of blood. The silhouette becomes longer and narrower during inspiration because the fibrous pericardium is attached to the diaphragm that descends during inspiration.

Right Atrium. This chamber forms the right border of the heart and receives venous blood from the SVC and IVC and the coronary sinus (Figs. 2.21*A* and *C* and 2.26). The earlike **right auricle** is a small, conical muscular pouch that projects from the **right atrium,** increasing the capacity of the atrium as it overlaps the ascending aorta. The primordial atrium is represented in the adult by the right auricle. The definitive atrium is enlarged by incorporation of most of the embryonic venous sinus (L. sinus venosus). The **coronary sinus** lies in the posterior part of the coronary groove and receives blood from the cardiac veins. The coronary si-

nus is also a derivative of the embryonic venous sinus. The part of the venous sinus incorporated into the primordial atrium becomes the smooth-walled **sinus venarum** of the adult right atrium. The separation between the primordial atrium—the adult auricle—and the sinus venarum—the derivative of the venous sinus—is indicated externally by the **terminal groove** and internally by the terminal crest (Figs. 2.26 and 2.32). The **interior of the right atrium** (Fig. 2.26) has

- A smooth, thin-walled posterior part—the **sinus venarum**—which the SVC, IVC, and coronary sinus open, bringing poorly oxygenated blood into the heart
- A rough, muscular wall composed of **pectinate muscles** (L. musculi pectinati)
- The **opening of the SVC** into its superior part, at the level of the right third costal cartilage
- The **opening of the IVC** into the inferior part, almost in line with the SVC at approximately the level of the 5th costal cartilage
- The **opening of the coronary sinus** between the right AV orifice and IVC orifice

- A **right AV orifice** through which the right atrium discharges the poorly oxygenated blood into the right ventricle
- The **interatrial septum,** separating the atria, has an oval, thumbprint-sized depression, the **oval fossa** (L. fossa ovalis), a remnant of the foramen ovale and its valve in the fetus (Moore and Persaud, 1998).

Right Ventricle. The right ventricle forms the largest part of the anterior surface of the heart, a small part of the diaphragmatic surface, and almost the entire inferior border of the heart. Superiorly the **right ventricle** tapers into an arterial cone—the **conus arteriosus** (infundibulum) that leads into the pulmonary

ATRIAL SEPTAL DEFECTS

Congenital anomalies of the interatrial septum—usually related to incomplete closure of the oval foramen—are atrial septal defects (**ASDs**). A probe-sized patency (defect) appears in the superior part of the oval fossa in 15% to 25% of people. These small ASDs, by themselves, are usually of no clinical significance; however, large ASDs allow oxygenated blood from the lungs to be shunted from the left atrium through the defect into the right atrium, causing enlargement of the right atrium and ventricle and dilation of the pulmonary trunk.

trunk (Fig. 2.26). The interior of the right ventricle has irregular muscular elevations called **trabeculae carneae.** A thick muscular ridge, the **supraventricular crest,** separates the ridged muscular wall of the inflow part of the

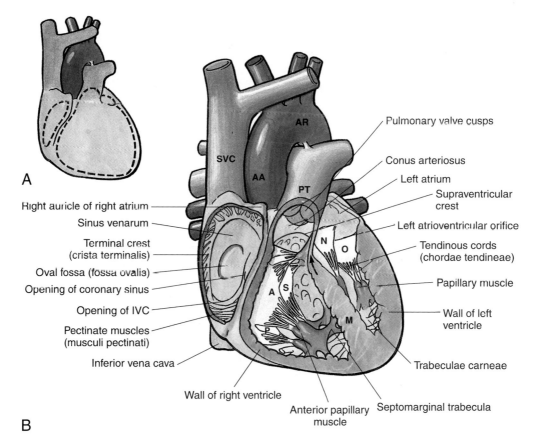

A

Right auricle of right atrium
Sinus venarum
Terminal crest (crista terminalis)
Oval fossa (fossa ovalis)
Opening of coronary sinus
Opening of IVC
Pectinate muscles (musculi pectinati)
Inferior vena cava

Wall of right ventricle

Anterior papillary muscle

Pulmonary valve cusps
Conus arteriosus
Left atrium
Supraventricular crest
Left atrioventricular orifice
Tendinous cords (chordae tendineae)
Papillary muscle
Wall of left ventricle
Trabeculae carneae

Septomarginal trabecula

B

FIGURE 2.26   Anterior view of interior of the heart. A. Parts of the wall of the heart that have been removed in **B.** Observe features of each chamber in **B.** Note three cusps of the tricuspid valve [anterior (*A*), posterior (*P*), septal (*S*)] and two cusps of the mitral valve [anterior (*N*) and posterior (*O*)]. *AA*, ascending aorta; *AR*, arch of aorta. *M*, muscular part of interventricular septum; *PT*, pulmonary trunk; *SVC*, superior vena cava. *Arrow*, membranous part of interventricular septum.

chamber from the smooth wall of the conus arteriosus or outflow part of the right ventricle. The *inflow part of the right ventricle* receives blood from the right atrium through the **right AV orifice,** located posterior to the body of the sternum at the level of the 4th and 5th intercostal spaces. The right AV orifice is surrounded by a fibrous ring (part of fibrous skeleton of heart) that resists the dilation that might otherwise result from blood being forced through it (Fig. 2.24).

The **tricuspid valve** (Figs. 2.26 and 2.27*A*) guards the right AV orifice. The bases of the valve cusps are attached to the fibrous ring around the orifice. **Tendinous cords** (L. chordae tendineae) attach to the free edges and ventricular surfaces of the anterior, posterior, and septal cusps—much like the cords attaching to a parachute. Because the cords are attached to adjacent sides of two cusps, they prevent separation of the cusps and their inversion when tension is applied to the cords throughout ventricular contraction (systole); that is, the cusps of the tricuspid valve are prevented from prolapsing (being driven into right atrium) as ventricular pressure rises. Thus, regurgitation of blood (backward flow of blood) from the right ventricle into the right atrium is blocked by the valve cusps. The **papillary muscles** form conical projections with their bases attached to the ventricular wall and tendinous cords arising from their apices. There are usually three papillary muscles (anterior, posterior, and septal) in the right ventricle that correspond in name to the cusps of the tricuspid valve. The papillary muscles begin to contract before contraction of the right ventricle, tightening the tendinous cords and drawing the cusps together. Contraction is maintained throughout systole. This prevents ventricular blood from passing back (regurgitating) into the right atrium.

The **interventricular (IV) septum**—composed of membranous and muscular parts—is a strong, obliquely placed partition between the right and left ventricles (Fig. 2.26), forming part of the walls of each. The superoposterior *membranous part of the IV septum is thin* and is continuous with the fibrous skeleton of the heart. The *muscular part of the IV septum*

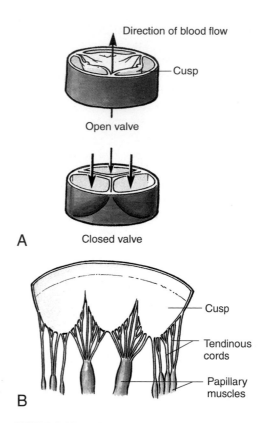

FIGURE 2.27 Tricuspid and pulmonary valves.
A. Tricuspid valve spread out. **B.** Pulmonary valve.

is thick and bulges into the cavity of the right ventricle because of the higher blood pressure in the left ventricle. The **septomarginal trabecula** (moderator band) is a curved muscular bundle that runs from the inferior part of the interventricular septum to the base of the anterior papillary muscle. This trabecula is important because it carries part of the **right bundle of the AV bundle** of the conducting system of the heart (p. 102), which takes a "short cut" across the chamber of the ventricle to reach the anterior papillary muscle.

The **right AV orifice** is large enough to admit the tips of three fingers. When the right atrium contracts, blood is forced through this orifice into the right ventricle, pushing the cusps of the tricuspid valve aside like curtains. The inflow of blood into the right ventricle (*inflow tract*) enters posteriorly, and the outflow of blood into the pulmonary trunk (*outflow tract*) leaves superiorly and to the left. Consequently, the blood takes a U-shaped path through the right ventricle. The inflow (AV) orifice and outflow (pulmonary) orifice are approximately 2 cm apart. The **pulmonary valve** at the apex of the **conus arteriosus** is at the level of the left 3rd costal cartilage (Figs. 2.26 and 2.27*B*). Each of the semilunar **cusps of the pulmonary valve** (anterior, right, and left), is concave when viewed superiorly. The *pulmonary sinuses* are the spaces at the origin of the pulmonary trunk between the dilated wall of the vessel and each cusp of the pulmonary valve. The blood in the pulmonary sinuses prevents the cusps from sticking to the wall of the pulmonary trunk and failing to close.

VENTRICULAR SEPTAL DEFECTS
The membranous part of the IV septum develops separately from the muscular part and has a complex embryological origin. Consequently, this part is the common site of ventricular septal defects (**VSDs**). These congenital anomalies rank first on all lists of cardiac defects. Isolated VSD accounts for approximately 25% of all forms of congenital heart disease (Moore and Persaud, 1998). The size of the defect varies from 1 to 25 mm. A VSD causes a left-to-right shunt of blood through the defect. A large shunt increases pulmonary bloodflow, which causes pulmonary disease (hypertension—increased blood pressure) and may cause cardiac failure.

Pulmonary Stenosis
With *pulmonary valve stenosis* (narrowing), the valve cusps are fused, forming a dome with a narrow central opening. In *infundibular pulmonary stenosis,* the conus arteriosus is underdeveloped producing a restriction of right ventricular outflow. Both types of pulmonary stenosis may occur together. The degree of hypertrophy of the right ventricle is variable.

Left Atrium. This heart chamber forms most of the base of the heart (Fig. 2.21*C*). The valveless pairs of right and left **pulmonary veins** enter the left atrium. The left auricle forms the superior part of the left border of the heart and overlaps the pulmonary trunk. The **interior of the left atrium** has

- A larger smooth-walled part and a smaller muscular auricle containing pectinate muscles.
- Four pulmonary veins (two superior and two inferior) entering its posterior wall

- A slightly thicker wall than that of the right atrium
- An interatrial septum that slopes posteriorly and to the right
- A left AV orifice through which the left atrium discharges the oxygenated blood it receives into the left ventricle.

The smooth-walled part of the left atrium is formed by absorption of parts of the embryonic pulmonary veins, whereas the rough-walled part, mainly in the auricle, represents the remains of the left part of the primordial atrium.

STROKES OR CARDIOVASCULAR ACCIDENTS
Thrombi (immobile blood clots) form on the walls of the left atrium in certain types of heart disease. If these thrombi become detached or pieces break off, the emboli (mobile blood clots) pass into the systemic circulation and occlude peripheral arteries. Occlusion of an artery in the brain by an embolus results in a stroke or cardiovascular accident (**CVA**) that paralyzes the parts of the body previously controlled by the now-damaged area of the brain.

Left Ventricle. This chamber forms the apex of the heart, nearly all of its left (pulmonary) surface and border, and most of the diaphragmatic surface (Fig. 2.21, *A* and *C*). Because arterial pressure is much higher in the systemic than in the pulmonary circulation, the **left ventricle** performs more work than the right ventricle. The **interior of the left ventricle** (Fig. 2.26) has

- A double-leaflet **mitral valve** that guards the left AV orifice (Fig. 2.28)
- Walls that are twice as thick as that of the right ventricle
- A conical cavity that is longer than that of the right ventricle
- Walls that are covered with thick muscular ridges—**trabeculae carneae**—that are more numerous than in the right ventricle
- Anterior and posterior **papillary muscles** that are larger than those in the right ventricle because this ventricle works harder
- A superoanterior outflow part formed by the smooth-walled *aortic vestibule* leading to the aortic orifice

- An *aortic orifice* that lies in its right posterosuperior part and is surrounded by a fibrous ring to which the right, posterior, and left **cusps of the aortic valve** are attached.

The **mitral valve** closing the orifice between the left atrium and left ventricle has two cusps, anterior and posterior (Figs. 2.26 and 2.28). "Mitral" derives from the valve's resemblance to a bishop's miter (headdress). The mitral valve is located posterior to the sternum at the level of the 4th costal cartilage. Each of its cusps receives **tendinous cords** from more than one papillary muscle. These muscles and their cords support the mitral valve, allowing the cusps to resist the pressure developed during contractions (pumping) of the left ventricle. The cords become taut, preventing the cusps from being forced (prolapsed) into the left atrium. The **ascending aorta,** approximately 2.5 cm in diameter, begins at the aortic orifice. The **aortic valve** (Figs. 2.24 and 2.29), obliquely placed, is located posterior to the left side of the

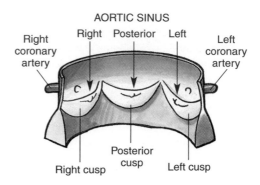

AORTIC SINUS

Right coronary artery — Right — Posterior — Left — Left coronary artery

Right cusp — Posterior cusp — Left cusp

FIGURE 2.29   **Aortic valve spread out.** It is between the left ventricle and ascending aorta.

sternum at the level of the 3rd intercostal space. Superior to each valve, dilations of the aortic wall form **aortic sinuses.** The mouth of the right coronary artery is in the right aortic sinus; the mouth of the left coronary artery is in the left aortic sinus; and no artery arises from the posterior aortic (noncoronary) sinus.

VALVULAR INSUFFICIENCY AND HEART MURMURS

The mitral valve is the most frequently diseased of the heart valves. Nodules form on the valve cusps causing irregular (turbulent) blood flow. Later, the diseased cusps undergo scarring and shortening, resulting in *mitral insufficiency*—defective functioning of the mitral valve. As a result, blood regurgitates into the left atrium when the left ventricle contracts, producing a characteristic heart murmur. *Aortic insufficiency*—defective functioning of the aortic valve—results in aortic regurgitation, a backrush of blood into the left ventricle, producing a *heart murmur* and a *collapsing pulse* (forcible impulse that rapidly diminishes).

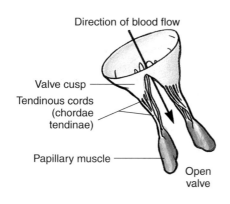

Direction of blood flow

Valve cusp

Tendinous cords (chordae tendinae)

Papillary muscle

Open valve

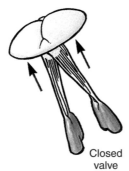

Closed valve

FIGURE 2.28   **Mitral valve.** It closes the orifice between the left atrium and left ventricle.

Arterial Supply of Heart. The coronary arteries—the 1st branches of the aorta—supply the myocardium and epicardium. The right and left **coronary arteries** arise from the corresponding **aortic sinuses** at the proximal part of the ascending aorta (Figs. 2.29 and 2.30, Table 2.6), just superior to the **aortic valve.** The coronary arteries supply both the atria and ventricles; however, the atrial branches are usually small.

The **right coronary artery** (RCA) arises from the **right aortic sinus** of the ascending aorta and runs in the coronary groove (sulcus). Near its origin, the RCA usually gives off an ascending **sinuatrial (SA) nodal branch**

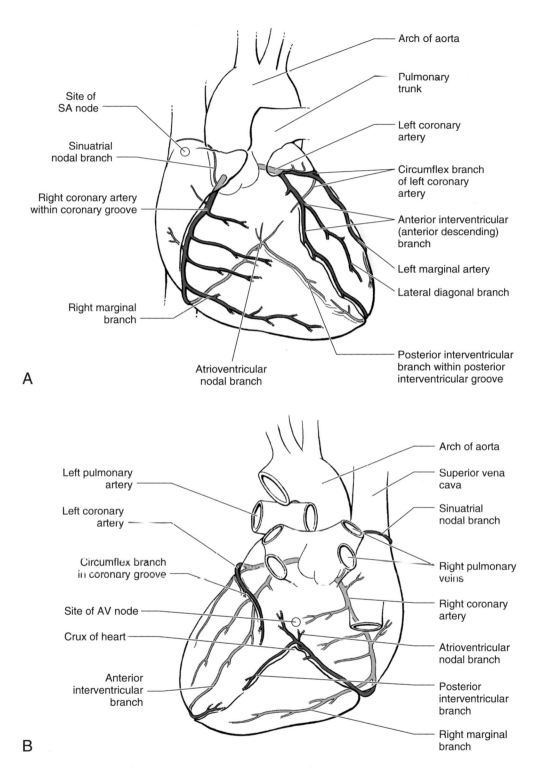

A

B

FIGURE 2.30 **Arterial supply of the heart. A.** Anterior view. **B.** Posteroinferior view.

TABLE 2.6.   ARTERIAL SUPPLY OF HEART

Artery/Branch	Origin	Course	Distribution	Anastomoses
Right coronary	Right aortic sinus	Follows coronary (AV) groove between the atria and ventricles	Right atrium, SA and AV nodes, and posterior part of IV septum	Circumflex and anterior IV branches of left coronary artery
SA nodal	Right coronary artery near its origin (in 60%)	Ascends to SA node	Pulmonary trunk and SA node	
Right marginal	Right coronary artery	Passes to inferior margin of heart and apex	Right ventricle and apex of heart	IV branches
Posterior interventricular	Right coronary artery	Runs from posterior IV groove to apex of heart	Right and left ventricles and IV septum	Circumflex and anterior IV branches of left coronary artery
AV nodal	Right coronary artery near origin of posterior IV artery	Passes to AV node	AV node	
Left coronary	Left aortic sinus	Runs in AV groove and gives off anterior interventricular and circumflex branches	Most of left atrium and ventricle, IV septum, and AV bundles; may supply AV node	Right coronary artery
SA nodal	Circumflex branch (in 40%)	Ascends on posterior surface of left atrium to SA node	Left atrium and SA node	
Anterior interventricular	Left coronary artery	Passes along anterior IV groove to apex of heart	Right and left ventricles and IV septum	Posterior IV branch of right coronary artery
Circumflex	Left coronary artery	Passes to left in AV groove and runs to posterior surface of heart	Left atrium and left ventricle	Right coronary artery
Left marginal	Circumflex branch	Follows left border of heart	Left ventricle	IV branches

(Fig. 2.30*A*) that supplies the *sinuatrial (SA) node*—the mass of specialized cardiac muscle fibers that normally act as the "pacemaker" of the cardiac conducting system. The RCA then descends in the coronary groove and gives off the **right marginal branch** that supplies the right border of the heart as it runs toward (but does not reach) the apex of the heart. After giving off this branch, the RCA turns to the left and continues in the coronary groove on the posterior aspect of the heart. At the **crux** (cross) of the heart, the junction of the septa and walls of the four heart chambers, the RCA gives rise to the **AV nodal**

branch, which supplies the *AV node,* a circumscribed mass of modified cardiac muscle fibers that gives rise to the AV bundle of the conduction system of the heart. The RCA then gives off the large posterior IV artery that descends in the posterior IV groove toward the apex of the heart (Fig. 2.30*B*). The **posterior IV artery** supplies both ventricles and sends perforating *IV septal branches* to the IV septum. Near the apex of the heart, the RCA anastomoses with the circumflex and anterior IV branches of the left coronary artery. **Typically, the RCA supplies:**

- The right atrium
- Most of right ventricle
- Part of left ventricle (diaphragmatic surface)
- Part of IV septum (usually posterior third)
- The SA node (in approximately 60% of people)
- The AV node (in approximately 80% of people).

The **left coronary artery** (LCA) arises from the *left aortic sinus* of the ascending aorta and passes between the left auricle and pulmonary trunk in the coronary groove. In approximately 40% of people, the **SA nodal branch** arises from the circumflex branch of the LCA and ascends on the posterior surface of the left atrium to the SA node. At the left end of the coronary groove—located just left of the pulmonary trunk (Fig. 2.30)—the LCA divides into two branches, an **anterior IV branch** (left anterior descending branch, LAD branch) and a **circumflex branch.** The anterior IV branch passes along the IV groove to the apex of the heart. Here it turns around the inferior border of the heart and anastomoses with the posterior IV branch of the right coronary artery. The anterior IV branch supplies both ventricles and the IV septum (Table 2.6). In many people, the anterior IV artery gives rise to a **lateral (diagonal) branch,** which descends on the anterior surface of the heart. The smaller **circumflex branch of the LCA** follows the coronary groove around the left border of the heart to the posterior surface of the heart. The **left marginal artery,** a branch of the cir-

cumflex branch, follows the left margin of the heart and supplies the left ventricle. The circumflex branch of the LCA terminates on the posterior aspect of the heart and often anastomoses with the posterior IV branch of the RCA. **Typically, the LCA supplies**

- The left atrium
- Most of left ventricle
- Part of right ventricle
- *Most of IV septum (usually its anterior two-thirds), including the AV bundle of conducting tissue, through its perforating IV septal branches*
- The SA node (in approximately 40% of people).

VARIATIONS OF CORONARY ARTERIES

Variations in the branching patterns of the coronary arteries are common. In most people the RCA and LCA share approximately equally in the blood supply to the heart. In approximately 15% of hearts the LCA is dominant in that the posterior IV branch is a branch of the circumflex artery. A few people have only a single coronary artery. In other people the circumflex artery arises from the right aortic sinus. Approximately 4% of people have an accessory coronary artery. The branches of coronary arteries are considered to be end arteries—ones that supply regions of the myocardium without functional overlap from other large branches. However, anastomoses do exist between small branches of the coronary arteries. The functional value of these anastomoses appears to be effective in slowly progressive coronary artery disease.

Myocardial Infarction

With sudden occlusion of a major artery by an embolus, the region of myocardium supplied by the occluded vessel becomes infarcted (rendered virtually bloodless) and soon degenerates. An area of myocardium that has undergone necrosis is a *myocardial infarct* (MI). The most common cause of *ischemic heart disease* (ischemia–lacking adequate blood supply) is *coronary insufficiency,* resulting from *atherosclerosis of the coronary arteries* (arteriosclerosis—hardening of the arteries—characterized by lipid deposits in the medium and large-sized arteries, causing narrowing of arterial lumens). A person with coronary arterial disease often suffers from *angina pectoris* (usually pain in the substernal region and down the medial side of the left arm and forearm). For a fuller discussion of the clinical anatomy of coronary artery disease, angina, and coronary bypass surgery, see Moore and Dalley (1999).

Venous Drainage of Heart. The heart is drained mainly by veins that empty into the **coronary sinus,** and partly by small **anterior car-**

diac veins that empty directly into the right atrium (Fig. 2.31) and the other heart chambers (smallest cardiac veins). The **coronary sinus,** the main vein of the heart, is a wide venous channel that runs from left to right in the posterior part of the coronary groove. The coronary sinus receives the **great cardiac vein**—the main tributary of the sinus—at its left end and the **middle** and **small cardiac veins** at its right end. The **left posterior vein** and **left marginal vein** also open into the coronary sinus. The *smallest cardiac veins* (L. venae cordis minimae) are minute vessels that begin in the capillary beds of the myocardium and open directly into the chambers of the heart, chiefly the atria. Although called veins, they are valveless communications with the capillary beds of the myocardium and may carry blood from the heart chambers to the myocardium; thus, they provide a collateral circulation to the heart musculature.

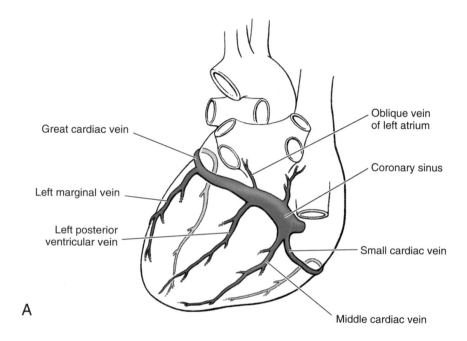

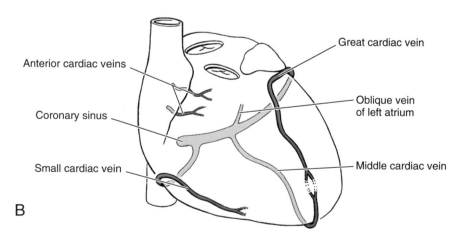

FIGURE 2.31   **Venous drainage of the heart. A.** Posteroinferior view. **B.** Anterior view.

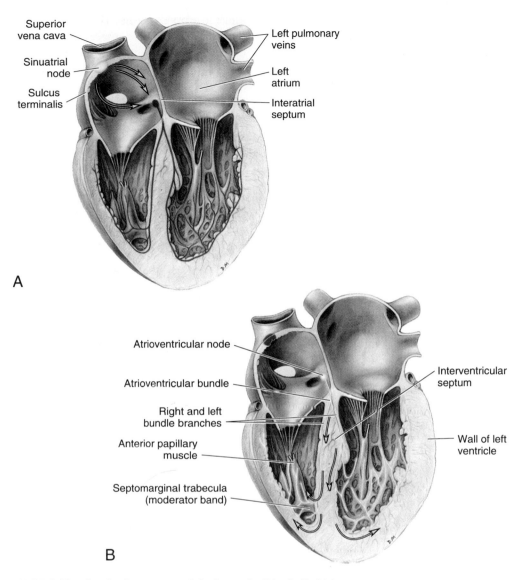

FIGURE 2.32 **Conducting system of the heart. A.** Atria. **B.** Ventricles.

Lymphatic Drainage of Heart. Lymphatic vessels in the myocardium and subendocardial connective tissue pass to the *subepicardial lymphatic plexus*. Vessels from this plexus pass to the coronary groove and follow the coronary arteries. A single lymphatic vessel, formed by the union of various vessels from the heart, ascends between the pulmonary trunk and left atrium and ends in the inferior **tracheobronchial lymph nodes** (Fig. 2.19*C*), usually on the right side.

Conducting System of Heart. The impulse-conducting system—which *coordinates the cardiac cycle* (Fig. 2.23)—consists of cardiac muscle cells and highly specialized conducting fibers for initiating impulses and conducting them rapidly through the heart (Fig. 2.32). *Nodal tissue initiates the heartbeat and coordinates the contractions of the four heart chambers.* The **sinuatrial (SA) node** gives off an impulse about 70 times per minute in most people. The SA node—*the pacemaker of the heart*—is located anterolaterally just deep to the epi-cardium at the junction of the SVC and right atrium. The **atrioventricular (AV) node** is a smaller collection of nodal tissue located in the posteroinferior region of the interatrial septum near the opening of the coronary sinus. The sig-nal generated by the SA node passes through the walls of the right atrium propagated by the cardiac muscle (*myogenic conduction*), which transmits the signal rapidly from the SA node to the AV node. The AV node then distributes the signal to the ventricles through the **atri-oventricular (AV) bundle**—a group of modified cardiac muscle fibers. *Sympathetic stimulation speeds up the rate at which impulses are gener-ated and conducted.* Parasympathetic stimula-tion slows down the rate at which impulses are generated and conducted. The *AV bundle,* the only bridge between the atrial and ventricular myocardium, passes from the AV node through the fibrous skeleton of the heart and along the membranous part of the IV septum. At the junction of the membranous and muscular parts of the septum, the AV bundle divides into **right** and **left bundle branches.** The bundles proceed on each side of the muscular IV sep-tum deep to the endocardium and then ramify into *subendocardial branches* (Purkinje fibers), which extend into the walls of the respective ventricles. The subendocardial branches of the right bundle stimulate the muscle of the IV sep-tum, the anterior papillary muscle (through the **septomarginal trabecula** or moderator band), and the wall of the right ventricle. The suben-docardial branches of the left bundle stimulate the IV septum, the anterior and posterior pap-illary muscles, and the wall of the left ventricle. **Summary of conducting system of heart:**

- The SA node initiates an impulse that is rapidly conducted to cardiac muscle fibers in the atria, causing them to contract.
- The impulse spreads by myogenic conduction that rapidly transmits the impulse from the SA node to the AV node.
- The signal is distributed from the AV node through the AV bundle and the right and left bundle branches, which pass on each side of the IV septum to supply subendocardial branches to the papillary muscles and the walls of the ventricles.

INJURY TO CONDUCTING SYSTEM OF HEART
When there is an *atrial septal defect* (ASD), the AV bundle 131 usually lies in the margin of the defect. Obviously this vital part of the conducting system must be preserved during surgical repair of the ASD because its destruction would cut the only physiological link between the atrial and ventricular musculature. Damage to the conducting system, often resulting from ischemia caused by *coronary artery disease,* produces disturbances of cardiac muscle contraction. Damage to the AV node results in a *heart block* because the atrial excitation does not reach the ventricles. As a result, the ventricles begin to contract in-dependently at their own rate, which is slower than that of the atria. Damage to one of the bundle branches results in a *bundle branch block,* in which excitation passes along the unaffected branch and causes systole of that ventricle. The impulse then spreads to the other ventricle, producing a late asynchronous contraction.

Electrocardiography
The passage of impulses over the heart from the SA node can be amplified and recorded as an *electrocardiogram* (ECG). Because many heart problems involve abnormal functioning of the conducting system, electrocardiograms are of considerable importance in detecting the cause of irregularities of the heartbeat.

INNERVATION OF HEART. The heart is supplied by autonomic nerve fibers from su-perficial and deep **cardiac plexuses** (Fig. 2.19*D*). These nerve networks lie anterior to the bifurcation of the trachea, posterior to the ascending aorta, and superior to the bifurca-tion of the pulmonary trunk. The **sympathetic supply of the heart** is from presynaptic fibers with cell bodies in the intermediolateral cell columns (lateral horns) of the superior five or six thoracic segments of the spinal cord, and from postsynaptic sympathetic fibers with cell bodies in the cervical and superior thoracic paravertebral ganglia of the sympathetic trunks. The postsynaptic fibers end in the SA and AV nodes and in relation to the termina-tions of parasympathetic fibers on the coronary arteries. *Sympathetic stimulation of the nodal tissue increases the heart's rate and the force of its contractions.* Sympathetic stimulation (indi-rectly) produces dilation of the coronary arter-ies by inhibiting their constriction. This sup-plies more oxygen and nutrients to the myocardium during periods of increased activ-ity. The **parasympathetic supply of the heart** is from presynaptic fibers of the *vagus nerves* (CN X). The postsynaptic parasympathetic fibers also end in the SA and AV nodes and directly on the coronary arteries. The cell bodies of the postsynaptic fibers constitute intrinsic ganglia in the vicinity of these structures. *Stimulation of parasympathetic nerves slows the heart rate, reduces the force of the heartbeat, and constricts the coronary arteries, saving energy between periods of increased demand.*

CARDIAC REFERRED PAIN

The heart is insensitive to touch, cutting, cold, and heat; however, ischemia and the accumulation of metabolic products stimulate pain endings in the myocardium. The afferent pain fibers run centrally in the middle and inferior cervical branches and especially in the thoracic cardiac branches of the sympathetic trunk. The axons of these primary sensory neurons enter spinal cord segments T1 through T4 or T5, especially on the left side. *Cardiac referred pain is a phenomenon whereby noxious stimuli originating in the heart are perceived by the person as pain arising from a superficial part of the body*—the skin on the medial aspect of the left upper limb, for example. Visceral pain is transmitted by visceral afferent fibers accompanying sympathetic fibers and is typically referred to somatic structures or areas such as the upper limb having afferent fibers with cell bodies in the same spinal ganglion, and central processes that enter the spinal cord through the same posterior roots.

Superior Mediastinum

The superior mediastinum is located superior to the transverse thoracic plane passing through the sternal angle and the junction (IV disc) of vertebrae T4 and T5 (Fig. 2.33). From anterior to posterior, **the main contents of the superior mediastinum** (Fig. 2.34) are:

- Thymus, a primary lymphoid organ
- Great vessels related to the heart and pericardium:
  - Brachiocephalic veins
  - Superior part of SVC
  - Arch of aorta, and roots of its major branches:
    - Brachiocephalic trunk
    - Left common carotid artery
    - Left subclavian artery
- Vagus and phrenic nerves
- Cardiac plexus of nerves
- Left recurrent laryngeal nerve
- Trachea

- Esophagus
- Thoracic duct
- Prevertebral muscles.

Thymus. This lymphoid organ is located in the lower part of the neck and the anterior part of the superior mediastinum. It lies posterior to the manubrium of the sternum and extends into the anterior mediastinum, anterior to the pericardium. After puberty the thymus undergoes gradual involution and is largely replaced by fat (see Fig. 2.36). A rich *arterial supply to the thymus* derives mainly from the anterior intercostal and anterior mediastinal branches of the **internal thoracic arteries.** The **veins of the thymus** end in the left brachiocephalic, internal thoracic, and inferior thyroid veins. The **lymphatic vessels of the thymus** end in the parasternal, brachiocephalic, and tracheobronchial lymph nodes (Fig. 2.19C).

Great Vessels in Mediastinum. The *brachiocephalic veins* form posterior to the sternoclavicular joints by the union of the internal jugular and subclavian veins (Fig. 2.35). At the level of

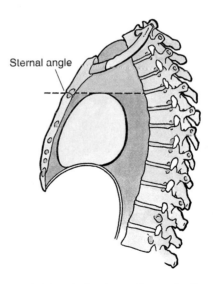

FIGURE 2.33 Mediastinum. The mediastinum is divided into superior and inferior parts. Superior mediastinum—*green.* Inferior mediastinum has three parts: anterior—*purple,* middle—*yellow,* and posterior—*blue.*

Surface Anatomy of Heart

The heart and great vessels are approximately in the middle of the thorax, surrounded laterally and posteriorly by the lungs and bounded anteriorly by the sternum and the central part of the thoracic cage. The *apex beat* is an impulse that results from the apex being forced against the anterior thoracic wall when the left ventricle contracts. The *location of the apex beat* varies in position and may be located in the 4th or 5th intercostal spaces, 6 to 10 cm from the midline of the thorax. The *outline of the heart* can be traced on the anterior surface of the thorax by using these guidelines:

- The *superior border of heart* corresponds to a line connecting the inferior border of the 2nd left costal cartilage to the superior border of the 3rd right costal cartilage
- The *right border of the heart* corresponds to a line drawn from the 3rd right costal cartilage to the 6th right costal cartilage; this border is slightly convex to the right
- The *inferior border of the heart* corresponds to a line drawn from the inferior end of the right border to a point in the 5th intercostal space close to the left midclavicular line; the left end of this line corresponds to the location of the apex of the heart and the apex beat
- The *left border of the heart* corresponds to a line connecting the left ends of the lines representing the superior and inferior borders
- The pulmonary, aortic, mitral, and tricuspid valves are located posterior to the sternum; however, the sounds produced by them are best heard at the **auscultatory areas** illustrated: [pulmonary (P), aortic (A), mitral (M), tricuspid (T)].

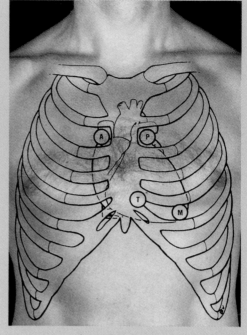

Auscultatory areas

Clinicians' interest in the surface anatomy of the heart and the location of the valves results from their need to listen to the valve sounds. Because the auscultatory areas are wide apart, the sounds produced at any given valve may be clearly distinguished from those produced at other valves. *Blood tends to carry the sound in the direction of its flow.* Each area is situated superficial to the chamber or vessel into which the blood has passed and in a direct line with the valve orifice.

the inferior border of the 1st right costal cartilage, *the brachiocephalic veins unite to form the SVC.* The **left brachiocephalic vein** is over twice as long as the right brachiocephalic vein because it passes from the left to the right side, passing across the anterior aspects of the roots of the three major branches of the **arch of the aorta,** and shunting blood from the head, neck, and left upper limb to the right atrium. The origin of the **right brachiocephalic vein** (i.e., by union of right internal jugular and subclavian veins—the right "venous angle") receives lymph from the *right lymphatic duct,* and the origin of the left brachiocephalic vein (the left "venous angle") receives lymph from the **thoracic duct** (see Fig. 2.40).

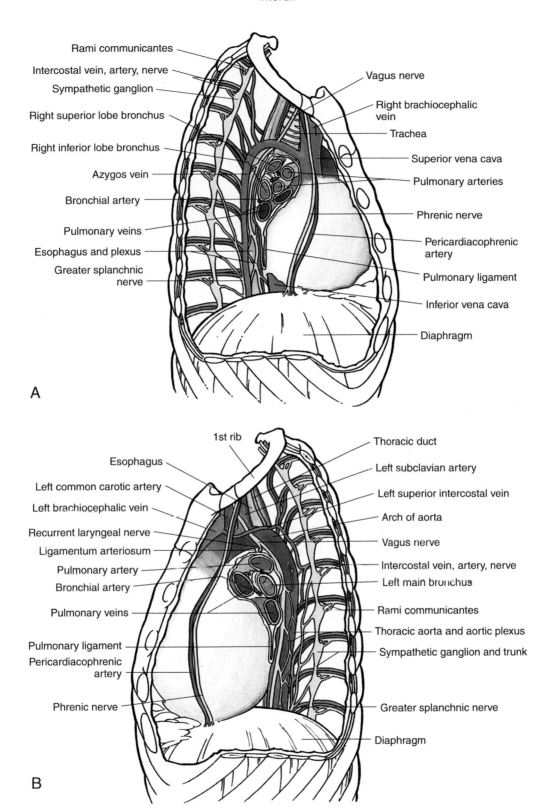

FIGURE 2.34 **Drawings of dissections of the mediastinum. A.** Right side. **B.** Left side.

The **SVC** returns blood from all structures superior to the diaphragm, except the lungs and heart. It passes inferiorly and ends at the level of the third costal cartilage, where it enters the right atrium. The SVC lies in the right side of the superior mediastinum, anterolateral to the trachea and posterolateral to the ascending aorta (Fig. 2.35). The **right phrenic nerve** lies between the SVC and the mediastinal pleura. The terminal half of the SVC is in the middle mediastinum, where it lies beside the ascending aorta and forms the posterior boundary of the transverse pericardial sinus (Fig. 2.21). The **arch of the aorta,** the curved continuation of the ascending aorta, begins posterior to the 2nd right sternocostal joint at the level of the sternal angle and arches superoposteriorly and to the left (Figs. 2.34 and 2.35; Table 2.7). The aortic arch ascends anterior to the right pulmonary artery and the bifurcation of the trachea to reach its apex at the left side of the trachea and esophagus, as it passes over the root of the left lung. The arch descends on

the left side of the body of T4 vertebra and ends by becoming the **thoracic aorta** posterior to the 2nd left sternocostal joint.

The **ligamentum arteriosum**—the remnant of the fetal ductus arteriosus (Moore and Persaud, 1998)—passes from the root of the left pulmonary artery to the inferior surface of the arch of the aorta. The **left recurrent laryngeal nerve** hooks beneath the arch adjacent to the ligamentum arteriosum and then ascends between the trachea and esophagus (Fig. 2.35). **The branches of the arch of the aorta** are the

- Brachiocephalic artery or trunk
- Left common carotid artery
- Left subclavian artery.

The **brachiocephalic artery or trunk,** the first and largest branch of the arch, arises posterior to the manubrium where it lies anterior to the trachea and posterior to the left brachiocephalic vein. It ascends superolaterally to

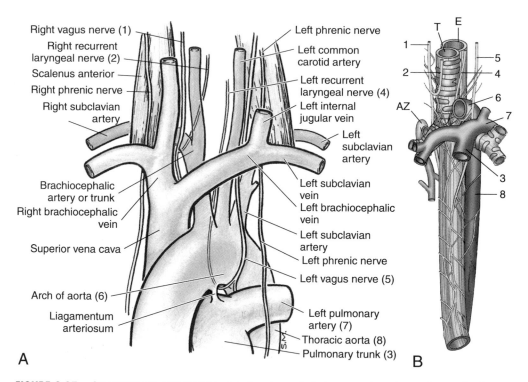

FIGURE 2.35 **Great vessels and nerves.** Anterior views. **A.** In lower neck and superior mediastinum. **B.** Relationships to trachea (*T*), esophagus (*E*), and azygos vein (*AZ*).

TABLE 2.7.   AORTA AND ITS BRANCHES IN THORAX

Artery	Origin	Course	Branches
Ascending aorta	Aortic orifice of left ventricle	Ascends approximately 5 cm to sternal angle where it becomes arch of aorta	Right and left coronary arteries
Arch of aorta	Continuation of ascending aorta	Arches posteriorly on left side of trachea and esophagus and superior to left main bronchus	Brachiocephalic, left common carotid, left subclavian arteries
Thoracic aorta	Continuation of arch of aorta	Descends in posterior mediastinum to left of vertebral column; gradually shifts to right to lie in median plane at aortic hiatus	Posterior intercostal arteries, subcostal, some phrenic arteries and visceral branches (e.g., esophageal)
Posterior intercostal	Posterior aspect of thoracic aorta	Pass laterally, and then anteriorly parallel to ribs	Lateral and anterior cutaneous branches
Bronchial (1–2 branches)	Anterior aspect of aorta or posterior intercostal artery	Run with the tracheobronchial tree	Bronchial and peribronchial tissue, visceral pleura
Esophageal (4–5 branches)	Anterior aspect of thoracic aorta	Run anteriorly to esophagus	To esophagus
Superior phrenic (vary in number)	Anterior aspect of thoracic aorta	Arise at aortic hiatus and pass to superior aspect of diaphragm	To diaphragm

reach the right side of the trachea and the right sternoclavicular joint, where it divides into the right common carotid and right subclavian arteries. The **left common carotid artery,** the 2nd branch of the aortic arch, arises posterior to the manubrium, slightly posterior and to the left of the brachiocephalic trunk. It ascends anterior to the left subclavian artery and at first anterior to the trachea and then is to its left. It enters the neck by passing posterior to the left sternoclavicular joint. The **left subclavian artery,** the 3rd branch of the aortic arch, arises from the posterior part of the arch, just posterior to the left common carotid artery. It ascends lateral to the trachea and the left common carotid artery through the superior mediastinum. *The left subclavian artery has no branches in the mediastinum.* As it leaves the thorax and enters the root of the neck, it passes posterior to the left sternoclavicular joint and lateral to the left common carotid artery.

Nerves in Superior Mediastinum. The **vagus nerves** (CN X) arise bilaterally from the medulla of the brain, exit the cranium, and descend through the neck posterolateral to the common carotid arteries. Each nerve enters the superior mediastinum posterior to the respective sternoclavicular joint and brachiocephalic vein (Figs. 2.35, 2.36 and 2.37; Table 2.8). The **right vagus nerve** enters the thorax anterior to the right subclavian artery, where it gives rise to the **right recurrent laryngeal nerve** (Fig. 2.35). This nerve hooks underneath the right subclavian artery and ascends between the trachea and esophagus to supply the larynx. The right vagus nerve runs posteroinferiorly through the superior mediastinum on the right side of the trachea. It then passes posterior to the right brachiocephalic vein, SVC, and root of the right lung. Here it breaks up into a number of branches that contribute to the **pulmonary plexus** (Fig.

2.37*B*). Usually the right vagus nerve leaves the pulmonary plexus as a single nerve and passes to the esophagus, where it again breaks up and contributes fibers to the **esophageal plexus** (Fig. 2.37*C*). The right vagus nerve also gives rise to nerves that contribute to the **cardiac plexus**.

The **left vagus nerve** descends in the neck (Fig. 2.35) and enters the thorax and mediastinum between the left common carotid and left subclavian arteries and posterior to the left brachiocephalic vein. When it reaches the left side of the arch of the aorta, the left vagus nerve diverges posteriorly from the left

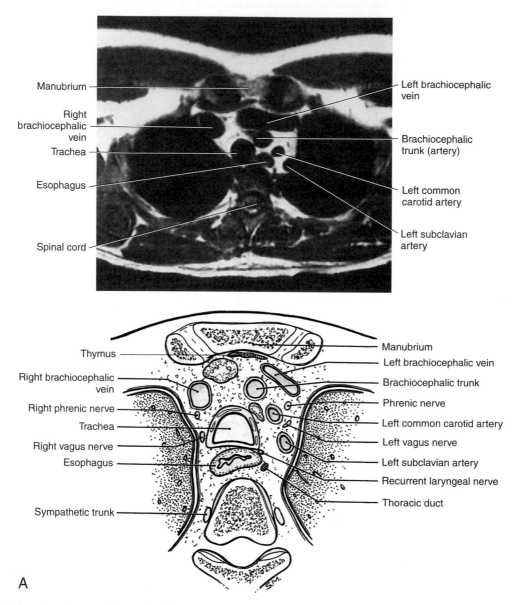

FIGURE 2.36 Superior mediastinum. A. Transverse magnetic resonance image (MRI) superior to arch of aorta. **B.** Transverse MRI at level of arch of aorta. **C.** *Broken lines* indicate level of MRIs in **A** and **B.** *BT,* brachiocephalic trunk (artery); *E,* esophagus; *LB,* left brachiocephalic vein; *LC,* left common carotid artery; *LS,* left subclavian artery; *RB,* right brachiocephalic vein; *T,* trachea.

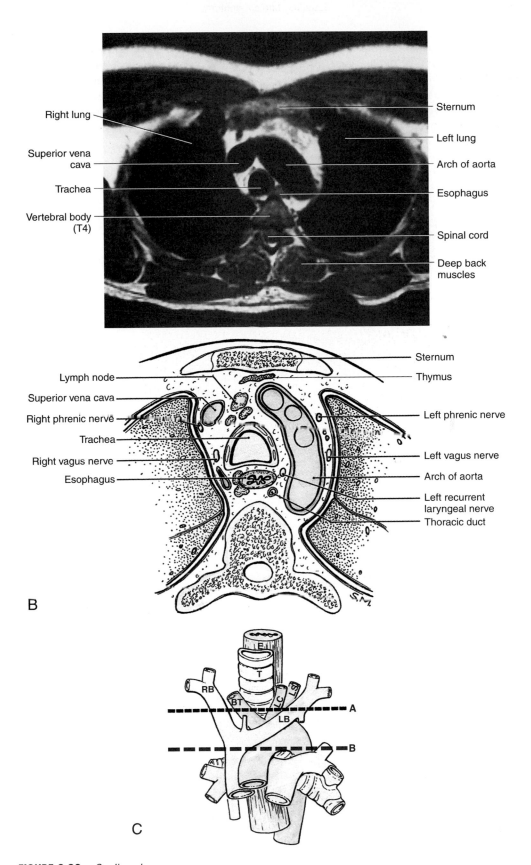

Right lung

Superior vena cava

Trachea

Vertebral body (T4)

Sternum

Left lung

Arch of aorta

Esophagus

Spinal cord

Deep back muscles

Lymph node

Superior vena cava

Right phrenic nerve

Trachea

Right vagus nerve

Esophagus

Sternum

Thymus

Left phrenic nerve

Left vagus nerve

Arch of aorta

Left recurrent laryngeal nerve

Thoracic duct

B

C

FIGURE 2.36   *Continued.*

phrenic nerve. It is separated laterally from the phrenic nerve by the left superior intercostal vein. As the left vagus nerve curves medially at the inferior border of the arch of the aorta, it gives off the **left recurrent laryngeal nerve** (Figs. 2.35 and 2.37, *A* and *B*). This nerve passes inferior to the arch of the aorta just posterolateral to the **ligamentum arteriosum** and ascends to the larynx in the

groove between the trachea and esophagus. The left vagus nerve continues on to pass posterior to the root of the left lung, where it breaks up into many branches that contribute to the **pulmonary and cardiac plexuses.** The nerve leaves these plexuses as a single trunk and passes to the esophagus, where it joins fibers from the right vagus in the **esophageal plexus.**

TABLE 2.8. NERVES OF THORAX

Nerve	Origin	Course	Distribution
Vagus (CN X)	8 to 10 rootlets from medulla of brainstem	Enters superior mediastinum posterior to sternoclavicular joint and brachiocephalic vein; gives rise to recurrent laryngeal nerve; continues into abdomen	Pulmonary plexus, esophageal plexus, and cardiac plexus
Phrenic	Ventral rami of C3–C5 nerves	Passes through superior thoracic aperture and runs between mediastinal pleura and pericardium	Central portion of diaphragm
Intercostals	Ventral rami of T1–T11 nerves	Run in intercostal spaces between internal and innermost layers of intercostal muscles	Muscles and skin over intercostal space; lower nerves supply muscles and skin of anterolateral abdominal wall
Subcostal	Ventral ramus of T12 nerve	Follows inferior border of 12th rib and passes into abdominal wall	Abdominal wall and skin of gluteal region
Recurrent laryngeal	Vagus nerve artery	Loops around subclavian artery on right; on left it runs around arch of aorta and ascends in tracheoesophageal groove	Intrinsic muscles of larynx (except cricothyroid); sensory inferior to level of vocal folds
Cardiac plexus	Cervical and cardiac branches of vagus nerve and sympathetic trunk	From arch of aorta and posterior surface of heart, fibers extend along coronary arteries and to SA node	Impulses pass to SA node; parasympathetic fibers slow rate; reduce force of heartbeat, and constrict coronary arteries; sympathetic fibers have opposite effect
Pulmonary plexus	Vagus nerve and sympathetic trunk	Forms on root of lung and extends along bronchial subdivisions	Parasympathetic fibers constrict bronchioles; sympathetic fibers dilate them
Esophageal plexus	Vagus nerve, sympathetic ganglia and greater splanchnic nerve	Distal to tracheal bifurcation, the vagus and sympathetic nerves form the plexus around the esophagus	Vagal and sympathetic fibers to smooth muscle and glands of inferior two thirds of esophagus

SA, sinuatrial; AV, atrioventricular.

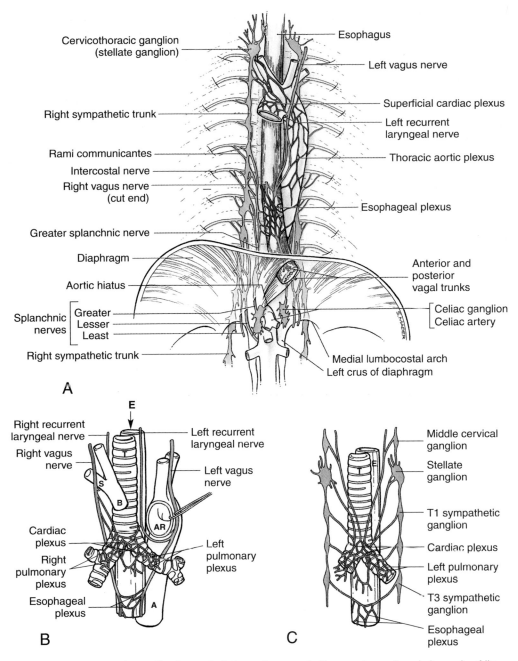

FIGURE 2.37 **Nerves in mediastinum. A.** Autonomic nerves in the superior and posterior parts of the mediastinum. *Orange,* sympathetic; *green,* parasympathetic; *blue,* plexus. **B.** Parasympathetic nerves. *A,* aorta; *AR,* arch of aorta; *B,* right brachiocephalic artery; *E,* esophagus; *S,* right subclavian artery; *T,* trachea. **C.** Sympathetic nerves.

The **phrenic nerves** are the sole motor supply to the diaphragm (Figs. 2.34 and 2.35); approximately one-third of their fibers are sensory to the diaphragm. Each phrenic nerve enters the superior mediastinum between the subclavian artery and the origin of the brachiocephalic vein (Table 2.8). The **right phrenic nerve** passes along the right side of the right brachiocephalic vein, SVC, and pericardium over the right atrium. It also passes anterior to the root of the right lung and descends on the right side of the IVC to the diaphragm, which it penetrates or passes through the caval opening (foramen). The **left phrenic nerve** descends between the left subclavian and left common carotid arteries. It crosses the left surface of the arch of the aorta anterior to the left vagus nerve and passes over the left superior intercostal vein. It then descends anterior to the root of the left lung and runs along the pericardium, superficial to the left atrium and ventricle of the heart, where it penetrates the diaphragm to the left of the pericardium.

Trachea. The trachea descends anterior to the esophagus and enters the superior mediastinum, inclining a little to the right of the median plane (Figs. 2.38 and 2.39). The posterior surface of the trachea is flat where its cartilaginous "rings" are incomplete and where it is related to the esophagus. The trachea ends at the level of the sternal angle by dividing into the right and left main bronchi.

Esophagus. The esophagus is a fibromuscular tube that extends from the pharynx to the stomach. It is usually flattened anteroposteriorly (Fig. 2.39). The esophagus enters the superior mediastinum between the trachea and vertebral column, where it lies anterior to the bodies of vertebrae T1 through T4. Initially, the esophagus inclines to the left but is moved by the aortic arch to the median plane opposite the root of the left lung. The **thoracic duct** (Fig. 2.40) usually lies on the left side of the esophagus and deep to the aortic arch. Inferior to the arch, the esophagus inclines to the left as it approaches and passes through the esophageal hiatus in the diaphragm.

Posterior Mediastinum

The posterior mediastinum is located anterior to vertebrae T5 through T12, posterior to the pericardium and diaphragm, and between the parietal pleura of the two lungs (Fig. 2.33). **The posterior mediastinum contains the:**

- Thoracic aorta
- Thoracic duct
- Posterior mediastinal lymph nodes (e.g., tracheobronchial nodes)
- Azygos and hemiazygos veins
- Esophagus
- Esophageal plexus
- Thoracic sympathetic trunks
- Thoracic splanchnic nerves.

Thoracic Aorta. The thoracic aorta—the thoracic part of the descending aorta—is the continuation of the **arch of the aorta** (Figs. 2.34*B* and 2.35, Table 2.7). It begins on the left side of the inferior border of the body of T4 vertebra and descends in the posterior mediastinum on the left sides of T5 through T12 vertebrae. As it descends, it approaches the median plane and displaces the esophagus to the right. The **thoracic aortic plexus,** an autonomic nerve network, surrounds it (Fig. 2.37*A*). The thoracic aorta lies posterior to the root of the left lung, the pericardium, and esophagus. It terminates—changes its name to abdominal aorta—anterior to the inferior border of T12 vertebra and enters the abdomen through the **aortic hiatus** (opening) in the diaphragm (Figs. 2.37 and 2.39). The **thoracic duct** and azygos vein descend on the right side of the thoracic aorta and accompany it

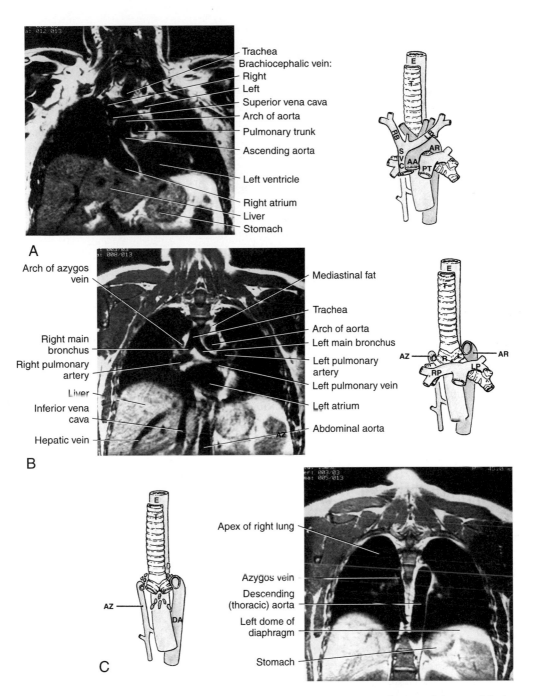

FIGURE 2.38 **Coronal magnetic resonance images (MRIs) of the thorax and upper abdomen.** Orientation drawings of main structures are shown. *AA,* ascending aorta; *AR,* arch of aorta; *AZ,* azygos vein; *DA,* descending aorta; *E,* esophagus; *L,* left main bronchus; *LB,* left brachiocephalic vein; *LP,* left pulmonary artery; *R,* right main bronchus; *RB,* right brachiocephalic vein; *RP,* right pulmonary vein; *T,* trachea.

through this hiatus (Fig. 2.40). **The branches of (arteries arising from) the thoracic aorta** (Fig. 2.41) are:

- Bronchial
- Pericardial
- Posterior intercostal
- Superior phrenic
- Esophageal
- Mediastinal
- Subcostal

The **bronchial arteries** consist of one right and two small left vessels. The bronchial arteries supply the trachea, bronchi, lung tissue, and lymph nodes. The **pericardial arteries** send twigs to the pericardium. The **posterior intercostal arteries** (nine pairs) pass into the 3rd through 11th intercostal spaces. The **superior phrenic arteries** pass to the posterior surface of the diaphragm, where they anastomose with the musculophrenic and pericardiacophrenic branches of the internal thoracic artery. Usually two **esophageal arteries** supply the middle third of the esophagus. The **medi-**

astinal arteries are small and supply the lymph nodes and other tissues of the posterior mediastinum. The **subcostal arteries** that course on the abdominal side of the origin of the diaphragm—paralleling it—are in series with the intercostal arteries.

Esophagus. The esophagus descends into the posterior mediastinum from the superior mediastinum, passing posterior and to the right of the arch of the aorta and posterior to the pericardium and left atrium. The esophagus constitutes the primary posterior relationship of the base of the heart. It then deviates to the left and passes through the **esophageal hiatus** in the diaphragm at the level of T10 vertebra, anterior to the aorta. The esophagus may have three impressions, or "constrictions," in its thoracic part. These may be observed as narrowings of the lumen in oblique chest radiographs that are taken as barium is swallowed. The esophagus is compressed by three structures: the aortic arch, left main bronchus and diaphragm. No constrictions are visible in the empty esophagus; however, as it expands during filling, the above structures compress its walls.

Thoracic Duct. In the posterior mediastinum, the thoracic duct lies on the bodies of the inferior seven thoracic vertebrae (Fig. 2.40). *The thoracic duct conveys most lymph of the body to the venous system* (that from the lower limbs, pelvic cavity, abdominal cavity, left side of thorax, left side of head, neck, and left upper limb). The thoracic duct originates from the **chyle cistern** (L. cisterna chyli) in the abdomen and ascends through the aortic hiatus in the diaphragm. The thoracic duct is usually thin-walled and dull white; often it is beaded because of its numerous valves. It ascends between the thoracic aorta on its left, the azygos vein on its right, the esophagus anteriorly, and the vertebral bodies posteriorly. At the level of T4, T5, or T6 vertebrae, *the thoracic duct crosses to the left*, posterior to the esophagus, and ascends into the superior mediastinum. The thoracic duct receives branches from the middle and upper intercostal spaces of both sides through several col-

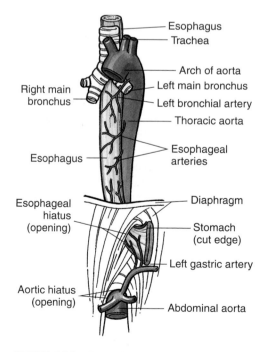

Esophagus
Trachea

Arch of aorta
Right main bronchus
Left main bronchus
Left bronchial artery
Thoracic aorta

Esophagus
Esophageal arteries

Esophageal hiatus (opening)
Diaphragm

Stomach (cut edge)

Left gastric artery

Aortic hiatus (opening)
Abdominal aorta

FIGURE 2.39   Posterior mediastinum: trachea, esophagus, and aorta. Anterior view.

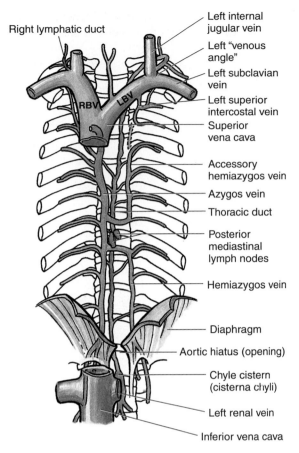

FIGURE 2.40 **Azygos system of veins and thoracic duct.** Anterior view. *RBV,* right brachiocephalic vein; *LBV,* left brachiocephalic vein.

lecting trunks. It also receives branches from posterior mediastinal structures. Near its termination it often receives the jugular, subclavian, and bronchomediastinal lymphatic trunks. The thoracic duct usually empties into the venous system near the union of the left internal jugular and subclavian veins—the left "venous angle" (Fig. 2.40) or origin of the left brachiocephalic vein.

LACERATION OF THORACIC DUCT

Because the thoracic duct is thin-walled and may be colorless, it may not be easily identified. Consequently, it is vulnerable to inadvertent injury during investigative and/or surgical procedures in the posterior mediastinum. Laceration of the thoracic duct results in chyle escaping into the thoracic cavity. Chyle may also enter the pleural cavity, producing *chylothorax.*

Vessels and Lymph Nodes of Posterior Mediastinum. The thoracic aorta and its branches were discussed previously. The **azygos system of veins,** on each side of the vertebral column, drains the back thoracoabdominal walls (Fig. 2.40), as well as the mediastinal viscera. The azygos system exhibits much variation, not only in its origin but also in its course, tributaries, anastomoses, and termination. The **azygos vein** (azygos means paired) and its main tributary, the **hemiazygos vein,** usually arise from "roots" or anastomoses with the posterior aspect of the IVC and/or renal vein, respectively, and the ascending lumbar veins. *The azygos vein forms a collateral pathway between the SVC and IVC and drains blood from the posterior walls of the thorax and abdomen.* The azygos vein ascends in the posterior mediastinum,

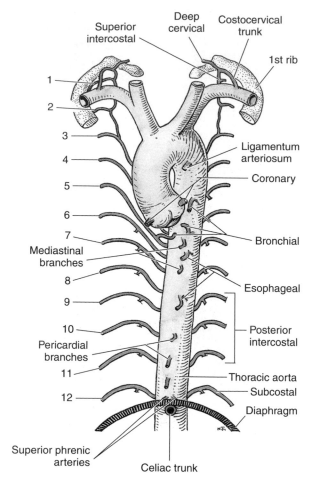

FIGURE 2.41   **Branches of the thoracic aorta.** Superior phrenic arteries arising from the inferior part of the thoracic aorta supply the diaphragm. The numbers 1 to 12 indicate posterior intercostal arteries.

passing close to the right sides of the bodies of the inferior eight thoracic vertebrae. It arches over the superior aspect of the root of the right lung to join the SVC. In addition to the **posterior intercostal veins,** the azygos vein communicates with the vertebral venous plexuses that drain the back, vertebrae, and structures in the vertebral canal (see Chapter 5). The azygos vein also receives the mediastinal, esophageal, and bronchial veins. For more information on the azygos system of veins, see Moore and Dalley (1999).

Posterior mediastinal lymph nodes lie posterior to the pericardium, where they are related to the esophagus and thoracic aorta (Fig. 2.40). There are several nodes posterior to the inferior part of the esophagus and more anterior and lateral to it. The posterior mediastinal lymph nodes receive lymph from the esophagus, the posterior aspect of the pericardium and diaphragm, and the middle posterior intercostal spaces.

COLLATERAL VENOUS ROUTES TO HEART

The azygos, hemiazygos, and accessory hemiazygos veins offer alternate means of venous drainage from the thoracic, abdominal, and back regions when *obstruction of the IVC* occurs. In some people, an accessory azygos vein parallels the main azygos vein on the right side. Other people have no hemiazygos system of veins. A clinically important variation, although uncommon, is when the azygos system receives all the blood from the IVC, except that from the liver. In these people, the azygos system drains nearly all the blood inferior to the diaphragm, except from the digestive tract. When *obstruction of the SVC* occurs superior to the entrance of the azygos vein, blood can drain inferiorly into the veins of the abdominal wall and return to the right atrium through the IVC and azygos system of veins.

Nerves of Posterior Mediastinum. The sympathetic trunks and their associated ganglia form a major portion of the ANS (Fig. 2.37, Table 2.8). The **thoracic sympathetic trunks** are in continuity with the cervical and lumbar sympathetic trunks. *The thoracic sympathetic trunks lie against the heads of the ribs in the superior part of the thorax, the costovertebral joints in the midthoracic level, and the sides of the vertebral bodies in the inferior part of the thorax.* The **lower thoracic splanchnic nerves**—also known as greater, lesser, and least splanchnic nerves—are part of the *abdominopelvic splanchnic nerves* because they supply viscera inferior to the diaphragm. They consist of presynaptic fibers from the 5th through 12th sympathetic ganglia, which pass through the diaphragm and synapse in prevertebral ganglia in the abdomen. They supply sympathetic innervation for most of the abdominal viscera. The splanchnic nerves are discussed further with the abdomen in Chapter 3.

Anterior Mediastinum

The anterior mediastinum (Fig. 2.33), the smallest subdivision of the mediastinum, lies between the body of the sternum and the transverse thoracic muscles (L. transversus thoracis) anteriorly and the pericardium posteriorly. The anterior mediastinum is continuous with the superior mediastinum at the *sternal angle* and is limited inferiorly by the diaphragm. The anterior mediastinum consists of loose connective tissue (*sternopericardial ligaments*–fibrous bands that pass from the pericardium to the sternum), fat, lymphatic vessels, a few lymph nodes, and branches of the internal thoracic vessels. In infants and children, the anterior mediastinum contains the inferior part of the thymus.

3 Abdomen

*T*he abdomen is the part of the trunk between the thorax and pelvis (Fig. 3.1). It has musculotendinous walls, except posteriorly where the wall includes the lumbar vertebrae and intervertebral (IV) discs. The abdominal wall encloses the abdominal cavity containing the peritoneal cavity and abdominal viscera such as the stomach.

ABDOMINAL CAVITY

The abdominal cavity is the space bounded by the abdominal walls, diaphragm, and pelvis. The abdominal cavity forms the major part of the **abdominopelvic cavity**—the combined and continuous abdominal and pelvic cavities. *The abdominal cavity is:*

- Surrounded on all sides by the abdominal wall

- Separated superiorly from the thoracic cavity by the diaphragm
- Extends superiorly into the thoracic cage to the 4th intercostal space (approximately the level of the male nipple)
- Continuous inferiorly with the pelvic cavity
- Lined with peritoneum, a serous membrane
- The location of most of the digestive organs, the spleen, kidneys, and the ureters for most of their course.

Clinicians subdivide the abdominal cavity into nine regions to locate abdominal organs or pains: right hypochondriac, right lumbar, right inguinal, epigastric, umbilical, hypogastric, left hypochondriac, left lumbar, and left inguinal. *The nine regions are delineated by four planes* (Fig. 3.2A):

- Two horizontal:
  - *Subcostal plane* passing through inferior border of 10th costal cartilage on each side

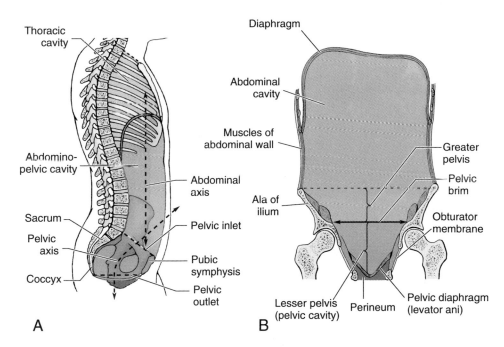

FIGURE 3.1 Thoracic and abdominopelvic cavities. A. Median section of the trunk. The pelvic inlet (superior pelvic aperture) is the opening into the lesser pelvis. The pelvic outlet (inferior pelvic aperture) is the lower opening of the lesser pelvis. **B.** Schematic coronal section of abdominopelvic cavity. Observe that the plane of the pelvic brim (*double-headed arrow*) separates the greater pelvis—part of the abdominal cavity—from the lesser pelvis, the pelvic cavity.

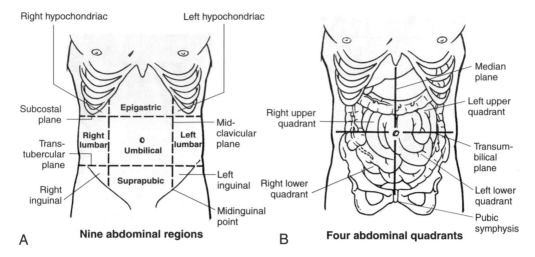

A   **Nine abdominal regions**   B   **Four abdominal quadrants**

FIGURE 3.2   **Subdivisions of the abdomen. A.** Regions. **B.** Quadrants.

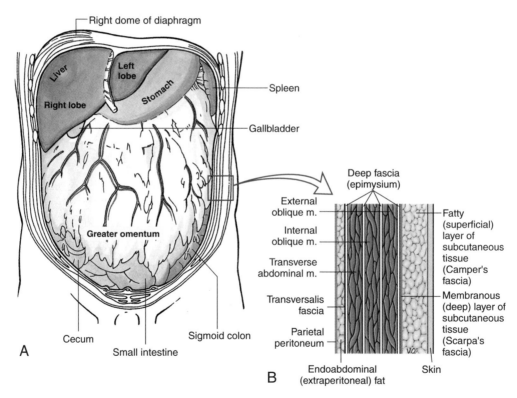

FIGURE 3.3   **Layers of the anterolateral abdominal wall. A.** Orientation drawing. Anterior view. The anterior abdominal wall is cut away. Most of the intestine is covered by the greater omentum. **B.** Longitudinal section showing the layers of the inferior part of the wall.

- *Transtubercular plane* passing through the iliac tubercles (p. 125) and the body of L5 vertebra
- Two vertical:
  - *Midclavicular planes* passing from the midpoints of clavicles to *midinguinal points*—midpoints of lines joining the anterior superior iliac spines and the superior edge of the pubic symphysis.

For general clinical descriptions, clinicians also use four quadrants of the abdominal cavity: right upper quadrant, right lower quadrant, left upper quadrant, and left lower quadrant. *The four quadrants are defined by two planes* (Fig. 3.2B).

- One horizontal:
  - *Transumbilical plane* passing through the umbilicus and IV disc between L3 and L4 vertebrae
- One vertical:
  - *Median plane* passing longitudinally through midline of the body, dividing it into right and left halves.

ANTEROLATERAL ABDOMINAL WALL

Although the abdominal wall is continuous, it is subdivided for descriptive purposes into the *anterior wall, right and left lateral walls* (flanks), and a *posterior wall*. The major part of the wall is musculoaponeurotic. The boundary between the anterior and lateral walls is indefinite. Consequently, the combined term *anterolateral abdominal wall*—extending from the thoracic cage to the pelvis—is often used because some structures, such as the muscles and cutaneous nerves, are continuous within the anterior and lateral walls. *The anterolateral abdominal wall is bounded* (see Fig. 3.4):

- Superiorly by cartilages of 7th through 10th ribs and the xiphoid process of sternum
- Inferiorly by inguinal ligament and pelvic bones.

The wall consists of skin, subcutaneous tissue (superficial fascia), muscles, deep fascia, endoabdominal fascia/fat, and parietal peritoneum (Fig. 3.3). The skin attaches loosely to the subcutaneous tissue except at the umbilicus (navel), where it attaches firmly.

FASCIA OF ANTEROLATERAL ABDOMINAL WALL

The **subcutaneous tissue** (superficial fascia, L. tela subcutanea) over most of the wall consists of a layer of connective tissue that contains a variable amount of fat (Fig. 3.3B). *In the inferior part of the anterolateral wall, the subcutaneous tissue is composed of two layers:*

- *Fatty layer* (Camper's fascia)
- *Membranous layer* (Scarpa's fascia).

The **deep fascia** in the abdomen is very thin, being represented by the epimysium (fibrous sheath), and invests the external oblique muscle. A relatively firm membranous sheet—the **transversalis fascia**—lines most of the abdominal wall. This fascial layer covers the deep surface of the transverse abdominal muscle (L. transversus abdominis) and its aponeurosis; the right and left sides of the transversalis fascia are continuous deep to the **linea alba** (Fig. 3.4, *A* and *B*). The **parietal peritoneum** is internal to the transversalis fascia and is separated from it by a variable amount of **endoabdominal (extraperitoneal) fat.**

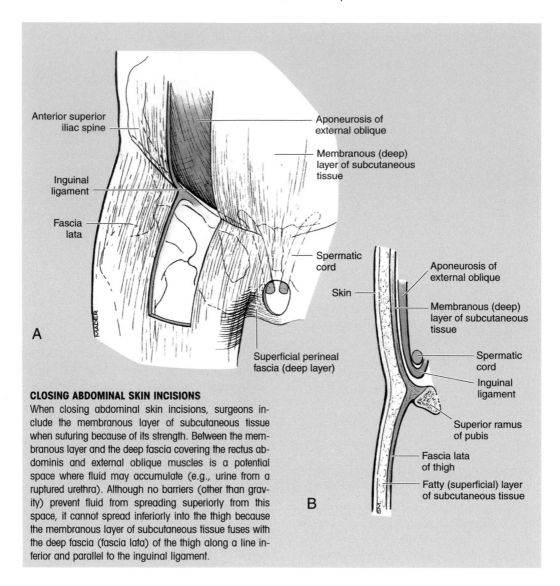

A

CLOSING ABDOMINAL SKIN INCISIONS
When closing abdominal skin incisions, surgeons include the membranous layer of subcutaneous tissue when suturing because of its strength. Between the membranous layer and the deep fascia covering the rectus abdominis and external oblique muscles is a potential space where fluid may accumulate (e.g., urine from a ruptured urethra). Although no barriers (other than gravity) prevent fluid from spreading superiorly from this space, it cannot spread inferiorly into the thigh because the membranous layer of subcutaneous tissue fuses with the deep fascia (fascia lata) of the thigh along a line inferior and parallel to the inguinal ligament.

B

MUSCLES OF ANTEROLATERAL ABDOMINAL WALL

There are five muscles in the anterolateral abdominal wall (Fig. 3.4): *three flat muscles* and *two vertical muscles*. Their attachments, nerve supply, and main actions are listed in Table 3.1.

The three flat muscles are the:

- **External oblique,** the superficial muscle; its fibers pass inferomedially and interdigitate with slips of the serratus anterior.

- **Internal oblique,** the intermediate muscle; its fibers run at right angles to those of the external oblique.

- **Transverse abdominal,** the innermost muscle; its fibers, except for the most inferior ones, run more or less horizontally.

All three flat muscles end anteriorly in a strong sheetlike **aponeurosis.** The fibers of each aponeurosis interlace at the **linea alba** (L. white line) with their fellows of the opposite side to form the **rectus sheath.**

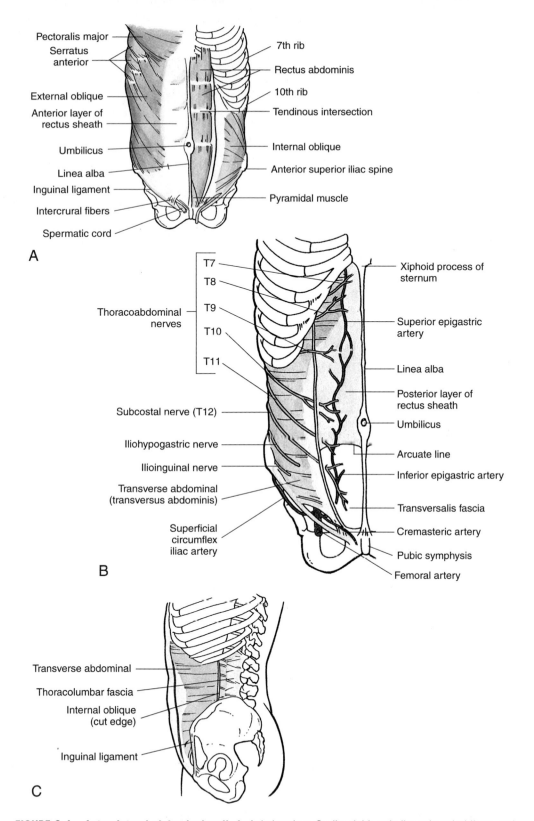

FIGURE 3.4 **Anterolateral abdominal wall. A.** Anterior view. On the right, note the external oblique and intact rectus sheath. On the left, note the internal oblique and opened rectus sheath revealing the rectus abdominis. **B.** Anterior view. Note the transverse abdominal muscle and cutaneous nerves. The rectus abdominis has been removed to show the extent of the posterior layer of the rectus sheath and the epigastric vessels. **C.** Lateral view. Observe the relationship of the transverse abdominal muscle and the thoracolumbar fascia.

TABLE 3.1.   PRINCIPAL MUSCLES OF ANTEROLATERAL ABDOMINAL WALL

Muscles	Origin	Insertion	Innervation	Action(s)
External oblique	External surfaces of 5th–12th ribs	Linea alba, pubic tubercle, and anterior half of iliac crest	Inferior six thoracic nerves and subcostal nerve	Compress and support abdominal viscera; flex and rotate trunk
Internal oblique	Thoracolumbar fascia, anterior two thirds of iliac crest, and lateral half of inguinal ligament	Inferior borders of 10th–12th ribs, linea alba, and pubis via conjoint tendon	Anterior rami of inferior six thoracic and first lumbar nerves	
Transverse abdominal	Internal surfaces of 7th–12th costal cartilages, thoracolumbar fascia, iliac crest, and lateral third of inguinal ligament	Linea alba with aponeurosis of internal oblique, pubic crest, and pecten pubis via conjoint tendon		Compresses and supports abdominal viscera
Rectus abdominis	Pubic symphysis and pubic crest	Xiphoid process and 5th–7th costal cartilages	Anterior rami of inferior six thoracic nerves	Flexes trunk and compresses abdominal viscera

Approximately 80% of people have a *pyramidal muscle,* which is located in the rectus sheath anterior to the most inferior part of the rectus abdominis. It extends from the pubic crest of the hip bone to the linea alba. This small muscle draws down on the linea alba.

The two vertical muscles are the:

- **Rectus abdominis,** a long, broad, straplike muscle that is the principal vertical muscle; most of it is enclosed in the **rectus sheath** (Figs. 3.4 and 3.5). The contractile (fleshy) fibers of the rectus do not run the length of the muscle; rather, they run between three or more **tendinous intersections** (Fig. 3.4A), which are typically located at the level of the xiphoid process, umbilicus, and a level halfway between these points. Each intersection is firmly attached to the anterior layer of the rectus sheath.

- **Pyramidal** (L. pyramidalis), a small triangular muscle that lies in the rectus sheath anterior to the inferior part of the rectus abdominis (Fig. 3.4A). It ends in the **linea alba,** a fibrous band running a variable distance superior to the pubic symphysis.

The **rectus sheath** (Fig. 3.5) has

- An *anterior layer* consisting (in the upper three-fourths of the sheath) of the interlaced aponeurosis of the external oblique and the anterior lamina of the internal oblique aponeurosis

- A *posterior layer* consisting of the fused posterior lamina of the internal oblique aponeurosis and the transverse abdominal aponeurosis; the inferior one-fourth of this layer is deficient because the entire aponeuroses of all three flat muscles pass anterior to the rectus abdominis, contributing to the anterior layer and leaving the posterior surface of the muscle in contact with the transversalis fascia

- A *crescentic line*—the **arcuate line**—that demarcates the lower limit of the aponeurotic posterior wall of the sheath covering the superior three-fourths of the muscle; below this line only the transversalis fascia covers the inferior one-fourth of the muscle.

The **contents of the rectus sheath** are the rectus abdominis and pyramidal muscles, the anastomosing superior and inferior epigastric vessels, lymphatic vessels, and the terminal portions of the anterior primary rami of spinal

Surface Anatomy of Anterolateral Abdominal Wall

The **umbilicus,** an obvious feature of this wall, is the reference point for the transumbilical plane. This indentation of skin in the center of the abdominal wall is where the umbilical cord entered in the fetus. It is typically at the level of the IV disc between L3 and L4 vertebrae; however, its position varies with the amount of fat in the subcutaneous tissue. The location of the **linea alba**—often indicated by a vertical skin groove—is a subcutaneous fibrous band extending from the **xiphoid process** to the **pubic symphysis.** This symphysis can be felt as a firm resistance in the median plane inferior to the linea alba. The bony **iliac crest** at the level of L4 vertebra can be easily palpated as it extends posteriorly from the **anterior superior iliac spine.** In a lean individual with good muscle definition, curved skin grooves—**semilunar lines** (L. lineae semilunares) at the lateral borders of the rectus abdominis—extend from the inferior tips of the costal margins near the ninth costal cartilages to the **pubic tubercles.** Three transverse skin grooves overlie the **tendinous intersections** of the rectus abdominis. The interdigitating bellies of the serratus anterior and external oblique muscles may also be visible. The location of the **inguinal ligament** is indicated by a skin crease just inferior and parallel to the ligament, marking the division between the anterolateral abdominal wall and thigh.

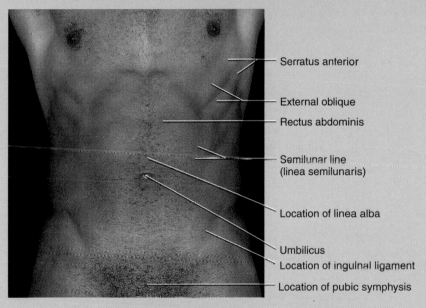

- Serratus anterior
- External oblique
- Rectus abdominis
- Semilunar line (linea semilunaris)
- Location of linea alba
- Umbilicus
- Location of inguinal ligament
- Location of pubic symphysis

Anterior abdominal wall

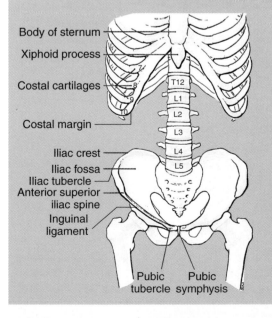

- Body of sternum
- Xiphoid process
- Costal cartilages
- Costal margin
- Iliac crest
- Iliac fossa
- Iliac tubercle
- Anterior superior iliac spine
- Inguinal ligament
- T12
- L1
- L2
- L3
- L4
- L5
- Pubic tubercle
- Pubic symphysis

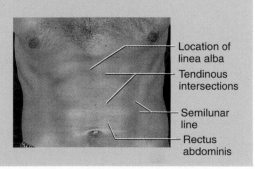

- Location of linea alba
- Tendinous intersections
- Semilunar line
- Rectus abdominis

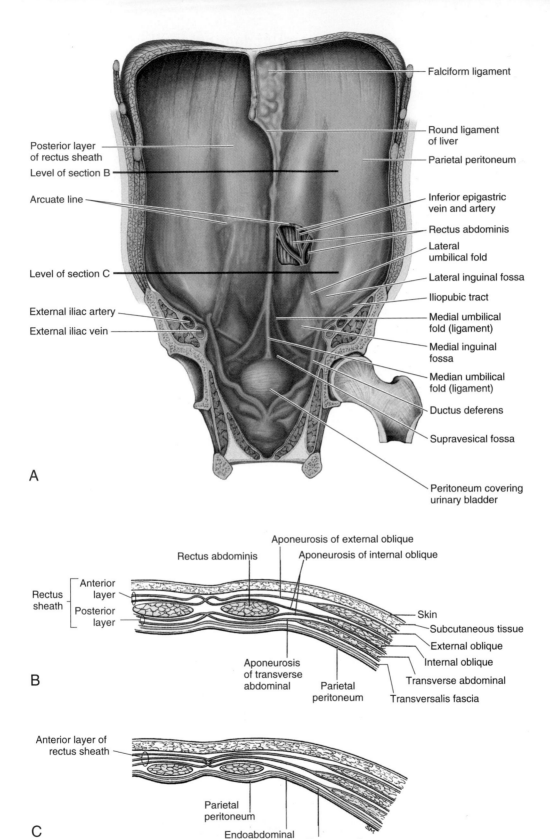

FIGURE 3.5 Anterolateral abdominal wall. A. Internal view of the infraumbilical part of the wall showing the umbilical peritoneal folds and fossae (supravesical, medial inguinal, and lateral inguinal). **B.** Rectus sheath. Schematic transverse section of the wall superior to the arcuate line. **C.** Rectus sheath. Transverse section inferior to the arcuate line.

nerves T7 through T12, which supply the muscle and overlying skin.

Functions and Actions of Anterolateral Abdominal Muscles

The muscles of the anterolateral abdominal wall:

- Provide strong yet flexible support for the anterolateral abdominal wall
- Contain the abdominal viscera and protect them from injury
- Oppose or assist the diaphragm in compressing the abdominal contents, maintaining or increasing intra-abdominal pressure to assist in the elimination of gas (in respiration, coughing, sneezing, eructation or flatulence), liquid and solid (in urination, defecation and vomiting)
- Move the trunk (by assisting in the rotation of thoracic vertebrae or by flexing lumbar vertebrae) and help to maintain posture.

NERVES OF ANTEROLATERAL ABDOMINAL WALL

The skin and muscles of the anterolateral abdominal wall (Fig. 3.6, Table 3.2) are supplied mainly by the:

- *Thoracoabdominal (former inferior intercostal) nerves*—the anterior abdominal (cutaneous) branches of anterior primary rami of the inferior six thoracic nerves (T7 through T11)
- *Subcostal nerves* (T12)
- *Iliohypogastric and ilioinguinal nerves* (T1).

The anterior abdominal cutaneous branches of thoracoabdominal nerves:

- Pierce the rectus sheath a short distance from the median plane, after the rectus muscle has been supplied
- T7 through T9 supply skin superior to umbilicus

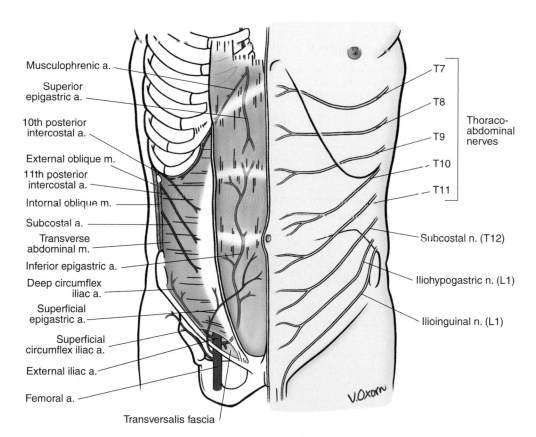

Musculophrenic a.
Superior epigastric a.
10th posterior intercostal a.
External oblique m.
11th posterior intercostal a.
Internal oblique m.
Subcostal a.
Transverse abdominal m.
Inferior epigastric a.
Deep circumflex iliac a.
Superficial epigastric a.
Superficial circumflex iliac a.
External iliac a.
Femoral a.
Transversalis fascia

T7
T8
T9
T10
T11
Thoraco-abdominal nerves

Subcostal n. (T12)
Iliohypogastric n. (L1)
Ilioinguinal n. (L1)

V.Oxorn

FIGURE 3.6 **Arteries and nerves of the anterolateral abdominal wall.** Anterior view.

TABLE 3.2. NERVES OF ANTEROLATERAL ABDOMINAL WALL

Nerve	Origin	Course	Distribution
Thoracoabdominal (T7–T11)	Continuation of lower intercostal nerves	Run between 2nd and 3rd layers of abdominal muscles	Anterior abdominal muscles and overlying skin; periphery of diaphragm
Subcostal (T12)	Anterior ramus of 12th thoracic nerve	Runs along inferior border of 12th rib	Lowest slip of external oblique muscle and skin over anterior superior iliac spine and hip
Iliohypogastric (L1)	Chiefly from anterior ramus of 1st lumbar nerve	Pierces transverse abdominal muscle; branches pierce external oblique aponeurosis	Skin of hypogastric region and over iliac crest; internal oblique and transverse abdominal
Ilioinguinal (L1)	Anterior ramus of 1st lumbar nerve	Passes between 2nd and 3rd layers of abdominal muscles and passes through inguinal canal	Skin of scrotum or labium majus, mons pubis, and adjacent medial aspect of thigh; internal oblique and transverse abdominal

- T10 innervates skin around umbilicus
- T11, plus cutaneous branches of the subcostal (T12), iliohypogastric, and ilioinguinal (L1), supply skin inferior to umbilicus.

VESSELS OF ANTEROLATERAL ABDOMINAL WALL

The blood vessels of the anterolateral abdominal wall (Fig. 3.6, Table 3.3) are the:

- *Superior epigastrics* from the internal thoracic arteries and veins
- *Inferior epigastrics* and *deep circumflex iliacs* from the external iliac arteries and veins
- *Superficial circumflex iliacs* and *superficial epigastrics* from the femoral artery and great saphenous vein
- *Anterior and collateral branches of the posterior intercostal vessels* in the 10th and 11th intercostal spaces, and from anterior branches of subcostal arteries and veins

- *Branches of the musculophrenic vessels* from the internal thoracic arteries and veins.

The **superior epigastric artery,** the direct continuation of the internal thoracic artery, enters the rectus sheath superiorly through its posterior layer (Fig. 3.4), supplies the upper part of the rectus abdominis, and anastomoses with the inferior epigastric artery. The **inferior epigastric artery** arises from the external iliac artery just proximal to its passage under the inguinal ligament. It runs superiorly in the transversalis fascia to enter the rectus sheath inferior to the arcuate line. Its branches enter the lower rectus abdominis and anastomose with those of the superior epigastric artery approximately in the umbilical region.

The **superficial lymphatic vessels** accompany the subcutaneous veins; those superior to the umbilicus drain mainly to the *axillary lymph nodes,* whereas those inferior to it drain to the *superficial inguinal lymph nodes.* The **deep lymphatic vessels** accompany the deep veins and drain to the external iliac, common iliac and lumbar (lateral aortic) lymph nodes (see Fig. 3.8).

TABLE 3.3. PRINCIPAL ARTERIES OF ANTEROLATERAL ABDOMINAL WALL

Artery	Origin	Course	Distribution
Superior epigastric (Fig. 3.6)	Internal thoracic artery	Descends in rectus sheath deep to rectus abdominis	Rectus abdominis and superior part of anterolateral abdominal wall
Inferior epigastric	External iliac artery	Runs superiorly and enters rectus sheath; runs deep to rectus abdominis	Rectus abdominis and medial part of anterolateral abdominal wall
Deep circumflex iliac		Runs on deep aspect of anterior abdominal wall, parallel to inguinal ligament	Iliacus muscle and inferior part of anterolateral abdominal wall
Superficial circumflex iliac	Femoral artery	Runs in superficial fascia along inguinal ligament	Subcutaneous tissue and skin over inferior portion of anterolateral abdominal wall
Superficial epigastric		Runs in superficial fascia toward umbilicus	Subcutaneous tissue and skin over suprapubic region

ABDOMINAL SURGICAL INCISIONS

Surgeons use various incisions to gain access to the abdominal cavity. The incision that allows adequate exposure and, secondarily, the best possible cosmetic effect, is chosen. The location of the incision also depends on the type of operation, the location of the organ(s), bony or cartilaginous boundaries, avoidance of (especially motor) nerves, maintenance of blood supply, and prevention of injury to muscles and fascia of the wall. Instead of transecting muscles, causing irreversible necrosis (death) of muscle fibers, the surgeon splits them between their fibers. Muscles and viscera are retracted toward, not away from, their neurovascular supply. Cutting a motor nerve paralyzes the muscle fibers supplied by it, thereby weakening the anterolateral abdominal wall. However, because of overlapping areas of innervation between nerves in the abdominal wall, one or two small branches of nerves may usually be cut without a noticeable loss of motor supply to the muscles or loss of sensation to the skin. *The most common surgical incisions* are illustrated (photograph).

Incisional Hernia

If the muscular and aponeurotic layers of the abdomen do not heal properly, a hernia may occur through the defect. An incisional hernia is a protrusion of omentum (fold of peritoneum) or an organ through a surgical incision or scar.

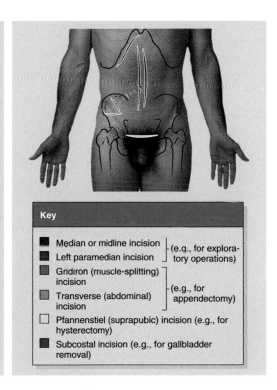

Key

- ■ Median or midline incision ⎤ (e.g., for exploratory operations)
- ■ Left paramedian incision ⎦
- ■ Gridiron (muscle-splitting) incision ⎤ (e.g., for appendectomy)
- ■ Transverse (abdominal) incision ⎦
- □ Pfannenstiel (suprapubic) incision (e.g., for hysterectomy)
- ■ Subcostal incision (e.g., for gallbladder removal)

INTERNAL SURFACE OF ANTEROLATERAL ABDOMINAL WALL

The internal surface of the anterolateral abdominal wall (Fig. 3.5, *A* and *B*) is covered with **parietal peritoneum.** The infraumbilical part of this surface of the wall exhibits several **peritoneal folds,** some of which contain remnants of vessels that carried blood to and from the fetus. **Five umbilical folds**—two on each side and one in the median plane—pass toward the umbilicus:

- The **median umbilical fold,** extending from the apex of the urinary bladder to the umbilicus, covers the **median umbilical ligament,** the remnant of the *urachus* that joined the apex of the fetal bladder to the umbilicus

- Two **medial umbilical folds,** lateral to the median umbilical fold, cover the **medial umbilical ligaments,** the remnants of the fetal umbilical arteries (Moore and Persaud, 1998)
- Two **lateral umbilical folds,** lateral to the medial umbilical folds, cover the **inferior epigastric vessels**, which are functional ones that bleed if cut.

The depressions lateral to the umbilical folds are **peritoneal fossae,** each of which is a potential site for a hernia. The location of a hernia in one of these fossae determines how the hernia is classified. *The shallow fossae between the umbilical folds are the:*

- **Supravesical fossae** between the median and medial umbilical folds, formed as the peritoneum reflects from the anterior abdominal wall onto the bladder. The level of the supravesical fossae rises and falls with filling and emptying of the bladder.
- **Medial inguinal fossae** between the medial and lateral umbilical folds (areas also commonly called *inguinal or Hesselbach triangles*). These are potential sites for direct inguinal hernias.
- **Lateral inguinal fossae,** lateral to the lateral umbilical folds, include the deep inguinal rings and are potential sites for the most common type of hernia in the lower abdominal wall—*indirect inguinal hernia.*

INGUINAL REGION

The inguinal region in the inferior part of the anterolateral abdominal wall includes an area of weakness, especially in males, because of the passage of the spermatic cord through the inguinal canal.

Inguinal Canal

The inguinal canal in adults is an oblique, inferomedially directed passage (between the su-perficial and deep inguinal rings) through the inferior part of the anterior abdominal wall (Fig. 3.7). The inguinal canal lies parallel and just superior to the medial half of the **inguinal ligament.** The main occupant of the inguinal canal is the **spermatic cord** in males and the **round ligament of the uterus** in females. The inguinal canal also contains blood and lymphatic vessels and the **ilioinguinal nerve** in both sexes. *The inguinal canal has an opening at each end.*

- The **deep (internal) ring**—entrance to inguinal canal—is an *outpouching of the transversalis fascia* approximately 1.25 cm superior to the middle of the inguinal ligament and *lateral to the inferior epigastric vessels* (Fig. 3.7*B*).
- The **superficial (external) inguinal ring**— exit from inguinal canal—is a slitlike opening between the diagonal fibers of the aponeurosis of the external oblique, *superolateral to the pubic tubercle* (Fig. 3.7*C*). The lateral and medial margins of the superficial ring formed by the split in the aponeurosis are the **lateral** and **medial crura** (L. leglike parts).

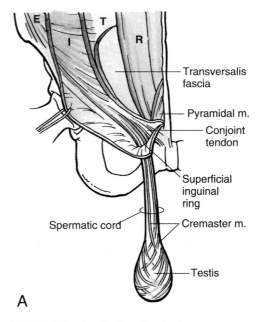

A

FIGURE 3.7   Inguinal region. A. Spermatic cord and inguinal canal. Anterior view. *E,* external oblique; *I,* internal oblique; *T,* transverse abdominal; *R,* rectus abdominis.

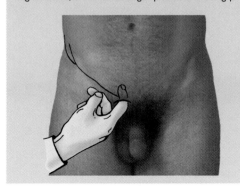

The deep and superficial inguinal rings do not overlap because of the oblique path of the inguinal canal through the aponeuroses of the abdominal muscles. Consequently, increases in intra-abdominal pressure force the posterior wall of the canal against the anterior wall, closing this passageway and thus strengthening this potential defect of the abdominal wall. Contraction of the external oblique also approximates the anterior wall of the canal to the posterior wall. Contraction of the internal oblique and transverse abdominal muscles makes the roof of the canal descend, which constricts the canal. All these events occur simultaneously during acts such as sneezing, coughing, and "bearing down" (Valsalva maneuver) to increase intra-abdominal pressure for elimination.

The inguinal canal has two walls (anterior and posterior), a roof, and a floor.

- **Anterior wall**—formed by *external oblique aponeurosis* throughout the length of the canal, with the anterior wall of the lateral part of the canal being reinforced by fibers of internal oblique.
- **Posterior wall**—formed by *transversalis fascia* (see iliopubic tract below) with the posterior wall of the medial part of the canal being reinforced by merging of the pubic attachments of the internal oblique and transverse abdominal aponeuroses into a common tendon—the **conjoint tendon** (Fig. 3.7, *A* and *B*).

- **Roof**—formed by *arching fibers of internal oblique* and *transverse abdominal muscles.*
- **Floor**—formed by *superior surface of inguinal ligament*—an in-curving of the thickened inferior border of the external oblique aponeurosis; the inguinal ligament thus forms a shallow trough. The most medial part of the floor is formed by part of the inguinal ligament that, rather than attaching directly to the **pubic tubercle** as most of the ligament does, reflects deeply and blindly to attach to the superior pubic ramus as the **lacunar ligament** (Fig. 3.7, *B* and *C*).

External oblique

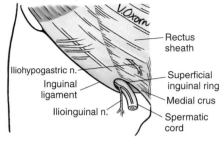

Internal oblique

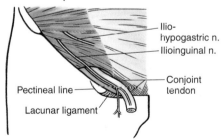

Transverse abdominal

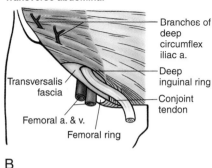

B

FIGURE 3.7 *Continued.* **B.** Progressive dissections of abdominal muscles showing the relationships of the inguinal canal.

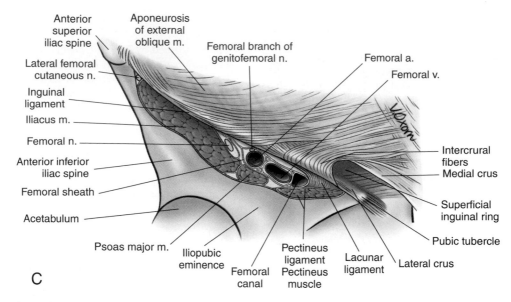

FIGURE 3.7 *Continued.* **C.** Inguinal ligament and superficial inguinal ring. Anterolateral view. Note the lacunar and pectineal ligaments.

The **iliopubic tract** (deep crural arch)—the thickened inferior margin of the transversalis fascia—is a fibrous band that runs parallel and posterior (deep) to the inguinal ligament. The iliopubic tract—seen only when the inguinal region is viewed from its internal aspect, as through an endoscope (Fig. 3.5*A*)—contributes to the posterior wall of the inguinal canal.

Spermatic Cord

The spermatic cord—the ropelike structure suspending the testis in the scrotum—is formed by the **ductus deferens** and its associated structures and the coverings they gain as they penetrate the deep inguinal ring through the inguinal canal to enter and extend into the scrotum (Figs. 3.7, *A* and *B* and 3.8). **The spermatic cord:**

- Begins as the ductus deferens and associated neurovascular structures pass through the deep inguinal ring, lateral to the inferior epigastric vessels
- Gains its coverings as it passes through the inguinal canal and exits the superficial inguinal ring
- Ends in the scrotum at the posterior border of the testis; it becomes surrounded by its fascial coverings derived from the

fascia of the layered anterolateral abdominal wall during its passage through them during development.

The fascial coverings of the spermatic cord (Table 3.4) include the:

- **Internal spermatic fascia**—derived from an extension of the transversalis fascia at the deep inguinal ring
- **Cremasteric fascia**—derived from the fascia covering the superficial and deep aspects of the internal oblique
- **External spermatic fascia**—derived from the external oblique aponeurosis.

The cremasteric fascia includes loops of the **cremaster muscle,** extensions of the lowermost fascicles of the part of the internal oblique that arises from the inguinal ligament. *The cremaster muscle reflexly draws the testis superiorly in the scrotum,* particularly when it is cold. In a warm environment such as a hot bath, the cremaster relaxes and the testis descends deeply in the scrotum, which also lengthens or expands as its **dartos muscle** (Table 3.4) relaxes. Both responses occur in an attempt to regulate the temperature of the testis for *spermatogenesis* (formation of sperms), which requires a

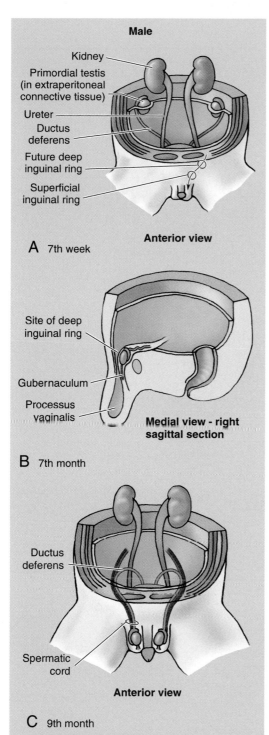

Male

Kidney

Primordial testis (in extraperitoneal connective tissue)

Ureter

Ductus deferens

Future deep inguinal ring

Superficial inguinal ring

A 7th week

Anterior view

Site of deep inguinal ring

Gubernaculum

Processus vaginalis

Medial view - right sagittal section

B 7th month

Ductus deferens

Spermatic cord

Anterior view

C 9th month

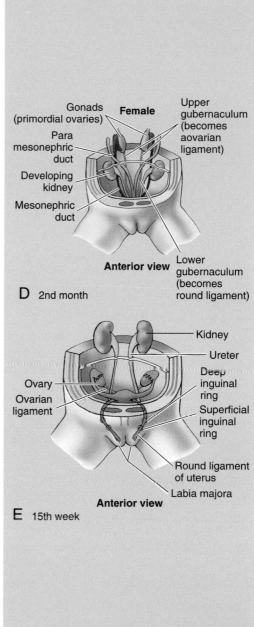

Gonads (primordial ovaries)

Para mesonephric duct

Developing kidney

Mesonephric duct

Female

Upper gubernaculum (becomes aovarian ligament)

Anterior view

Lower gubernaculum (becomes round ligament)

D 2nd month

Kidney

Ureter

Deep inguinal ring

Superficial inguinal ring

Ovary

Ovarian ligament

Round ligament of uterus

Labia majora

Anterior view

E 15th week

Descent of Gonads

The **fetal testes** descend from the dorsal abdominal wall in the superior lumbar region to the deep inguinal rings during the 9th to 12th fetal weeks. This movement probably results from growth of the vertebral column and pelvis. The male *gubernaculum,* attached to the caudal pole of the testis and accompanied by an outpouching of peritoneum, the *processus vaginalis,* projects into the scrotum. The testis descends posterior to the processus vaginalis. The inferior remnant of the processus vaginalis forms the *tunica vaginalis* covering the testis. The ductus deferens, testicular vessels, nerves, and lymphatics accompany the testes. The final descent of the testis usually occurs before or shortly after birth. The **fetal ovaries** also descend from the dorsal abdominal wall in the superior lumbar region during the 12th week but pass into the lesser pelvis. The female gubernaculum also attaches to the caudal pole of the ovary and projects into the labia majora, attaching *en route* to the uterus; the part passing from the uterus to the ovary forms the *ovarian ligament* and the remainder of it becomes the *round ligament of the uterus.* For a complete description of the embryology of the inguinal region, see Moore and Persaud (1998).

**TABLE 3.4.   CORRESPONDING LAYERS OF THE ANTERIOR ABDOMINAL WALL,
SPERMATIC CORD, AND SCROTUM**

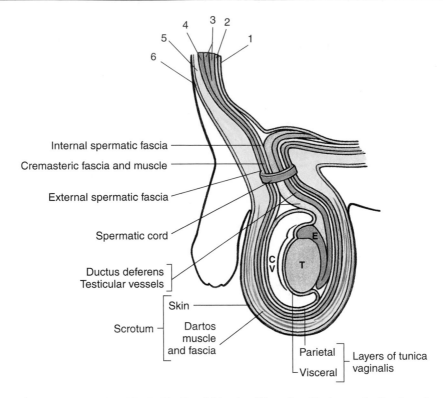

Coverings of spermatic cord and testis (T). *E,* epididymis; *CV,* cavity of tunica vaginalis; *1,* peritoneum; *2,* transversalis fascia; *3,* transverse abdominal, internal oblique; *4,* external oblique; *5,* subcutaneous fat; *6,* skin

Layers of Anterior Abdominal Wall	Scrotum and Coverings of Testis	Coverings of Spermatic Cord
Skin	Skin	
Subcutaneous tissue (superficial fascia)	Superficial (dartos) fascia and dartos muscle	Scrotum (and scrotal septum)
External oblique aponeurosis	External spermatic fascia	External spermatic fascia
Internal oblique muscle	Cremaster muscle	Cremaster muscle
Fascia of both superficial and deep surfaces of internal oblique muscle	Cremasteric fascia	Cremasteric fascia
Transverse abdominal muscle		
Transversalis fascia	Internal spermatic fascia	Internal spermatic fascia
Extraperitoneal fat		
Peritoneum	Tunica vaginalis	Obliterated processus vaginalis

constant temperature approximately one degree cooler than core temperature. The cremaster is innervated by the genital branch of the *genitofemoral nerve* (L1, L2), a derivative of the lumbar plexus.

Constituents of the spermatic cord (Fig. 3.8) are the:

- **Ductus deferens** (deferent duct, vas deferens), a muscular tube that *conveys sperms from the epididymis to the ejaculatory duct* (p. 226), which courses through the substance of the prostate to open into the prostatic part of the urethra
- **Testicular artery** arising from the aorta and supplying the testis and epididymis
- **Artery of ductus deferens** arising from the inferior vesical artery
- **Cremasteric artery** arising from the inferior epigastric artery
- **Pampiniform plexus,** a venous network formed by up to 12 venous channels, draining into the right or left testicular veins
- **Sympathetic nerve fibers** on arteries and sympathetic and parasympathetic fibers on the ductus deferens
- **Genital branch of genitofemoral nerve** supplying the cremaster muscle
- **Lymphatic vessels** draining the testis and closely associated structures to the lumbar and preaortic lymph nodes (Fig. 3.8*B*).

Scrotum

The scrotum is a musculocutaneous sac consisting of two layers: heavily pigmented skin and closely related **dartos fascia**—a layer of smooth muscle fibers (Table 3.4)—responsible for the rugose (wrinkled) appearance of the scrotum. Because the **dartos muscle** attaches to the skin, its contraction causes the scrotum to wrinkle and thus become smaller when cold, which helps to regulate the loss of heat through its skin.

The **arteries of the scrotum** (Fig. 3.8*B*) are the:

- *Posterior scrotal arteries,* terminal branches of perineal branch of *internal pudendal artery*

- *Anterior scrotal arteries,* terminal branches of external pudendal branches of *femoral artery.*

The **veins of the scrotum** accompany the arteries. The **lymphatic vessels** drain into the **superficial inguinal lymph nodes** (Fig. 3.8*B*). The **nerves of the scrotum** are the:

- *Genital branch of the genitofemoral nerve* (L1, L2) supplying the anterolateral surface of the scrotum
- *Anterior scrotal nerves*—branches of the *ilioinguinal nerve* (L1)—supplying the anterior surface of the scrotum.
- *Posterior scrotal nerves*—branches of the perineal branch of the *pudendal nerve* (S2 to S4) supplying the posterior surface of the scrotum
- Perineal branches of the *posterior femoral cutaneous nerve* (S2, S3) supplying the lateral surface of the scrotum.

Testes

The ovoid testes are suspended in the scrotum by the spermatic cords (Figs. 3.7*A* and 3.8*A*). The testes produce sperms (spermatozoa) and hormones, principally testosterone. The sperms are formed in the **seminiferous tubules** that are joined by **straight tubules** to the **rete testis.** The surface of each testis is covered by the visceral layer of the tunica vaginalis, except where the testis attaches to the epididymis and spermatic cord. The **tunica vaginalis** is a closed peritoneal sac surrounding the testis (Table 3.4). The **visceral layer of the tunica vaginalis**—a glistening, transparent serous membrane—is closely applied to the testis, epididymis, and inferior part of the ductus deferens. The **parietal layer of the tunica vaginalis,** adjacent to the internal spermatic fascia, is more extensive than the visceral layer and extends superiorly for a short distance into the distal part of the spermatic cord. The small amount of fluid in the cavity of the tunica vaginalis separates the visceral and parietal layers, allowing the testis to move freely within its side of the scrotum.

The **testicular arteries** (Fig. 3.8*B*) arise from the abdominal aorta just inferior to the renal arteries. The long, slender testicular ar-

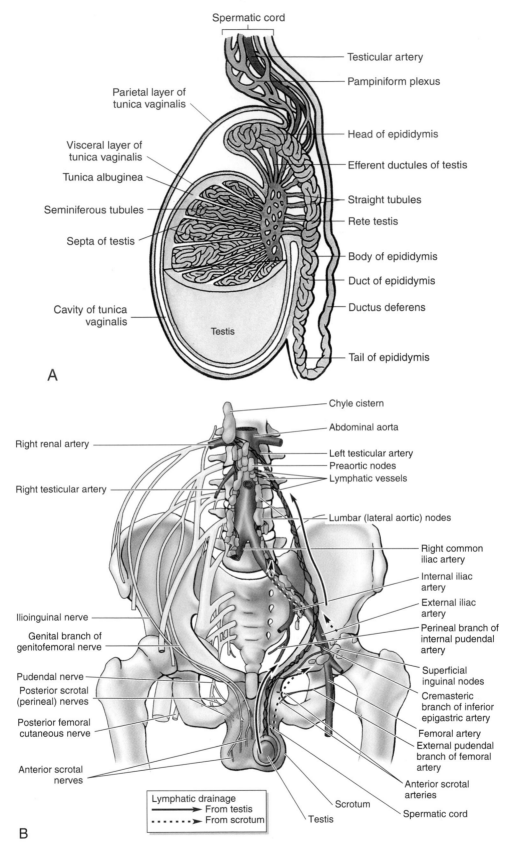

FIGURE 3.8 Testis, epididymis, and spermatic cord. A. Schematic vertical section. **B.** Blood supply, innervation, and lymphatic drainage. Anterior view. *Arrows,* direction of flow of lymph to lymph nodes.

teries pass retroperitoneally (external or posterior to the peritoneum) in an oblique direction, crossing over the ureters and the inferior parts of the external iliac arteries. They traverse the inguinal canals becoming part of the spermatic cords to reach and supply the testes.

The **testicular veins** emerge from the testis and epididymis and join to form a venous network, the **pampiniform plexus,** consisting of 8 to 12 anastomosing veins lying anterior to the ductus deferens and surrounding the testicular artery in the spermatic cord (Fig. 3.8*A*). The cooler venous blood within the pampiniform plexus absorbs heat from the arterial blood, providing a *thermoregulatory system for the testis,* helping to keep this gland at a constant temperature—one degree lower than that of the trunk. The **left testicular vein** originates as the veins of the pampiniform plexus coalesce; it empties into the left renal vein. The **right testicular vein** has a similar origin and course but enters the inferior vena cava (IVC).

The **lymphatic drainage of the testis** is to the *lumbar* and *preaortic lymph nodes* (Fig. 3.8*B*). **The autonomic nerves of the testis** arise as the *testicular plexus of nerves* on the testicular artery, which contains vagal parasympathetic fibers and sympathetic and visceral afferent fibers from T7 segment of the spinal cord.

Epididymis

The epididymis is formed by minute convolutions of the **duct of the epididymis,** so tightly compacted that they appear solid (Fig. 3.8*A*). The **epididymis** lies on the posterior surface of the testis, which is covered by the tunica vaginalis except at its posterior margin where the epididymis lies. The **ductus deferens** begins at the tail of the epididymis as a relatively thick-walled continuation of the duct of the epididymis. The **efferent ductules** transport newly formed sperms from the rete testis to the epididymis where they are stored until mature. The **rete testis** is a network of canals at the termination of the seminiferous tubules. **The epididymis consists of:**

- A **head** that is the superior expanded part composed of lobules formed by the *coiled ends of 12 to 14 efferent ductules*
- A **body** that consists of the *convoluted duct of the epididymis*
- A **tail** that is continuous with the ductus deferens, the duct that transports sperms from the epididymis to the ejaculatory duct for expulsion into the prostatic urethra (p. 234).

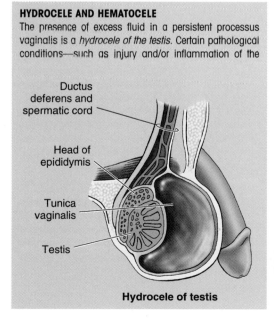

HYDROCELE AND HEMATOCELE

The presence of excess fluid in a persistent processus vaginalis is a *hydrocele of the testis*. Certain pathological conditions—such as injury and/or inflammation of the epididymis—may also produce a hydrocele of the spermatic cord. A *hematocele of the testis* is a collection of blood in the cavity of the tunica vaginalis.

Ductus deferens and spermatic cord

Head of epididymis

Tunica vaginalis

Testis

Hydrocele of testis

Hemorrhage into tunica vaginalis due to injury to the spermatic vessels

Hematocele of testis

Inguinal Hernias

An inguinal hernia ("rupture") is a protrusion of parietal peritoneum and viscera such as part of the intestine through a normal or abnormal opening from the abdominal cavity. *There are two major categories of inguinal hernia:* indirect and direct; approximately 75% are indirect hernias.

An indirect (congenital) inguinal hernia:

- *Leaves the abdominal cavity lateral to the inferior epigastric vessels* and enters the deep inguinal ring
- Passes through the inguinal canal

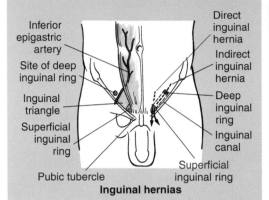

Inguinal hernias

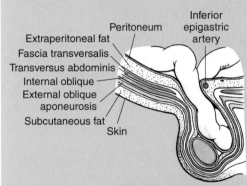

Indirect inguinal hernia

- *Has a hernial sac formed by the persistent processus vaginalis*
- Exits the superficial inguinal ring and commonly enters the scrotum.

If the entire stalk of the processus vaginalis persists, the hernia extends into the scrotum superior to the testis.

An indirect inguinal hernia can occur in women; however, it is about 20 times more common in males of all ages.

A direct (acquired) inguinal hernia:

- *Leaves the abdominal cavity medial to the inferior epigastric artery,* protruding through an area of relative weakness in the posterior wall of the inguinal canal—the *inguinal (Hesselbach) triangle* between the inferior epigastric artery superolaterally, the rectus abdominis medially, and the inguinal ligament inferiorly

- *Has a hernial sac formed by transversalis fascia*
- Does not traverse the entire inguinal canal—usually only its most medial part (lower end) adjacent to the superficial inguinal ring
- Emerges through or around the conjoint tendon to reach the superficial inguinal ring, gaining an outer covering of external spermatic fascia, inside or parallel to that on the cord itself

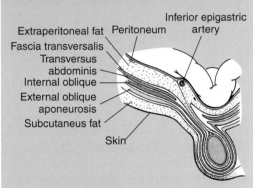

Direct inguinal hernia

- Lies outside the processes vaginalis, which is usually obliterated, parallel to the spermatic cord, and outside the inner one or two fascial coverings of the cord
- Almost never enters the scrotum; however, when it does it passes lateral to the spermatic cord, deep to the skin and dartos fascia.

Vasectomy

The *ductus deferens* is ligated bilaterally when sterilizing a man. To perform a vasectomy, also called a *deferentectomy,* the duct is isolated on each side and transected, or a small section of it is removed. Sperms can no longer pass to the urethra; they degenerate in the epididymis and proximal end of the ductus deferens. However the secretions of the *auxiliary genital glands* (seminal vesicles, bulbourethral glands, and prostate) can still be ejaculated. The testis continues to function as an endocrine gland for the production of testosterone.

Varicocele

The pampiniform plexus of veins may become varicose (dilated) and tortuous. These varicose vessels often result from defective valves in the testicular vein. The palpable enlargement, which feels like a bundle of worms, usually drains and thus seems to disappear when the person lies down.

Testicular Cancer
Because the testes descend from the dorsal abdominal wall into the scrotum during fetal development, their lymphatic drainage differs from that of the scrotum, which is an out-pouching of the anterolateral abdominal skin. Consequently,

- *Cancer of the testis* metastasizes directly to the **lumbar lymph nodes**
- *Cancer of the scrotum* metastasizes initially to the **superficial inguinal nodes.**

Cremasteric Reflex
The cremasteric reflex is the rapid elevation of the testis on the same side; this reflex is extremely active in children. Contraction of the cremaster muscle—producing the reflex—can be induced by lightly stroking the skin on the medial aspect of the superior part of the thigh with an applicator stick or tongue depressor. This area is supplied by the *ilioinguinal nerve.*

PERITONEUM AND PERITONEAL CAVITY

The **peritoneum**—a continuous, glistening, transparent serous membrane—consists of two continuous layers (Fig. 3.9):

- *Parietal peritoneum,* lining the internal surface of the abdominopelvic wall
- *Visceral peritoneum,* investing viscera (organs) such as the spleen and stomach.

The peritoneum and viscera are in the abdominal cavity. *The peritoneal cavity is a potential space of capillary thinness between the parietal and visceral layers of peritoneum.* **There are no viscera in the peritoneal cavity,** which is normally empty except for a thin layer of peritoneal fluid that keeps the peritoneal surfaces moist. The smooth glistening peritoneum, lubricated with **peritoneal fluid,** enables the viscera to move over each other essentially without friction, allowing the movements of digestion. In addition to lubricating the surfaces of the viscera, the peritoneal fluid contains leukocytes and antibodies that resist infection. *The peritoneal cavity is completely closed in males;* however, there is a communication pathway in females to the exterior of the body through the uterine tubes, uterine cavity, and vagina (see Chapter 4).

This communication constitutes a potential pathway of infection. *The relationship of the viscera to the peritoneum is as follows:*

- **Intraperitoneal organs** are almost completely covered with visceral peritoneum (e.g., the spleen and stomach); *they are not in the peritoneal cavity.*
- **Extraperitoneal** (outside peritoneal cavity) or **retroperitoneal organs** are external or posterior to the parietal peritoneum and are only partially covered with peritoneum (usually on one surface). Organs such as the kidneys are between the parietal peritoneum and the posterior abdominal wall (Fig. 3.9) and have parietal peritoneum only on their anterior surfaces, often with a considerable amount of fatty tissue (*endoabdominal fascia*) intervening.

PERITONEAL VESSELS AND NERVES

Parietal peritoneum is:

- Supplied by blood vessels of the abdominopelvic wall
- Innervated by somatic nerves
- Drained by lymphatic vessels that are continuous with those in the abdominopelvic wall.

Visceral peritoneum is:

- Supplied by branches of blood vessels of the viscera
- Innervated by visceral afferent (autonomic) nerves
- Drained by lymphatic vessels that join those from the viscera.

PERITONITIS
Inflammation of the peritoneum causes pain in the overlying skin and an increase in the tone of the anterolateral abdominal muscles. A person with an *acute abdomen* (intense abdominal pain) has spasms of the anterolateral abdominal muscles—*guarding*—a boardlike muscular rigidity that cannot be willfully suppressed.

Peritoneal Adhesions
If the peritoneum is injured by a stab wound, for example, and peritonitis develops, parts of the inflamed parietal and

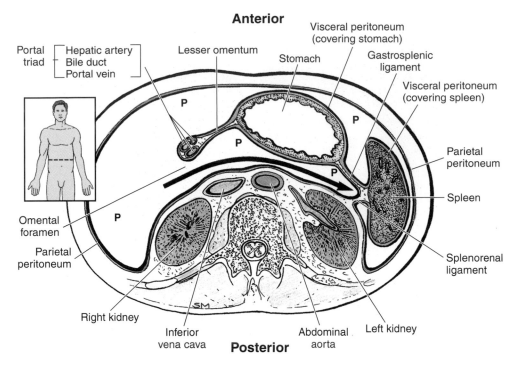

FIGURE 3.9   Transverse section of the abdomen. The orientation drawing shows the level of the section through the upper abdomen. Observe the omental foramen and the horizontal extent of the omental bursa (lesser sac). The *black arrow* passes from the greater sac through the omental foramen across the full extent of the omental bursa. *P,* peritoneal cavity.

Continued
visceral layers of the peritoneum may adhere, forming an *adhesion* that interferes with the movement of the viscera. The surgical separation of adhesions is *adhesiotomy*.

Ascites and Paracentesis
Under certain pathological conditions such as *peritonitis,* the peritoneal cavity may be distended with abnormal fluid (*ascites*). Widespread *metastases* (spread) of cancer cells to the abdominal viscera cause exudation (escape) of fluid that is often blood stained. *Paracentesis of the abdomen* may be performed to analyze or remove an excess of fluid. After injection of a local anesthetic agent, a needle or trochar and a cannula are inserted into the peritoneal cavity through the linea alba, for example.

TERMS DESCRIBING PARTS OF PERITONEUM

Various terms are used to describe the parts of the peritoneum that connect organs with other organs or to the abdominal wall. The disposition of peritoneum in the adult is easier to un-

derstand when developmental changes are considered (see description of the embryology of the peritoneal cavity and viscera in Moore and Persaud (1998) and Moore and Dalley (1999)).

A **mesentery** (Figs. 3.10, 3.11*A*, and 3.12) *is a double layer of peritoneum reflecting away from the abdominal wall to enclose part or all of one of the viscera* (e.g., mesentery of transverse colon or transverse mesocolon). A mesentery constitutes a continuity of the visceral and parietal peritoneum that *provides a means for neurovascular communication between the organ and the body wall*. A mesentery has a core of connective tissue containing blood vessels, lymphatic vessels, nerves, fat, and lymph nodes. Viscera with a mesentery are mobile; the degree of mobility depends on the length of the mesentery.

A **peritoneal ligament** consists of a *double layer of peritoneum* (more limited than, or a specific part or subdivision of, a mesentery) that connects an organ with another organ or to the abdominal wall. For example, the liver is connected to the anterior abdominal wall by the **falciform ligament** (Figs. 3.5*A* and 3.10*A*); the stomach is connected to the inferior surface of the diaphragm by the **gastrophrenic lig-** **ament** and to the spleen by the **gastrosplenic ligament** (Fig. 3.10*B*).

An **omentum** is a broad, double-layered sheet of peritoneum passing from the stomach to another abdominal organ. The **greater omentum** (gastrocolic ligament) hangs down

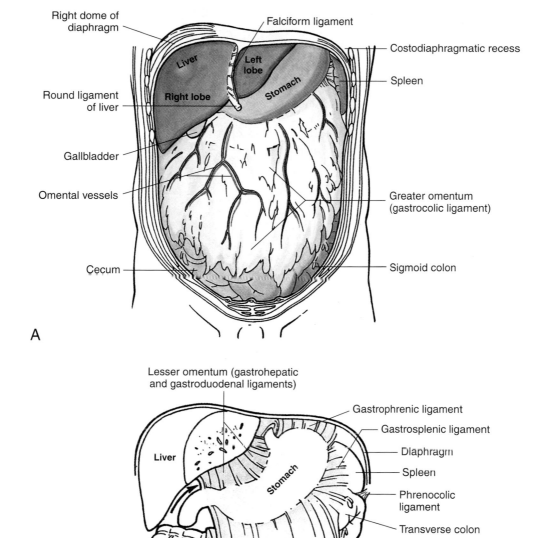

FIGURE 3.10 **Abdominal contents and peritoneum. A.** Anterior thoracic and abdominal walls are cut away to show undisturbed contents. **B.** Stomach and lesser and greater omenta and associated peritoneal ligaments. *Arrow,* site of omental foramen.

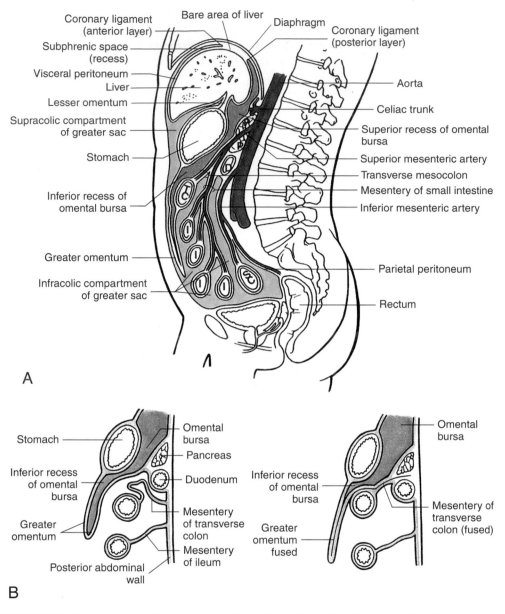

FIGURE 3.11 **Mesenteries and blood vessels. A.** Sagittal section of the abdomen and pelvis showing the viscera and the arrangement of the peritoneum. *P,* pancreas; *D,* duodenum; *TC,* transverse colon; *I,* jejunum and ileum; *SC,* sigmoid colon. **B.** Sagittal section through the inferior recess of the omental bursa. Formation of the transverse mesocolon and fusion of the layers of the greater omentum are illustrated.

from the greater curvature of the stomach and the proximal part of the duodenum (Fig. 3.10*A*). After descending, it folds back and attaches to the anterior surface of the transverse colon and its mesentery. The **lesser omentum** (gastrohepatic and gastroduodenal ligaments) connects the lesser curvature of the stomach

and the proximal part of the duodenum to the liver (Fig. 3.10*B*). The gastrohepatic and hepatoduodenal ligaments are continuous parts of the lesser omentum and are separated only for descriptive convenience. The stomach is connected to the liver by the **gastrohepatic ligament**—the membranous part of the lesser omentum. The **hepatoduodenal ligament**—the thickened free edge of the lesser omentum—conducts the **portal triad:** portal vein, hepatic artery, and bile duct.

A **peritoneal fold,** such as the *medial* and *lateral umbilical folds* (Fig. 3.5*A*), is a reflection of peritoneum that is raised from the body wall by underlying blood vessels, ducts, and obliterated fetal vessels.

A **peritoneal recess** is a pouch or concavity lined with peritoneum, and often formed by a peritoneal fold, such as the **subphrenic space (recess)** between the liver and the diaphragm and the **inferior recess of the omental bursa** between the layers of the greater omentum (Fig. 3.11).

GREATER SAC AND OMENTAL BURSA

The peritoneal cavity is divided into a greater sac and an omental bursa (Figs. 3.11 and 3.12).

- The **greater sac** is the main and larger part of the peritoneal cavity

- The **omental bursa** (lesser sac), an extensive saclike cavity, is the smaller part of the peritoneal cavity that lies posterior to the stomach and adjoining omenta.

The omental bursa permits free movement of the stomach because the anterior and posterior walls of the omental bursa slide smoothly over each other. *The omental bursa has two recesses* (Fig. 3.11*A*):

- A **superior recess** that is limited superiorly by the diaphragm and the posterior layer of the coronary ligament of the liver
- An **inferior recess** between the superior part of the layers of the greater omentum.

Most of the inferior recess of the omental bursa is a potential space sealed off from the main part of the omental bursa posterior to the stomach following adhesion of the anterior and posterior layers of the greater omentum (Fig. 3.11*B*). The omental bursa communicates with the greater sac through the **omental foramen** (epiploic foramen, foramen of

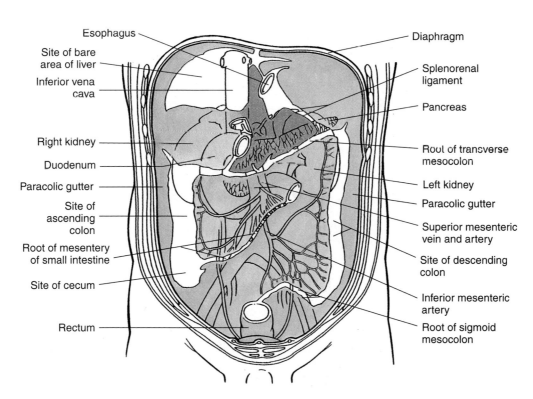

FIGURE 3.12   **Posterior wall of the peritoneal cavity showing the roots of the peritoneal reflection.** Anterior view.

Winslow), an opening situated posterior to the free edge of the lesser omentum forming the hepatoduodenal ligament (Figs. 3.9 and 3.10B). *The boundaries of the omental foramen are:*

- *Anteriorly*—portal vein, hepatic artery, and bile duct
- *Posteriorly*—IVC and right crus of the diaphragm, covered with parietal peritoneum; they are retroperitoneal
- *Superiorly*—caudate lobe of the liver, covered with visceral peritoneum
- *Inferiorly*—superior or first part of the duodenum, portal vein, hepatic artery, and bile duct.

FUNCTIONS OF GREATER OMENTUM

The large, fat-laden greater omentum usually prevents the visceral peritoneum from adhering to the parietal peritoneum lining the anterolateral abdominal wall. The apronlike greater omentum has considerable mobility and moves around the peritoneal cavity with both changes of position relative to gravity (standing, lying, and turning over) and peristaltic movements of the viscera. It is capable of wrapping itself around an inflamed organ such as the appendix, "walling it off" and thereby protecting other viscera from the infected organ.

Spread of Pathological Fluids

Peritoneal recesses are of clinical importance in connection with the spread of pathological fluids such as pus, a product of inflammation. The recesses determine the extent and direction of the spread of fluids that may enter the peritoneal cavity when an organ is diseased or injured.

ABDOMINAL VISCERA

The principal viscera of the abdomen are the esophagus (terminal part), stomach, intestines, spleen, pancreas, liver, gallbladder, kidneys, and suprarenal glands. The **transverse mesocolon**—mesentery of transverse colon (Fig. 3.11A)—divides the abdominal cavity into a:

- **Supracolic compartment** containing the stomach, liver, and spleen
- **Infracolic compartment** containing the small intestine and ascending and descending colon. The infracolic compartment lies posterior to the greater

omentum and is divided into right and left **infracolic spaces** by the mesentery of the small intestine. Most commonly, free communication occurs between the supracolic and infracolic compartments through the **paracolic gutters**—the grooves between the lateral aspect of the ascending or descending colon and the posterolateral abdominal wall (Fig. 3.12).

While **peristalsis** causing the propulsion of the ingested food mass occurs all along the alimentary or digestive tract, from pharynx to rectum, digestion mostly occurs in the stomach and duodenum. A specific type of "non-motile" peristalsis—ringlike contraction waves that begin around the middle of the stomach and move slowly toward the pyloric part of the stomach (see Fig. 3.15B)—is responsible for churning and mixing of the masticated food mass with gastric juices. "Nonmotile" peristalsis is followed by *motile peristalsis* for emptying the contents of the stomach into the duodenum. Absorption of chemical compounds occurs principally in the small intestine—**duodenum, jejunum,** and **ileum** (Fig. 3.13). The stomach is continuous with the duodenum, which receives the openings of the **pancreas** and **liver**—major glands of the alimentary tract. The **large intestine** consists of the **cecum,** which receives the terminal part of the ileum, **appendix, colon** (ascending, transverse, and descending), **rectum,** and **anal canal,** which ends at the **anus.** Most reabsorption of water occurs in the ascending colon. The stool (semi-solid feces or excrement) is formed in the descending and sigmoid colon and accumulates in the rectum before *defecation* (a bowel movement).

The **arterial supply to the abdominal part of the alimentary tract,** spleen, pancreas, gallbladder, and liver is from the **abdominal aorta** (Fig. 3.14A). The three major branches of the abdominal aorta are the **celiac trunk** and the **superior** and **inferior mesenteric arteries.**

The **portal vein**—formed by the union of the superior mesenteric and splenic veins (Fig. 3.14B)—is the main channel of the **portal system of veins** that collects blood from the abdominal part of the gastrointestinal (GI) tract, pancreas, spleen, and most of the gallbladder and carries it to the liver.

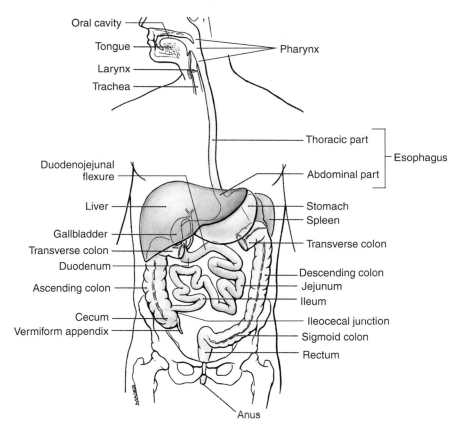

FIGURE 3.13 **Overview of the alimentary tract and abdominal viscera.** Anterior view.

ESOPHAGUS

The esophagus is a muscular tube that extends from the pharynx to the stomach (Figs. 3.13 and 3.15). The **esophagus:**

- Follows the concavity of the vertebral column as it descends through the neck and *posterior mediastinum* (see Chapter 2)
- Passes through the elliptical *esophageal hiatus* in the diaphragm, just to the left of the median plane at the level of T10 vertebra (see Fig. 3.38)
- Terminates at the *esophagogastric junction* where ingested matter enters the stomach through its *cardial orifice* to the left of the midline at the level of the 7th left costal cartilage and T11 vertebrae
- Is retroperitoneal during its very short abdominal course but is covered anteriorly and laterally by peritoneum.

The **esophagogastric junction** is marked internally by the abrupt transition from esopha-geal to gastric mucosa, referred to clinically as the Z-line (Fig. 3.15C), which is readily apparent during endoscopy on a living person, but often it is not apparent on the embalmed cadaver. At this junction, the diaphragmatic musculature forming the esophageal hiatus functions as a physiological **esophageal sphincter** that contracts and relaxes. Food or liquid may be stopped here momentarily and the sphincter mechanism is normally efficient in preventing reflux of gastric contents into the esophagus.

The *arterial supply of the abdominal part of the esophagus* is from the **left gastric artery** (Fig. 3.14A), a branch of the *celiac trunk*, and the **left inferior phrenic artery** (see also Chapter 2). The *venous drainage of the abdominal part of the esophagus is primarily to the portal venous system* through the **left gastric vein** (Fig. 3.14B), while the proximal *thoracic part of the esophagus* drains primarily into the *systemic venous system* through the esophageal veins entering the **azygos vein**

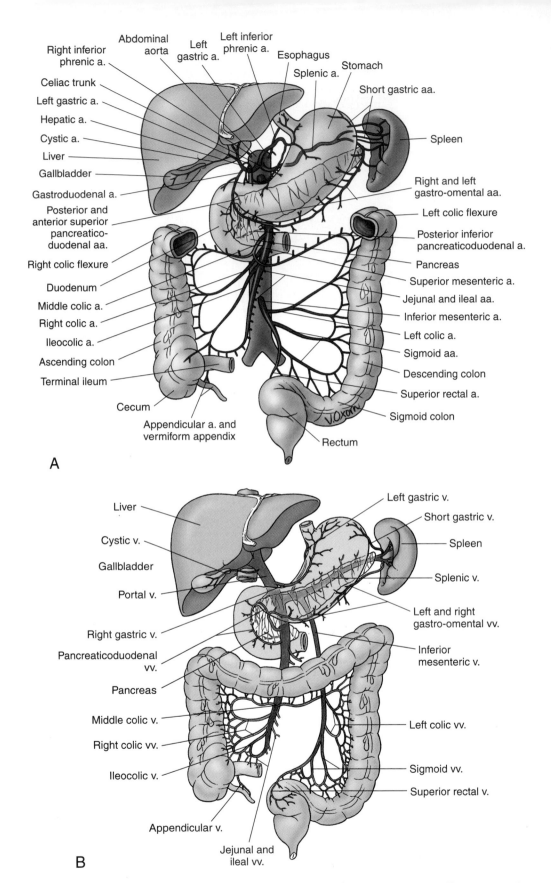

FIGURE 3.14 **Arterial supply and venous drainage of the abdominal part of the alimentary tract.**
A. Arterial supply. **B.** Venous drainage. The portal vein drains poorly oxygenated, nutrient-rich blood
from the GI tract, spleen, pancreas, and gallbladder to the liver.

(see Chapter 2). However, the veins of these two parts of the esophagus communicate and provide a clinically important portal-systemic anastomosis (p. 180).

The *lymphatic drainage of the abdominal part of the esophagus* is into the **left gastric lymph nodes** (Fig. 3.16*C*); efferent lymphatic vessels from these nodes drain mainly to the **celiac lymph nodes.** *The innervation of the abdominal part of the esophagus* (Fig. 3.16*D*) is from the **vagal trunks** (becoming anterior and posterior gastric nerves), the **thoracic sympathetic trunks,** the greater and lesser **splanchnic nerves,** and the **esophageal nerve plexus** around the **left gastric artery** and **left**

inferior phrenic artery (Fig. 3.14*A*, see also Chapter 2).

STOMACH

The stomach acts as a food blender and reservoir; its chief function is enzymatic digestion. The *gastric juice* gradually converts a mass of food into a liquid mixture—*chyme*—that passes into the duodenum.

Parts and Curvature of Stomach

The shape of the stomach is dynamic (changing in shape as it functions) and highly vari-

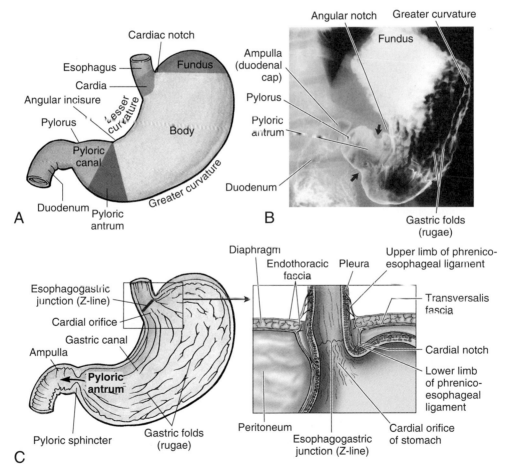

FIGURE 3.15 **Esophagus (terminal part), stomach, and proximal duodenum. A.** External surface, anterior view. **B.** Radiograph of the stomach and small intestine after barium ingestion. Anterior view. *Arrows,* peristaltic wave. **C.** Internal surface (mucous membrane), anterior wall removed. *Arrow* passes through the pyloric canal. The gastroesophageal junction is illustrated in the inset drawing.

able from person to person. *The stomach has four parts and two curvatures* (Fig. 3.15):

- The **cardia** is the part immediately adjacent to the Z-line—esophagogastric junction (Fig. 3.15*C*). The **cardial (cardiac) orifice** is the trumpet-shaped opening of the esophagus into the stomach. This part is primarily distinguished from the remainder of the stomach on an histological basis (presence of cardiac glands).
- The **fundus** of the stomach is the dilated superior part that is related to the left dome of the diaphragm and is limited inferiorly by the horizontal plane of the cardial orifice. The superior part of the fundus usually reaches the level of the left 5th intercostal space. The **cardial (cardiac) notch** is between the esophagus and fundus. The fundus may be dilated by gas, fluid, food, or any combination of these.
- The **body** of the stomach lies between the fundus and the pyloric antrum.
- The **pyloric part** of the stomach is the funnel-shaped region; its wide part, the **pyloric antrum,** leads into the **pyloric canal,** its narrow part. The primary distinction of the pyloric part is the histological presence of pyloric glands. The **pylorus**—the distal sphincteric region—is thickened to form the **pyloric sphincter,** which controls discharge of the stomach contents through the **pyloric orifice** into the duodenum.
- The **lesser curvature** forms the shorter concave border of the stomach; the **angular incisure** is the sharp indentation approximately two-thirds of the distance along the lesser curvature that approximates the junction of the body and pyloric part of the stomach.
- The **greater curvature** forms the longer convex border of the stomach.

Interior of Stomach

When contracted (empty), the gastric mucosa is thrown into longitudinal **gastric folds** (Fig. 3.15, *B* and *C*). A **gastric canal** (furrow) forms temporarily during swallowing between the gastric folds along the lesser curvature. Saliva and small quantities of masticated food and other fluids pass along the gastric canal to the pyloric canal.

Relations of Stomach

The stomach is covered by peritoneum except where blood vessels run along its curvatures and in a small area posterior to the cardial orifice. The two layers of the lesser omentum separate to extend around the stomach and come together again to leave its greater curvature as the greater omentum.

- *Anteriorly,* the stomach is related to the **diaphragm,** the left lobe of the liver, and the anterior abdominal wall (Fig. 3.10*A*).
- *Posteriorly,* the stomach is related to the **omental bursa** and **pancreas;** the posterior surface of the stomach forms most of the anterior wall of the omental bursa (Figs. 3.11 and 3.12).

The **stomach bed** on which the stomach rests when a person is in the supine position is formed by the structures forming the posterior wall of the omental bursa (see Table 3.6). *From superior to inferior, the stomach bed is formed by the:*

- Left dome of the diaphragm
- Spleen
- Left kidney and suprarenal gland
- Splenic artery
- Pancreas
- Transverse mesocolon and colon.

Vasculature and Nerves of Stomach

The gastric arteries arise from the celiac trunk and its branches (Fig. 3.16*A*, Table 3.5):

- **Left gastric artery** arises directly from the celiac trunk and runs in the lesser omentum to the cardia of the stomach. It gives off the esophageal artery and then turns abruptly to course along the lesser curvature and anastomose with the right gastric artery.
- **Right gastric artery** is highly variable in its origin, but it most often arises from the **hepatic artery** and runs to the left along the lesser curvature to anastomose with the left gastric artery.
- **Right gastro-omental artery** (gastroepiploic artery) arises as one of two terminal branches of the **gastroduodenal artery,** runs to the left along the greater curvature, and anastomoses with the left gastro-omental artery.

Surface Anatomy of Stomach

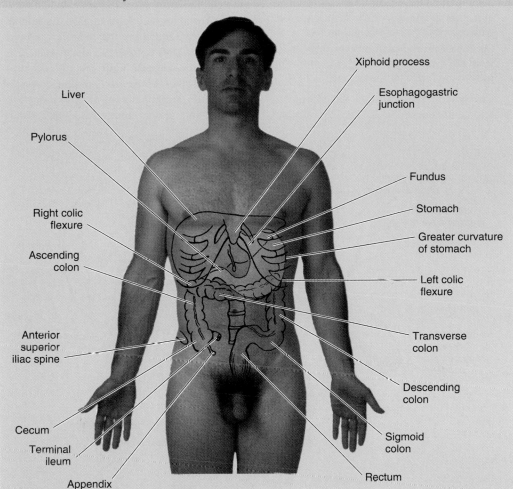

Liver

Pylorus

Right colic flexure

Ascending colon

Anterior superior iliac spine

Cecum

Terminal ileum

Appendix

Xiphoid process

Esophagogastric junction

Fundus

Stomach

Greater curvature of stomach

Left colic flexure

Transverse colon

Descending colon

Sigmoid colon

Rectum

The surface markings of the stomach vary because its size and position change under various circumstances (e.g., after a heavy meal).

- The **esophagogastric junction** lies to *the left of T11 vertebra* on the horizontal plane that passes through the tip of the xiphoid process
- The **cardial orifice** usually lies *posterior to 7th left costal cartilage,* 2 to 4 cm from the median plane at the *level of T10 or T11 vertebra*
- The **fundus** usually lies posterior to the *5th left rib* in the midclavicular plane
- The **greater curvature** passes inferiorly to the left as far as the *10th left costal*

cartilage before turning medially to reach the pyloric antrum

- The *lesser curvature* passes from the right side of the cardia to the pyloric antrum; the most inferior part of the curvature is marked by the *angular incisure* (Fig. 3.15*A*), which lies just to the left of the midline
- The *pyloric part of the stomach* usually lies at the level of the 9th costal cartilage at the level of L1 vertebra; the *pyloric orifice* is approximately 1.25 cm left of the midline
- *In the erect position, the pylorus usually lies on the right side;* its location varies from L2 through L4 vertebrae.

- **Left gastro-omental artery** arises from the distal part of the **splenic artery** and courses along the greater curvature to anastomose with the right gastro-omental artery.
- **Short gastric arteries** (four to five) also arise from the distal part of the **splenic artery** and pass to the fundus of the stomach.

The **gastric veins** parallel the arteries in position and course (Fig. 3.16*B*). The left and right gastric veins drain directly into the **portal vein** while the **short gastric veins** and the **left gastro-omental vein** drain into the **splenic vein,** which then joins the **superior mesenteric vein** (SMV) to form the portal vein. The **right gastro-omental vein** usually empties into the SMV. The **gastric lymphatic vessels** (Fig. 3.16C) accompany the arteries along the greater and lesser curvatures. They drain

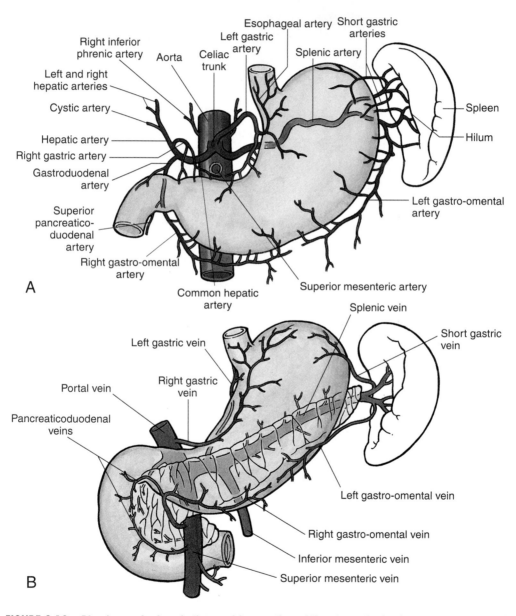

FIGURE 3.16 **Blood vessels, lymphatics, and innervation of the stomach, duodenum, pancreas, and spleen. A.** Arteries. **B.** Portal venous drainage.

TABLE 3.5. ARTERIAL SUPPLY TO ESOPHAGUS, STOMACH, DUODENUM, LIVER, GALLBLADDER, PANCREAS, AND SPLEEN

Artery	Origin	Course	Distribution
Celiac	Abdominal aorta just distal to aortic hiatus of diaphragm	Soon divides into left gastric, splenic, and common hepatic arteries	Supplies esophagus, stomach, duodenum (proximal to bile duct), liver and biliary apparatus, and pancreas
Left gastric	Celiac trunk	Ascends retroperitoneally to esophageal hiatus, where it passes between layers of hepatogastric ligament	Distal portion of esophagus and lesser curvature of stomach
Splenic	Celiac trunk	Runs retroperitoneally along superior border of pancreas; it then passes between the layers of splenorenal ligament to the hilum of spleen	Body of pancreas, spleen, and greater curvature of stomach
Left gastro-omental (gastroepiploic)	Splenic artery in hilum of spleen	Passes between layers of the gastrosplenic ligament to the greater curvature of stomach	Left portion of greater curvature of stomach
Short gastric (*n* = 4–5)	Splenic artery in hilum of spleen	Pass between the layers of the gastrosplenic ligament to the fundus of stomach	Fundus of stomach
Hepatic[a]	Celiac trunk	Passes retroperitoneally to reach hepatoduodenal ligament and passes between its layers to porta hepatis; divides into right and left hepatic arteries	Liver, gallbladder, stomach, pancreas, duodenum, and respective lobes of liver
Cystic	Right hepatic artery	Arises within hepatoduodenal ligament	Gallbladder and cystic duct
Right gastric	Hepatic artery	Runs between layers of hepatogastric ligament	Right portion of lesser curvature of stomach
Gastroduodenal	Hepatic artery	Descends retroperitoneally posterior to gastroduodenal junction	Stomach, pancreas, first part of duodenum, and distal part of bile duct
Right gastro-omental (gastroepiploic)	Gastroduodenal artery	Passes between layers of greater omentum to greater curvature of stomach	Right portion of greater curvature of stomach
Anterior and posterior superior pancreaticoduodenal	Gastroduodenal artery	Descend on head of pancreas	Proximal portion of duodenum and head of pancreas
Anterior and posterior inferior pancreaticoduodenal	Superior mesenteric artery	Ascend retroperitoneally on head of pancreas	Distal portion of duodenum and head of pancreas

[a]For descriptive purposes, the hepatic artery is often divided into the common hepatic artery from its origin to the origin of gastroduodenal artery, and the remainder of the vessel is called hepatic artery proper.

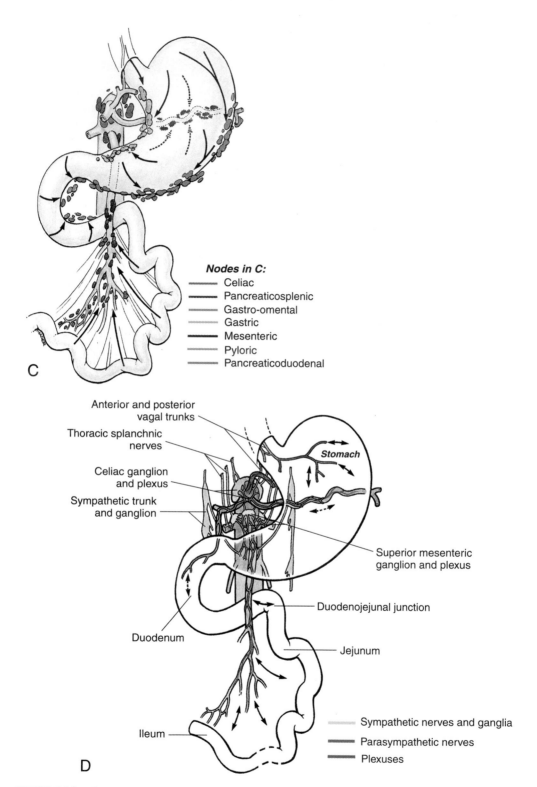

FIGURE 3.16 *Continued.* **C.** Lymphatic drainage. *Arrows,* direction of lymph flow to lymph nodes. **D.** Innervation. *Arrows,* afferent and efferent nerves.

lymph from its anterior and posterior surfaces toward its curvatures, where the **gastric and gastro-omental lymph nodes** are located. The efferent vessels from these nodes accompany the large arteries to the **celiac lymph nodes.**

The **parasympathetic nerve supply of the stomach** (Fig. 3.16*D*) is from the anterior and posterior **vagal trunks** and their branches, which enter the abdomen through the esophageal hiatus. The **sympathetic nerve supply of the stomach** from T6 through T9 segments of the spinal cord passes to the **celiac plexus** via the greater splanchnic nerves and is distributed as plexuses around the gastric and gastro-omental arteries.

SMALL INTESTINE

The small intestine—consisting of the duodenum, jejunum, and ileum—*extends from the pylorus of the stomach to the ileocecal junction,* where the ileum joins the cecum, the first part of the large intestine (Fig. 3.13).

Duodenum

The duodenum—*the first and shortest part of the small intestine*—is also the widest and most fixed part. The duodenum *begins at the* pylorus on the right side and *ends at the duode-*nojejunal junction on the left side. Four parts of the duodenum are described (Fig. 3.17):

- **Superior (1st) part** is short (approximately 5 cm long), mostly horizontal, and lies anterolateral to the body of L1 vertebra.
- **Descending (2nd) part** is longer (7–10 cm long) and runs inferiorly along the right sides of L2 and L3 vertebrae, curving around the head of the pancreas. Initially it lies to the right and parallel to the IVC.
- **Horizontal (3rd) part** (6–8 cm long) crosses anterior to the IVC and aorta and posterior to the SMA and SMV at the level of L3 vertebra
- **Ascending (4th) part** is short (approximately 5 cm long) and begins at the left of L3 vertebra and rises superiorly as far as the superior border of L2 vertebra. It passes on the left side of the aorta to reach the inferior border of the body of the pancreas. Here it curves anteriorly to join the jejunum at the **duodenojejunal junction** that takes the form of an acute angle—the **duodenojejunal flexure** (Fig. 3.13)—which is supported by the attachment of the *suspensory muscle of the duodenum* (ligament of Treitz). This muscle is commonly composed of a slip of skeletal muscle from the diaphragm and a fibromuscular band of smooth muscle from the third and fourth parts of the

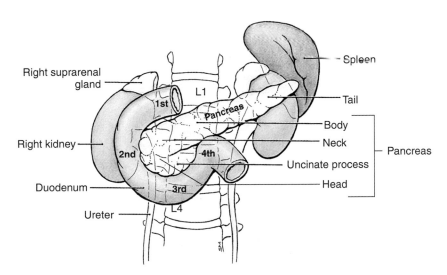

FIGURE 3.17 **Relations of the duodenum.** Schematic anterior view.

TABLE 3.6.   RELATIONSHIPS OF THE DUODENUM, SPLEEN, AND PANCREAS

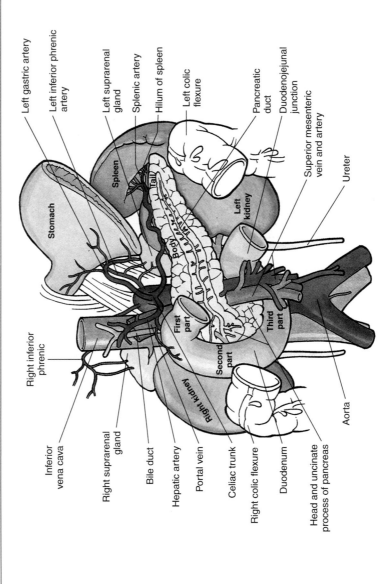

Organ	Anterior	Posterior	Medial	Superior	Inferior	Level
Superior (1st part) of duodenum	Peritoneum Gallbladder Quadrate lobe of liver	Bile duct Gastroduodenal artery Portal vein IVC		Neck of gallbladder	Neck of pancreas	Anterolateral to L1 vertebra
Descending (2nd part) of duodenum	Transverse colon Transverse mesocolon Coils of small intestine	Hilum of right kidney Renal vessels Ureter Psoas major	Head of pancreas Pancreatic duct Bile duct			Right of L2–L3 vertebrae
Horizontal (3rd part) of duodenum	SMA SMV Coils of small intestine	Right psoas major IVC Aorta Right ureter		Head and uncinate process of pancreas Superior mesenteric vessels		Anterior to L3 vertebra
Ascending (4th part) of duodenum	Beginning of root of mesentery Coils of jejunum	Left psoas major Left margin of aorta	Head of pancreas	Body of pancreas		Left of L3 vertebra
Spleen	Stomach	Left part of diaphragm	Left kidney		Left colic flexure	Left upper quadrant between 9–11 ribs
Head of pancreas		IVC, right renal artery and vein				
Neck of pancreas	Pylorus of stomach	SMA and SMV				
Body of pancreas	Omental bursa	Aorta, SMA, left suprarenal gland, left kidney and renal vessels				L2 vertebra
Tail of pancreas		Left kidney				

SMA, superior mesenteric artery; SMV, superior mesenteric vein; IVC, inferior vena cava.

duodenum. Contraction of this suspensory muscle widens the angle of the duodenojejunal flexure, facilitating movement of the intestinal contents. The suspensory muscle passes posterior to the pancreas and splenic vein and anterior to the left renal vein.

The first 2 cm of the superior part of the duodenum has a mesentery and is mobile. This free part—relatively dilated and smooth-walled—is the **ampulla** or duodenal cap (Fig. 3.15, *B* and *C*). The distal 3 cm of the superior part and the other three parts of the duodenum have no mesentery and are immobile because they are retroperitoneal (Fig. 3.12). The principal relations of the duodenum are outlined in Table 3.6.

An important transition in the blood supply of the alimentary tract occurs over the course of the descending (2nd) part of the duodenum, approximately where the bile duct enters. Consequently, the **duodenal arteries** arise from two different sources (Fig. 3.16*A*; see Fig. 3.23*A*):

- Proximally, the abdominal part of the alimentary tract is supplied by the **celiac trunk,** with the 1st and 2nd parts of the duodenum being supplied via the gastroduodenal artery and its branch, the **superior pancreaticoduodenal artery.**
- Distally, a major part of the alimentary canal (extending as far distally as the left colic flexure) is supplied by the **SMA,** with the 3rd and 4th parts of the duodenum being supplied by its branch, the **inferior pancreaticoduodenal artery.**

The pancreaticoduodenal arteries form an anastomotic loop between the celiac trunk and SMA; consequently, there is potential for collateral circulation here. The **duodenal veins** follow the arteries and drain into the **portal vein** (Fig. 3.16*B*)—some veins drain directly and others indirectly through the superior mesenteric and splenic veins. The **duodenal lymphatic vessels** follow the arteries in a retrograde direction. The anterior lymphatic vessels drain into the **pancreaticoduodenal lymph nodes** located along the superior and inferior pancreaticoduodenal arteries, and into the **py-**loric lymph nodes** that lie along the gastro-duodenal artery (Fig. 3.16*C*). The posterior lymphatic vessels pass posterior to the head of the pancreas and drain into the **superior mesenteric lymph nodes.** Efferent lymphatic vessels from the duodenal lymph nodes drain into the **celiac lymph nodes.** The **nerves of the duodenum** derive from the **vagus** and **sympathetic nerves** through the **celiac** and **superior mesenteric plexuses** on the pancreaticoduodenal arteries (Fig. 3.16*D*).

DUODENAL ULCERS

Most inflammatory erosions of the duodenal wall—*duodenal ulcers*—are in the posterior wall of the superior part of the duodenum. Occasionally an ulcer perforates the duodenal wall permitting its contents to enter the peritoneal cavity and produce *peritonitis.* Because the superior part of the duodenum closely relates to the liver and gallbladder, either of them may adhere to and be ulcerated by a duodenal ulcer. *Erosion of the gastroduodenal artery,* a posterior relation of the superior part of the duodenum, by a duodenal ulcer results in severe hemorrhage into the peritoneal cavity.

Jejunum and Ileum

The jejunum begins at the **duodenojejunal junction** and the ileum ends at the **ileocecal junction**—the union of the terminal ileum and cecum (Fig 3.13). Together, the jejunum and ileum are 6 to 7 meters long in cadavers; however, tonic contraction makes them substantially shorter in living persons. The jejunum constitutes approximately two-fifths of the length and the ileum the remainder. The terminal ileum usually lies in the pelvis from which it ascends to end in the medial aspect of the cecum. Although no clear line of demarcation between the jejunum and ileum exists, they have distinctive characteristics for most of their lengths (Table 3.7).

The **mesentery**—a fan-shaped fold of peritoneum—attaches the jejunum and ileum to the posterior abdominal wall. The **root (origin) of the mesentery** (approximately 15 cm long) is directed obliquely, inferiorly, and to the right (Fig. 3.18). It extends from the duodenojejunal junction on the left side of L2 vertebra to the ileocolic junction and the right

TABLE 3.7.   DISTINGUISHING CHARACTERISTICS OF JEJUNUM AND ILEUM IN LIVING PERSONS

Characteristic	Jejunum	Ileum
Color	Deeper red	Paler pink
Caliber	2–4 cm	2–3 cm
Wall	Thick and heavy	Thin and light
Vascularity	Greater	Less
Vasa recta	Long	Short
Arcades	A few large loops	Many short loops
Fat in mesentery	Less	More
Circular folds (plicae circulares)	Large, tall, and closely packed	Low and sparse; absent in distal part
Lymphoid nodules (Peyer's patches)	Few	Many

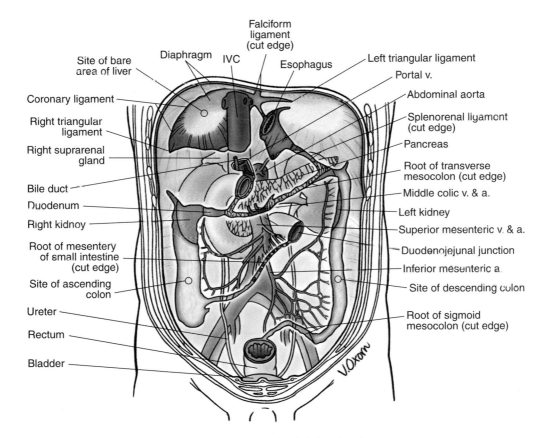

FIGURE 3.18   Posterior wall of the peritoneal cavity. Anterior view.

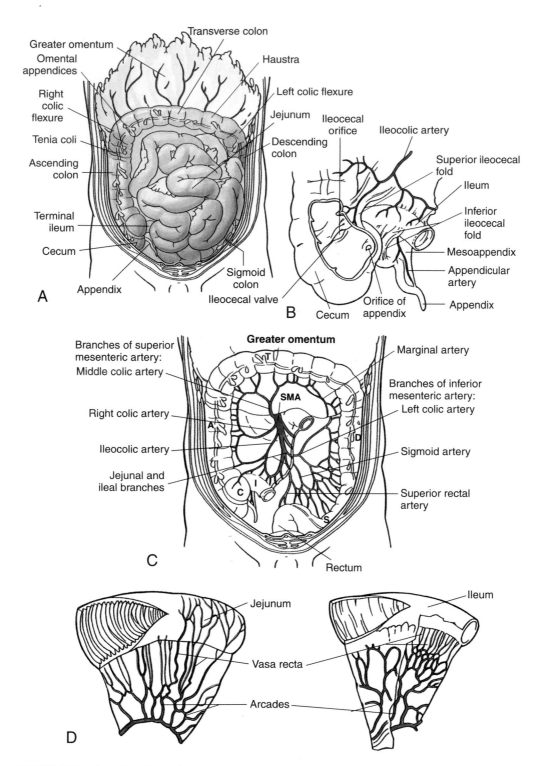

FIGURE 3.19 **Small and large intestine, arteries, and mesenteries. A.** Greater omentum has been pulled superiorly to show the intestine. Anterior view. **B.** Cecum and appendix showing their blood supply. Anterior view. A window has been cut in the wall of the cecum to show the ileocecal orifice and the orifice of the appendix. **C.** Most of the small intestine has been removed to show the blood supply of the large intestine. Anterior view. *T*, transverse colon; *SMA*, superior mesenteric artery; *A*, ascending colon; *D*, descending colon; *I*, terminal ileum; *C*, cecum; *S*, sigmoid colon. **D.** Blood supply of jejunum and ileum.

sacroiliac joint. *The root of the mesentery crosses (successively) the:*

- Ascending and horizontal parts of duodenum
- Abdominal aorta
- Inferior vena cava
- Right ureter
- Right psoas major
- Right testicular or ovarian vessels.

The *superior mesenteric artery* (SMA) supplies the jejunum and ileum (Fig. 3.19*C*, Table 3.8). The **SMA** runs between the layers of the mesentery and sends many branches to the jejunum and ileum. The arteries unite to form loops or arches—**arterial arcades**—that give rise to straight arteries—the **vasa recta** (Fig. 3.19*D*). The **superior mesenteric vein** (SMV) drains the jejunum and ileum (Fig. 3.16*B*). The **SMV** lies anterior and to the right of the SMA in the root of the mesentery. The SMV ends posterior to the neck of the pancreas where it unites with the splenic vein to form the portal vein.

The **lymphatic vessels of the jejunum and ileum** pass between the layers of the mesen-

TABLE 3.8. ARTERIAL SUPPLY TO INTESTINES

Artery	Origin	Course	Distribution
Superior mesenteric	Abdominal aorta	Runs in root of mesentery to ileocecal junction	Part of gastrointestinal tract derived from midgut
Intestinal (*n*=15–18)	Superior mesenteric artery	Passes between the two layers of mesentery	Jejunum and ileum
Middle colic	Superior mesenteric artery	Ascends retroperitoneally and passes between layers of transverse mesocolon	Transverse colon
Right colic	Superior mesenteric artery	Passes retroperitoneally to reach ascending colon	Ascending colon
Ileocolic	Terminal branch of superior mesenteric artery	Runs along root of mesentery and divides into ileal and colic branches	Ileum, cecum, and ascending colon
Appendicular	Ileocolic artery	Passes between layers of mesoappendix	Appendix
Inferior mesenteric	Abdominal aorta	Descends retroperitoneally to left of abdominal aorta	Supplies part of gastrointestinal tract derived from hindgut
Left colic	Inferior mesenteric artery	Passes retroperitoneally toward left to descending colon	Descending colon
Sigmoid (*n*=3–4)	Inferior mesenteric artery	Passes retroperitoneally toward left to descending colon	Descending and sigmoid colon
Superior rectal	Terminal branch of inferior mesenteric artery	Descends retroperitoneally to rectum	Proximal part of rectum
Middle rectal	Internal iliac artery	Passes retroperitoneally to rectum	Midpart of rectum
Inferior rectal	Internal pudendal artery	Crosses ischioanal fossa to reach rectum	Distal part of rectum and anal canal

tery (Fig. 3.16C); the **mesenteric lymph nodes** are located:

- Close to the intestinal wall
- Among the arterial arcades
- Along the proximal part of the SMA.

Efferent lymphatic vessels from the mesenteric nodes drain into the **superior mesenteric lymph nodes.** Lymphatic vessels from the terminal ileum follow the ileal branch of the ileocolic artery to the **ileocolic lymph nodes.**

The SMA and its branches are surrounded by a dense **perivascular nerve plexus** through which the nerve fibers are conducted to the parts of the intestine supplied by the SMA. The **sympathetic fibers** in the nerves to the jejunum and ileum originate in the T5 through T9 segments of the spinal cord and reach the **celiac plexus** through the *sympathetic trunks* and *thoracic (greater and lesser) splanchnic nerves* (Figs. 3.16D and 3.20). The presynaptic sympathetic fibers synapse on cell bodies of postsynaptic sympathetic neurons in the *celiac and superior mesenteric (prevertebral) ganglia.* **The parasympathetic fibers** in the nerves to the jejunum and ileum derive from the **posterior vagal trunk.** The presynaptic parasympa-

thetic fibers synapse with postsynaptic parasympathetic neurons in the *myenteric and submucous plexuses* in the intestinal wall. In general,

- *Sympathetic stimulation reduces motility of the intestine and secretion and acts as a vasoconstrictor,* reducing or stopping digestion and making blood (and energy) available for "fleeing or fighting."
- *Parasympathetic stimulation increases motility of the intestine and secretion, restoring digestive activity following a sympathetic reaction.* The small intestine also has sensory (visceral afferent) fibers. The intestine is insensitive to most pain stimuli, including cutting and burning; however, it is sensitive to sudden distention ("gas pains") and transient ischemia from abnormally long contractions that are perceived as **colic** (spasmodic abdominal pains—"intestinal cramps").

ISCHEMIA OF SMALL INTESTINE

Occlusion of vasa recta by thrombi (blood clots) results in *ischemia*—deficiency of blood supply—of the part of the intestine concerned. If the ischemia is severe, *necrosis* (pathologic death) *of the part of the intestine concerned results* and *ileus*—a severe colicky pain of the paralytic type, accompanied by distention, vomiting, and often fever and dehydration—occurs.

Ileal Diverticulum

An *ileal diverticulum* (Meckel diverticulum of ileum) is a congenital anomaly that occurs in 1 to 2% of people. A remnant of the proximal part of the embryonic yolk stalk, the diverticulum usually appears as a fingerlike pouch (3 to 6 cm long). *It is always on the antimesenteric border of the ileum*—the border of the intestine opposite the mesenteric attachment. An ileal diverticulum may become inflamed and produce pain mimicking the pain produced by appendicitis.

LARGE INTESTINE

The large intestine consists of the **cecum, colon** (ascending transverse, descending, and sigmoid), **rectum,** and **anal canal** (Fig. 3.19, *A* to *C*). *The large intestine can be distinguished from the small intestine by:*

- **Teniae coli**—three thickened bands of longitudinal muscle fibers

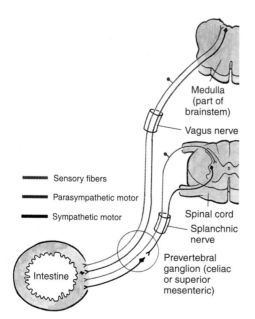

Sensory fibers
Parasympathetic motor
Sympathetic motor

Medulla (part of brainstem)
Vagus nerve

Spinal cord
Splanchnic nerve
Prevertebral ganglion (celiac or superior mesenteric)

Intestine

FIGURE 3.20   Innervation of intestine.

- **Haustra**—sacculations or pouches of the colon between the teniae
- **Omental appendices**—fatty appendices of colon
- **Caliber**—the internal diameter is much larger.

The three teniae coli comprise most of the longitudinal muscle of the large intestine, except in the rectum. Because the teniae are shorter than the large intestine, the colon has the typical sacculated shape formed by the haustra. *There are no teniae in the appendix or rectum;* they begin at the base of the appendix and run through the colon to the rectosigmoid junction.

Cecum and Appendix

The **cecum**—the first part of the large intestine that is continuous with the ascending colon—is a *blind intestinal pouch* in the right lower quadrant where it lies in the iliac fossa inferior to the junction of the terminal ileum and cecum. The cecum is usually almost entirely enveloped by peritoneum and can be lifted freely; however, *the cecum has no mesentery* (Fig. 3.12). The ileum enters the cecum obliquely and partly invaginates into it, forming folds (lips) superior and inferior to the **ileocecal orifice** (Fig. 3.19*B*). These folds form the **ileocecal valve.** The vermiform (L. wormlike) **appendix,** a blind intestinal diverticulum, extends from the posteromedial aspect of the cecum inferior to the ileocecal junction. The appendix varies in length and has a short triangular mesentery— the **mesoappendix**—which derives from the posterior side of the mesentery of the terminal ileum. The mesoappendix attaches to the cecum and the proximal part of the appendix. The position of the appendix is variable but it is usually retrocecal (posterior to cecum). The base of the appendix most often lies deep to a point that is one-third of the way along the oblique line joining the right anterior superior iliac spine to the umbilicus (*spinoumbilical* or *McBurney point*).

The cecum is supplied by the **ileocolic artery,** the terminal branch of the SMA. The appendix is supplied by the **appendicular artery,** a *branch* of the ileocolic artery (Fig. 3.19, *B* and

C, Table 3.8). A tributary of the SMV, the **ileocolic vein,** drains blood from the cecum and appendix (Fig. 3.14). The **lymphatic vessels** from the cecum and appendix pass to nodes in the mesoappendix and to the **ileocolic lymph nodes** that lie along the ileocolic artery (Fig. 3.21*A*). Efferent lymphatic vessels pass to the **superior mesenteric lymph nodes.** The *nerve supply to the cecum and appendix* derives from sympathetic and parasympathetic nerves from the **superior mesenteric plexus** (Fig. 3.21*B*). The **sympathetic nerve fibers** originate in the lower thoracic part of the spinal cord, and the **parasympathetic nerve fibers** derive from the **vagus nerves.** Afferent nerve fibers from the appendix accompany the sympathetic nerves to T10 segment of the spinal cord.

APPENDICITIS

Acute inflammation of the appendix is a common cause of an *acute abdomen*—severe abdominal pain arising suddenly. Digital pressure over the spinoumbilical (McBurney point) registers the maximum abdominal tenderness. *The pain of appendicitis usually commences as a vague pain in the periumbilical region because afferent pain fibers enter the spinal cord at the T10 level. Later, severe pain in the right lower quadrant results from irritation of the parietal peritoneum lining the posterior abdominal wall.*

Colon

The colon is described in four parts—ascending, transverse, descending, and sigmoid—that succeed one another in an arch (Fig. 3.19, *A* and *C*). The **ascending colon** passes superiorly on the right side of the abdominal cavity from the cecum to the right lobe of the liver, where it turns to the left as the **right colic flexure** (hepatic flexure). *The ascending colon—narrower than the cecum—lies retroperitoneally along the right side of the posterior abdominal wall.* The ascending colon is covered by peritoneum anteriorly and on its sides; however, in approximately 25% of people it has a short mesentery. The ascending colon is separated from the anterior abdominal wall by the greater omentum. **The arterial supply to the ascending colon** and right colic flexure is from branches of the SMA—the **ileocolic** and **right colic arteries** (Fig. 3.19*C*, Table 3.8). Tributaries of the SMV,

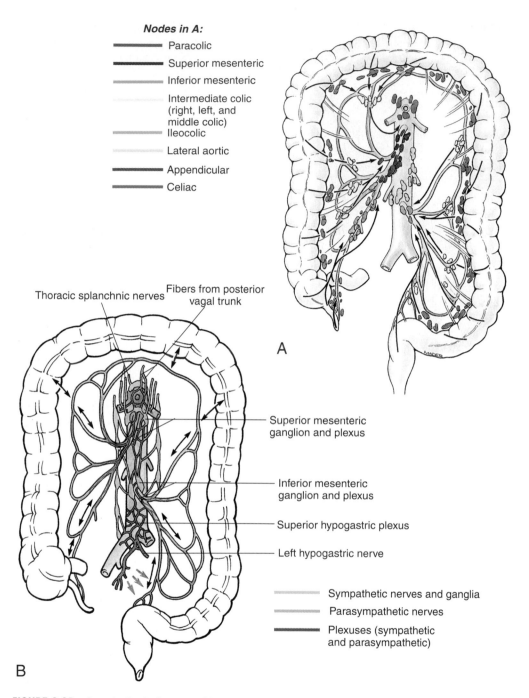

Nodes in A:

Paracolic

Superior mesenteric

Inferior mesenteric

Intermediate colic
(right, left, and
middle colic)

Ileocolic

Lateral aortic

Appendicular

Celiac

Thoracic splanchnic nerves

Fibers from posterior
vagal trunk

A

Superior mesenteric
ganglion and plexus

Inferior mesenteric
ganglion and plexus

Superior hypogastric plexus

Left hypogastric nerve

Sympathetic nerves and ganglia

Parasympathetic nerves

Plexuses (sympathetic
and parasympathetic)

B

FIGURE 3.21   Lymphatic drainage and innervation of the large intestine. A. Lymphatic drainage. *Arrows,* direction of lymph flow to lymph nodes. **B.** Innervation. *Black arrows,* afferent and efferent nerves; *green arrows,* pelvic splanchnic nerves (S2 through S4).

the **ileocolic** and **right colic veins,** drain blood from the ascending colon. The **lymphatic vessels** pass to the **epicolic and paracolic lymph nodes** and from them to the **superior mesenteric nodes** (Fig. 3.21*A*). The **nerves to the ascending colon** derive from the **superior mesenteric plexus** (Fig. 3.21*B*).

The **transverse colon**—the largest and most mobile part of the large intestine—*crosses the abdomen from the right colic flexure to the left colic flexure,* where it bends inferiorly to become the descending colon (Fig. 3.19*A*). The **left colic flexure** (splenic flexure)—usually more superior, more acute, but less mobile than the right colic flexure—lies anterior to the inferior part of the left kidney and attaches to the diaphragm through the **phrenicocolic ligament** (Fig. 3.10*B*). The mesentery of the transverse colon—the *transverse mesocolon*—loops down, often inferior to the level of the iliac crests, and is adherent to the posterior wall of the omental bursa. The **root of the transverse mesocolon** (Fig. 3.18) lies along the inferior border of the pancreas and is continuous with the parietal peritoneum posteriorly. The **arterial supply** of the transverse colon is mainly from the **middle colic artery** (Fig. 3.19*C,* Table 3.8), a branch of the SMA; however, it may also be supplied to variable degrees by the *right* and *left colic arteries.* **Venous drainage** of the transverse colon is through the **SMV.** *Lymphatic drainage* is to the **middle colic lymph nodes,** which in turn drain to the **superior mesenteric lymph nodes** (Fig. 3.21*A*). The *nerves of the transverse colon* arise from the **superior mesenteric plexus** and follow the right and middle colic arteries (Fig. 3.21*B*). These nerves transmit sympathetic and parasympathetic (vagal) nerve fibers. The nerves that derive from the **inferior mesenteric plexus** follow the left colic artery.

The **descending colon** passes retroperitoneally from the left colic flexure into the left iliac fossa, where it is continuous with the sigmoid colon. Peritoneum covers the colon anteriorly and laterally and binds it to the posterior abdominal wall. Although retroperitoneal, the descending colon, especially in the iliac fossa, has a short mesentery in approximately 33% of people. As it descends, the colon passes ante-

rior to the lateral border of the left kidney (Fig. 3.18). As with the ascending colon, the descending colon has a **paracolic gutter** on its lateral aspect (Fig. 3.12).

The **sigmoid colon,** characterized by its S-shaped loop of variable length, links the descending colon and the rectum (Fig. 3.19*A*). The sigmoid colon extends from the iliac fossa to the third sacral segment where it joins the rectum. *The termination of the teniae coli indicates the rectosigmoid junction.* The sigmoid colon usually has a long mesentery (*sigmoid mesocolon*) and therefore has considerable freedom of movement, especially its middle part. The **root of the sigmoid colon** has an inverted V-shaped attachment (Fig. 3.18), extending first medially and superiorly along the external iliac vessels and then medially and inferiorly from the bifurcation of the common iliac vessels to the anterior aspect of the sacrum. *The left ureter and the division of the left common iliac artery lie retroperitoneally posterior to the apex of the root of the sigmoid mesocolon.*

The second important transition in the blood supply to the abdominal portion of the alimentary tract occurs approximately at the left colic flexure. Proximal to this point (back to mid-duodenum), the blood is supplied to the alimentary tract by the **SMA;** distal to this point, blood is supplied by the **IMA.** The *arterial supply of the descending and sigmoid colon* is from the **left colic** and **sigmoid arteries,** branches of the IMA (Fig. 3.19*C,* Table 3.8). The left colic and sigmoid arteries pass to the left where they divide into ascending and descending branches. Usually all or most of the branches of the arteries supplying blood to the colon (ileocolic; right, middle, and left colic; and sigmoid arteries) anastomose with each other as they approach the colon, thus forming a continuous anastomotic channel, the **marginal artery** (of Drummond), which may provide important collateral circulation (Fig. 3.19*C*).

The **IMV** returns blood from the sigmoid and descending colon, flowing into the splenic vein and then the portal vein on its way to the liver (Fig. 3.14*B*). The *lymphatic vessels from the descending and sigmoid colon* pass to the epicolic and **paracolic lymph nodes** and then through the **intermediate colic lymph nodes** along the left colic artery (Fig. 3.21*A*). Lymph from these nodes passes to **inferior mesenteric lymph nodes** that lie around the IMA; however, lymph from the left colic main flexure also drains to the *superior mesenteric lymph nodes.* The **sympathetic nerve supply** of the descending and sigmoid colon is from the lumbar part of the sympathetic trunk and the **superior hypogastric plexus** through the plexuses on the IMA and its branches (Fig. 3.21*B*). The **parasympathetic nerve supply** is from the **pelvic splanchnic nerves,** which convey presynaptic fibers from the sacral part of the spinal cord (Table 3.9).

Rectum and Anal Canal

The rectum—the fixed terminal part of the large intestine—is continuous with the sigmoid colon at the level of S3 vertebra. The junction is at the lower end of the mesentery of the sigmoid colon (Fig. 3.18). The rectum is continuous inferiorly with the anal canal. These parts of the large intestine are described with the pelvis in Chapter 4.

COLITIS, COLECTOMY, AND ILEOSTOMY

Chronic inflammation of the colon (*ulcerative colitis*) is characterized by severe inflammation and ulceration of the colon and rectum. In some patients a *colectomy* is performed, during which the terminal ileum and colon, as well as the rectum and anal canal, are removed. An *ileostomy* is then constructed to establish an opening between the ileum and the skin of the anterior abdominal wall.

Colonoscopy

The interior of the colon can be observed with an elongated *endoscope,* usually with a flexible, fiberoptic *colonoscope.* The endoscope is a tube that inserts into the colon through the anus and rectum. Most tumors of the large intestine occur in the rectum; approximately 12% of them appear near the rectosigmoid junction.

TABLE 3.9.   SPLANCHNIC NERVES

Splanchnic Nerves	Autonomic Fiber Type[a]	System	Origin	Destination
A. Cardiopulmonary	Postsynaptic	Sympathetic	Cervical and upper thoracic sympathetic trunk	Thoracic cavity (viscera above level of diaphragm)
B. Abdominopelvic			Lower thoracic and abdominal sympathetic trunk	Abdominopelvic cavity (prevertebral ganglia serving viscera below level of diaphragm)

1. Lower thoracic:
    a. Greater
    b. Lesser
    c. Least
	Presynaptic	Sympathetic	Thoracic sympathetic trunk:
			  a. T5–T9 or T10 level
			  b. T10–T11 level
			  c. T12 level
				Prevertebral ganglia:
				  a. Celiac ganglia
				  b. Superior mesenteric ganglia
				  c. Aorticorenal ganglia

2. Lumbar	Presynaptic	Sympathetic	Abdominal sympathetic trunk	Inferior mesenteric ganglia and ganglia of intermesenteric and hypogastric plexuses
C. Pelvic	Presynaptic	Parasympathetic	Anterior rami of S2–S4 spinal nerves	Intrinsic ganglia of descending and sigmoid colon, rectum, and pelvic viscera

[a]Splanchnic nerves also convey visceral afferent fibers.

SPLEEN

The spleen, a mobile lymphatic organ, lies intraperitoneally in the left upper quadrant (Table 3.6). The spleen is entirely surrounded by peritoneum except at the **hilum** (Fig. 3.9), where the splenic branches of the splenic artery and vein enter and leave. It is associated posteriorly with the left 9th through 11th ribs and separated from them by the diaphragm and the **costodiaphragmatic recess**—the cleft-like extension of the pleural cavity between the diaphragm and the lower part of the thoracic cage (Fig. 3.10A). The spleen normally does not descend inferior to the costal (rib) region; it rests on the left colic flexure. The spleen varies considerably in size, weight, and shape; however, it is usually about 12 cm long and 7 cm wide—roughly the size and shape of a clenched fist. The *diaphragmatic surface of the spleen* is convexly curved to fit the concavity of the diaphragm. The anterior and superior borders of the spleen are sharp and often notched, whereas its posterior and inferior borders are rounded. The spleen contacts the posterior wall of the stomach and is connected to its greater curvature by the **gastrosplenic ligament** and to the left kidney by the **splenorenal ligament** (Figs. 3.9 and 3.10B). These ligaments, containing splenic vessels, are attached to the hilum of the spleen on its medial aspect. Except at the hilum where these peritoneal reflections occur, the spleen is intimately covered with peritoneum. The **hilum of the spleen** is often in contact with the tail of the pancreas and constitutes the left boundary of the omental bursa.

The **splenic artery**—the largest branch of the celiac trunk—follows a tortuous course posterior to the omental bursa, anterior to the left kidney, and along the superior border of the pancreas (Fig. 3.16A). Between the layers of the splenorenal ligament, the splenic artery divides into five or more "proper splenic" branches that enter the hilum of the spleen. The **splenic vein** is formed by several tributaries that emerge from the hilum (Fig. 3.16B). It is joined by the IMV and runs posterior to the body and tail of the pancreas throughout most of its course. The splenic vein unites with the superior mesenteric vein posterior to the neck

of the pancreas to form the **portal vein.** The *splenic lymphatic vessels* leave the lymph nodes in the hilum and pass along the splenic vessels to the **pancreaticosplenic lymph nodes** (Fig. 3.22A). These nodes relate to the posterior surface and superior border of the pancreas. The **nerves of the spleen** derive from the **celiac plexus** (Fig. 3.22B). They are distributed mainly along branches of the splenic artery and are vasomotor in function.

RUPTURE OF SPLEEN

Although well protected by the 9th through 12th ribs, the spleen is the most frequently injured organ in the abdomen when severe blows are received on the left side to one or more of the adjacent ribs. Blunt trauma to other regions of the abdomen that cause a sudden, marked increase in intra-abdominal pressure (e.g., by impalement on the handlebars of a bicycle) can also rupture the spleen. If ruptured, the spleen bleeds profusely because its capsule is thin and its parenchyma (essential substance) is soft and pulpy. *Rupture of the spleen causes severe intraperitoneal hemorrhage and shock.* Repair of a ruptured spleen is difficult; consequently, *splenectomy* is often performed to prevent the patient from bleeding to death.

PANCREAS

The pancreas—an elongated accessory digestive gland—*lies retroperitoneally and transversely across the posterior abdominal wall,* posterior to the stomach between the duodenum on the right and the spleen on the left (Figs. 3.17 and 3.19). The root of the transverse mesocolon lies along its anterior margin. The pancreas produces exocrine secretion (*pancreatic juice from the acinar cells*) that enters the duodenum and endocrine secretions (*glucagon* and *insulin* from the *pancreatic islets*) that enter the blood. For descriptive purposes the pancreas is divided into four parts: head, neck, body, and tail (Fig. 3.17). The **head of the pancreas**—the expanded part of the gland—is embraced by the C-shaped curve of the duodenum. The **uncinate process,** a projection from the inferior part of the head, extends medially to the left, posterior to the SMA. The **neck of the pancreas** is short and overlies the superior mesenteric vessels, which form a groove in its posterior aspect. The **body of the pancreas** continues from the neck and lies to the left of

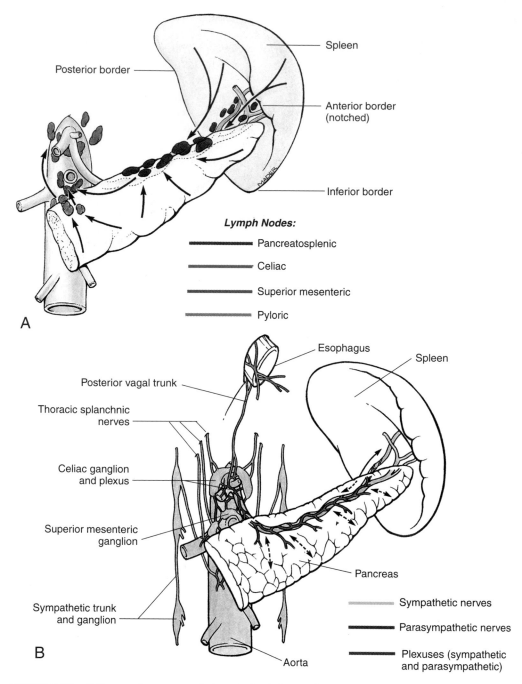

FIGURE 3.22   Spleen and pancreas. A. Lymphatic drainage. *Arrows,* direction of lymph flow to lymph nodes. **B.** Innervation. *Arrows,* afferent and efferent nerves.

the SMA and SMV. The **tail of the pancreas** is closely related to the hilum of the spleen and the *left colic flexure* (Table 3.6). The tail is relatively mobile and passes between the layers of the **splenorenal ligament** with the splenic vessels. The **pancreatic duct** begins in the tail of the pancreas and runs through the parenchyma (substance) of the gland to the head, where it turns inferiorly and merges with the bile duct (Fig. 3.23, *B* and *C*, Table 3.5).

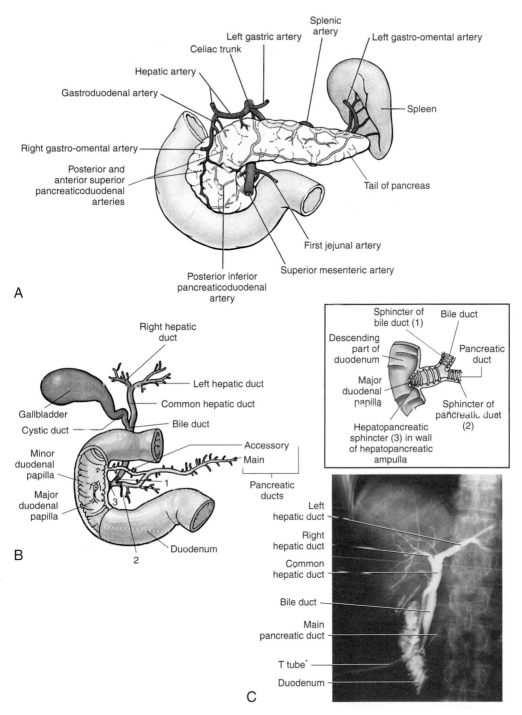

FIGURE 3.23   Pancreas and biliary system. A. Pancreatic arteries. **B.** Extrahepatic bile passages and pancreatic ducts. Sphincters are illustrated in the inset drawing. **C.** Endoscopic retrograde cholangiography and pancreatography of the bile and pancreatic ducts. *A T-shaped tube, the top of which is placed within the bile duct and the stem of the tube is placed through the skin.

The **bile duct** (common bile duct) crosses the posterosuperior surface of the head of the pancreas or is embedded in its substance. The pancreatic and bile ducts unite to form a short, dilated **hepatopancreatic ampulla** (Fig. 3.23*B*), which opens into the descending part of the duodenum at the summit of the **major duodenal papilla**. The **sphincter of the pancreatic duct** (around the terminal part of the pancreatic duct), the **sphincter of the bile duct** (*choledochal sphincter*, around the termination of the bile duct), and the **hepatopancreatic sphincter** (sphincter of Oddi)—around the hepatopancreatic ampulla—are smooth muscle sphincters that control the flow of bile and pancreatic juice into the duodenum. The **accessory pancreatic duct** drains the uncinate process and the inferior part of the head of the pancreas and opens into the duodenum at the **minor duodenal papilla** (Fig. 3.23*B*). Usually the accessory duct communicates with the main pancreatic duct but in some people it is a separate duct.

The **pancreatic arteries** derive mainly from the branches of the splenic artery (Fig. 3.23*A*, Table 3.5). The anterior and posterior **superior pancreaticoduodenal arteries,** branches of the gastroduodenal artery, and the anterior and posterior **inferior pancreaticoduodenal arteries,** branches of the SMA, supply the head. The **pancreatic veins** are tributaries of the splenic and superior mesenteric parts of the portal vein; however, most of them empty into the **splenic vein** (Fig. 3.16*B*). The **pancreatic lymphatic vessels** follow the blood vessels (Fig. 3.22*A*). Most of them end in the **pancreaticosplenic nodes** that lie along the splenic artery, but some vessels end in the **pyloric lymph nodes.** Efferent vessels from these nodes drain to the **celiac, hepatic,** and **superior mesenteric lymph nodes.** The *nerves of the pancreas* are derived from the **vagus** and **thoracic splanchnic nerves** passing through the diaphragm (Fig. 3.22*B*, Table 3.9). The **parasympathetic** and **sympathetic nerve fibers** reach the pancreas by passing along the arteries from the **celiac plexus** and **superior mesenteric plexuses.** They are vasomotor (sympathetic) and parenchymal (sympathetic and parasympathetic—to pancreatic acinar cells and islets) in their distribution.

RUPTURE OF PANCREAS

Pancreatic injury can result from sudden, severe, forceful compression of the abdomen such as the force of a seat belt in an automobile accident. Because the pancreas lies transversely, the vertebral column acts like an anvil and the traumatic force may rupture the pancreas. Rupture of the pancreas frequently tears its duct system, allowing pancreatic juice to enter the parenchyma of the gland and to invade adjacent tissues. Digestion of pancreatic and other tissues by pancreatic juice is painful.

Pancreatic Cancer

Cancer involving the pancreatic head accounts for most cases of extrahepatic obstruction of the biliary system. Because of the posterior relationships of the pancreas, cancer of the head often compresses and obstructs the bile duct and/or the hepatopancreatic ampulla. This condition causes *obstructive jaundice,* resulting in the retention of bile pigments, enlargement of the gallbladder, and jaundice (yellow staining of most body tissues). Cancer of the neck and body of the pancreas may cause portal or IVC obstruction because the pancreas overlies these large veins.

LIVER

The liver—the largest internal organ and largest gland in the body—weighs about 1500 g (Fig. 3.24*A*). It lies inferior to the diaphragm, which separates it from the pleura, lungs, pericardium, and heart. With the exception of lipids, every substance absorbed by the alimentary tract is received first by the liver. In addition to its many metabolic activities, the liver stores glycogen and secretes bile.

Surfaces of Liver

The liver has a convex *diaphragmatic surface* located anteriorly, superiorly, and somewhat posteriorly, and a relatively flat or even concave *visceral surface* located posteroinferiorly. The **diaphragmatic surface of the liver** is separated anteriorly from the visceral surface by the sharp inferior border of the liver (Fig. 3.24*A*). The diaphragmatic surface is smooth and dome-shaped where it is related to the concavity of the inferior surface of the diaphragm. The diaphragmatic surface is largely separated from the diaphragm by the **subphrenic space** between the anterior part of the liver and the diaphragm (Fig. 3.25). The subphrenic space is separated by the **falciform ligament** into right and left spaces. The **hepatorenal recess** (Morrison pouch) is a

Surface Anatomy of Spleen and Pancreas

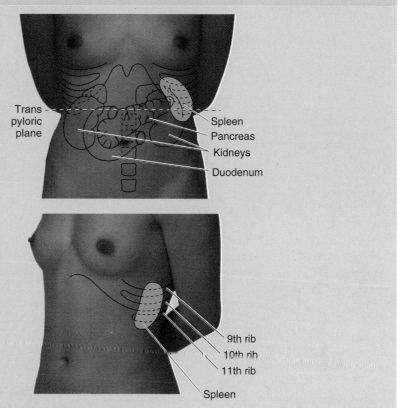

The spleen lies superficially in the left upper abdominal quadrant between the 9th to 11th ribs; its convex, costal surface fits the curved bodies of these elongated, flattened bones. In the supine position, the long axis of the spleen is roughly parallel to the long axis of the 10th rib. The *neck of the pancreas* overlies the 1st and 2nd lumbar vertebrae in the *transpyloric plane.*

Its head is to the right and inferior to this plane, and its body and tail are to the left and superior to this level. Because the spleen does not normally extend inferior to the left costal margin, the pancreas is deep in the abdominal cavity and lies posterior to the stomach and omental bursa. The spleen is seldom palpable through the anterolateral abdominal wall unless it is enlarged.

deep recess of the peritoneal cavity on the right side inferior to the liver and anterior to the kidney and suprarenal gland. The hepatorenal recess is a gravity-dependent part of the peritoneal cavity when a person is in the supine position; fluid draining from the omental bursa flows into this recess. The hepatorenal recess communicates anteriorly with the right subphrenic space. The diaphragmatic surface is covered with peritoneum except posteriorly in the **bare area of the liver,** where it lies in direct contact with the diaphragm (Fig. 3.24). The **visceral surface of**

the liver is covered with peritoneum, except at the *bed of the gallbladder* and the *porta hepatis* where vessels and ducts enter and leave the liver. *The visceral surface of the liver is related to the:*

- Right side of the anterior aspect of the stomach—the *gastric and pyloric areas*
- Superior part of the duodenum—the *duodenal area*
- Lesser omentum
- Gallbladder

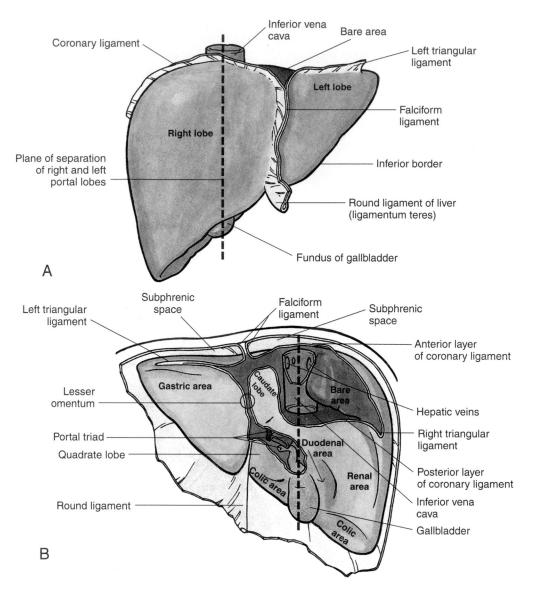

FIGURE 3.24 **Liver and gallbladder. A.** Diaphragmatic surface. **B.** Visceral surface. Gastric, duodenal, colic, and renal areas indicate where these organs are related to the liver. The bare area is demarcated by the reflection of peritoneum from the diaphragm to the liver as the anterior (upper) and posterior (lower) layers of the **coronary ligament**. These layers meet at the right to form the **right triangular ligament** and diverge toward the left to enclose the bare area. The anterior layer of the coronary ligament is continuous on the left with the right layer of the falciform ligament, and the posterior layer is continuous with the right layer of the lesser omentum. The left layers of the falciform ligament and lesser omentum meet to form the **left triangular ligament**.

- Right colic flexure and right transverse colon—the *colic area*
- Right kidney and suprarenal gland—the *renal and suprarenal areas.*

The **lesser omentum** passes from the liver to the lesser curvature of the stomach and the first

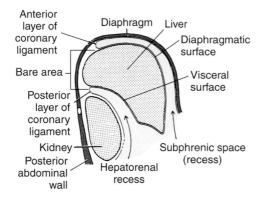

FIGURE 3.25   Bare area, surfaces, spaces, and recesses of the liver. Sagittal section through the diaphragm, liver, and right kidney showing that the bare area is situated between the posterior ends of two peritoneal recesses.

2 cm of the superior part of the duodenum (Fig. 3.26*A*). The **porta hepatis** or hepatic portal is a transverse fissure in the middle visceral surface of the liver, where the portal vein and hepatic artery enter the liver and the hepatic ducts leave. *The porta hepatis gives passage to the:*

- Portal vein
- Hepatic artery
- Hepatic nerve plexus
- Hepatic ducts
- Lymphatic vessels.

The thickened free edge of the lesser omentum extending between the porta hepatis and the duodenum is the **hepatoduodenal ligament** (Fig. 3.26*B*); it encloses the **portal triad**—portal vein, hepatic artery, and bile duct—a few lymph nodes and lymphatic vessels, and the hepatic plexus of nerves.

SUBPHRENIC ABSCESSES

Peritonitis may result in the formation of abscesses (localized collections of pus) in various parts of the peritoneal cavity. A common site for an abscess is in a subphrenic

Surface Anatomy of Liver

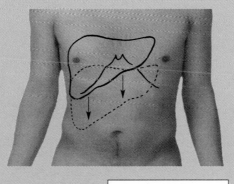

Position of liver
——————— Full expiration
- - - - - - - Full inspiration

The liver lies mainly in the right upper quadrant where it is hidden and protected by the thoracic cage and diaphragm. The normal liver lies deep to ribs 7 through 11 on the right side and crosses the midline toward the left nipple. The liver is located more inferi-

orly when one is erect because of gravity. Its sharp inferior border follows the right costal margin. When the person is asked to inspire deeply, the liver may be palpated because of the inferior movement of the diaphragm and liver.

Continued
space. Subphrenic abscesses occur much more frequently on the right side because of the frequency of ruptured appendices and perforated duodenal ulcers. Because the right and left subphrenic spaces are continuous with the hepatorenal recess (Fig. 3.25), pus from a subphrenic abscess may drain into one of the hepatorenal recesses, especially when persons are bedridden. A subphrenic abscess is often drained by an incision inferior to, or through, the bed of the 12th rib.

Lobes and Segments of Liver
Anatomically—based only on external features—the liver is described as having four

"lobes": right, left, caudate, and quadrate; however, functionally in terms of blood supply and glandular secretion the liver is divided into independent right and left parts—portal lobes (Fig. 3.24). The anatomical left lobe is demarcated from the caudate and quadrate lobes by the fissure for the round ligament of the liver and the fissure for the ligamentum venosum on the visceral surface and by the attachment of the falciform ligament on the diaphragmatic surface. The round ligament (ligamentum teres) is the obliterated remains of the umbilical vein (Fig. 3.27), which carried

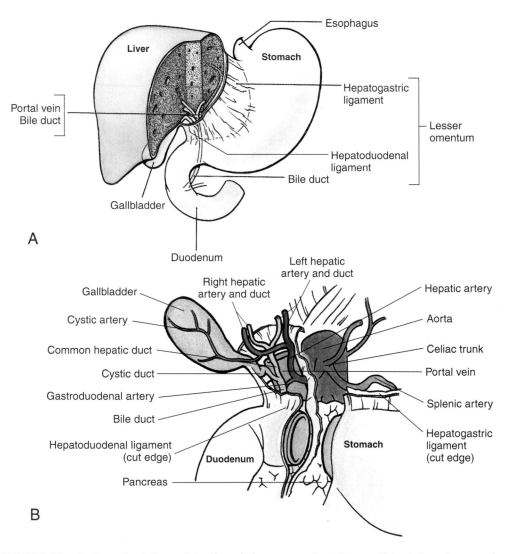

FIGURE 3.26   Peritoneal relations of the liver. A. Lesser omentum. Two sagittal cuts have been made through the liver, and these cuts have been joined by a coronal cut. **B.** Portal triad (bile duct, hepatic artery, and portal vein) within the hepatoduodenal ligament.

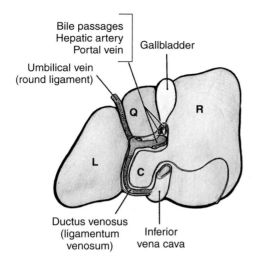

Bile passages
Hepatic artery
Portal vein   Gallbladder

Umbilical vein
(round ligament)

Q   R

L

C

Ductus venosus
(ligamentum   Inferior
venosum)   vena cava

FIGURE 3.27   Schematic view of the posteroinferior surface of the liver. The round ligament (ligamentum teres) is the occluded remains of the fetal umbilical vein. The ligamentum venosum is the fibrous remnant of the fetal ductus venosus. *R,* right lobe; *Q,* quadrate lobe; *C,* caudate lobe; *L,* left lobe.

well-oxygenated blood from the placenta to the fetus (Moore and Persaud, 1998). The ligamentum venosum is the fibrous remnant of the fetal ductus venosus that shunted blood from the umbilical vein to the IVC, short-circuiting the liver (Fig. 3.27).

The **portal lobes** are approximately equal in mass. The division between *right* and *left portal lobes* is approximated by the sagittal plane passing through the gallbladder fossa and the fossa for the IVC on the visceral surface of the liver (Fig. 3.24) and an imaginary line over the diaphragmatic surface that runs from the fundus of the gallbladder to the IVC. The left portal lobe includes the anatomical caudate and most of the quadrate lobes. Each portal lobe has its own blood supply from the hepatic artery and portal vein and its own venous and biliary drainage. *The portal lobes of the liver are further subdivided into eight segments* (Fig. 3.28). The segmentation is based on the principal branches of the right and left hepatic arteries, portal veins, and hepatic ducts. Each segment is supplied by a branch of the right or left hepatic artery and portal vein and drained by a branch of the right or left hepatic duct. *Intersegmental hepatic veins* pass

between and thus further demarcate segments on their way to the IVC.

HEPATIC LOBECTOMIES AND SEGMENTECTOMY
When it was discovered that the right and left hepatic arteries and ducts, as well as branches of the right and left portal veins, do not communicate significantly, it became possible to perform *hepatic lobectomies*—removal of the right or left (part of the) liver—with a minimal amount of bleeding. If a severe injury or tumor involves one segment or adjacent segments, it may be possible to resect (remove) only the affected segment(s): *segmentectomy.* The intersegmental hepatic veins serve as guides to the interlobular planes.

Vasculature and Nerves of Liver

The liver receives blood from two sources (Figs. 3.26*B* and 3.28*A*):

- The portal vein (70%)
- The hepatic artery (30%).

The **portal vein** carries poorly oxygenated blood from the abdominopelvic portion of the gastrointestinal tract. The **hepatic artery,** a branch of the celiac trunk, carries well-oxygenated blood from the aorta. At or close to the porta hepatis, the hepatic artery and portal vein terminate by dividing into right and left branches, which supply the right and left parts of the liver, respectively. Within each lobe the primary branches of the portal vein and hepatic artery are consistent enough to form **vascular segments** (Fig 3.28). Between the segments are the hepatic veins that drain parts of adjacent segments. The **hepatic veins,** formed by the union of the central veins of the liver, open into the IVC just inferior to the diaphragm (Fig. 3.24*B*). The attachment of these veins to the IVC helps to hold the liver in position.

The liver is a major lymph-producing organ; between one-quarter and one-half of the lymph received by the thoracic duct comes from the liver. The **lymphatic vessels of the liver** occur as *superficial lymphatics* in the subperitoneal fibrous capsule of the liver (Glisson capsule), which form its outer surface, and as *deep lymphatics* in the connective tissue that accompanies the ramifications of the portal triad and hepatic veins. Superficial lymphatics from the anterior aspects of the diaphragmatic and visceral surfaces and the deep

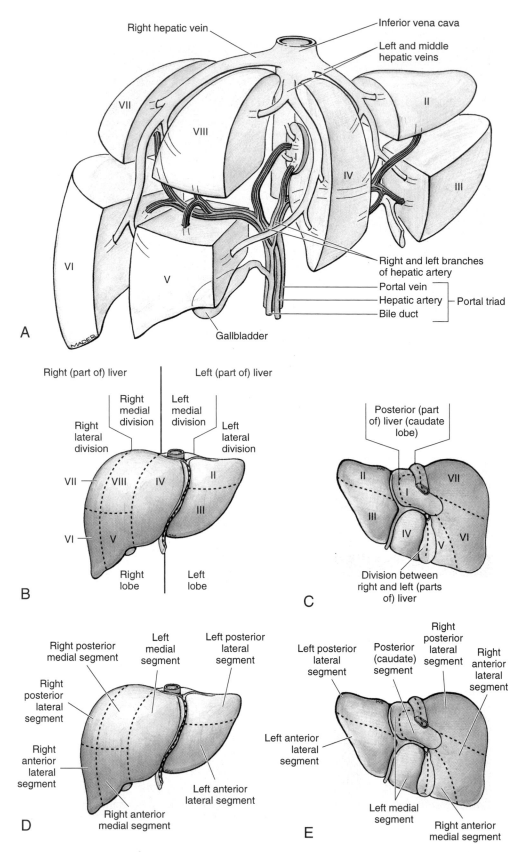

FIGURE 3.28 **Hepatic segmentation A.** Anterior view showing that segmentation is based on the principal divisions of the hepatic artery and portal vein and the accompanying hepatic duct. **B** and **D.** Anterior views. **C** and **E.** Posteroinferior views.

lymphatic vessels accompanying the portal triads converge toward the porta hepatis and drain to the **hepatic lymph nodes** scattered along the hepatic vessels and ducts in the lesser omentum (Fig. 3.29*A*). Efferent lymphatic vessels from these lymph nodes drain into the **celiac lymph nodes,** which in turn drain into the **chyle cistern** (L. cisterna chyli) at the inferior end of the thoracic duct (p. 202). Superficial lymphatics from the posterior aspects of the diaphragmatic and visceral surfaces of the liver drain toward the bare area of the liver.

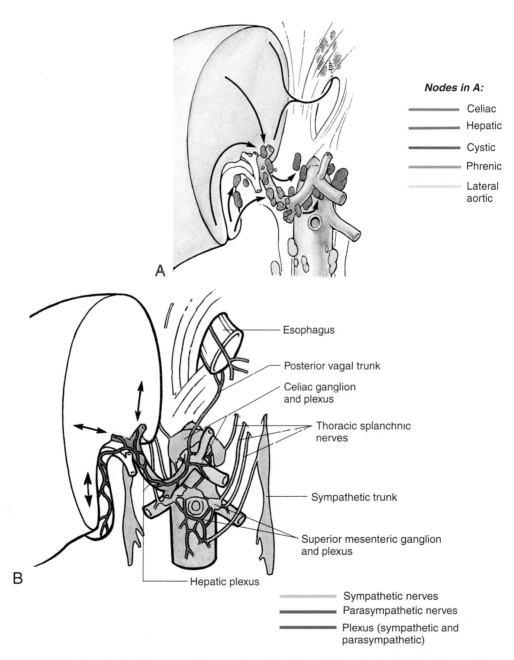

Nodes in A:

— Celiac
— Hepatic
— Cystic
— Phrenic
— Lateral aortic

— Esophagus
— Posterior vagal trunk
— Celiac ganglion and plexus
— Thoracic splanchnic nerves
— Sympathetic trunk
— Superior mesenteric ganglion and plexus
— Hepatic plexus

— Sympathetic nerves
— Parasympathetic nerves
— Plexus (sympathetic and parasympathetic)

FIGURE 3.29 **Lymphatic drainage and innervation of the liver. A.** Lymphatic drainage. *Arrows,* direction of lymph flow to lymph nodes. **B. Innervation.** *Arrows,* afferent and efferent nerves.

Here they drain into **phrenic lymph nodes,** or join deep lymphatics that have accompanied the hepatic veins converging on the IVC, and pass with this large vein through the diaphragm to drain into the **posterior mediastinal lymph nodes.** Efferent vessels from these nodes join the right lymphatic and thoracic ducts. The **nerves of the liver** derive from the **hepatic nerve plexus** (Fig. 3.29*B*), the largest derivative of the celiac plexus. The hepatic plexus accompanies the branches of the *hepatic artery and portal vein to the liver.* It consists of *sympathetic fibers* from the **celiac plexus** and *parasympathetic fibers* from the anterior and posterior **vagal trunks.**

LIVER BIOPSY

Hepatic tissue may be obtained for diagnostic purposes by liver biopsy. The *needle puncture* is commonly made through the right 10th intercostal space in the midaxillary line. Before the physician takes the biopsy, the person is asked to hold his or her breath in full expiration to reduce the *costodiaphragmatic recess* and to lessen the possibility of damaging the lung and contaminating the pleural cavity.

Rupture of Liver

Although less so than the spleen, the liver is vulnerable to rupture because it is large, fixed in position, and friable (easily crumbled). Often the liver is torn by a fractured rib that perforates the diaphragm. Because of the liver's great vascularity and friability, liver lacerations often cause considerable hemorrhage and right upper quadrant pain.

Cirrhosis of Liver

There is progressive destruction of hepatocytes in cirrhosis of the liver and replacement of them by fibrous tissue. This tissue surrounds the intrahepatic blood vessels and biliary ducts, making the liver very firm and impeding circulation of blood through it. Cirrhosis, the most common of many causes of *portal hypertension,* frequently develops in persons suffering from chronic alcoholism.

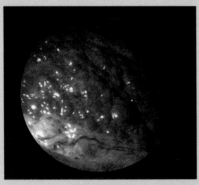

Cirrhosis of liver

BILIARY DUCTS AND GALLBLADDER

Bile is produced in the liver and stored in the gallbladder. In addition to storing bile, the gallbladder concentrates it by absorbing water and salts. When food enters the duodenum, the gallbladder sends concentrated bile through the cystic and bile ducts to the duodenum. The hepatocytes (liver cells) secrete bile into the **bile canaliculi** formed between them (Fig. 3.30*A*). The canaliculi drain into the small *interlobular biliary ducts* and then into large collecting bile ducts of the intrahepatic portal triad, which merge to form the right and left hepatic ducts. The **right and left hepatic ducts** drain the right and left functional (portal) lobes of the liver, respectively. Shortly after leaving the *porta hepatis,* the right and left hepatic ducts unite to form the **common hepatic duct,** which is joined on the right side by the **cystic duct** to form the **bile duct** (Fig. 3.30, *B* and *C*).

Bile Duct

The bile duct (common bile duct) forms in the free edge of the lesser omentum by the union of the **cystic duct** and **common hepatic duct** (Figs. 3.26 and 3.30*B*). The bile duct descends posterior to the superior part of the duodenum and lies in a groove on the posterior surface of the head of the pancreas. On the left side of the descending part of the duodenum, the bile duct comes into contact with the **main pancreatic duct** (Fig. 3.23, *B* and *C*). The two ducts run obliquely through the wall of this part of the duodenum, where they unite to form the **hepatopancreatic ampulla** (ampulla of Vater). The distal end of the ampulla opens into the duodenum through the **major duodenal papilla.** The muscle around the distal end of the bile duct is thickened to form the **sphincter of the bile duct** (choledochal sphincter). When this sphincter contracts, bile cannot enter the ampulla and/or the duodenum; hence, bile backs up and passes along the *cystic duct* to the **gallbladder** for concentration and storage. The **arteries supplying the bile duct** (Figs. 3.23*A* and 3.26*B*) include the:

- **Posterior superior pancreaticoduodenal artery** and **gastroduodenal artery,** supplying the retroduodenal part of the duct

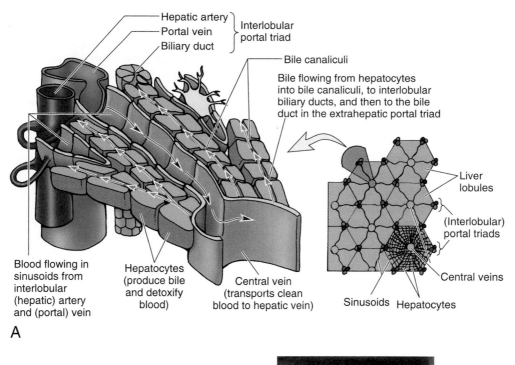

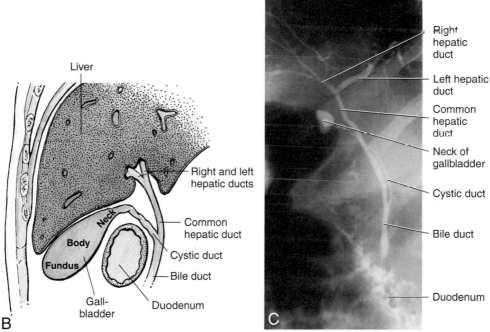

FIGURE 3.30   **Biliary ducts and gallbladder. A.** Flow of blood and bile in the liver. Schematic drawing of a small part of a liver lobule, illustrating the components of the interlobular portal triad and the positioning of the sinusoids and bile canaliculi. To the right of this drawing is a schematic view of the cut surface of the liver, showing the hexagonal pattern of the lobes. **B.** Extrahepatic bile passages and gallbladder. Schematic sagittal section. **C.** Endoscopic retrograde cholangiography of the gallbladder and biliary passages. The cystic duct usually lies on the right of the common hepatic duct and joins it just superior to the first part of the duodenum.

- **Cystic artery,** supplying the proximal part of the duct
- **Right hepatic artery,** supplying the middle part of the duct.

The *veins from the proximal part of the bile duct and the hepatic ducts generally enter the liver directly.* The **posterior superior pancreaticoduodenal vein** drains the distal part of the bile duct and empties into the **portal vein** or one of its tributaries (Fig. 3.31*A*). The **lymphatic vessels from the bile duct** pass to the **cystic lymph node** near the neck of the gallbladder, the **node of the omental foramen,** and the **hepatic lymph nodes** (Fig. 3.29*A*). Efferent lymphatic vessels pass to the **celiac lymph nodes.** Nerves are prominent along the bile duct. The posterior **hepatic plexus** is related to the bile duct and its nerves arise in the **right celiac plexus** and from the celiac division of the **posterior vagal trunk** (Fig. 3.29*B*).

Gallbladder

The pear-shaped gallbladder (7–10 cm long) lies in the **gallbladder fossa** on the visceral surface of the liver (Fig. 3.24*B*). Peritoneum completely surrounds the fundus of the gallbladder and binds its body and neck to the liver. The hepatic surface of the gallbladder attaches to the liver by connective tissue of the fibrous capsule of the liver. *The gallbladder has three parts* (Fig. 3.30*B*).

- The **fundus,** the wide end, projects from the inferior border of the liver and is usually located at the tip of the right 9th costal cartilage in the midclavicular line.
- The **body** contacts the visceral surface of the liver, the transverse colon, and the superior part of the duodenum.
- The **neck** is narrow, tapered, and directed toward the *porta hepatis.* The neck makes an S-shaped bend and joins the **cystic duct.** Internally, the mucosa of the neck spirals into a fold—the **spiral valve—** which keeps the cystic duct open so that bile can easily divert into the gallbladder when the distal end of the bile duct is closed by the sphincter of the bile duct and/or the hepatopancreatic sphincter, or

when bile passes to the duodenum as the gallbladder contracts. The **cystic duct** (approximately 4 cm long) connects the **neck of the gallbladder** to the common hepatic duct. The cystic duct passes between the layers of the lesser omentum, usually parallel to the **common hepatic duct**, which it joins to form the bile duct.

The **cystic artery** (Fig. 3.26*B*) that supplies the gallbladder and cystic duct commonly arises from the **right hepatic artery** in the angle between the common hepatic duct and the cystic duct. *Variations in the origin and course of the cystic artery are common.* The **cystic veins** draining the biliary ducts and the neck of the gallbladder may pass to the liver directly or drain through the portal vein to the liver (Fig. 3.31*A*). The veins from the fundus and body pass directly into the visceral surface of the liver and drain into the hepatic sinusoids. The **lymphatic drainage** of the gallbladder is to the **hepatic lymph nodes** (Fig. 3.29*A*), often by way of the **cystic lymph node** located near the neck of the gallbladder. Efferent lymphatic vessels from these nodes pass to the **celiac lymph nodes.** The *nerves to the gallbladder and cystic duct* (Fig. 3.29*B*) pass along the cystic artery from the **celiac plexus** (sympathetic), the **vagus nerve** (parasympathetic), and the *right phrenic nerve* (sensory).

IMPACTION OF GALLSTONES

The distal end of the hepatopancreatic ampulla is the narrowest part of the biliary passages and is the common site for impaction of a gallstone. Gallstones may also lodge in the hepatic ducts or in the cystic duct, causing **biliary colic** (pain in the epigastric region). When the gallbladder relaxes, the stone in the cystic duct may pass back into the gallbladder. If a stone blocks the cystic duct, *cholecystitis* (inflammation of the gallbladder) occurs because of bile accumulation, causing enlargement of the gallbladder. Pain develops in the epigastric region and later shifts to the right hypochondriac region at the junction of the 9th costal cartilage and the lateral border of the rectus sheath. Inflammation of the gallbladder may cause pain in the posterior thoracic wall or right shoulder as a result of irritation of the diaphragm. If bile cannot leave the gallbladder, it enters the blood and causes *obstructive jaundice* (discussed on p. 168).

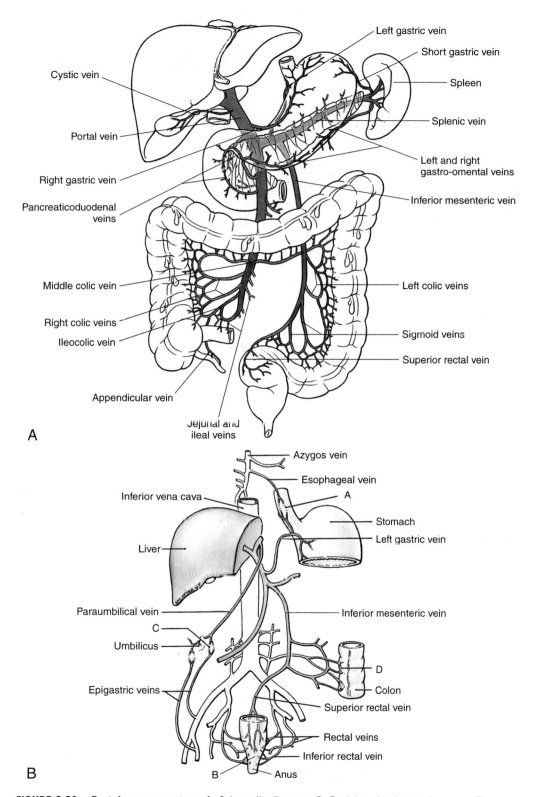

Cystic vein

Portal vein

Right gastric vein

Pancreaticoduodenal veins

Left gastric vein

Short gastric vein

Spleen

Splenic vein

Left and right gastro-omental veins

Inferior mesenteric vein

Middle colic vein

Right colic veins

Ileocolic vein

Left colic veins

Sigmoid veins

Superior rectal vein

Appendicular vein

Jejunal and ileal veins

A

Azygos vein

Esophageal vein

A

Inferior vena cava

Stomach

Left gastric vein

Liver

Paraumbilical vein

C

Umbilicus

Inferior mesenteric vein

D

Colon

Superior rectal vein

Epigastric veins

Rectal veins

Inferior rectal vein

B

Anus

FIGURE 3.31 **Portal venous system. A.** Schematic diagram. **B.** Portal-systemic anastomoses. These communications provide collateral circulation in cases of obstruction in the liver or portal vein. In this diagram, portal tributaries are darker blue and systemic tributaries are lighter blue. **A-D** indicate sites of anastomoses. *A,* between esophageal veins. *B,* between rectal veins. *C,* paraumbilical veins (portal) anastomosing with small epigastric veins of the anterior abdominal wall. *D,* twigs of colic veins (portal) anastomosing with the retroperitoneal veins.

PORTAL VEIN AND PORTAL-SYSTEMIC ANASTOMOSES

The **portal vein** is the main channel of the **portal venous system** (Fig. 3.31*A*). It collects poorly oxygenated but nutrient-rich blood from the abdominal part of the GI tract, including the gallbladder, pancreas, and spleen and carries it to the liver. There it branches to end in expanded capillaries—the **venous sinusoids of the liver** (Fig. 3.30*A*). *The portal venous system communicates with the systemic venous system in the following locations* (Fig. 3.31*B*):

- Between the **esophageal veins** draining into either the **azygos vein** (systemic system) or the **left gastric vein** (portal system); when dilated these are *esophageal varices.*
- Between the **rectal veins,** the inferior and middle veins draining into the IVC (systemic system) and the superior rectal vein continuing as the inferior mesenteric vein (portal system); *when abnormally dilated within subluxated mucosa these are hemorrhoids.*
- **Paraumbilical veins** of the anterior abdominal wall (portal system) anastomosing with **superficial epigastric veins** (systemic system); *when dilated these veins produce caput medusae*—varicose veins radiating from the umbilicus. These dilated veins were called caput medusae because of their resemblance to the serpents on the head of Medusa, a character in Greek mythology.
- Twigs of **colic veins** (portal system) anastomosing with retroperitoneal veins (systemic system).

Portal Hypertension
When scarring and fibrosis from *cirrhosis of the liver* (p. 176) obstruct the portal vein, pressure rises in the portal vein and its tributaries—producing *portal hypertension.* At the sites of anastomoses between portal and systemic veins, portal hypertension produces enlarged *varicose veins* and blood flow from the portal to the systemic system of veins. The veins may become so dilated that their walls rupture, resulting in hemorrhage. *Bleeding from esophageal varices* (dilated esophageal veins) at the distal end of the esophagus is often severe and may be fatal.

KIDNEYS, URETERS, AND SUPRARENAL GLANDS

The **kidneys** lie retroperitoneally on the posterior abdominal wall, one on each side of the vertebral column at the level of T12 to L3 vertebrae (Fig. 3.32). These *urinary organs* remove excess water, salts, and wastes of protein metabolism from the blood while returning nutrients and chemicals to the blood. The kidneys convey the waste products from the blood into the urine, which drains through the ureters to the urinary bladder. The **ureters** run inferiorly from the kidneys, passing over the pelvic brim at the bifurcation of the common iliac arteries. They then run along the lateral wall of the pelvis and enter the **urinary bladder.** The superomedial aspect of each kidney normally contacts a suprarenal gland. A weak septum of renal fascia separates these glands from the kidneys. The **suprarenal glands** function as part of the endocrine system, completely separate in function from the kidneys. They secrete corticosteroids and androgens and make epinephrine and norepinephrine hormones.

Kidneys

The *right kidney lies at a slightly lower level than the left kidney* because of the large size of the right lobe of the liver. Each kidney has anterior and posterior surfaces, medial and lateral margins, and superior and inferior poles (Fig. 3.33). The lateral margin is convex and the medial margin is concave where the renal sinus and renal pelvis are located. The indented medial margin gives the kidney a somewhat kidney-bean-shaped appearance. Superiorly, *the kidneys are related to the di-*

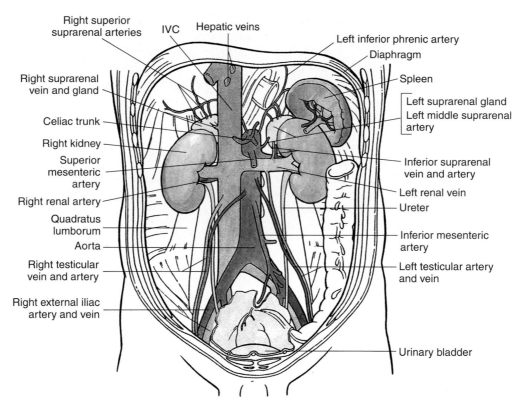

FIGURE 3.32 **Retroperitoneal viscera and vessels of the posterior abdominal wall.** Anterior view.

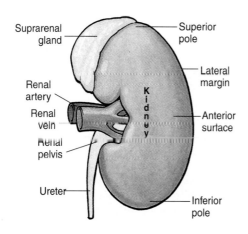

FIGURE 3.33 **Right kidney and suprarenal gland.** Anterior view.

hypogastric and ilioinguinal nerves descend diagonally across the posterior surfaces of the kidneys. The liver, duodenum, and ascending colon are anterior to the right kidney. The left kidney is related to the stomach, spleen, pancreas, jejunum, and descending colon. At the concave medial margin of each kidney is a vertical cleft—the **renal hilum** (see Fig. 3.35). The hilum is the entrance to the space within the kidney—the **renal sinus**—that is occupied mostly by fat in which the renal pelvis, calices, vessels, and nerves are embedded. The left hilum lies in the transpyloric plane, about 5 cm from the median plane at the level of L1 vertebra. At the hilum, the **renal vein** is anterior to the **renal artery,** which is anterior to the renal pelvis (Fig. 3.33).

Ureters

The **ureters** are muscular ducts with narrow lumina that carry urine from the kidneys to the urinary bladder (Fig. 3.32). The superior ex-

aphragm, which separates them from the pleural cavities and the 12th pair of ribs. More inferiorly, the posterior surface of the kidney is related to the quadratus lumborum muscle. The subcostal nerve and vessels and the ilio-

panded end of the ureter—the **renal pelvis** —is formed through the merging of two or three **major calices** (calyces), each of which was formed by the merging of two or three **minor calices** (Fig. 3.34). Each minor calix (calyx) is indented by the apex of the **renal pyramid**—the **renal papilla.** The abdominal parts of the ureters adhere closely to the parietal peritoneum and are retroperitoneal throughout their course. The ureters run inferomedially along the transverse processes of the lumbar vertebrae and cross the external iliac artery just beyond the bifurcation of the common iliac artery. They then run along the lateral wall of the pelvis to enter the urinary bladder.

Renal Fascia and Fat

The fibrous tissue surrounding the kidney—the **renal fascia**—is separated from the fibrous capsule of the kidney by **perirenal fat,** derived from extraperitoneal fat (Fig. 3.35), which is continuous at the hilum of the kidney with the fat in the **renal sinus.** External to the renal fascia is **pararenal fat,** which is most obvious posterior to the kidney. Movement of the kidneys during respiration is accommodated by the perirenal and pararenal fat. The renal fascia

sends collagen bundles through the fat, which, along with the renal vessels and ureter, hold the kidney in position. The renal fascia ascends to envelop the suprarenal glands. Inferior to the kidney the renal fascia is replaced by loose connective tissue, which connects the parietal peritoneum to the posterior abdominal wall.

PERINEPHRIC ABSCESS
The attachments of the renal fascia determine the path of extension of a *perinephric abscess*. For example, the fascia at the renal hilum firmly attaches to the renal vessels and ureter, usually preventing spread of pus to the contralateral side. However, pus from an abscess (or blood from an injured kidney) may force its way into the pelvis between the loosely attached anterior and posterior layers of the pelvic fascia.

Renal Transplantation
Renal transplantation is now an established operation for the treatment of selected cases of chronic renal failure. The site for the transplanted kidney is in the iliac fossa of the greater pelvis (Chapter 4) where it is firmly supported, and where only short lengths of renal vessels and ureters are required for transplantation. The renal artery and vein are joined to the adjacent external iliac artery and vein, respectively, and the ureter is sutured into the nearby urinary bladder.

Suprarenal Glands

The suprarenal (adrenal) glands are located between the superomedial aspects of the kidneys and the diaphragmatic crura (Figs. 3.32 and 3.33), where they are surrounded by connective tissue containing considerable perinephric fat. The glands are enclosed by renal fascia by which they are attached to the diaphragmatic crura; however, they are separated from the kidneys by fibrous tissue. *The shape and relations of the suprarenal glands differ on the two sides.*

- The *triangular right gland* lies anterior to the diaphragm and makes contact with the IVC anteromedially and the liver anterolaterally.
- The *semilunar left gland* is related to the spleen, stomach, pancreas, and the left crus of the diaphragm (see Fig. 3.38*B*).

Each suprarenal gland has two parts: the **suprarenal cortex** and **suprarenal medulla** (Fig. 3.34). These parts have different embryological origins, different functions, and usually somewhat different coloration (Moore and Persaud, 1998; Moore and Dalley, 1999).

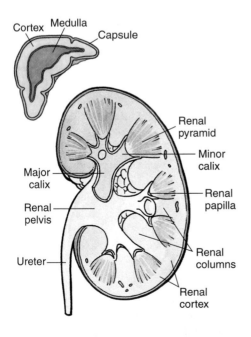

Cortex   Medulla
             Capsule

Renal pyramid

Minor calix

Major calix

Renal papilla

Renal pelvis

Renal columns

Ureter

Renal cortex

FIGURE 3.34   Coronal section of the kidney and suprarenal gland.

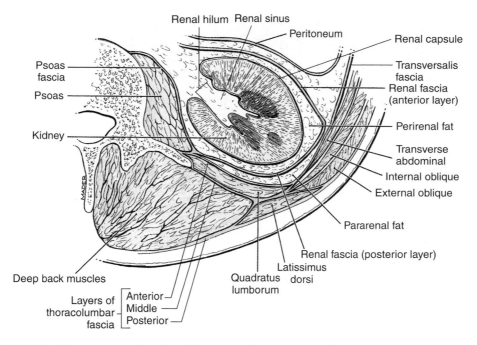

FIGURE 3.35 Transverse section of the kidney showing the relationships of muscle and fascia.

Vasculature of Kidneys, Ureters, and Suprarenal Glands

The **renal arteries** arise at the level of the IV disc between L1 and L2 vertebrae (Fig. 3.32). The longer **right renal artery** passes posterior to the IVC. Typically each artery divides close to the hilum into five **segmental arteries** that are end arteries; i.e., they do not anastomose (Fig. 3.36). Segmental arteries are distributed to the **segments of the kidney**. Several veins drain the kidney and unite in a variable fashion to form the renal vein. The **renal veins** lie anterior to the renal arteries, and the *longer left renal vein passes anterior to the aorta.* Each renal vein drains into the IVC. The **arteries to the ureters** (Fig. 3.32) arise mainly from three sources: the *renal artery, testicular or ovarian arteries,* and *abdominal aorta.* The **veins of the ureters** drain into the renal and testicular or ovarian veins. The endocrine function of the suprarenal glands makes their abundant blood supply necessary. The **suprarenal arteries** are (Fig. 3.32):

- **Superior suprarenal arteries** (six to eight) from the *inferior phrenic artery*
- **Middle suprarenal arteries** (one or more) from the *abdominal aorta* near the origin of the SMA

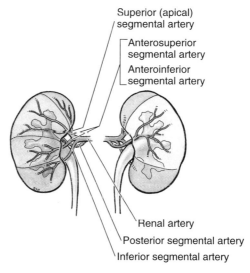

FIGURE 3.36 **Segments and segmental arteries of the kidneys.** Only the superior and inferior arteries supply the whole thickness of the kidney.

- **Inferior suprarenal arteries** (one or more) from the *renal artery.*

The *venous drainage of the suprarenal gland* is into a large **suprarenal vein** (see Fig. 3.39*B*). The short *right suprarenal vein drains into the*

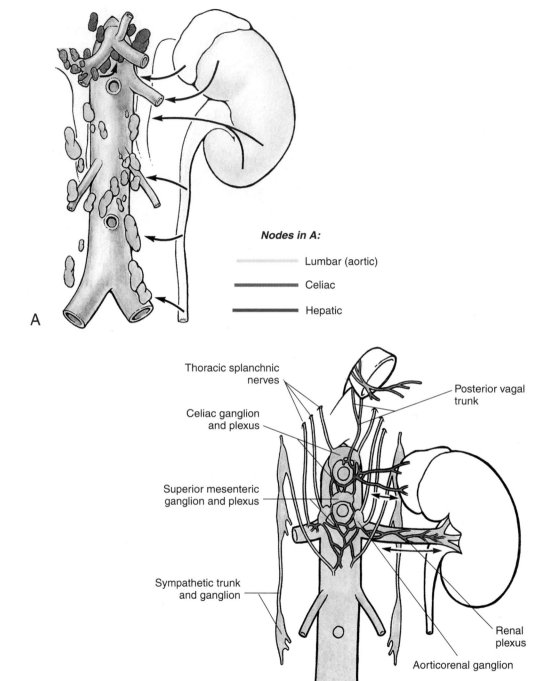

Nodes in A:

Lumbar (aortic)

Celiac

Hepatic

FIGURE 3.37 **Suprarenal gland, kidney, and proximal ureter. A.** Lymphatic drainage. *Arrows,* direction of lymph flow to lymph nodes. **B.** Innervation. *Arrows,* afferent and efferent nerves.

IVC, whereas the longer *left suprarenal vein,* often joined by the inferior phrenic vein, *empties into the left renal vein.*

The **renal lymphatic vessels** follow the renal veins and drain into the **lumbar lymph nodes** (Fig. 3.37*A*). Lymphatic vessels from the superior part of the ureter may join those from the kidney or pass directly to the lumbar nodes. Lymphatic vessels from the middle part of the ureter usually drain into the **common iliac lymph nodes,** whereas vessels from its inferior part drain into the common, external, or internal **iliac lymph nodes.** The **suprarenal lymphatic vessels** arise from a plexus deep to the capsule of the gland and from one in its medulla. The lymph passes to the **lumbar lymph nodes.**

Nerves of Kidneys, Ureters, and Suprarenal Glands

The **nerves to the kidneys and ureters** arise from the **renal plexus** and consist of sympathetic, parasympathetic, and visceral afferent fibers (Fig. 3.37*B*). The **renal plexus** is supplied by fibers from the thoracic (especially the least) splanchnic nerves (Table 3.9). The **suprarenal glands** have a rich nerve supply from the **celiac plexus** and **thoracic splanchnic nerves**. The nerves are mainly myelinated presynaptic sympathetic fibers that derive from the lateral horn of the spinal cord and are distributed to the chromaffin cells in the suprarenal medulla.

ACCESSORY RENAL VESSELS
During their "ascent" to their final site, the embryonic kidneys receive their blood supply and venous drainage from successively more superior vessels. Usually the inferior vessels degenerate as superior ones take over the blood supply and venous drainage. Failure of some of these vessels to degenerate results in *accessory (or polar) renal arteries and veins.* Variations in the number and position of these vessels occur in about 25% of people (Moore and Persaud, 1998).

Renal and Ureteric Calculi
Excessive distention of the ureter due to an *ureteric calculus* (kidney stone) causes severe rhythmic pain— *ureteric colic*—as it is gradually forced down the ureter by waves of contraction. These stones cause complete or intermittent obstruction of urinary flow. Ureteric colic is usually a sharp, stabbing pain (accompanied by nausea and

vomiting and other visceral responses) that follows the course of the ureter. The pain is referred to the cutaneous areas innervated by the spinal cord segments and sensory ganglia, which supply the ureter—mainly T11 through L2.

THORACIC DIAPHRAGM

The diaphragm is a dome-shaped, musculotendinous partition separating the thoracic and abdominal cavities. The diaphragm—*the chief muscle of inspiration*—forms the convex floor of the thoracic cavity and the concave roof of the abdominal cavity (Fig. 3.38). The diaphragm descends during inspiration; however, only its central part moves because its periphery, as the fixed origin of the muscle, attaches to the inferior margin of the thoracic cage and the superior lumbar vertebrae. The diaphragm curves superiorly into **right** and **left domes;** normally the right dome is higher than the left because of the large size of the liver. During expiration the right dome reaches as high as the 5th rib and the left dome ascends to the 5th intercostal space. *The level of the domes of the diaphragm varies according to the:*

- Phase of respiration (inspiration or expiration)
- Posture (e.g., supine or standing)
- Size and degree of distention of the abdominal viscera.

The muscular part of the diaphragm is situated peripherally with fibers that converge radially on the trifoliate central aponeurotic part—the **central tendon.** This tendon has no bony attachments and is incompletely divided into three leaves, resembling a wide cloverleaf. Although it lies near the center of the diaphragm, the central tendon is closer to the anterior part of the thorax. The surrounding muscular part of the diaphragm forms a continuous sheet; however, for descriptive purposes it is divided into three parts, based on the peripheral attachments:

- A **sternal part,** consisting of two muscular slips that attach to the posterior aspect of

Surface Anatomy of Kidneys and Ureters

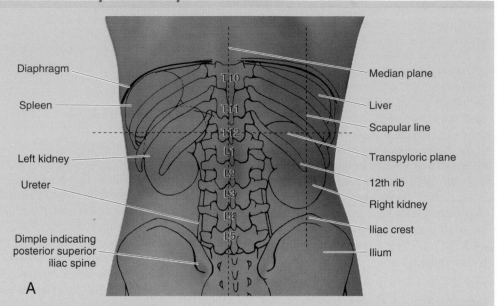

Diaphragm

Spleen

Left kidney

Ureter

Dimple indicating posterior superior iliac spine

T10
T11
T12
L1
L2
L3
L4
L5

Median plane

Liver

Scapular line

Transpyloric plane

12th rib

Right kidney

Iliac crest

Ilium

A

The hilum of the left kidney lies near the transpyloric plane, approximately 5 cm from the median plane. The transpyloric plane passes through the superior pole of the right kidney, which is approximately 2.5 cm lower than the left pole. Posteriorly, the superior parts

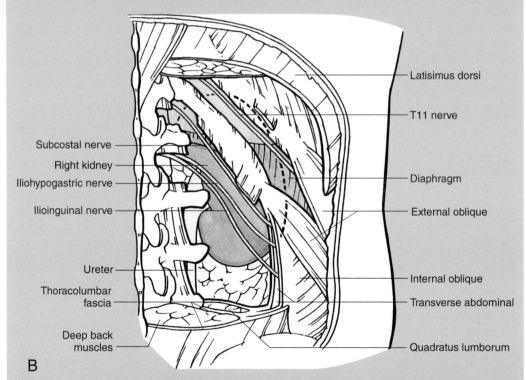

Subcostal nerve

Right kidney

Iliohypogastric nerve

Ilioinguinal nerve

Ureter

Thoracolumbar fascia

Deep back muscles

Latisimus dorsi

T11 nerve

Diaphragm

External oblique

Internal oblique

Transverse abdominal

Quadratus lumborum

B

of the kidneys lie deep to the 11th and 12th ribs. The levels of the kidneys change during respiration and with changes in posture. Each kidney moves approximately 3 cm in a vertical direction during the movement of the diaphragm that occurs with deep breathing. In extremely muscular and/or obese people, the kidneys may be impalpable. In most adults, the inferior pole of the right kidney is palpable by bimanual examination as a firm, smooth, somewhat rounded mass that descends during inspiration. The left kidney is usually not palpable unless it is enlarged.

the xiphoid process of the sternum; this part is not always present

- A **costal part,** consisting of wide muscular slips that attach to the internal surfaces of the inferior six costal cartilages and their adjoining ribs on each side; the costal part forms the domes of the diaphragm

- A **lumbar part,** arising from two aponeurotic arches—the medial and lateral **arcuate ligaments**—and the three superior lumbar vertebrae; the lumbar part forms right and left muscular crura that ascend to the central tendon.

The **crura of the diaphragm** are musculo-tendinous bundles that arise from the anterior surfaces of the bodies of the superior three lumbar vertebrae, the anterior longitudinal ligament, and the IV discs. The **right crus,** larger and longer than the left crus, arises from the first three of four lumbar vertebrae, whereas the **left crus** arises from only the first two or three. The crura are united by the **median arcuate ligament**, which passes over the anterior surface of the aorta. The diaphragm is also attached on each side to the **medial and lateral arcuate ligaments,** which are thickenings of the fascia covering the psoas and quadratus lumborum muscles, respectively.

DIAPHRAGMATIC APERTURES

The diaphragmatic apertures permit structures (e.g., esophagus, vessels, nerves, and lymphatics) to pass between the thorax and abdomen (Fig. 3.38). The three large apertures for the IVC, esophagus, and aorta are the caval opening, esophageal hiatus, and aortic hiatus.

Caval Opening

The caval opening (caval foramen) is an aperture in the central tendon primarily for the IVC. Also passing through the caval opening are terminal branches of the right phrenic nerve and some lymphatic vessels on their way from the liver to the middle phrenic and mediastinal lymph nodes. The caval opening is located to the right of the median plane at the junction of the tendon's right and middle leaves. The most superior of the three diaphragmatic apertures, *the caval opening lies at the level of the IV disc between the T8 and T9 vertebrae.* The IVC is adherent to the margin of the opening: consequently, when the diaphragm contracts during inspiration, it widens the opening and dilates the IVC. These changes facilitate bloodflow to the heart through this large vein.

Esophageal Hiatus

The esophageal hiatus is an oval aperture for the esophagus in the muscle of the right crus of the diaphragm at the level of T10 vertebra. The esophageal hiatus also transmits the anterior and posterior vagal trunks, esophageal branches of the left gastric vessels, and a few lymphatic vessels. In most cases, a superficial muscular bundle from the left crus contributes to the formation of the right margin of the hiatus.

Aortic Hiatus

The aortic hiatus is the opening posterior to the diaphragm. The aortic hiatus transmits the aorta, azygos vein, and the thoracic duct. Because the aorta does not pierce the diaphragm, bloodflow through it is not affected by its movements during respiration. The **aorta** passes between the crura of the diaphragm posterior to the median arcuate ligament, which is at the level of T12 vertebra.

Other Apertures in Diaphragm

There is a small opening, the *sternocostal foramen,* between the sternal and costal attachments of the diaphragm. This foramen transmits lymphatic vessels from the diaphragmatic surface of the liver and the superior epigastric vessels. The sympathetic trunks pass deep to the medial arcuate ligament. There are two small apertures in each crus of the diaphragm; one transmits the greater and the other the lesser splanchnic nerve.

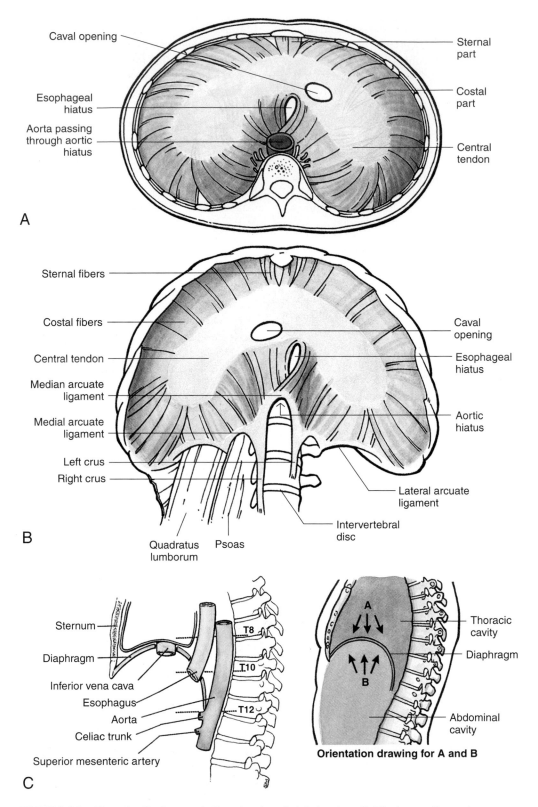

FIGURE 3.38 **Thoracic diaphragm. A.** Superior view. **B.** Inferior view. **C.** Diaphragmatic apertures. *Caval foramen* for the IVC is most anterior at the T8 level to the right of the midline. *Esophageal hiatus* is intermediate at T10 level and to the left. *Aortic hiatus* is in the midline at the T12 level.

VASCULATURE AND NERVES OF DIAPHRAGM

The **arteries of the diaphragm** form a branchlike pattern on both its superior and inferior surfaces. *The arteries supplying the superior surface of the diaphragm* (Fig. 3.39, Table 3.10) are the:

- **Pericardiacophrenic and musculophrenic arteries**—branches of internal thoracic artery
- **Superior phrenic arteries**—arising from thoracic aorta.

The arteries supplying the inferior surface of the diaphragm are the **inferior phrenic arteries,** which typically are the first branches of the *abdominal aorta;* however, they may arise from the celiac trunk. The veins draining the superior surface of the diaphragm are the **pericardiacophrenic** and **musculophrenic veins,** which empty into the *internal thoracic veins* and, on the right side, a *superior phrenic vein* that drains into the IVC. The inferior phrenic veins drain blood from the inferior surface of the diaphragm. The **right inferior phrenic vein** usually opens into the IVC, whereas the **left inferior phrenic vein** is usually double, with one branch passing anterior to the esophageal hiatus to end in the IVC and the other, more posterior branch usually joining the left suprarenal vein.

The **lymphatic plexuses** on the thoracic and abdominal surfaces of the diaphragm communicate freely (Fig. 3.39C). The anterior and posterior **diaphragmatic lymph nodes** are on the thoracic surface of the diaphragm. Lymph from these nodes drains into the **parasternal, posterior mediastinal,** and **phrenic lymph nodes.** Lymph vessels from the abdominal surface of the diaphragm drain into the anterior diaphragmatic, phrenic, and **superior lumbar lymph nodes.** Lymphatic vessels are dense on the inferior surface of the diaphragm, constituting the primary means for absorption of peritoneal fluid and substances introduced by IP injection. *The entire motor supply to the diaphragm is from the phrenic nerves,* each of which is distributed to half of the diaphragm and arises from the ventral rami of C3 through C5 segments of the spinal cord. The phrenic

nerves also supply fibers (pain and proprioception) to most of the diaphragm. Peripheral parts of the diaphragm receive their sensory nerve supply from the **intercostal nerves** (lower 6 or 7) and the **subcostal nerves.**

Actions of Diaphragm

When the diaphragm contracts, its domes move inferiorly so that the convexity of the diaphragm is somewhat flattened. Although this movement is often described as the "descent of the diaphragm," only the domes of the diaphragm descend; its periphery remains attached to the ribs and cartilages of the inferior six ribs. As the diaphragm descends, it pushes the abdominal viscera inferiorly. This increases the volume of the thoracic cavity and decreases the intrathoracic pressure, resulting in air being taken into the lungs. In addition, the volume of the abdominal cavity decreases slightly and the intra-abdominal pressure increases somewhat. Movements of the diaphragm are also important in circulation because the increased intra-abdominal pressure and decreased intrathoracic pressure help to return venous blood to the heart. When the diaphragm contracts, compressing the abdominal viscera, blood in the IVC is forced superiorly into the heart.

REFERRED PAIN FROM DIAPHRAGM

Pain from the diaphragm radiates to two different areas because of the difference in the sensory nerve supply of the diaphragm (Table 3.10). Pain resulting from irritation of the diaphragmatic pleura or diaphragmatic peritoneum is referred to the shoulder region, the area of skin supplied by the C3 through C5 segments of the spinal cord. These segments also contribute anterior rami to the phrenic nerves. Irritation of peripheral regions of the diaphragm, innervated by the inferior intercostal nerves, is more localized, being referred to the skin over the costal margins of the anterolateral abdominal wall.

Section of Phrenic Nerve

Section of a phrenic nerve in the neck results in complete paralysis and eventual atrophy of the muscular part of the corresponding half of the diaphragm, except in persons who have an accessory phrenic nerve (see Chapter 9). *Paralysis of a hemidiaphragm* can be recognized radiographically by its permanent elevation and paradoxical movement. Instead of descending on inspiration, it is forced superiorly by the increased intra-abdominal pressure secondary to descent of the opposite unparalyzed hemidiaphragm.

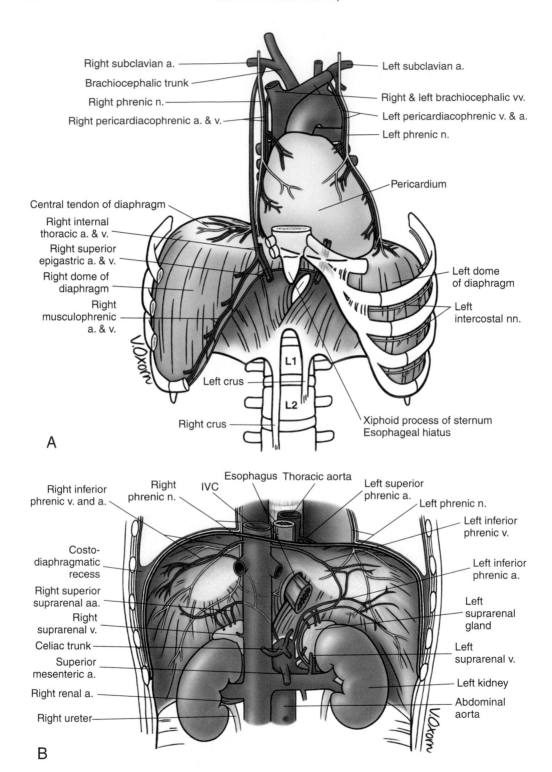

Right subclavian a.

Brachiocephalic trunk

Right phrenic n.

Right pericardiacophrenic a. & v.

Left subclavian a.

Right & left brachiocephalic vv.

Left pericardiacophrenic v. & a.

Left phrenic n.

Pericardium

Central tendon of diaphragm

Right internal thoracic a. & v.

Right superior epigastric a. & v.

Right dome of diaphragm

Right musculophrenic a. & v.

Left dome of diaphragm

Left intercostal nn.

L1

L2

Left crus

Right crus

Xiphoid process of sternum
Esophageal hiatus

A

Esophagus   Thoracic aorta

Right inferior phrenic v. and a.

Right phrenic n.

IVC

Left superior phrenic a.

Left phrenic n.

Left inferior phrenic v.

Costo-diaphragmatic recess

Right superior suprarenal aa.

Right suprarenal v.

Celiac trunk

Superior mesenteric a.

Right renal a.

Right ureter

Left inferior phrenic a.

Left suprarenal gland

Left suprarenal v.

Left kidney

Abdominal aorta

B

FIGURE 3.39   **Blood vessels and lymphatics of the diaphragm. A.** Arteries and veins of the superior surface. Posterior view. **B.** Arteries and veins of the inferior surface. Anterior view.

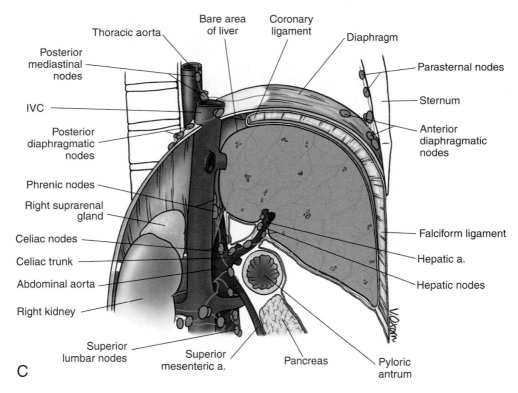

FIGURE 3.39 *Continued.* **O.** Lymphatics. Schematic lateral view

TABLE 3.10. VESSELS AND NERVES OF DIAPHRAGM

Vessels and Nerves	Superior Surface of Diaphragm	Inferior Surface of Diaphragm
Arterial supply	Superior phrenic arteries from thoracic aorta Musculophrenic and pericardiacophrenic arteries from internal thoracic arteries	Inferior phrenic arteries from abdominal aorta
Venous drainage	Musculophrenic and pericardiacophrenic veins drain into internal thoracic veins; superior phrenic vein (right side) drains into IVC	Inferior phrenic veins: right vein drains into IVC; left vein is doubled and drains into IVC and left suprarenal vein
Lymphatic drainage	Diaphragmatic lymph nodes to phrenic nodes then to parasternal and posterior mediastinal nodes	Superior lumbar lymph nodes; lymphatic plexuses on superior and inferior surfaces communicate freely
Innervation	Motor supply: phrenic nerves (C3–C5) Sensory supply: centrally by phrenic nerves (C3–C5); peripherally by intercostal nerves (T5–T11) and subcostal nerves (T12)	

POSTERIOR ABDOMINAL WALL

The posterior abdominal wall (Figs. 3.40 and 3.41) is composed mainly—from deep (posterior) to superficial (anterior)—of the:

- Five lumbar vertebrae and associated IV discs
- Posterior abdominal wall muscles—psoas, quadratus lumborum, iliacus, transverse abdominal, and oblique muscles
- Lumbar plexus, composed of the anterior rami of lumbar spinal nerves
- Fascia, including thoracolumbar fascia
- Diaphragm, contributing to the superior part of the posterior wall
- Fat, nerves, vessels, and lymph nodes.

FASCIA OF POSTERIOR ABDOMINAL WALL

The posterior abdominal wall is covered with a continuous layer of endoabdominal fascia that lies between the parietal peritoneum and the muscles. The fascia lining the posterior abdominal wall is continuous with the transversalis fascia that lines the transverse abdominal muscle (Fig. 3.35). It is customary to name the fascia according to the structure it covers. The **psoas fascia** covering the psoas major (psoas sheath) is attached medially to the lumbar vertebrae and pelvic brim. The psoas fascia is thickened superiorly to form the **medial arcuate ligament** (Fig. 3.38B). The psoas fascia fuses laterally with the quadratus lumborum and anterior layer of the **thoracolumbar fascia**. The thoracolumbar fascia is an extensive fascial sheet that splits into anterior, middle, and posterior layers, enclosing the quadratus lumborum and deep muscles of the back (Fig. 3.35). It is thin and transparent where it covers thoracic parts of the deep muscles but is thick and strong in the lumbar region. The lumbar part of the thoracolumbar fascia, extending between the 12th rib and the iliac crest, attaches laterally to the internal oblique and transverse abdominal muscles. Inferior to the iliac crest, the psoas fascia is continuous with the part of the iliac fascia covering the iliacus muscle. The **anterior layer of the tho-racolumbar fascia** (quadratus lumborum fascia) covering the quadratus lumborum muscle is a dense membranous layer that attaches to the anterior surfaces of the transverse processes of the lumbar vertebrae, the iliac crest, and the 12th rib and is continuous with the transversalis fascia. The anterior layer of the thoracolumbar fascia is thickened superiorly to form the **lateral arcuate ligaments** (Fig. 3.38B) and is adherent inferiorly to the iliolumbar ligaments.

PSOAS ABSCESS

An abscess resulting from tuberculosis in the lumbar region tends to spread from the vertebrae into the psoas fascia (psoas sheath), where it produces a *psoas abscess*. As a consequence, the psoas fascia thickens to form a strong stockinglike tube. Pus from the psoas abscess passes inferiorly along the psoas within this fascial tube over the pelvic brim and deep to the inguinal ligament. The pus usually surfaces in the superior part of the thigh. Pus can also reach the psoas sheath by passing from the posterior mediastinum when the thoracic vertebrae are diseased.

MUSCLES OF POSTERIOR ABDOMINAL WALL

The main paired muscles in the posterior abdominal wall (Fig. 3.40) are the:

- **Psoas major,** passing inferolaterally
- **Iliacus,** lying along the lateral sides of the inferior part of the psoas major
- **Quadratus lumborum,** lying adjacent to the transverse processes of the lumbar vertebrae and lateral to the superior parts of the psoas major.

The attachments, nerve supply, and main actions of these muscles are summarized in Table 3.11.

POSTERIOR ABDOMINAL PAIN

The *iliopsoas* (compound muscle—iliacus and psoas major) has extensive and clinically important relations to the kidneys, ureters, cecum, appendix, sigmoid colon, pancreas, lumbar lymph nodes, and nerves of the posterior abdominal wall. When any of these structures is diseased, movement of the iliopsoas usually causes pain. When intra-abdominal inflammation is suspected, the **iliopsoas test** is performed. The person is asked to lie on the unaffected side and to extend the thigh on the affected side against the resistance of the examiner's hand. Pain resulting from this maneuver is a *positive psoas sign*. An acutely inflamed appendix, for example, will produce a positive sign.

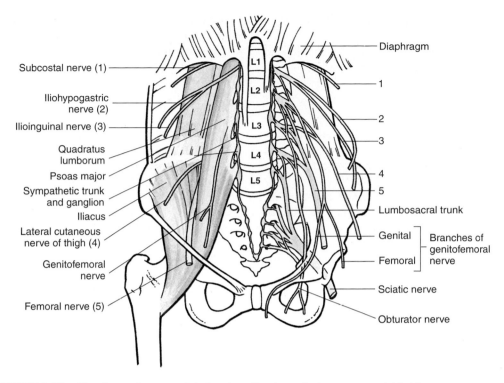

Subcostal nerve (1)

Iliohypogastric nerve (2)

Ilioinguinal nerve (3)

Quadratus lumborum

Psoas major

Sympathetic trunk and ganglion

Iliacus

Lateral cutaneous nerve of thigh (4)

Genitofemoral nerve

Femoral nerve (5)

Diaphragm

L1

L2

L3

L4

L5

1

2

3

4

5

Lumbosacral trunk

Genital

Femoral

Branches of genitofemoral nerve

Sciatic nerve

Obturator nerve

FIGURE 3.40   Muscles and nerves. Anterior view. *Numbers* refer to nerves on right side.

TABLE 3.11.   MAIN MUSCLES OF POSTERIOR ABDOMINAL WALL

Muscle	Superior Attachments	Inferior Attachment(s)	Innervation	Action(s)
Psoas major[a]	Transverse processes of lumbar vertebrae; sides of bodies of T12–L5 vertebrae and intervening IV discs	By a strong tendon to lesser trochanter of femur	Lumbar plexus via anterior branches of L1, L2, and L3 nerves	Acting inferiorly with iliacus, it flexes thigh; acting superiorly it flexes vertebral column laterally; it is used to balance the trunk; when sitting it acts inferiorly with iliacus to flex trunk
Iliacus[a]	Superior two thirds of iliac fossa, ala of sacrum, and anterior sacroiliac ligaments	Lesser trochanter of femur and shaft inferior to it, and to psoas major tendon	Femoral nerve (**L2** and L3)	Flexes thigh and stabilizes hip joint; acts with psoas major
Quadratus lumborum	Medal half of inferior border of 12th rib and tips of lumbar transverse processes	Iliolumbar ligament and internal lip of iliac crest	Anterior branches of T12 and L1–L4 nerves	Extends and laterally flexes vertebral column; fixes 12th rib during inspiration

[a]Psoas major and iliacus muscles are often described together as the iliopsoas muscle when flexion of the thigh is discussed (Chapter 6). *The iliopsoas is the chief flexor of the thigh,* and when thigh is fixed, it is a strong flexor of the trunk (e.g., during situps).

NERVES OF POSTERIOR ABDOMINAL WALL

There are somatic and autonomic nerves in the posterior abdominal wall.

Somatic Nerves of Posterior Abdominal Wall

The **subcostal nerves**—the anterior rami of T12—arise in the thorax, pass posterior to the lateral arcuate ligaments into the abdomen, and run inferolaterally on the anterior surface of the quadratus lumborum muscle (Fig. 3.40). They pass through the transverse abdominal and internal oblique muscles to supply the external oblique and skin of the anterolateral abdominal wall. The **lumbar nerves** pass from the spinal cord through the IV foramina inferior to the corresponding vertebrae, where they divide into posterior and anterior primary rami. Each ramus contains sensory and motor fibers. The posterior primary rami pass posteriorly to supply the muscles and skin of the back, whereas the anterior primary rami pass into the psoas major, and are connected to the *sympathetic trunks* by rami communicantes (communicating branches). The **lumbar plexus of nerves** is in the posterior part of the psoas major, anterior to the lumbar transverse processes. This nerve network is composed of the anterior rami of L1 through L4 nerves. All rami receive gray rami communicantes from the sympathetic trunks, and the superior two send white rami communicantes to these trunks. The following nerves are **branches of the lumbar plexus**; the three largest are listed first:

- The **obturator nerve** (L2 through L4) emerges from the medial border of the psoas major and passes through the pelvis to the medial thigh, supplying the adductor muscles.
- The **femoral nerve** (also L2 through L4) emerges from the lateral border of the psoas major and innervates the iliacus and passes deep to the inguinal ligament to the anterior thigh, supplying the flexors of the hip and extensors of the knee.
- The **lumbosacral trunk** (L4, L5) passes over the ala (wing) of the sacrum and descends into the pelvis to participate in the formation of the **sacral plexus** along with the anterior rami of S1 through S4 nerves.

- The **ilioinguinal and iliohypogastric nerves** (L1) arise from the anterior ramus of L1 and enter the abdomen posterior to the *medial arcuate ligaments* and pass inferolaterally, anterior to the quadratus lumborum. They pierce the transverse abdominal muscles near the anterior superior iliac spines and pass through the internal and external oblique muscles to supply the skin of the suprapubic and inguinal regions (both nerves also supply branches to the abdominal musculature).
- The **genitofemoral nerve** (L1, L2) pierces the anterior surface of the psoas major and runs inferiorly on it deep to the psoas fascia; it divides lateral to the common and external iliac arteries into femoral and genital branches.
- The **lateral femoral cutaneous nerve** (L2, L3) runs inferolaterally on the iliacus muscle and enters the thigh posterior to the inguinal ligament, just medial to the anterior superior iliac spine; it supplies the skin on its anterolateral surface of the thigh.

Autonomic Nerves of Posterior Abdominal Wall

The autonomic nerves of the abdomen consist of one cranial nerve (the vagus) and several different splanchnic nerves that deliver presynaptic sympathetic and parasympathetic fibers to the nerve plexuses and sympathetic ganglia along the abdominal aorta. The periarterial extensions of these plexuses reach the abdominal viscera, where intrinsic parasympathetic ganglia occur (Fig. 3.41, Table 3.9).

The sympathetic part of the autonomic nervous system in the abdomen consists of:

- Abdominopelvic splanchnic nerves: *lower thoracic splanchnic nerves* (greater, lesser, and least) from the thoracic part of the sympathetic trunks and *lumbar splanchnic nerves* from the lumbar part of the sympathetic trunks
- Prevertebral sympathetic ganglia
- Abdominal autonomic plexuses
- Periarterial plexuses. The plexuses are mixed, shared with the parasympathetic nervous system and visceral afferent fibers.

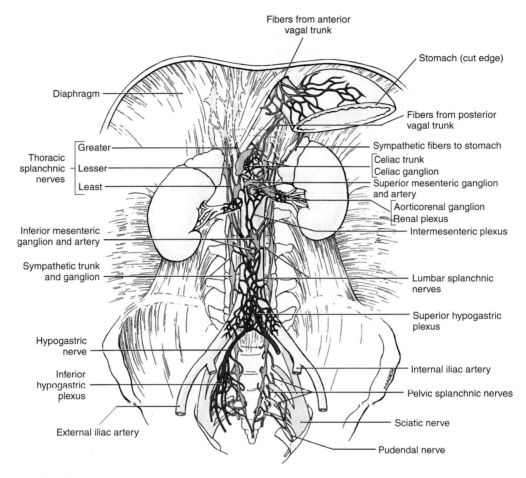

Fibers from anterior
vagal trunk

Stomach (cut edge)

Diaphragm

Fibers from posterior
vagal trunk

Thoracic
splanchnic
nerves
Greater
Lesser
Least

Sympathetic fibers to stomach
Celiac trunk
Celiac ganglion
Superior mesenteric ganglion
and artery
Aorticorenal ganglion
Renal plexus
Intermesenteric plexus

Inferior mesenteric
ganglion and artery

Sympathetic trunk
and ganglion

Lumbar splanchnic
nerves

Superior hypogastric
plexus

Hypogastric
nerve

Inferior
hypogastric
plexus

Internal iliac artery

Pelvic splanchnic nerves

External iliac artery

Sciatic nerve

Pudendal nerve

FIGURE 3.41   Autonomic nerve supply of the abdomen. Anterior view. *Orange,* sympathetic; *green,* parasympathetic; *blue,* plexus; *yellow,* nerves of sacral plexus.

The **abdominopelvic splanchnic nerves** are the source of sympathetic innervation in the abdominopelvic cavity. The presynaptic sympathetic fibers they convey originated from cell bodies in the intermediolateral cell column, or lateral horn, of gray substance (matter) of spinal cord segments T7 through L2 or L3. The fibers pass successively through the anterior roots, anterior rami, and white rami communicantes of thoracic and upper lumbar spinal nerves to reach the sympathetic trunks. They pass through the paravertebral ganglia of these trunks without synapsing to enter the abdominopelvic splanchnic nerves that convey them to the prevertebral ganglia of the abdominal cavity.

The **lower thoracic splanchnic nerves** are the main source of presynaptic sympathetic fibers serving abdominal viscera. The **greater** (from the sympathetic trunk at T5 through T9 or T10 vertebral levels), **lesser** (from T10 and T11 levels), and **least** (from the T12) level **splanchnic nerves** are the specific thoracic splanchnic nerves that arise from the thoracic part of the sympathetic trunks and pierce the corresponding crus of the diaphragm to convey the presynaptic sympathetic fibers to the celiac, superior mesenteric, and aorticorenal (prevertebral) sympathetic ganglia.

The **lumbar splanchnic nerves** arise from the abdominal part of the sympathetic trunks. The sympathetic trunks extend into the abdomen from the thorax by passing posterior to the medial arcuate ligaments. They lie on the anterolateral aspects of the bodies of the lumbar vertebrae in a groove formed by the adjacent psoas muscle. The abdominal part of the trunks is composed of four **lumbar (paravertebral) sympathetic ganglia** and interconnecting fibers. Laterally, the trunks receive white rami communicantes from the anterior rami of the L1, L2, and occasionally L3 spinal nerves, and send gray rami communicantes back to the adjacent ventral rami. Medially, the abdominal sympathetic trunks give off three to four lumbar splanchnic nerves, which pass to the **intermesenteric, inferior mesenteric,** and **superior hypogastric plexuses,** conveying presynaptic sympathetic fibers to the associated prevertebral ganglia.

The cell bodies of postsynaptic sympathetic neurons constitute the major prevertebral ganglia that cluster about the roots of the major branches of the abdominal aorta—the celiac, aorticorenal, superior mesenteric, and inferior mesenteric ganglia—and minor, unnamed prevertebral ganglia that occur within the intermesenteric and superior hypogastric plexuses. The synapse between presynaptic and postsynaptic neurons occurs in the prevertebral ganglia. Postsynaptic sympathetic nerve fibers pass from the prevertebral ganglia to the abdominal visceral through the periarterial plexuses associated with the branches of the abdominal aorta. Sympathetic innervation in the abdomen, as elsewhere, is primarily involved in producing vasoconstriction. With regard to the GI tract, it acts to inhibit (slow down or stop) peristalsis. The sympathetic supply to the suprarenal gland is an exception. The secretory cells of the medulla are postsynaptic sympathetic neurons that lack axons or dendrites. Consequently, the **suprarenal medulla** is supplied directly by presynaptic sympathetic neurons (Fig. 3.42).

Visceral afferent fibers conveying pain sensations accompany the sympathetic (visceral motor) fibers. The pain impulses pass retrograde to those of the motor fibers along the splanchnic nerves to the sympathetic trunk. The fibers then pass through white rami communicantes to the anterior rami of the spinal nerves, and then enter into the root and pass into the spinal sensory ganglia.

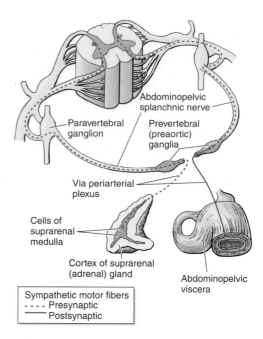

FIGURE 3.42   **Sympathetic motor innervation of the suprarenal gland and abdominopelvic viscera.**

The parasympathetic part of the autonomic nervous system in the abdomen (Fig. 3.41, Table 3.9) consists of the:

- Anterior and posterior vagal trunks
- Pelvic splanchnic nerves
- Abdominal and periarterial autonomic nerve plexuses; the nerve plexuses are mixed, shared with the sympathetic nervous system and visceral afferent fibers
- Intrinsic (enteric) parasympathetic ganglia.

The **anterior and posterior vagal trunks** are the continuation of the left and right vagus nerves that emerge from the esophageal plexus and pass through the esophageal hiatus on the anterior and posterior aspects of the esophagus and stomach. The vagus nerves convey presynaptic parasympathetic and visceral afferent fibers (mainly for unconscious sensations associated with reflexes) to the abdominal aortic plexuses and the periarterial plexuses, which extend along the branches of the aorta.

The **pelvic splanchnic nerves** are distinct from other splanchnic nerves in that they:

- Have nothing to do with the sympathetic trunks

- Derive directly from anterior rami of spinal nerves S2 through S4
- Convey presynaptic parasympathetic fibers to the inferior hypogastric (pelvic) plexus.

Presynaptic fibers terminate on the isolated and widely scattered cell bodies of postsynaptic neurons lying on or within the abdominal viscera, constituting intrinsic ganglia. The presynaptic parasympathetic and visceral afferent reflex fibers conveyed by the vagus nerves extend to intrinsic ganglia of the lower esophagus, stomach, small intestine (including the duodenum), ascending and most of the transverse parts of the colon; those conveyed by the pelvic splanchnic nerves supply the descending and sigmoid parts of the colon, rectum, and pelvic organs. That is, in terms of the GI tract, the vagus nerves provide parasympathetic innervation of the smooth muscle and glands of the gut as far as the left colic flexure; the pelvic splanchnic nerves provide the remainder.

The **abdominal autonomic plexuses** are networks consisting of both sympathetic and parasympathetic fibers that surround the abdominal aorta and its major branches. The celiac, superior mesenteric, and inferior mesenteric plexuses are interconnected. The **prevertebral sympathetic ganglia** are scattered among the celiac and mesenteric plexuses. The **intrinsic parasympathetic ganglia,** such as the *myenteric plexus* (Auerbach plexus) in the muscular coat of the stomach and intestine, are in the walls of the viscera.

The **celiac plexus** (solar plexus), surrounding the root of the celiac arterial trunk, contains irregular right and left *celiac ganglia* (approximately 2 cm long) that unite superior and inferior to the celiac trunk. The *parasympathetic root of the celiac plexus* is a branch of the *posterior vagal trunk* that contains fibers from the right and left vagus nerves. The *sympathetic roots of the celiac plexus* are the greater and lesser splanchnic nerves. The **superior mesenteric plexus** and ganglion or ganglia surround the origin of the SMA. The plexus has one median and two lateral branches. The median branch is from the celiac plexus and the lateral branches arise from the lesser and least splanchnic nerves, sometimes with a contribution from

the first lumbar ganglion of the sympathetic trunk. The **inferior mesenteric plexus** surrounds the inferior mesenteric artery and gives off shoots to its branches. It receives a medial root from the intermesenteric plexus and lateral roots from the lumbar ganglia of the sympathetic trunks. An *inferior mesenteric ganglion* may also appear just inferior to the root of the inferior mesenteric artery. The **intermesenteric plexus** is part of the aortic plexus of nerves between the superior and inferior mesenteric arteries. It gives rise to renal, testicular or ovarian, and ureteric plexuses. The **superior hypogastric plexus** is a continuation of the *para-aortic plexus* inferior to the bifurcation of the aorta. Right and left **hypogastric nerves** join the superior and inferior hypogastric plexuses. The superior hypogastric plexus supplies *ureteric* and *testicular plexuses* and a plexus on each common iliac artery. The **inferior hypogastric plexus** is formed on each side by a hypogastric nerve from the superior hypogastric plexus. The right and left plexuses are situated on the sides of the rectum, uterine cervix, and urinary bladder. The plexuses receive small branches from the superior sacral sympathetic ganglia and the sacral parasympathetic outflow from S2 through S4 (*pelvic parasympathetic splanchnic nerves*). Extensions of the inferior hypogastric plexus send autonomic fibers along the blood vessels, which form visceral plexuses on the walls of the pelvic viscera (e.g., *the rectal and vesical plexuses).*

VASCULATURE OF POSTERIOR ABDOMINAL WALL

Most arteries supplying the posterior abdominal wall arise from the **abdominal aorta** (Fig. 3.43); however, the **subcostal arteries** arise from the thoracic aorta and distribute inferior to the 12th rib. The abdominal aorta—approximately 13 cm in length—begins at the aortic hiatus in the diaphragm at the level of T12 vertebra and ends at the level of L4 vertebra by dividing into two common iliac arteries. The **level of the aortic bifurcation** is 2 to 3 cm inferior and to the left of the umbilicus at the level of the iliac crests. Four or five pairs of **lumbar arteries** arise from the abdominal aorta and supply the lumbar vertebrae, back muscles, and posterior abdominal wall. The **common iliac arteries**—terminal

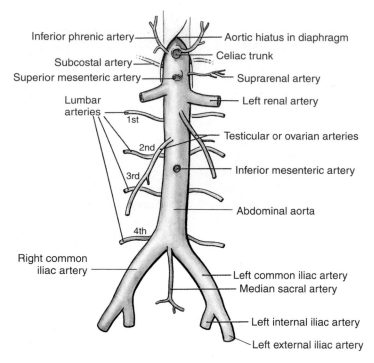

FIGURE 3.43   Abdominal aorta and its branches.

branches of the abdominal aorta—diverge and run inferolaterally, following the medial border of the psoas muscles to the pelvic brim. Here each common iliac artery divides into the **internal** and **external iliac arteries**. The internal iliac artery enters the pelvis; its course and branches are described in Chapter 4. The external iliac artery follows the iliopsoas muscle. Just before leaving the abdomen, the external iliac artery gives rise to the **inferior epigastric** and **deep iliac circumflex arteries** that supply the anterolateral abdominal wall. From superior to inferior the important **anterior relations of the abdominal aorta** are the (Table 3.6):

- Celiac plexus and ganglion
- Body of pancreas
- Splenic and left renal veins
- Horizontal part of duodenum
- Coils of small intestine.

The abdominal aorta descends anterior to the bodies of T12 through L4 vertebrae. The left lumbar veins pass posterior to the aorta to reach the IVC. *On the right,* the aorta is related to the

azygos vein, chyle cistern, right crus of diaphragm, and right celiac ganglion. *On the left,* the aorta is related to the left crus of diaphragm and left celiac ganglion. The branches of the abdominal aorta may be described as visceral or parietal and paired or unpaired (Fig. 3.43).

The **paired visceral branches** are the:

- Suprarenal arteries (L1)
- Renal arteries (L1)
- Gonadal arteries, the ovarian or testicular arteries (L2).

The **unpaired visceral branches** arise at the following vertebral levels:

- Celiac trunk (T12)
- Superior mesenteric artery (L1)
- Inferior mesenteric artery (L3).

The **paired parietal branches** are the:

- Inferior phrenic arteries that arise just inferior to the aortic hiatus and supply the inferior surface of the diaphragm and the suprarenal glands

VISCERAL REFERRED PAIN

Pain arising from a viscus such as the stomach varies from dull to very severe; however, the pain is poorly localized. It radiates to the dermatome level, which receives visceral sensory fibers from the organ concerned.

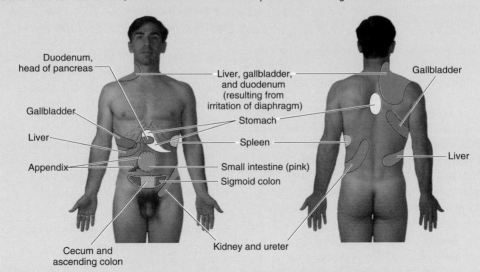

Organ	Nerve Supply	Spinal Cord	Referred Site and Clinical Example
Stomach	Anterior and posterior vagal trunks. Presynaptic sympathetic fibers reach celiac and other ganglia through greater splanchnic nerves.	T6–T9 or T10	Epigastric and left hypochondriac regions (e.g., gastric peptic ulcer)
Duodenum	Vagus nerves. Presynaptic sympathetic fibers reach celiac and superior mesenteric ganglia through greater splanchnic nerves.	T5–T9 or T10	Epigastric region (e.g., duodenal peptic ulcer) Right shoulder if ulcer perforates
Pancreatic head	Vagus and thoracic splanchnic nerves.	T8–T9	Inferior part of epigastric region (e.g., pancreatitis)
Small intestine (jejunum and ileum)	Posterior vagal trunks. Presynaptic sympathetic fibers reach celiac ganglion through greater splanchnic nerves.	T5–T9	Periumbilical region (e.g., acute intestinal obstruction)
Colon	Vagus nerves. Presynaptic sympathetic fibers reach celiac, superior mesenteric, and inferior mesenteric ganglia through greater splanchnic nerves. Parasympathetic supply to distal colon is derived from pelvic splanchnic nerves through hypogastric nerves and inferior hypogastric plexus.	T10–T12 (proximal colon) L1–L3 (distal colon)	Hypogastric region (e.g., ulcerative colitis) Left lower quadrant (e.g., sigmoiditis)
Spleen	Celiac plexus, especially from greater splanchnic nerve.	T6–T8	Left hypochondriac region (e.g., splenic infarct)
Appendix	Sympathetic and parasympathetic nerves from superior mesenteric plexus. Afferent nerve fibers accompany sympathetic nerves to T10 segment of spinal cord.	T10	Periumbilical region and later to right lower quadrant (e.g., appendicitis)
Gallbladder and liver	Nerves are derived from celiac plexus (sympathetic), vagus nerve (parasympathetic), and right phrenic nerve (sensory).	T6–T9	Epigastric region and later to right hypochondriac region; may cause pain on posterior thoracic wall or right shoulder owing to diaphragmatic irritation
Kidneys and ureters	Nerves arise from the renal plexus and consist of sympathetic, parasympathetic, and visceral afferent fibers from thoracic and lumbar splanchnics and the vagus nerve.	T11–T12	Small of back, flank (lumbar quadrant), extending to groin (inguinal region) and genitals (e.g., renal or ureteric calculi)

Pain is perceived as originating in areas supplied by the somatic nerves entering the spinal cord at the same segment as the sensory nerves from the organ producing the pain. Although the areas of pain are not always as shown, they provide clues for the clinician when determining which organ may be affected.

- Lumbar arteries that pass around the sides of the superior four lumbar vertebrae to supply the posterior abdominal wall.

The unpaired parietal branch is the **median sacral artery** that arises from the aorta at its bifurcation and descends into the lesser pelvis.

The **veins of the posterior abdominal wall** are tributaries of the **inferior vena cava (IVC)**, except for the **left testicular** or **ovarian vein** that enters the **renal vein** before entering the IVC (Fig. 3.44). The IVC, the largest vein in the body, has no valves except for a variable, nonfunctional one at its orifice in the right atrium of the heart. The IVC returns poorly oxygenated blood from the lower limbs, most of the back, the abdominal walls, and the abdominopelvic viscera. Blood from the viscera passes through the *portal venous system* and the liver before entering the IVC via the hepatic veins. The IVC begins anterior to L5 vertebra by the union of the common iliac veins. This union occurs approximately 2.5 cm to the right of the median plane, inferior to the bifurcation of the aorta

and posterior to the proximal part of the right *common iliac artery*. The IVC ascends on the right side of the bodies of L3 through L5 vertebrae and on the psoas major muscle to the right of the aorta. The IVC leaves the abdomen by passing through the caval opening in the diaphragm to enter the thorax. The **tributaries of the IVC** correspond to branches of the aorta:

- Common iliac veins, formed by union of external and internal iliac veins
- 3rd (L3) and 4th (L4) lumbar veins
- Right testicular or ovarian veins
- Renal veins
- Ascending lumbar (azygos/hemiazygos) veins
- Right suprarenal vein
- Inferior phrenic veins
- Hepatic veins.

The left testicular or ovarian vein and the left suprarenal vein usually drain into the left renal vein. The ascending lumbar and azygos veins connect the IVC and superior vena cava (SVC), either directly or indirectly.

ABDOMINAL AORTIC ANEURYSM

Rupture of an aneurysm (localized enlargement) of the abdominal aorta causes severe pain in the abdomen or back. If unrecognized, a ruptured aneurysm has a mortality rate of nearly 90% because of heavy blood loss. Surgeons can repair an aneurysm by opening it, inserting a prosthetic graft (such as one made of Dacron), and sewing the wall of the aneurysmal aorta over the graft to protect it.

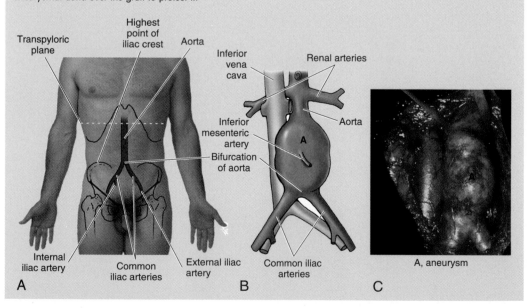

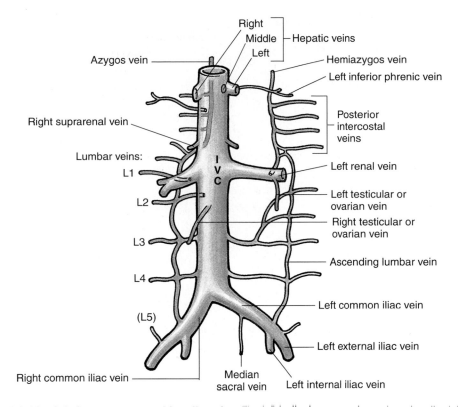

FIGURE 3.44 **Inferior vena cava and its tributaries.** The left testicular or ovarian vein enters the left renal vein.

The labels in the figure are:

- Azygos vein
- Right / Middle / Left — Hepatic veins
- Hemiazygos vein
- Left inferior phrenic vein
- Right suprarenal vein
- Posterior intercostal veins
- Left renal vein
- Lumbar veins: L1
- Left testicular or ovarian vein
- Right testicular or ovarian vein
- L2
- Ascending lumbar vein
- L3
- L4
- Left common iliac vein
- (L5)
- Left external iliac vein
- IVC
- Right common iliac vein
- Median sacral vein
- Left internal iliac vein

COLLATERAL ROUTES FOR ABDOMINOPELVIC VENOUS BLOOD

Three collateral routes, formed by valveless veins of the trunk, are available for venous blood to return to the heart when the IVC is obstructed or ligated.

- The *inferior epigastric veins*, tributaries of the external iliac veins of the inferior caval system, anastomose in the rectus sheath with *superior epigastric veins*, which drain in sequence through the internal thoracic veins of the superior caval system.

- The second collateral route involves the *superficial epigastric* or *superficial circumflex iliac veins*, normally tributaries of the great saphenous vein of the inferior caval system, which anastomose in the subcutaneous tissues of the anterolateral body wall with one of the tributaries of the axillary vein, commonly the *lateral thoracic vein*. When the IVC is obstructed, this subcutaneous collateral pathway—called the *thoracoepigastric vein*—becomes particularly conspicuous.

- The third collateral route involves the *epidural venous plexus* inside the vertebral column (illustrated and discussed in Chapter 4), which communicates with the *lumbar veins* of the inferior caval system, and the tributaries of the *azygos system of veins* that is part of the superior caval system.

Lymphatic vessels and lymph nodes lie along the aorta, IVC, and iliac vessels. The **common iliac lymph nodes** receive lymph from the external and internal iliac lymph nodes. Lymph from the common iliac lymph nodes passes to the **lumbar lymph nodes** (Fig. 3.45A). These nodes receive lymph directly from the posterior abdominal wall, kidneys, ureters, testes or ovaries, uterus, and uterine tubes. They also receive lymph from the descending colon, pelvis, and lower limbs through the **inferior mesenteric** and **common iliac lymph nodes.** Efferent lymphatic vessels from the large lymph nodes form the right and left **lumbar lymph trunks.** Lymphatic vessels from the intestine, liver, spleen, and pancreas pass along the celiac, superior, and inferior mesenteric arteries to **preaortic lymph nodes** (celiac and superior and inferior mesenteric nodes) scattered around the origins of these arteries from the aorta (Fig. 3.23A). Efferent vessels from these nodes form the **intestinal lymphatic trunks,**

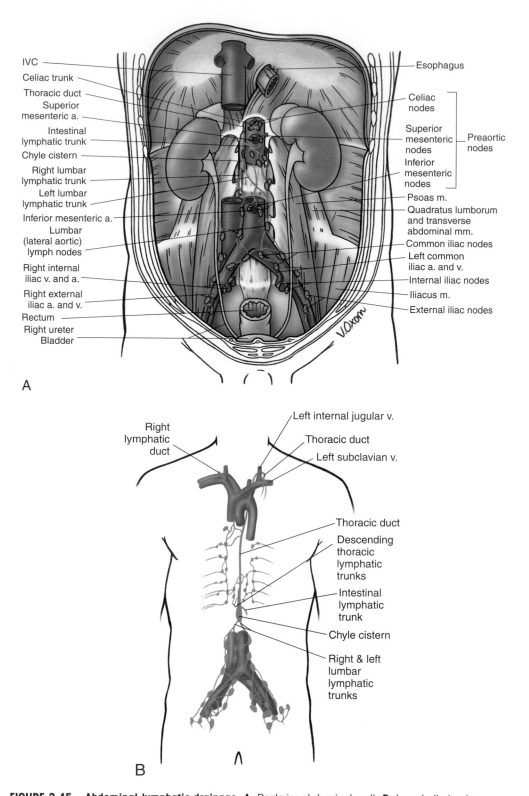

FIGURE 3.45 **Abdominal lymphatic drainage. A.** Posterior abdominal wall. **B.** Lymphatic trunks.

which may be single or multiple, and participate in the confluence of lymphatic trunks that gives rise to the thoracic duct.

The **chyle cistern** (cisterna chyli)—variable in size and shape—is a thin-walled sac at the inferior end of the **thoracic duct,** located anterior to the bodies of L1 and L2 vertebrae between the right crus of the diaphragm and the aorta (Fig. 3.45*B*). A pair of **descending thoracic lymphatic trunks** carry lymph from the lower six intercostal spaces on each side. Consequently, essentially all the lymphatic drainage from the lower half of the body (deep lymphatic drainage inferior to the level of the diaphragm, and all superficial drainage inferior to the level of the umbilicus) converges in the abdomen to enter the beginning of the thoracic duct. *The thoracic duct begins with the convergence of the main lymphatic ducts of the abdomen,* which only in a small proportion of individuals takes the form of the commonly depicted, thin-walled sac—the **chyle cistern.** More often there is merely a simple or plexiform convergence at this level of the lymphatic trunks. The thoracic duct ascends through the *aortic hiatus* in the diaphragm into the posterior mediastinum where it collects more parietal and visceral drainage, particularly from the left upper quadrant of the body, and ultimately ends by entering the venous system at the junction of the **left subclavian and internal jugular veins** (the left venous angle).

MEDICAL IMAGING OF ABDOMEN

Radiographs of the abdomen demonstrate normal and abnormal anatomical relationships of the stomach and duodenum, for example (Fig. 3.15B). Magnetic resonance imaging (MRI), ultrasound, and computerized tomography scans (CT) of the abdomen are also used to examine the abdominal viscera (Figs. 3.46 to 3.48). MRIs provide the best differentiation between soft tissues.

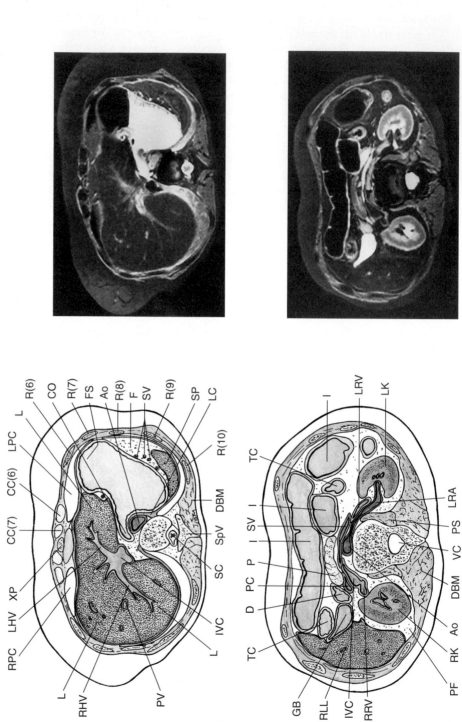

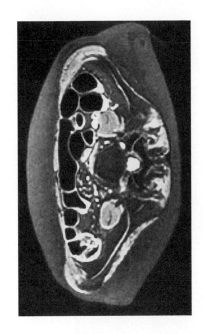

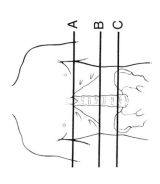

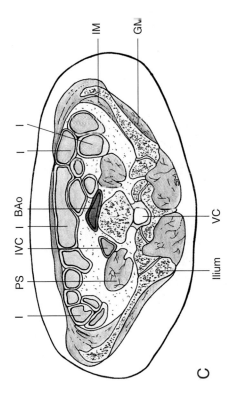

Ao	Aorta	GB	Gallbladder	CC	Costal cartilage
BAo	Bifurcation of aorta	P	Pancreas	R	Rib
LRA	Left renal artery	FS	Fundus of stomach	RPC	Right pleural cavity
IVC	Inferior vena cava	CO	Cardial orifice of stomach	LPC	Left pleural cavity
LHV	Left hepatic vein	D	Duodenum	VB	Vertebral body
RHV	Right hepatic vein	TC	Transverse colon	SpV	Spinous process of vertebra
PV	Portal vein (triad)	DC	Descending colon	VC	Vertebral canal
PC	Portal confluence	I	Intestine	SC	Spinal cord
SV	Splenic vein	RK	Right kidney	PS	Psoas muscle
LRV	Left renal vein	LK	Left kidney	IM	Iliacus muscle
RRV	Right renal vein	SP	Spleen	GM	Gluteus medius muscle
L	Liver	PF	Perirenal fat	DBM	Deep back muscles
RLL	Right lobe of liver	F	Fat	LC	Left crus
		XP	Xiphoid process		

FIGURE 3.46 Transverse magnetic resonance images (MRIs) of the abdomen.

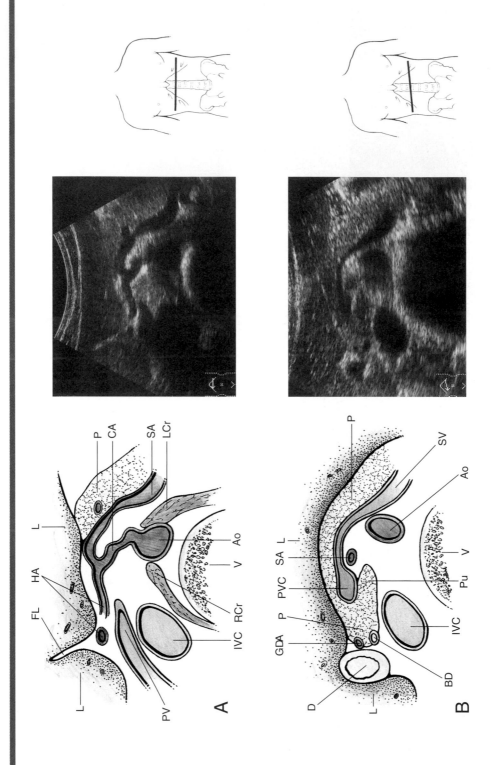

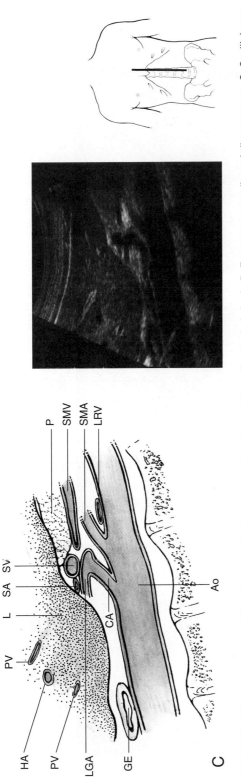

FIGURE 3.47 Ultrasound scans of the abdomen. A. Transverse section through the aorta. **B.** Transverse scan through the pancreas. **C.** Sagittal scan through the aorta. *Ao,* aorta; *BD,* bile duct; *CA,* celiac artery; *D,* duodenum; *FL,* falciform ligament; *GDA,* gastroduodenal artery; *GE,* gastroesophageal junction; *HA,* hepatic artery; *IVC,* inferior vena cava; *L,* liver; *LCA,* left gastric artery; *LCr,* left crus of diaphragm; *LGA,* left gastric artery; *LRV,* left renal vein; *P,* pancreas; *Pu,* uncinate process of pancreas; *PV,* portal vein; *PVC,* portal venous confluence; *RCr,* right crus of diaphragm; *SA,* splenic artery; *SMA,* superior mesenteric artery; *SMV,* superior mesenteric vein; *SV,* splenic vein; *V,* vertebra.

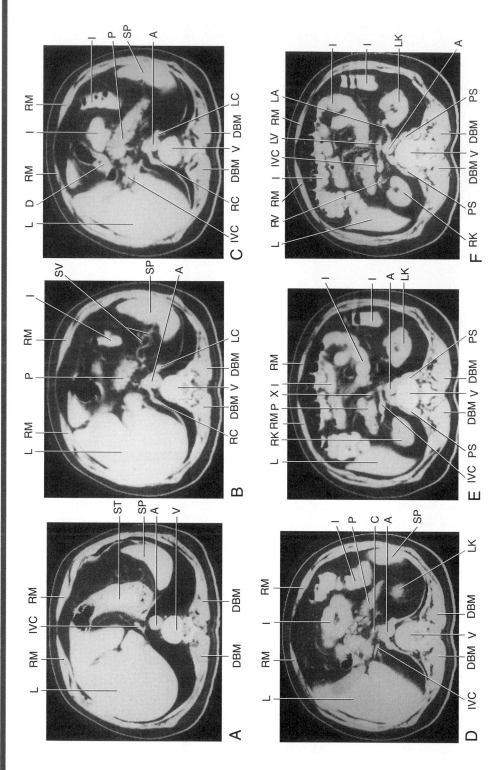

FIGURE 3.48   Computerized tomography (CT) scans of the abdomen at progressively lower levels showing viscera and blood vessels. *A,* aorta; *C,* celiac trunk; *D,* duodenum; *BDM,* deep back muscles; *I,* intestine, *IVC,* inferior vena cava; *L,* liver; *LA,* left renal artery; *LC,* left crus of diaphragm; *LK,* left kidney; *LV,* left renal vein; *P,* pancreas; *PS,* psoas major; *RA,* renal artery; *RC,* right crus of diaphragm; *RK,* right kidney; *RM,* rectus abdominis; *RV,* right renal vein; *SP,* spleen; *ST,* stomach; *SV,* splenic vessels; *V,* vertebral body; *X,* superior mesentery artery.

4 PELVIS AND PERINEUM

*T*he **pelvis** (L. basin) is the part of the trunk inferoposterior to the abdomen and is the area of transition between the trunk and the lower limbs (Fig. 4.1). *The pelvis is enclosed by walls with bony, ligamentous, and muscular portions.* The funnel-shaped **pelvic cavity**—the space bounded at the sides by the bones of the pelvis—is continuous with the abdominal cavity and is angulated posteriorly from it. The pelvic cavity contains the urinary bladder, terminal parts of the ureters, pelvic genital organs, rectum, blood vessels, lymphatics, and nerves. Although continuous (as the abdominopelvic cavity), the abdominal and pelvic cavities are usually described separately for descriptive and regional purposes. The **bony pelvis** (pelvic skeleton) is the basin-shaped ring of bones that protects the distal parts of the intestinal and urinary tracts and the internal genital organs.

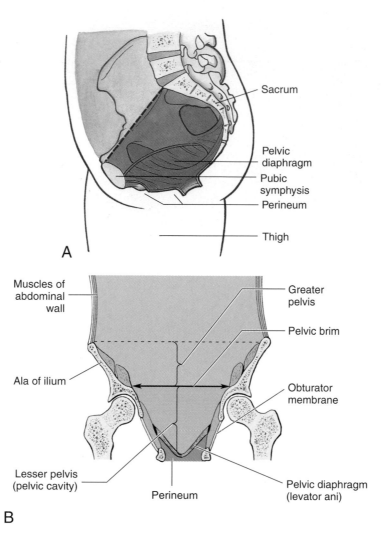

FIGURE 4.1   Abdominopelvic cavity. A. Lateral view. Note the pelvic diaphragm separating the pelvic cavity from the perineum. *Green,* greater (false) pelvis; *red,* lesser (true) pelvis. *Superior broken line,* plane of pelvic brim surrounding the superior pelvic aperture. **B.** Schematic coronal section. Observe that the plane of the pelvic brim of the pelvic inlet (*double-headed arrow*) separates the greater pelvis—part of the abdominal cavity—from the lesser pelvis, the pelvic cavity. The pelvic diaphragm is mainly formed by the levator ani.

The **perineum** refers to the:

- *Area of the trunk between the thighs and buttocks* extending from the pubis to the coccyx
- Shallow *compartment lying between this diamond shaped area* and the **pelvic floor** formed by the **pelvic diaphragm** (Fig. 4.1). In the male the perineum includes the penis, scrotum, and anus, and in the female, the vulva (external genitalia) and anus.

PELVIS

The superior boundary of the **pelvic cavity** is the **pelvic inlet**—the superior pelvic aperture (Figs. 4.1 and 4.2, Table 4.1). The pelvis is limited inferiorly by the **pelvic outlet**—the inferior pelvic aperture, which is closed by the musculofascial **pelvic diaphragm** and bounded anteriorly by the **pubic symphysis** (L. symphysis pubis) and posteriorly by the **coccyx.**

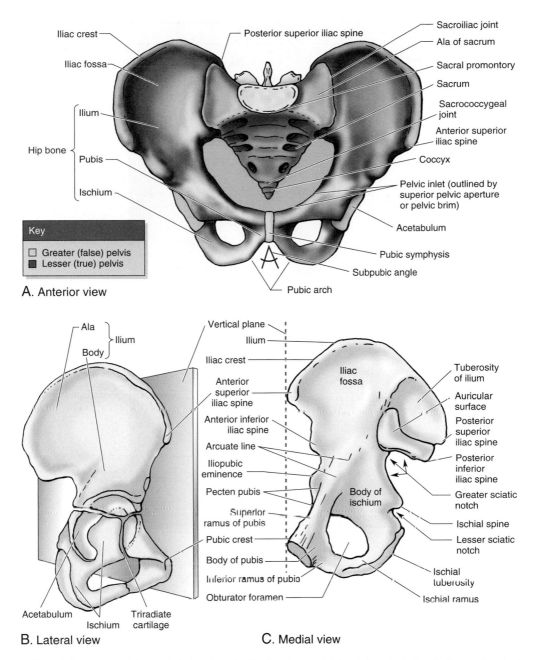

FIGURE 4.2 **Bony pelvis. A.** Anterior view. **B.** Child's hip bone, lateral view. Note that in the anatomical position the anterior superior iliac spine and the anterior aspect of the pubis lie in the same vertical plane. **C.** Medial view.

The **pelvic inlet** is bounded by the **linea terminalis** of the pelvis, which is formed by the:

- Superior margin of pubic symphysis anteriorly
- Posterior border of pubic crest

- Pecten pubis, the continuation of the superior ramus of the pubis that forms a sharp ridge
- Arcuate line of ilium
- Anterior border of ala of sacrum
- Sacral promontory.

TABLE 4.1.   COMPARISON OF MALE AND FEMALE PELVES

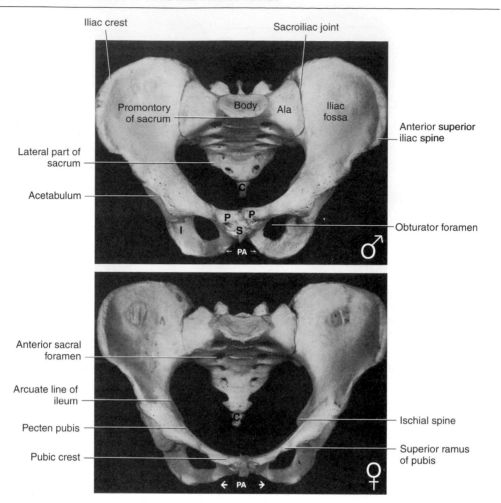

P, pubis; *S,* pubic symphysis; *C,* coccyx; *I,* ramus of ischium; *PA,* pubic arch.

Bony Pelvis	Male (♂)	Female (♀)
General structure	Thick and heavy	Thin and light
Greater pelvis (pelvis major)	Deep	Shallow
Lesser pelvis (pelvis minor)	Narrow and deep	Wide and shallow
Pelvic inlet (superior pelvic aperture)	Heart-shaped	Oval or rounded
Pelvic outlet (inferior pelvic aperture)	Comparatively small	Comparatively large
Pubic arch and subpubic angle	Narrow	Wide
Obturator foramen	Round	Oval
Acetabulum	Large	Small

The **pelvic outlet** is bounded by the:

- Inferior margin of pubic symphysis anteriorly
- Inferior rami of pubis and ischial tuberosities anterolaterally
- Sacrotuberous ligaments posterolaterally (Fig. 4.3*B*)
- Tip of coccyx posteriorly.

BONY PELVIS

The main functions of the strong bony pelvis are to transfer the weight of the upper body from the axial to the lower appendicular skeleton and to withstand compression and other forces resulting from its support of body weight. *The bony pelvis is formed by four bones* (Fig. 4.2, Table 4.1):

- **Hip bones,** two large, irregularly shaped bones, each of which forms at puberty by fusion of three bones—*ilium, ischium,* and *pubis*
- **Sacrum,** formed by the fusion of five originally separate sacral vertebrae
- **Coccyx,** formed by the fusion of four rudimentary coccygeal vertebrae.

The hip bones are joined at the **pubic symphysis** anteriorly and to the sacrum posteriorly at the **sacroiliac joints** to form a bony ring, the **pelvic girdle.**

The **ilium** is the superior, flattened, fan-shaped part of the hip bone (Fig. 4.2). The **ala** (L. wing) of the ilium represents the spread of the fan and the **body** of the ilium, the handle of the fan. The body of the ilium forms the superior part of the **acetabulum**—the cup-shaped depression on the external surface of the hip bone with which the head of the femur articulates. The **iliac crest,** the rim of the ilium, has a curve that follows the contour of the ala between the anterior and posterior **superior iliac spines.** The anterior concave part of the ala forms the **iliac fossa.**

The **ischium** has a body and ramus (L. branch). The **body** of the ischium forms the posterior part of the acetabulum and the **ramus** forms part of the inferior boundary of the **obturator foramen.** The large posteroinferior

protuberance of the ischium is the **ischial tuberosity** (Fig. 4.2*B*). The small pointed posterior projection near the junction of the ramus and body is the **ischial spine.**

The **pubis** is an angulated bone with a **superior ramus** that forms the anterior part of the acetabulum and an **inferior ramus** that forms part of the inferior boundary of the **obturator foramen.** The superior ramus has an oblique ridge—the **pecten pubis**—on its superior aspect. A thickening on the anterior part of the **body of the pubis** is the **pubic crest.**

The bony pelvis is divided into greater (false) and lesser (true) pelves (Figs. 4.1 and 4.2, Table 4.1). The **pelvic inlet** separates the greater pelvis from the lesser pelvis. The boundary or rim of the pelvic inlet—the *pelvic brim*—is obstetrically important.

The **greater pelvis** (L. pelvis major) is:

- Superior to the pelvic inlet
- Bounded by the abdominal wall anteriorly, the iliac alae laterally, and L5 and S1 vertebrae posteriorly
- The location of some abdominal viscera such as the sigmoid colon and some loops of ileum.

The cavity of the greater pelvis is the inferior part of the abdominal cavity.

The **lesser pelvis** (L. pelvis minor) is:

- Between the pelvic inlet and the pelvic diaphragm
- The location of the pelvic viscera—urinary bladder and reproductive organs such as the uterus and ovaries
- Bounded by the pelvic surfaces of the hip bones, sacrum, and coccyx
- Limited inferiorly by the musculofascial pelvic diaphragm.

The cavity of the lesser pelvis is the true pelvic cavity, forming the inferior part of the abdominopelvic cavity.

SEXUAL DIFFERENCES IN PELVES

The male and female bony pelves differ in several respects (Table 4.1). These sexual differences are linked to function. In both sexes the primary pelvic function is locomotor (pertaining to locomotion)—the ability to move

Continued

from one place to another. The sexual differences are related mainly to the heavier build and larger muscles of men and to the adaptation of the pelvis, particularly the lesser pelvis in women for childbearing. Hence, the **male pelvis** is heavier and thicker than the female pelvis and usually has more prominent bone markings. In contrast, the **female pelvis** is wider, shallower, and has a larger pelvic inlet and outlet. The size of the female lesser pelvis is important in obstetrics because it is the bony *pelvic canal* ("birth canal") through which the fetus passes during a vaginal birth. The *shape and size of the pelvic inlet (pelvic brim) is significant* because it is through this opening that the fetal head enters the lesser pelvis during labor. To determine the capacity of the pelvis for childbirth, the diameters of the lesser pelvis are noted radiographically or during a pelvic examination. The *ischial spines* face each other, and the interspinous distance between them is the narrowest part of the pelvic cavity.

Pelvic Fractures

Pelvic fractures can result from direct trauma to the pelvic bones such as occurs during an automobile accident or be caused by forces transmitted to these bones from the lower limbs during falls on the feet. Pelvic fractures may cause injury to pelvic soft tissues, blood vessels, nerves, and organs.

PELVIC JOINTS AND LIGAMENTS

The joints of the pelvis are the lumbosacral joints, the sacrococcygeal joint, the sacroiliac joints, and the pubic symphysis (Fig. 4.2). Strong ligaments support and strengthen these joints (Fig. 4.3).

Lumbosacral Joints

L5 and S1 vertebrae articulate at the anterior **intervertebral (IV) joint** formed by the IV disc between their bodies and at two posterior **zygapophysial joints** (facet joints) between the auricular (articular) processes of these vertebrae. The facets on S1 vertebra face posteromedially, thereby preventing L5 vertebra from sliding anteriorly. **Iliolumbar ligaments** unite the ilia and L5 vertebra.

Sacrococcygeal Joint

This secondary cartilaginous joint has an IV disc. Fibrocartilage and ligaments join the apex of the sacrum to the base of the coccyx. The anterior and posterior **sacrococcygeal ligaments** are long strands that reinforce the joint, much like the anterior and posterior longitudinal ligaments do for superior vertebrae.

Sacroiliac Joints

These articulations are strong, weightbearing synovial joints between the ear-shaped auricular surfaces of the sacrum and ilium (Figs. 4.2 and 4.4). These surfaces have irregular elevations and depressions that produce some interlocking of the bones. The sacrum is suspended between the iliac bones and is firmly attached to them by **interosseous** and **sacroiliac ligaments.** The sacroiliac joints differ from most synovial joints in that they allow very little mobility because of their role in transmitting the weight of most of the body to the hip bones. *Movement of the sacroiliac joints is limited because of the interlocking of the articulating bones* and the thick **interosseous** and **posterior sacroiliac ligaments** (Fig. 4.4). Movement is limited to slight gliding and rotary movements, except when subject to considerable force such as occurs following a high jump. The weight of the body is transmitted through the sacrum anterior to the rotation axis, tending to push the upper sacrum inferiorly and thus causing the inferior sacrum to rotate superiorly. This tendency is resisted by the strong sacrotuberous and sacrospinous ligaments. Weight is transferred from the axial skeleton to the ilia and then to the femurs during standing and to the ischial tuberosities during sitting. The **sacrotuberous** and **sacrospinous ligaments** allow only limited upward movement of the inferior end of the sacrum, thereby providing resilience to the sacroiliac region when the vertebral column sustains sudden weight increases (Figs. 4.3 and 4.4).

Pubic Symphysis

This secondary cartilaginous joint is formed by the union of the bodies of the pubic bones in the median plane (Figs. 4.2 and 4.3). The fibrocartilaginous *interpubic disc* of the symphysis is generally thicker in women than in men. The ligaments joining the pubic bones are thickened superiorly and inferiorly to form the **superior pubic ligament** and the **inferior (arcuate) pubic ligament,** respectively.

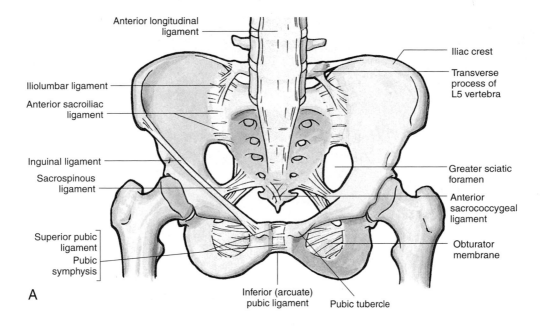

A

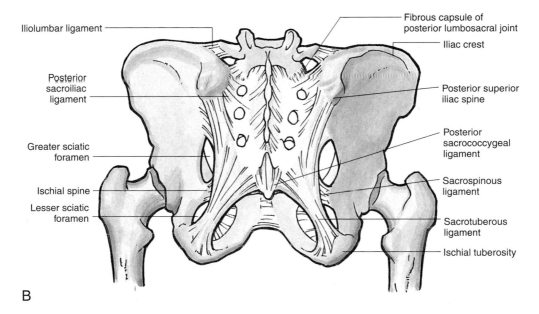

B

FIGURE 4.3   **Ligaments of the pelvis. A.** Anterior view. **B.** Posterior view.

RELAXATION OF PELVIC JOINTS AND LIGAMENTS DURING PREGNANCY

During pregnancy, the pelvic joints and ligaments relax and pelvic movements increase. The relaxation, caused by the *increase in sex hormones* and the presence of the hormone *relaxin,* permits freer movements between the inferior parts of the vertebral column and the pelvis. The sacroiliac interlocking mechanism is less effective because the relaxation permits greater rotation of the pelvis and a small increase in pelvic diameters during childbirth. Loosening of the interpubic disc also occurs, resulting in an increase in the distance between the pubic bones. The coccyx also moves posteriorly during childbirth. All these changes result in as much as a 10 to 15% increase in diameters (mostly transverse), which facilitate passage of the fetus through the pelvic canal.

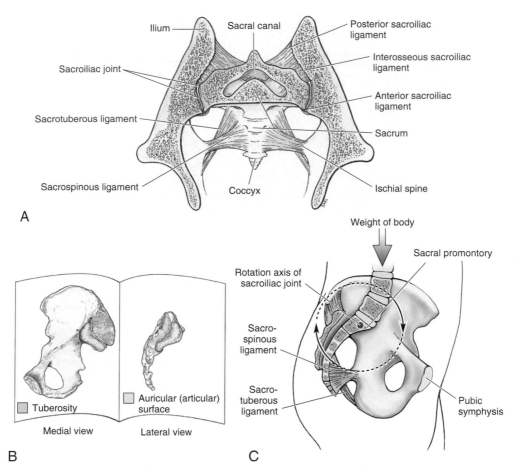

FIGURE 4.4 Sacroiliac joints and ligaments. A. Coronal section of the pelvis illustrating the sagittally oriented joints. **B.** Auricular surfaces of the sacroiliac joint. **C.** Axis of rotation of the sacroiliac joint.

PELVIC WALLS AND FLOOR

The pelvic walls are divided into an anterior wall, two lateral walls, and a posterior wall (Fig. 4.5). Muscles of the pelvic walls are summarized in Table 4.2.

The anterior pelvic wall:

- Is formed primarily by the bodies and rami of the pubic bones and the pubic symphysis
- Is anteroinferiorly placed in the anatomical position.

The lateral pelvic walls:

- Have a bony framework formed by the hip bones, including the obturator foramen (Fig. 4.2*A*); the *obturator foramen* is closed by the *obturator membrane* (Fig. 4.3*A*).

- Are covered and padded by the **obturator internus muscles** (Fig. 4.5, *B* and *C*). Each obturator internus passes posteriorly from its origin within the lesser pelvis, exits through the *lesser sciatic foramen,* and turns sharply laterally to attach to the femur (see Chapter 6).
- Have the obturator nerves and vessels and other branches of the internal iliac vessels located on their medial aspects (medial to obturator internus muscles).

The posterior pelvic wall:

- Is rooflike and formed by the sacrum and coccyx, adjacent parts of the ilia, and the sacroiliac joints and their associated ligaments.
- Is padded posterolaterally by the **piriformis muscles.** Each muscle leaves the

lesser pelvis through the *greater sciatic foramen* to attach to the femur (see Chapter 6).

- Is the site of the nerves of the **sacral plexus;** the piriformis muscles form a "muscular bed" for this nerve network (Fig. 4.5, *B* and *C*).

The **pelvic floor** is formed by the funnel-shaped **pelvic diaphragm,** which consists of the levator ani and coccygeus muscles and the fascia covering the superior and inferior aspects of these muscles (Fig. 4.5*A*). *The pelvic diaphragm stretches between the pubis anteriorly and the coccyx posteriorly and from one lateral pelvic wall to the other.* The levator ani—a broad muscular sheet—is the larger and more important muscle of the pelvic floor. *The levator ani:*

- Forms a muscular sling for supporting the abdominopelvic viscera
- Resists increases in intra-abdominal pressure
- Helps to hold the pelvic viscera in position.

The **levator ani** is attached to the internal surface of the lesser pelvis. *The levator ani—forming most of the pelvic floor—consists of two parts, one of which is further subdivided.* All parts are named according to the attachment of its fibers (Fig. 4.5, Table 4.2). *The parts of the levator ani are:*

- The **pubococcygeus,** the main anterior part of the levator ani, arises from the posterior aspect of the body of the pubis and passes almost horizontally. The lateral part of this muscle attaches posteriorly to the coccyx and anococcygeal raphe. *The medial part of the muscle is described as having two subdivisions:*
- In males, the most medial and anterior fibers pass across the side of the prostate to insert into the perineal body, forming the **puboprostaticus** (levator prostatae); comparable fibers in the female extend from the pubis into the lateral walls of the vagina forming the **pubovaginalis.**
- The **puborectalis,** consisting of the thicker, larger remainder of the medialmost part

TABLE 4.2. MUSCLES OF PELVIC WALLS

Muscle	Proximal Attachment	Distal Attachment	Innervation	Main Action
Obturator internus	Pelvic surfaces of ilium and ischium; obturator membrane	Greater trochanter of femur	Nerve to obturator internus (L5, S1, and S2)	Rotates thigh laterally; assists in holding head of femur in acetabulum
Piriformis	Pelvic surface of 2nd–4th sacral segments; superior margin of greater sciatic notch and sacrotuberous ligament		Anterior rami of S1 and S2	Rotates thigh laterally; abducts thigh; assists in holding head of femur in acetabulum
Levator ani (pubococcygeus and iliococcygeus)	Body of pubis, tendinous arch of obturator fascia, and ischial spine	Perineal body, coccyx, anococcygeal ligament, walls of prostate or vagina, rectum, and anal canal	Nerve to levator ani (branches of S4) and inferior anal (rectal) nerve and coccygeal plexus	Helps to support the pelvic viscera and resists increases in intra-abdominal pressure
Coccygeus (ischiococcygeus)	Ischial spine	Inferior end of sacrum	Branches of S4 and S5 nerves	Forms small part of pelvic diaphragm that supports pelvic viscera; flexes coccyx

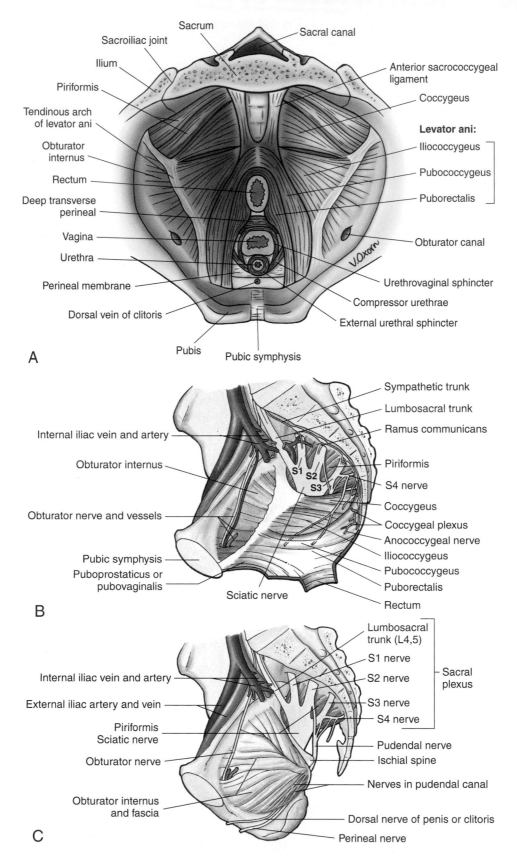

FIGURE 4.5 **Pelvic walls. A.** Floor of the female pelvis. **B.** Lateral wall of the lesser pelvis showing the pelvic diaphragm and its relationship to the sacral and coccygeal plexuses. **C.** Lateral wall of the lesser pelvis showing the obturator internus and piriformis muscles, sacral plexus, obturator nerve and vessels, and pudendal canal.

of the pubococcygeus, is formed by continuous fibers passing from one pubic bone to the other around the posterior aspect of the anorectal junction, forming a U-shaped muscular sling (Fig. 4.5*B*).

- The **iliococcygeus,** the posterior part of the levator ani, arising from the inner surface of the ilium, is thin and often poorly developed.

Acting together, the parts of the levator ani raise the pelvic floor, following its descent when relaxed to allow defecation and urination, restoring its normal position. Further contraction occurs when the thoracic diaphragm and anterolateral abdominal wall muscles contract to compress the abdominal and pelvic contents; thus, it can resist the increased intra-abdominal pressure that would otherwise force the abdominopelvic contents (gas, solid and liquid wastes, as well as the viscera) through the pelvic outlet. This action occurs reflexively during forced expiration, coughing, sneezing, vomiting, and fixation of the trunk during strong movements of the upper limbs, as occurs when lifting a heavy object. The levator ani also has important functions in the voluntary control of urination, fecal continence (via the puborectalis), and support of the uterus.

INJURY TO PELVIC FLOOR

During childbirth the pelvic floor supports the fetal head while the cervix of the uterus is dilating to permit delivery of the fetus. *The perineum, levator ani, and pelvic fascia may be injured during childbirth;* it is the pubococcygeus, the main part of the levator ani, that is usually torn. This part of the muscle is important because it encircles and supports the urethra, vagina, and anal canal. Weakening of the levator ani and pelvic fascia resulting from stretching or tearing during childbirth may alter the position of the neck of the bladder and urethra. These changes cause *urinary stress incontinence,* characterized by dribbling of urine when intra-abdominal pressure is raised during coughing and lifting, for example.

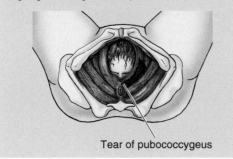

Tear of pubococcygeus

PELVIC NERVES

Pelvic structures are innervated mainly by the *sacral* (S1-S4) *and coccygeal nerves* and the pelvic part of the *autonomic nervous system.* The piriformis and coccygeus muscles form a bed for the sacral and coccygeal nerve plexuses (Fig. 4.5*B*). The anterior rami of S2 and S3 nerves emerge between the digitations of these muscles. The descending part of L4 nerve unites with the anterior ramus of L5 nerve to form the thick, cordlike **lumbosacral trunk.** It passes inferiorly, anterior to the ala of the sacrum to join the sacral plexus.

Sacral Plexus

The sacral plexus (Fig. 4.5, *B* and *C,* Table 4.3) *is located on the posterior wall of the lesser pelvis,* where it is closely related to the anterior surface of the piriformis. *The two main nerves of the sacral plexus are the sciatic and pudendal.* Most branches of the sacral plexus leave the pelvis through the greater sciatic foramen.

The **sciatic nerve**—the largest and broadest nerve in the body—is formed by the anterior rami of L4 to S3 that converge on the anterior surface of the piriformis. Most commonly, the sciatic nerve passes through the *greater sciatic foramen* inferior to the piriformis to enter the gluteal (buttock) region.

The **pudendal nerve**—*the main nerve of the perineum and the chief sensory nerve of the external genitalia*—is derived from the anterior divisions of the anterior rami of S2 through S4. It accompanies the internal pudendal artery and leaves the pelvis through the greater sciatic foramen between the piriformis and coccygeus muscles. The pudendal nerve hooks around the ischial spine and sacrospinous ligament (Fig. 4.5*C*) and enters the perineum through the lesser sciatic foramen. It supplies the skin and muscles of the perineum, ending as the dorsal nerve of the penis or of the clitoris.

The **superior gluteal nerve** (Table 4.3) arises from the posterior divisions of the anterior rami of L4 through S1 and leaves the pelvis through the greater sciatic foramen, superior to the piriformis. It supplies two muscles in the gluteal region—the gluteus medius and minimus—and the tensor of fascia lata (see Chapter 6).

TABLE 4.3. NERVES OF SACRAL AND COCCYGEAL PLEXUSES

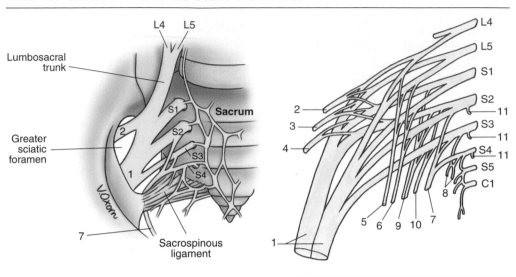

Nerve	Segmental Origin	Distribution
1. Sciatic	L4, L5, S1, S2, S3	Articular branches to hip joint and muscular branches to flexors of knee (hamstring muscles), and all muscles in leg and foot
2. Superior gluteal	L4, L5, S1	Gluteus medius and gluteus minimus muscles
3. Inferior gluteal	L5, S1, S2	Gluteus maximus muscle
4. Nerve to piriformis	S1, S2	Piriformis muscle
5. Nerve to quadratus femoris and inferior gemellus	L4, L5, S1	Quadratus femoris and inferior gemellus muscles
6. Nerve to obturator internus and superior gemellus	L5, S1, S2	Obturator internus and superior gemellus muscles
7. Pudendal	S2, S3, S4	Structures in perineum: sensory to genitalia, muscular branches to perineal muscles, sphincter urethrae and external anal sphincter
8. Nerves to levator ani and coccygeus	S3, S4	Levator ani and coccygeus muscles
9. Posterior femoral cutaneous	S2, S3	Cutaneous branches to buttock and uppermost medial and posterior surfaces of thigh
10. Perforating cutaneous	S2, S3	Cutaneous branches to medial part of buttock
11. Pelvic splanchnic	S2, S3, S4	Pelvic viscera via inferior hypogastric and pelvic plexus

The **inferior gluteal nerve** arises from the posterior divisions of the anterior rami of L5 through S2 and leaves the pelvis through the greater sciatic foramen, inferior to the piriformis and superficial to the sciatic nerve. It accompanies the inferior gluteal artery and breaks up into several branches that supply the overlying gluteus maximus muscle (see Chapter 6).

Obturator Nerve

The obturator nerve arises from the lumbar plexus (anterior divisions of anterior rami of L2 through L4) in the abdomen (greater pelvis) and enters the lesser pelvis (Fig. 4.5, *A–C*). It runs in the extraperitoneal fat along the lateral wall of the pelvis to the **obturator canal**—the opening in the obturator membrane—where it divides into anterior and posterior branches that leave the pelvis through this canal and supply the medial thigh muscles (see Chapter 6).

INJURY TO PELVIC NERVES

During childbirth the fetal head may compress the mother's sacral plexus, producing pain in her lower limbs. The obturator nerve is vulnerable to injury during surgery (e.g., during removal of cancerous lymph nodes from the lateral pelvic wall). *Injury to the obturator nerve* may cause painful spasms of the adductor muscles of the thigh (see Chapter 6) and sensory deficits in the medial thigh region.

Coccygeal Plexus

The coccygeal plexus is a small nerve network formed by the anterior rami of S4 and S5 and the coccygeal nerves. It lies on the pelvic surface of the coccygeus and supplies this muscle, part of the levator ani, and the sacrococcygeal joint (Fig. 4.5*B*). The **anococcygeal nerves** arising from this plexus pierce the sacrotuberous ligament and supply a small area of skin in the coccygeal region.

Pelvic Autonomic Nerves

The sacral sympathetic trunks are the inferior continuation of the lumbar sympathetic trunks (Fig. 4.6). Each sacral trunk usually has four sympathetic ganglia. The **sacral sympathetic trunks** descend on the pelvic surface of the sacrum just medial to the pelvic sacral foramina, and commonly converge to form the small median **ganglion impar** anterior to the coccyx. The sympathetic trunks descend posterior to the rectum in the extraperitoneal connective tissue and send communicating branches (gray rami communicantes) to each of the anterior rami of the sacral and coccygeal nerves. They also send branches to the median sacral artery and the inferior hypogastric plexus. The primary function of the sacral sympathetic trunks is to provide postsynaptic fibers to the sacral plexus for sympathetic innervation of the lower limb.

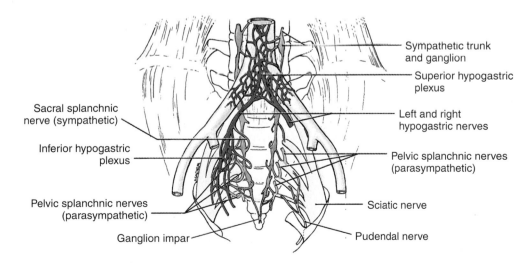

FIGURE 4.6 **Autonomic nerves of the pelvis.** Anterior view. *Orange,* sympathetic trunk and nerves; *green,* parasympathetic nerves; *purple,* plexuses; *yellow,* sciatic and pudendal nerves.

The **hypogastric plexuses**—superior and inferior—are networks of autonomic nerves (Fig. 4.6). The main part of the **superior hypogastric plexus** lies just inferior to the bifurcation of the aorta and descends into the pelvis. This plexus is the inferior prolongation of the *intermesenteric plexus* (see Chapter 3), which also receives the L3 and L4 splanchnic nerves. Branches from the superior hypogastric plexus enter the pelvis and descend anterior to the sacrum as the left and right **hypogastric nerves.** These nerves descend lateral to the rectum and then spread to form the **inferior hypogastric plexuses.** Extensions of the inferior hypogastric plexuses (pelvic plexuses) in both sexes pass to the lateral surfaces of the rectum and to the inferolateral surfaces of the urinary bladder, and in males to the prostate and seminal glands (vesicles) and in females to the cervix of the uterus and lateral parts of the fornix of the vagina.

The **pelvic splanchnic nerves** (Fig. 4.6, Table 4.3) contain parasympathetic and visceral afferent fibers derived from S2, S3, and S4 spinal cord segments and visceral afferent fibers from cell bodies in the spinal ganglia of the corresponding spinal nerves. The pelvic splanchnic nerves merge with the hypogastric nerves to form the inferior hypogastric (and pelvic) plexuses. The inferior hypogastric plexuses therefore contain both sympathetic and parasympathetic fibers, which pass along the branches of the internal iliac arteries and form subplexuses (such as the rectal plexus) on the pelvic viscera. Parasympathetic fibers from the inferior hypogastric plexuses also ascend to supply the descending and sigmoid colon.

PELVIC ARTERIES AND VEINS

Four main arteries enter the lesser pelvis in females, three in males:

- The paired internal iliac arteries
- The paired ovarian arteries
- The median sacral artery
- The superior rectal artery.

The origin, course, and distribution of these arteries and their branches are summarized in Table 4.4.

The pelvis is drained:

- Mainly by the internal iliac veins and their tributaries
- Superior rectal veins (see portal venous system, p. 180)
- Median sacral vein
- Gonadal veins
- Internal vertebral venous plexus (p. 292)

Pelvic venous plexuses are formed by the interjoining of veins in the pelvis (Table 4.4). The various plexuses (rectal, vesical, prostatic, uterine, and vaginal) unite and drain mainly into the **internal iliac vein,** but some drain through the superior rectal vein into the inferior mesenteric vein or through lateral sacral veins into the internal vertebral venous plexus.

PELVIC CAVITY AND VISCERA

The pelvic viscera include the inferior part of the intestinal tract (rectum), the urinary bladder, and parts of the ureters and reproductive system (Figs. 4.7 and 4.8). Although the sigmoid colon and parts of the small bowel extend into the pelvic cavity, they are mobile at their abdominal attachments; therefore, they are not pelvic viscera.

URINARY ORGANS

The pelvic urinary organs (Fig. 4.9) *are the:*

- Ureters, which carry urine from the kidneys
- Urinary bladder, which temporarily stores urine
- Urethra, which conducts urine from the urinary bladder to the exterior.

Ureters

The ureters are muscular tubes that connect the kidneys to the urinary bladder. The ureters run inferiorly from the kidneys, passing over the pelvic brim at the bifurcation of the common iliac arteries (Figs. 4.7 and 4.8). The ureters then run posteroinferiorly on the lateral walls of the pelvis, external to the parietal

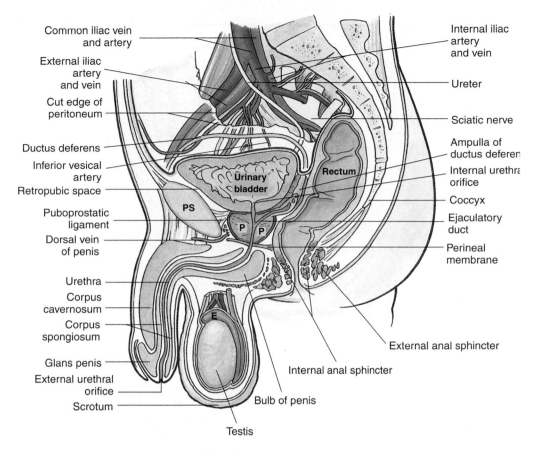

FIGURE 4.7 **Median section of the male pelvis.** *PS,* pubic symphysis; *P,* prostate; *E,* epididymis.

Common iliac vein and artery

External iliac artery and vein

Cut edge of peritoneum

Ductus deferens

Inferior vesical artery

Retropubic space

Puboprostatic ligament

Dorsal vein of penis

Urethra

Corpus cavernosum

Corpus spongiosum

Glans penis

External urethral orifice

Scrotum

Testis

Urinary bladder

Rectum

PS

P   P

E

Internal iliac artery and vein

Ureter

Sciatic nerve

Ampulla of ductus deferen

Internal urethra orifice

Coccyx

Ejaculatory duct

Perineal membrane

External anal sphincter

Internal anal sphincter

Bulb of penis

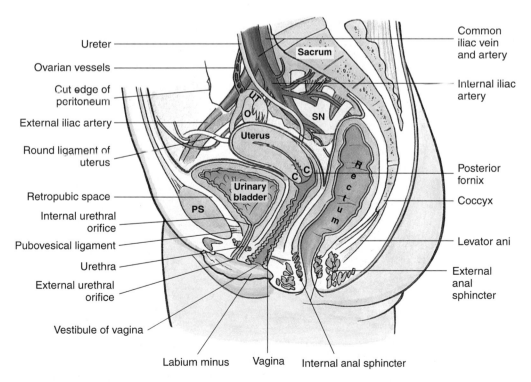

FIGURE 4.8 **Median section of the female pelvis.** *UT,* uterine tube; *O,* ovary; *SN,* sciatic nerve; *C,* cervix of uterus; *PS,* pubic symphysis.

Ureter

Ovarian vessels

Cut edge of peritoneum

External iliac artery

Round ligament of uterus

Retropubic space

Internal urethral orifice

Pubovesical ligament

Urethra

External urethral orifice

Vestibule of vagina

Labium minus

Vagina

Internal anal sphincter

Sacrum

UT

O

SN

Uterus

C   C

Rectum

Urinary bladder

PS

Common iliac vein and artery

Internal iliac artery

Posterior fornix

Coccyx

Levator ani

External anal sphincter

TABLE 4.4. ARTERIES AND VEINS OF PELVIS

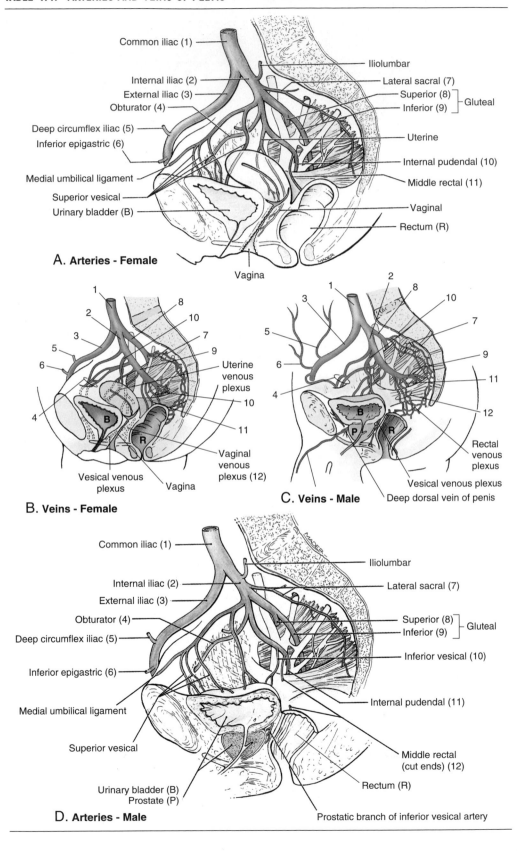

A. Arteries - Female

Common iliac (1)
Internal iliac (2)
External iliac (3)
Obturator (4)
Deep circumflex iliac (5)
Inferior epigastric (6)
Medial umbilical ligament
Superior vesical
Urinary bladder (B)
Vagina

Iliolumbar
Lateral sacral (7)
Superior (8)
Inferior (9) Gluteal
Uterine
Internal pudendal (10)
Middle rectal (11)
Vaginal
Rectum (R)

B. Veins - Female

1
2
3
5
6
8
10
7
9
4
B
R
Uterine venous plexus
10
11
Vesical venous plexus
Vagina
Vaginal venous plexus (12)

C. Veins - Male

1
3
5
6
4
2
8
10
7
9
11
12
B
P
R
Rectal venous plexus
Vesical venous plexus
Deep dorsal vein of penis

D. Arteries - Male

Common iliac (1)
Internal iliac (2)
External iliac (3)
Obturator (4)
Deep circumflex iliac (5)
Inferior epigastric (6)
Medial umbilical ligament
Superior vesical
Urinary bladder (B)
Prostate (P)

Iliolumbar
Lateral sacral (7)
Superior (8)
Inferior (9) Gluteal
Inferior vesical (10)
Internal pudendal (11)
Middle rectal (cut ends) (12)
Rectum (R)
Prostatic branch of inferior vesical artery

TABLE 4.4. *CONTINUED*

Artery	Origin	Course	Distribution
Internal iliac	Common iliac artery	Passes over pelvic brim to reach pelvic cavity	Main blood supply to pelvic organs, gluteal muscles, and perineum
Anterior division of internal iliac artery	Internal iliac artery	Passes anteriorly and divides into visceral branches and obturator artery	Pelvic viscera and muscles in medial compartment of thigh
Umbilical	Anterior division of internal iliac artery	Short pelvic course and ends as superior vesical artery in females	Superior aspect of urinary bladder in females; ductus deferens in males
Obturator		Runs anteroinferiorly on lateral pelvic wall	Pelvic muscles, nutrient artery to ilium, and head of femur
Superior vesical artery	Patent part of umbilical artery	Passes to superior aspect of urinary bladder	Superior aspect of urinary bladder
Artery to ductus deferens	Superior or inferior vesical artery	Runs retroperitoneally to ductus deferens	Ductus deferens
Inferior vesical		Passes retroperitoneally to inferior aspect of male urinary bladder	Urinary bladder, pelvic part of ureter, seminal gland, and prostate
Middle rectal		Descends in pelvis to rectum	Seminal gland, prostate, and rectum
Internal pudendal	Anterior division of internal iliac artery	Leaves pelvis through greater sciatic foramen and enters perineum (ischioanal fossa) by passing through lesser sciatic foramen	Main artery to perineum including muscles of anal canal and perineum; skin and urogenital triangle; erectile bodies
Inferior gluteal		Leaves pelvis through greater sciatic foramen	Piriformis, coccygeus, levator ani, and gluteal muscles
Uterine		Runs medially on levator ani; crosses ureter to reach base of broad ligament	Pelvic part of ureter, uterus, ligament of uterus, uterine tube, and vagina
Vaginal	Uterine artery	At junction of body and cervix of uterus, it descends to vagina	Vagina and branches to inferior part of urinary bladder
Gonadal (testicular and ovarian)	Abdominal aorta	Descends retroperitoneally; testicular artery passes into deep inguinal ring; ovarian artery crosses brim of pelvis and runs medially in suspensory ligament to ovary	Testis and ovary, respectively
Posterior division of internal iliac artery	Internal iliac artery	Passes posteriorly and gives rise to parietal branches	Pelvic wall and gluteal region
Iliolumbar	Posterior division of internal iliac artery	Ascends anterior to sacroiliac joint and posterior to common iliac vessels and psoas major	Iliacus, psoas major, quadratus lumborum muscles, and cauda equina in vertebral canal
Lateral sacral (superior and inferior)		Run on superficial aspect of piriformis	Piriformis and vertebral canal

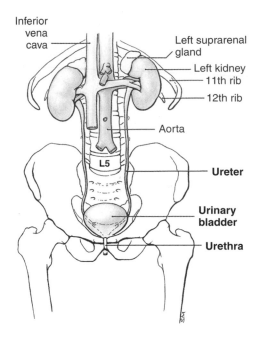

FIGURE 4.9 **Urinary organs.** The kidneys in the abdomen are connected by the ureters to the urinary bladder in the pelvis.

peritoneum (i.e., retroperitoneally) and anterior to the internal iliac arteries. They then curve anteromedially, superior to the levator ani, and enter the bladder. *In males* the only structure that passes between the ureter and the peritoneum is the **ductus deferens** (vas deferens). The ureter lies posterolateral to the ductus deferens and enters the posteroinferior part of the bladder (Fig. 4.8). *In females* the ureter passes medial to the origin of the uterine artery and continues to the level of the ischial spine, where it is crossed superiorly by the uterine artery and inferiorly by the vaginal artery. The ureter then passes close to the lateral part of the fornix of the vagina and enters the posteroinferior aspect of the bladder.

Vasculature of Ureters. Branches of the common and internal **iliac arteries** supply the pelvic part of the ureters (Table 4.4). The most constant arteries supplying this part of the ureters in females are branches of the **uterine arteries.** The sources of similar branches in males are the **inferior vesical arteries.** Veins from the ureters accompany the arteries and

have corresponding names. **Lymph** drains into the lumbar (lateral aortic), common iliac, external iliac, and internal iliac lymph nodes (see Fig. 4.12*A*).

Innervation of Ureters. The nerves to the ureters derive from adjacent *autonomic plexuses* (renal, aortic, superior and inferior hypogastric). Afferent (pain) fibers from the ureters follow sympathetic fibers retrogradely to reach the spinal ganglia and spinal cord segments T11 through L1 or L2 (see Fig. 4.12*B*).

URETERIC CALCULI

Ureteric calculi (stones) may cause complete or intermittent *obstruction of urinary flow.* The obstruction may occur anywhere along the ureter; however, it occurs most often where the ureter crosses the external iliac artery and the pelvic brim and where it passes through the wall of the bladder. The severity of the pain associated with calculi can be extremely intense; it depends on the location, type, size, and texture of the calculus.

Urinary Bladder

The urinary bladder, a hollow viscus with strong muscular walls, is in the lesser pelvis when empty, posterior and slightly superior to the pubic bones. It is separated from these bones by the **retropubic space** and lies inferior to the peritoneum where it rests on the pelvic floor (Figs. 4.7 and 4.8). The bladder is relatively free within the extraperitoneal fatty tissue except for its neck, which is held firmly by the **puboprostatic ligaments** in males and the **pubovesical ligaments** in females. As the bladder fills, it ascends superiorly into the extraperitoneal fatty tissue of the anterior abdominal wall and enters the greater pelvis. A full bladder may ascend to the level of the umbilicus. The bladder always contains some urine and is usually more or less rounded. The empty, contracted bladder in a cadaver has four surfaces (Fig. 4.10): a superior surface, two inferolateral surfaces, and a posterior surface. The bladder has an apex, body, fundus, neck, and uvula.

The **apex of the bladder** (anterior end) points toward the superior edge of the pubic symphysis. The **body of the bladder** is the part between the apex and fundus. The **fundus of the bladder** is formed by the posterior wall,

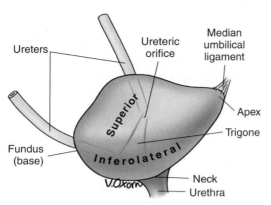

Ureters

Ureteric orifice

Median umbilical ligament

Apex

Trigone

Fundus (base)

Superior

Inferolateral

V.Oxorn

Neck

Urethra

A

FIGURE 4.10   **Urinary bladder. A.** Location of the urinary bladder in the pelvis, lateral view. **B.** Coronal section of male pelvis. **C.** Coronal section of female pelvis.

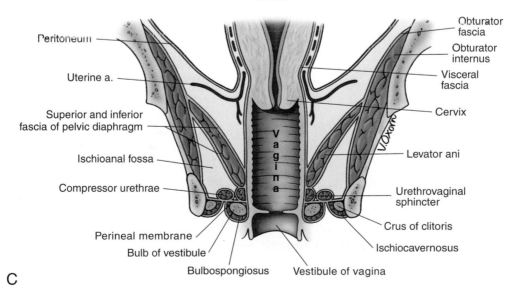

Ureteric orifices

Peritoneum

Detrusor muscle

Trigone

Superior and inferior fascia of pelvic diaphragm

Ischioanal fossa

External urethral sphincter

Compressor urethrae

Perineal membrane

Bulbospongiosus

Spongy urethra

Urinary bladder

Obturator fascia

Obturator internus

Visceral fascia

Internal urethral orifice

Levator ani

Prostate

Prostatic urethra

Bulbourethral gland

Crus of penis

Ischiocavernosus

Bulb of penis

B

Peritoneum

Uterine a.

Superior and inferior fascia of pelvic diaphragm

Ischioanal fossa

Compressor urethrae

Perineal membrane

Bulb of vestibule

Bulbospongiosus

Vestibule of vagina

Vagina

Obturator fascia

Obturator internus

Visceral fascia

Cervix

Levator ani

Urethrovaginal sphincter

Crus of clitoris

Ischiocavernosus

C

which is somewhat convex. *In females* the fundus is closely related to the anterior wall of the vagina; *in males* it is related to the rectum. The **neck of the bladder** is where the fundus and inferolateral surfaces converge (Fig. 4.11*A*). The **uvula of the bladder** is a slight projection of the **trigone of the bladder** situated posterior to the **internal urethral orifice** (Figs. 4.7 and 4.8).

The **bladder bed** is formed on each side by the pubic bones and the obturator internus and levator ani muscles and posteriorly by the rectum or vagina. The bladder is enveloped by loose connective tissue—*vesical fascia.* The wall of the bladder is composed chiefly of the **detrusor muscle** (Fig. 4.10*B*). Toward the neck of the male bladder, its muscle fibers form the involuntary **internal sphincter.** Some fibers run radially and assist in opening the **internal urethral orifice.** *In males* the muscle fibers in the neck of the bladder are continuous with the fibromuscular tissue of the prostate. *There is no internal sphincter in the female* at the neck of the bladder. The muscle fibers are longitudinal and are continuous with muscle fibers in the wall of the urethra. The **ureteric orifices** and the internal urethral orifice are at the angles of the **trigone of the bladder.** The ureters pass obliquely through the bladder wall in an inferomedial direction. An increase in bladder pressure presses the walls of the ureters together, preventing the pressure in the bladder from forcing urine up the ureters.

The peritoneal reflections in the pelvis are illustrated in Fig. 4.11.

Vasculature of Bladder. The main arteries supplying the bladder are branches of the **internal iliac arteries** (Table 4.4). The **superior**

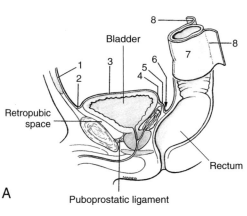

Male

Peritoneum passes:
• From the anterior abdominal wall (1)
• Superior to the pubic bone (2)
• On the superior surface of the urinary bladder (3)
• 2 cm inferiorly on the posterior surface of the urinary bladder (4)
• On the superior ends of the seminal glands (5)
• Posteriorly to line the rectovesical pouch (6)
• To cover the rectum (7)
• Posteriorly to become the sigmoid mesocolon (8)

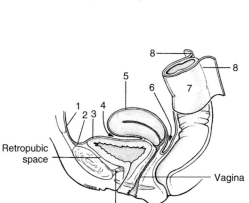

Female

Peritoneum passes:
• From the anterior abdominal wall (1)
• Superior to the pubic bone (2)
• On the superior surface of the urinary bladder (3)
• From the bladder to the uterus, forming the vesicouterine pouch (4)
• On the fundus and body of the uterus, posterior fornix, and all of the vagina (5)
• Between the rectum and uterus, forming the rectouterine pouch (6)
• On the anterior and lateral sides of the rectum (7)
• Posteriorly to become the sigmoid mesocolon (8)

FIGURE 4.11   Peritoneal reflections in the pelvis. A. Male. **B.** Female.

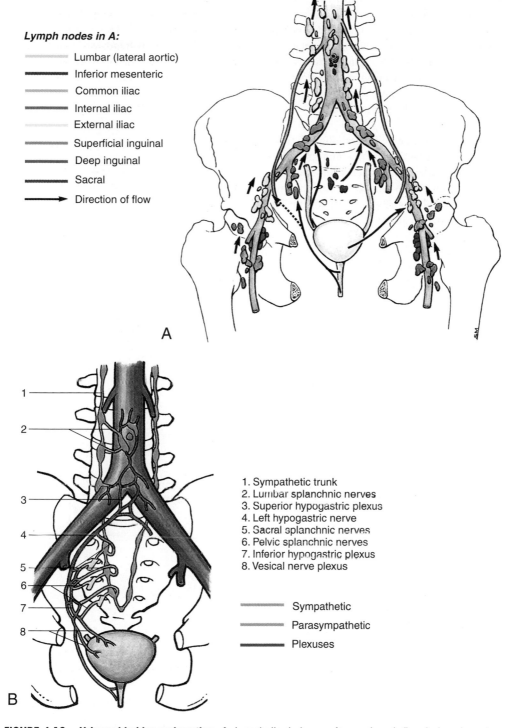

Lymph nodes in A:

Lumbar (lateral aortic)
Inferior mesenteric
Common iliac
Internal iliac
External iliac
Superficial inguinal
Deep inguinal
Sacral
Direction of flow

A

1. Sympathetic trunk
2. Lumbar splanchnic nerves
3. Superior hypogastric plexus
4. Left hypogastric nerve
5. Sacral splanchnic nerves
6. Pelvic splanchnic nerves
7. Inferior hypogastric plexus
8. Vesical nerve plexus

Sympathetic
Parasympathetic
Plexuses

B

FIGURE 4.12   Urinary bladder and urethra. A. Lymphatic drainage. *Arrows,* lymph flow to lymph nodes.
B. Autonomic innervation.

vesical arteries supply anterosuperior parts of the bladder. *In males,* the fundus and neck of the bladder are supplied by the **inferior vesical arteries.** *In females,* the inferior vesical arteries are replaced by the **vaginal arteries** that send small branches to posteroinferior parts of the bladder. The obturator and inferior gluteal arteries also supply small branches to the bladder.

The names of the veins draining the bladder correspond to the arteries and are tributaries of the internal iliac veins. In males the vesical venous plexus combines with the **prostatic venous plexus** (Fig. 4.13B) to envelop the fundus of the bladder and prostate, the seminal glands (vesicles), the ductus deferentes (plural of ductus deferens), and the inferior ends of the ureters. The prostatic venous plexus, a dense network of veins, also receives blood from the dorsal vein of the penis. The **vesical venous plexus** mainly drains through the inferior vesical veins into the internal iliac veins (Table 4.4); however, it may drain through the sacral veins into the *internal vertebral venous plexuses* (see p. 292). *In females* the **vesical venous plexus** envelops the pelvic part of the urethra and the neck of the bladder and receives blood from the dorsal vein of the clitoris and communicates with the **vaginal or uterine venous plexus** (Table 4.4). In both sexes, lymphatic vessels leave the superior surface of the bladder and pass to the **external iliac lymph nodes** (Fig. 4.10A), whereas those from the fundus pass to the **internal iliac lymph nodes.** Some vessels from the neck of the bladder drain into the sacral or common iliac lymph nodes.

Innervation of Bladder. Parasympathetic fibers to the bladder are derived from the **pelvic splanchnic nerves** (Fig. 4.10B). They are motor to the detrusor muscle in the bladder wall and inhibitory to the internal sphincter of males. Hence, when the visceral afferent fibers are stimulated by stretching, the bladder contracts, the internal sphincter relaxes in the male, and urine flows into the urethra. Adults suppress this reflex until it is convenient to void. *Sympathetic fibers* to the bladder are derived from T11 through L2 nerves. The nerves

supplying the bladder form the **vesical nerve plexus**, which consists of both sympathetic and parasympathetic fibers. This plexus is continuous with the **inferior hypogastric plexus**. Sensory fibers from the bladder are visceral and transmit pain sensations such as those from overdistention.

> **SUPRAPUBIC CYSTOTOMY**
> As the bladder fills, it extends superiorly in the extraperitoneal fatty tissue of the anterior abdominal wall. The bladder then lies adjacent to this wall without the intervention of peritoneum. Consequently the distended bladder may be punctured (*suprapubic cystostomy*) or approached surgically for the introduction of in-dwelling catheters or instruments without traversing the peritoneum and entering the peritoneal cavity.
>
> **Rupture of Bladder**
> Because of the superior position of a distended bladder, it may be ruptured by injuries to the inferior part of the anterior abdominal wall or by fractures of the pelvis. The rupture may result in the passage (extravasation) of urine retroperitoneally. Posterior rupture of the bladder usually results in passage of urine subperitoneally into the perineum.
>
> **Cystoscopy**
> The interior of the bladder and its three orifices can be examined with a *cystoscope,* a lighted tubular endoscope that is inserted through the urethra. The cystoscope consists of a light, observing lens, and various attachments for grasping, removing, cutting, and cauterizing.

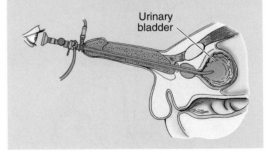

Urinary bladder

Male Urethra

The male urethra is a muscular tube that conveys urine from the internal urethral orifice of the urinary bladder (Fig. 4.13A) to the exterior through the external urethral orifice at the tip of the glans penis. The urethra also provides an exit for semen (sperms and glandular secretions). For descriptive purposes, *the urethra is divided into four parts:* urethra in the bladder neck (preprostatic urethra), prostatic

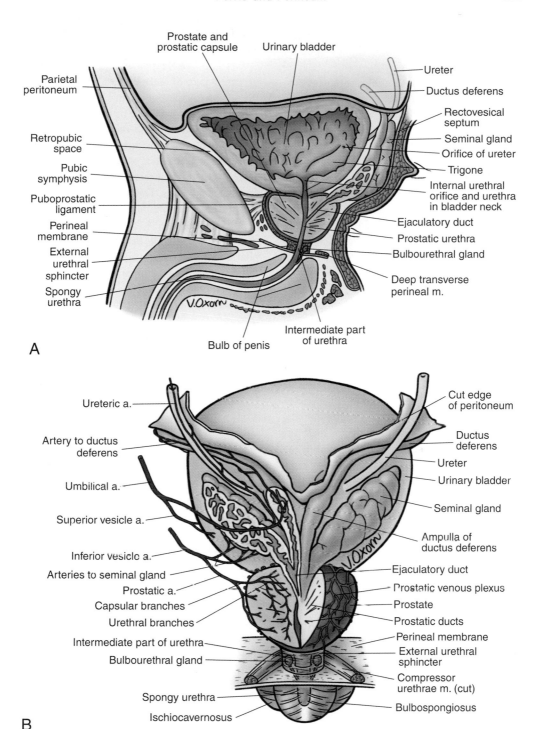

FIGURE 4.13   Urinary bladder, seminal glands, ductus deferentes, and prostate. A. Median section of the male pelvis showing the relationship of bladder, prostate, ductus deferens, and ejaculatory duct. **B.** Posterior view of the urinary bladder, ductus deferentes, and prostate. Left seminal gland and ampulla of ductus deferens have been opened, and the prostate has been cut away to expose the ejaculatory duct.

urethra, intermediate part of the urethra (membranous urethra), and spongy (penile) part of the urethra.

The **urethra in the bladder neck** (preprostatic urethra) extends almost vertically from the neck of the bladder to the superior aspect of the prostate. The **prostatic urethra** is continuous with the urethra in the bladder neck and *descends through the prostate,* forming a gentle curve that is concave anteriorly. The prostatic urethra—the widest and most dilatable part of the urethra—ends as the urethra becomes completely encircled by the external urethral sphincter. The internal surface of the posterior wall of the prostatic urethra has notable features (Fig. 4.14). The most prominent structure is the **urethral crest,** a median ridge that has a groove—**prostatic sinus**—on each side. Most prostatic ducts open into these sinuses. In the middle part of this crest is the **seminal colliculus,** a rounded eminence with a slitlike orifice, which opens into a small, vestigial cul-de-sac—the *prostatic utricle* ("little uterus"—the male homolog of the uterus). On each side of this orifice is the minute **opening of an ejaculatory duct** on or just within the prostatic utricle. The **intermediate part of the urethra** (membranous part) is the section passing through the external urethral sphincter and perineal membrane (Fig. 4.13A). The short, intermediate part extending from the prostatic urethra to the **spongy part of the urethra** in the penis is the narrowest and least dis

tensible part of the urethra because of the surrounding external urethral sphincter.

Vasculature of Male Urethra. The urethra in the bladder neck and the prostatic urethra are supplied by the prostatic branches of the **inferior vesical and middle rectal arteries** (Table 4.4). The intermediate and spongy parts of the urethra are supplied by the **internal pudendal artery**. The **veins** accompany the artery and have similar names. The **lymphatic vessels** from the urethra drain mainly into the **internal iliac lymph nodes** (Fig. 4.15A), but some lymph passes to the *external iliac lymph nodes.* Lymphatic vessels from the spongy urethra pass to the deep **inguinal lymph nodes.**

Innervation of Male Urethra. The nerves are derived from branches of the **pudendal nerve** (Fig. 4.6) and the **prostatic plexus** of the autonomic nervous system (Fig. 4.15B). This plexus arises from the inferior part of the inferior hypogastric plexus.

URETHRAL CATHETERIZATION

Urethral catheterization is done to remove urine from the bladder of a person who is unable to urinate. The circular investment of the external urethral sphincter makes the intermediate part of the urethra the least distensible part. Because of its thin wall, the inferior part of it is vulnerable to penetration by a urethral catheter or to rupture during an accident.

Urethral Stricture

Urethral stricture may result from external trauma of the penis or from infection of the urethra. Instruments— *urethral sounds*—are used to dilate the urethra for insertion of a *cystoscope* for example, to examine the interior of the bladder.

Rupture of Spongy Urethra

Rupture of the spongy part of the urethra in the bulb of the penis is common in "straddle injuries." The urethra is torn when it is caught between a hard object such as a steel beam and the person's pubic arch. Urine escapes into the *superficial perineal pouch* and passes from there inferiorly into the scrotum and superiorly into the fatty layer of subcutaneous connective tissue of the anterior abdominal wall (see p. 261).

Female Urethra

The short female urethra passes anteroinferiorly from the **internal urethral orifice** of the urinary bladder, posterior and then infe

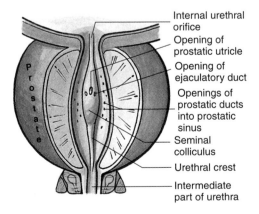

FIGURE 4.14   Posterior wall of the prostatic urethra. Observe the openings of the ejaculatory and prostatic ducts.

Internal urethral orifice
Opening of prostatic utricle
Opening of ejaculatory duct
Openings of prostatic ducts into prostatic sinus
Seminal colliculus
Urethral crest
Intermediate part of urethra

Prostate

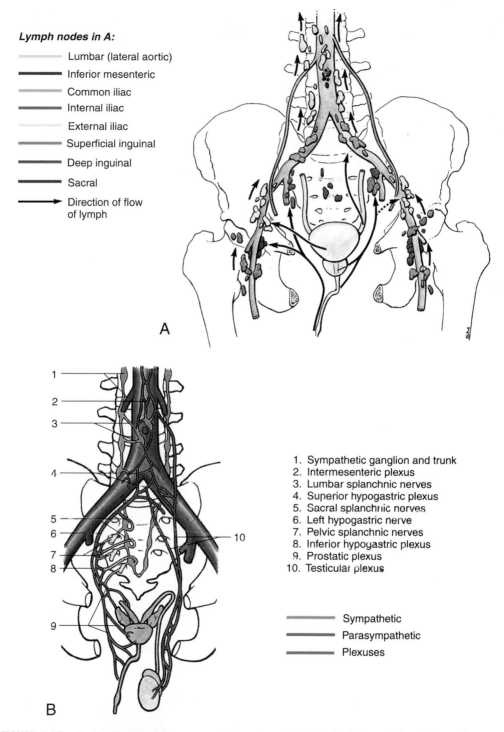

Lymph nodes in A:

Lumbar (lateral aortic)

Inferior mesenteric

Common iliac

Internal iliac

External iliac

Superficial inguinal

Deep inguinal

Sacral

Direction of flow
of lymph

A

B

1. Sympathetic ganglion and trunk
2. Intermesenteric plexus
3. Lumbar splanchnic nerves
4. Superior hypogastric plexus
5. Sacral splanchnic nerves
6. Left hypogastric nerve
7. Pelvic splanchnic nerves
8. Inferior hypogastric plexus
9. Prostatic plexus
10. Testicular plexus

Sympathetic

Parasympathetic

Plexuses

FIGURE 4.15 **Testis, ductus deferens, prostate, and seminal glands. A.** Lymphatic drainage. *Arrows,* lymph flow to lymph nodes. **B.** Autonomic innervation.

rior to the pubic symphysis (Fig. 4.8). The **external urethral orifice** is in the vestibule of the vagina. The urethra lies anterior to the vagina; its axis is parallel with the vagina. The urethra passes with the vagina through the pelvic diaphragm, external urethral sphincter, and perineal membrane. *Urethral glands* are present, particularly in the superior part of the urethra; the *paraurethral glands* are homologues to the prostate. These glands have a common paraurethral duct, which opens (one on each side) near the external urethral orifice. The inferior half of the urethra is in the perineum and is discussed subsequently with this section.

Vasculature of Female Urethra. Blood is supplied by the internal pudendal and vaginal arteries (Table 4.4). The veins follow the arteries and have similar names. Most lymphatic vessels from the urethra pass to the **sacral** and **internal iliac lymph nodes** (Fig. 4.12*A*). A few vessels drain into the inguinal lymph nodes.

Innervation of Female Urethra. The nerves to the urethra arise from the **pudendal nerve** (Fig. 4.6). Most afferents from the urethra are in the **pelvic splanchnic nerves** (Fig. 4.12*B*).

MALE INTERNAL GENITAL ORGANS

The male internal genital organs include the testes, epididymides (plural of epididymis), ductus deferentes (plural of ductus deferens), seminal glands (vesicles), ejaculatory ducts, prostate, and bulbourethral glands (Fig. 4.13). The testes and epididymides are described in Chapter 3.

Ductus Deferens

The ductus deferens (deferent duct, vas deferens) is the continuation of the duct of the epididymis (see Chapter 3). *The ductus deferens* (Figs. 4.7 and 4.13):

- Begins in the tail of the epididymis
- Ascends in the spermatic cord
- Passes through the inguinal canal

- Crosses over the external iliac vessels and enters the pelvis
- Passes along the lateral wall of the pelvis where it lies external to the parietal peritoneum
- Ends by joining the duct of the seminal gland to form the ejaculatory duct.

During its course no other structure intervenes between the ductus deferens and the peritoneum. The ductus crosses superior to the ureter near the posterolateral angle of the bladder, running between the ureter and peritoneum to reach the fundus of the urinary bladder. Posterior to the bladder, the ductus at first lies superior to the seminal gland, then descends medial to the ureter and the gland. Here the ductus enlarges to form the **ampulla of the ductus deferens** as it passes posterior to the bladder. The ductus then narrows and joins the duct of the seminal gland to form the **ejaculatory duct**.

Vasculature of Ductus Deferens. A long slender vessel, the **artery of the ductus deferens,** accompanies the ductus as far as the testis. The artery of the ductus, a branch of either the **superior** or **inferior vesical artery** (Table 4.4), terminates by anastomosing with the *testicular artery,* posterior to the testis. The veins accompany the arteries and have similar names. The lymphatic vessels from the ductus drain into the **external iliac lymph nodes** (Fig. 4.15*A*).

Innervation of Ductus Deferens. The nerves of the ductus are derived from the **inferior hypogastric plexus** (Fig. 4.15*B*). The ductus is richly innervated by autonomic nerve fibers, thereby facilitating its rapid contraction for expulsion of sperms during ejaculation.

STERILIZATION OF MALES

The common method of sterilizing males is **deferentectomy,** popularly called a *vasectomy*. During this procedure part of the ductus deferens is ligated and/or excised through an incision in the superior part of the scrotum. Hence, the ejaculated fluid from the seminal glands, prostate, and bulbourethral glands contains no sperms. The unexpelled sperms degenerate in the epididymis and the proximal part of the ductus deferens.

Seminal Glands

Each seminal gland (vesicle) is an elongated structure that lies between the fundus of the bladder and the rectum (Fig. 4.13). The seminal glands, obliquely placed structures superior to the prostate, *do not store sperms* as was once thought. They secrete a thick alkaline fluid that mixes with the sperms as they pass into the ejaculatory ducts and urethra. The superior ends of the seminal glands are covered with peritoneum and lie posterior to the ureters, where the peritoneum of the **rectovesical pouch** separates them from the rectum (Fig. 4.11). The inferior ends of the seminal glands are closely related to the rectum and are separated from it only by the **rectovesical septum**. The duct of the seminal gland joins the ductus deferens to form the ejaculatory duct (Fig. 4.13A).

Vasculature of Seminal Glands. The arteries to the seminal glands derive from the inferior vesical and middle rectal arteries (Table 4.4). The veins accompany the arteries and have similar names. The iliac lymph nodes, especially the **internal iliac lymph nodes,** receive lymph from the seminal glands (Fig. 4.15A).

Innervation of Seminal Glands. The walls of these glands contain a plexus of nerve fibers (Fig. 4.15B). *Sympathetic fibers* traverse the superior **lumbar and hypogastric nerves,** and parasympathetic fibers traverse the **pelvic splanchnic nerves** to reach the **inferior hypogastric plexuses**.

Ejaculatory Ducts

Each ejaculatory duct is a slender tube that arises by the union of the duct of a seminal gland with the ductus deferens (Fig. 4.13). The ejaculatory ducts arise near the neck of the bladder and run close together as they pass anteroinferiorly through the posterior part of the prostate and along the sides of the prostatic utricle. The ejaculatory ducts traverse the main part of the prostate and converge to open by slitlike apertures on, or just within, the opening of the prostatic utricle (Fig. 4.14).

Vasculature of Ejaculatory Ducts. The *arteries to the ductus deferentes,* usually branches of the inferior vesical arteries, supply the ejaculatory ducts (Table 4.4). The veins join the *prostatic and vesical venous plexuses.* The lymphatic vessels drain into the **external iliac lymph nodes** (Fig. 4.15A).

Innervation of Ejaculatory Ducts. The nerves of the ejaculatory ducts derive from the **inferior hypogastric plexus** (Fig. 4.15B).

Prostate

The walnut-sized prostate surrounds the prostatic urethra (Figs. 4.13–4.16). The prostate has a dense **prostatic capsule** that is surrounded by a fibrous *prostatic sheath,* which is continuous with the **puboprostatic ligaments**. The posterior part of the sheath, the **rectovesical septum,** passes from the perineal body to the floor of the rectovesical pouch. The rectovesical septum lies between the ampulla of the rectum posteriorly and the prostate, seminal glands, and ductus deferentes anteriorly (Fig. 4.13).

The prostate is like an inverted pyramid that has:

- A **base** (superior aspect) closely related to the neck of the bladder
- An **apex** (inferior aspect) that is in contact with fascia on the superior aspect of the urethral sphincter and deep perineal muscles
- A muscular **anterior surface,** featuring mostly transversely oriented muscle fibers continuous inferiorly with the urethral sphincter, that is separated from the pubic symphysis by retroperitoneal fat in the retropubic space
- A **posterior surface** that is related to the ampulla of the rectum
- **Inferolateral surfaces** that are related to the levator ani.

Although not clearly distinct anatomically, the following **lobes of the prostate** are traditionally described.

- The *anterior lobe* lies anterior to the urethra. It is fibromuscular, the muscle fibers representing a superior continuation

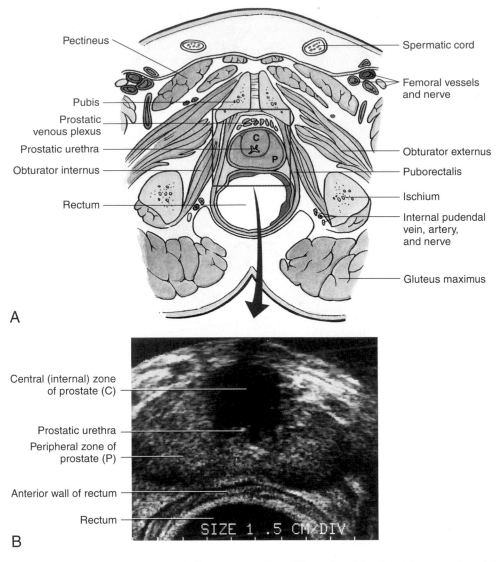

FIGURE 4.16 **Relations of prostate. A.** Transverse section of the male pelvis. *C* and *P,* zones of prostate in an ultrasound scan. **B.** Transverse (transrectal) ultrasound scan.

of the urethral sphincter and contains little, if any, glandular tissue. The *isthmus of the prostate* is the narrow middle part of the prostate anterior to the urethra.

- The *posterior lobe* lies posterior to the urethra and inferior to the ejaculatory ducts; it is readily palpable by digital rectal examination.
- The *lateral lobes* on either side of the urethra form the major part of the prostate.
- The *middle (median) lobe* lies between the urethra and the ejaculatory ducts and is

closely related to the neck of the bladder. It is indistinct unless hypertrophied.

Urologists and sonographers usually divide the prostate into peripheral and central (internal) zones (Fig. 4.16). The central zone is comparable to the middle lobe. The **prostatic ducts** (20 to 30) open chiefly into the **prostatic sinuses** that lie on either side of the seminal colliculus on the posterior wall of the prostatic urethra (Fig. 4.14). Prostatic fluid provides about 20% of the volume of semen.

Vasculature of Prostate. The prostatic arteries are mainly branches of the internal iliac artery (Table 4.4), especially the **inferior vesical arteries** but also the internal pudendal and **middle rectal arteries**. The *veins* join to form the **prostatic venous plexus** around the sides and base of the prostate (Fig. 4.13). This plexus, between the fibrous capsule of the prostate and the prostatic sheath, drains into the **internal iliac veins.** The plexus also communicates superiorly with the vesical venous plexus and posteriorly with the internal vertebral venous plexus (see Chapter 5). The *lymphatic vessels* (Fig. 4.15A) drain chiefly into the **internal iliac and sacral lymph nodes.**

Innervation of Prostate. The parasympathetic fibers arise from the **pelvic splanchnic nerves** (S2 through S4). The sympathetic fibers derive from the **inferior hypogastric plexus** (Fig. 4.15B).

PROSTATIC ENLARGEMENT AND CANCER

The prostate is of medical interest because benign enlargement—*hypertrophy of the prostate*—is common after middle age. An enlarged prostate compresses the prostatic urethra and impedes the passage of urine. *Prostatic cancer* is common in men older than 55. In most cases, prostatic cancer develops in the posterolateral region, which allows palpation of the prostate during a digital rectal examination. A malignant prostate feels hard and often irregular. In advanced stages cancer cells metastasize (spread) to the iliac and sacral lymph nodes and later to distant nodes and bone. Clinically, the most important fact about the innervation of the prostate is that the prostatic plexus, closely associated with the prostatic sheath, gives passage to parasympathetic fibers which give rise to the cavernous nerves that convey the fibers that cause penile erection. A major concern regarding **prostatectomy**—a common procedure for older males—is that impotency may be a consequence.

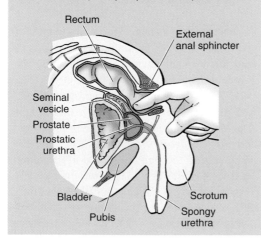

Rectum

External anal sphincter

Seminal vesicle

Prostate

Prostatic urethra

Bladder

Scrotum

Spongy urethra

Pubis

Bulbourethral Glands

The two pea-sized bulbourethral glands lie posterolateral to the intermediate (membranous) part of the urethra (Fig. 4.13, *A* and *B*). The ducts of these glands pass through the inferior fascia of the urethral sphincter (**perineal membrane**) with the urethra and open through minute apertures into the proximal part of the spongy urethra in the **bulb of the penis**. Their mucuslike secretion enters the urethra during sexual arousal.

FEMALE INTERNAL GENITAL ORGANS

The female internal genital organs include the vagina, uterus, uterine tubes, and ovaries.

Vagina

The vagina, a musculomembranous tube, extends from the cervix of the uterus to the **vestibule of the vagina**—the cleft between the labia minora into which the urethra also opens (Fig. 4.17). The superior end of the vagina surrounds the **cervix of the uterus**; the inferior end passes anteroinferiorly through the pelvic floor to open into the vestibule. *The vagina:*

- Serves as the excretory duct for menstrual fluid
- Forms the inferior part of the pelvic (birth) canal
- Receives the penis and ejaculate during sexual intercourse
- Communicates superiorly with the *cervical canal*—extending from the isthmus of the uterus to the external os (opening) of the uterus (Fig. 4.17)—and inferiorly with the vestibule of the vagina.

The vagina is normally collapsed so its anterior and posterior walls are in contact except at its superior end, where the cervix holds them open. The vagina pierces the perineal membrane. The **vaginal fornix,** the recess around the protruding cervix, is usually described as having anterior, posterior, and lateral parts. The **posterior part of the fornix** is the deepest and is closely related to the **rectouterine pouch** (Fig. 4.17B). This part of the vagina is very distensible and allows accommodation of the enlarged, erect penis dur-

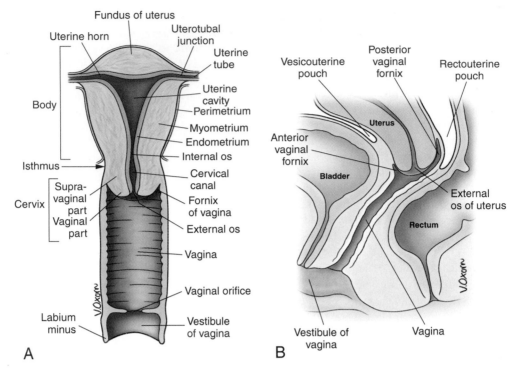

FIGURE 4.17 **Uterus and vagina. A.** Schematic coronal section. **B.** Median section of vagina.

ing intercourse, and palpation of the sacral promontory during a physical exam to determine the diameter of the pelvis (diagonal conjugate). Four muscles compress the vagina and act like sphincters: pubovaginalis, external urethral sphincter, urethrovaginal sphincter, and bulbospongiosus (Table 4.5). *The relations of the vagina are:*

- Anteriorly—the base of the bladder and urethra
- Laterally—the levator ani, visceral pelvic fascia, and ureters
- Posteriorly (inferior to superior)—the anal canal, rectum, and rectouterine pouch.

Vasculature of Vagina. The blood vessels supplying the superior part of the vagina derive from the **uterine arteries** (see Fig. 4.18*A*, Table 4.4). The **vaginal arteries** supplying the middle and inferior parts of the vagina derive from the *middle rectal artery* and the *internal pudendal artery.* The vaginal veins form **vaginal venous plexuses** along the sides of the vagina and within the vaginal mucosa (Fig. 4.18*B*). These veins communicate with the

vesical, uterine, and rectal venous plexuses and drain into the internal iliac veins. The **vaginal lymphatic vessels** (Fig. 4.19*A*) drain from the vagina as follows:

- Superior part into the internal and external iliac lymph nodes
- Middle part into the internal iliac lymph nodes
- Inferior part into the sacral and common iliac nodes, as well as into the superficial inguinal lymph nodes.

Innervation of Vagina. The nerves to most of the vagina derive from the **uterovaginal plexus** that lies with the uterine artery between the layers of the broad ligament of the uterus (Fig. 4.19, *B* and *C*). Sympathetic, parasympathetic, and afferent fibers pass through this plexus. *The uterovaginal plexus is an extension of the inferior hypogastric plexus.* Most afferent fibers ascend through the plexus to the spinal cord via T10 through T11 thoracic nerves and the subcostal nerve (T12). Only the lower one-fifth to one-fourth of the vagina is somatic in terms of innervation. Innervation of this lower

TABLE 4.5.   MUSCLES SUPPORTING AND CONNECTING MALE AND FEMALE PELVIC ORGANS: COMPRESSOR MUSCLES OF URETHRA AND VAGINA

Male

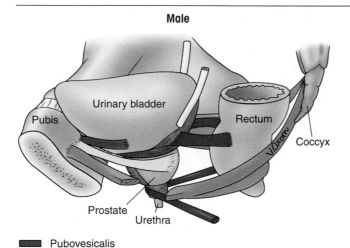

Muscles Compressing Urethra
- Internal urethral sphincter
- Pubovesicalis
- External urethral sphincter
- Compressor urethrae

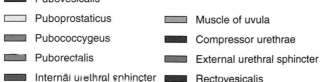

Pubovesicalis
Puboprostaticus   Muscle of uvula
Pubococcygeus   Compressor urethrae
Puborectalis   External urethral sphincter
Internal urethral sphincter   Rectovesicalis

Female

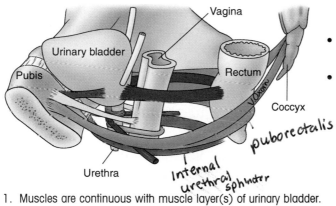

Muscles Compressing:

Urethra	Vagina
• Compressor urethrae	• Pubovaginalis
• External urethral sphincter	• Urethrovaginal sphincter (part of external urethral sphincter)
	• Bulbospongiosus

1. Muscles are continuous with muscle layer(s) of urinary bladder.
2. Part of levator ani (p. 217)
3. Muscle of deep perineal pouch (p. 260)
4. Muscle of superficial perineal pouch (p. 159)

part is from the deep perineal branch of the **pudendal nerve,** which conveys sympathetic and somatic afferent fibers (from the S2-S4 sensory ganglia) but no parasympathetic fibers. *Only this somatically innervated part of the vagina is sensitive to touch and temperature.*

DISTENTION AND EXAMINATION OF VAGINA
The vagina can be markedly distended by the fetus during childbirth, particularly in an anteroposterior direction. Distention of the vagina is limited laterally by the *ischial spines,* which project posterolaterally, and the *sacrospinous ligaments* extending from these spines to the lateral margins of the sacrum and coccyx. The interior of the vagina can be

Continued

distended for examination using a *vaginal speculum*. The cervix can also be palpated with the digits in the vagina or rectum.

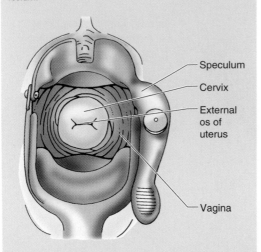

Speculum

Cervix

External os of uterus

Vagina

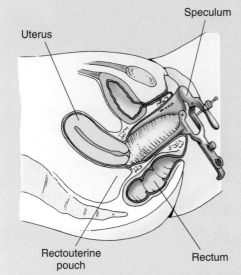

Uterus

Speculum

Rectouterine pouch

Rectum

Pelvic Abscess

A pelvic abscess (collection of pus) in the rectouterine pouch can be drained through an incision made in the thin vaginal wall separating the posterior part of the vaginal fornix from the rectouterine pouch (*colpotomy*). Similarly, fluid in this part of the perineal cavity (e.g., blood) can be aspirated at this site (*culdocentesis*).

Uterus

The uterus—a thick-walled, pear-shaped, hollow muscular organ—is in the lesser pelvis normally with its body lying over the urinary bladder and its cervix between the bladder and rectum (Fig. 4.17*B*). In the adult the uterus is usually *anteverted*—tipped anteriorly relative to the axis of the vagina—and an *anteflexed* uterine body is flexed or bent anteriorly relative to the cervix so that its mass lies over the bladder (Fig. 4.8). The position of the uterus changes with the degree of fullness of the bladder and rectum. *The uterus is divisible into two main parts—the body and cervix* (Fig. 4.17*A*):

- **Body,** forming the upper two-thirds of the uterus, has two parts: the **fundus**—the rounded part of the body that lies superior to the orifices of the uterine tubes and the **isthmus**—the relatively constricted region of the body just above the cervix
- **Cervix**—the cylindrical, narrow inferior part of the uterus that protrudes into the uppermost part of the vagina.

The **body of the uterus** lies between the layers of the broad ligament and is freely movable (Fig. 4.20*A*). It has two surfaces: vesical (related to the bladder) and intestinal. The **uterine horns** (L. cornua) are the superolateral regions where the uterine tubes enter. The **cervix of the uterus** is divided into vaginal and supravaginal parts (Fig. 4.17*A*). The rounded *vaginal part of the cervix* communicates with the vagina via the external os. The *supravaginal part of the cervix* is separated from the bladder anteriorly by loose connective tissue and from the rectum posteriorly by the **rectouterine pouch** (Fig. 4.17*B*). The **ligament of ovary** attaches to the uterus posteroinferior to the uterotubal junction (Fig. 4.20*A*). The **round ligament of uterus** attaches anteroinferiorly to this junction. Collectively, these ligaments are vestiges of the ovarian gubernaculum, homologous to the testicular gubernaculum (for more information, see Moore and Persaud, 1998).

The wall of the body of the uterus consists of three layers:

- The **perimetrium**—the outer serous coat—consists of peritoneum supported by a thin layer of connective tissue
- The **myometrium**—the middle muscular coat—typically a thick layer that becomes greatly distended during pregnancy; the main branches of the blood vessels and

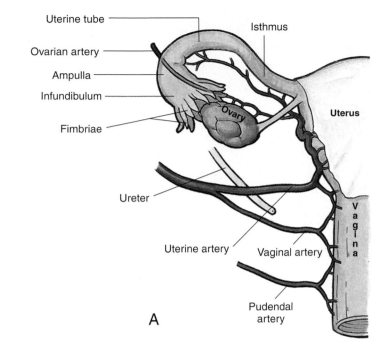

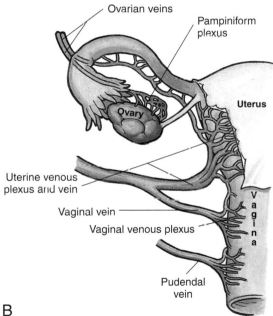

FIGURE 4.18 **Vasculature of vagina, uterus, uterine tube, and ovary. A.** Arterial supply. **B.** Venous drainage.

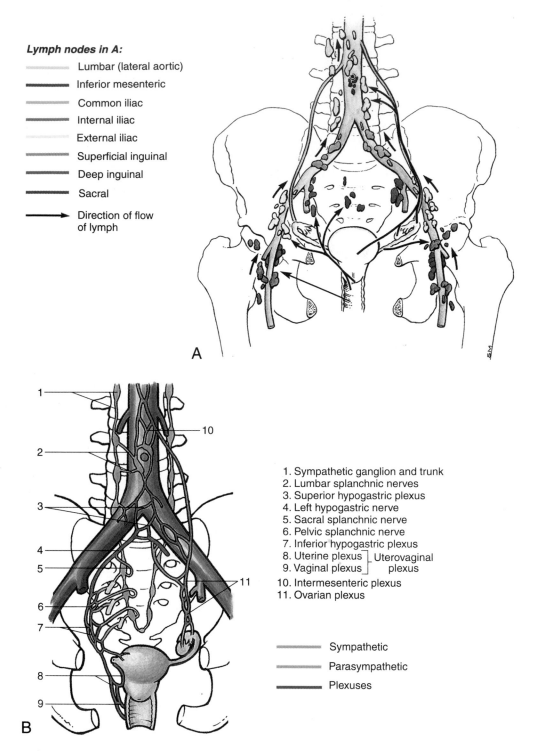

Lymph nodes in A:

Lumbar (lateral aortic)
Inferior mesenteric
Common iliac
Internal iliac
External iliac
Superficial inguinal
Deep inguinal
Sacral
→ Direction of flow of lymph

A

1. Sympathetic ganglion and trunk
2. Lumbar splanchnic nerves
3. Superior hypogastric plexus
4. Left hypogastric nerve
5. Sacral splanchnic nerve
6. Pelvic splanchnic nerve
7. Inferior hypogastric plexus
8. Uterine plexus ⎤ Uterovaginal
9. Vaginal plexus ⎦ plexus
10. Intermesenteric plexus
11. Ovarian plexus

Sympathetic
Parasympathetic
Plexuses

B

FIGURE 4.19   Uterus, vagina, and ovaries. Anterior views. **A.** Lymphatic drainage. *Arrows,* lymph flow to lymph nodes. **B** and **C.** Autonomic innervation.

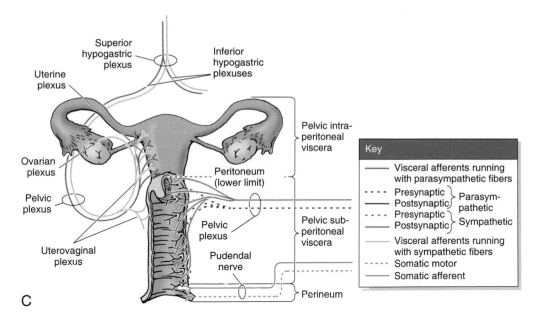

Superior
hypogastric
plexus

Inferior
hypogastric
plexuses

Uterine
plexus

Ovarian
plexus

Pelvic
plexus

Uterovaginal
plexus

Pelvic intra-
peritoneal
viscera

Peritoneum
(lower limit)

Pelvic
plexus

Pudendal
nerve

Pelvic sub-
peritoneal
viscera

Perineum

Key

—— Visceral afferents running
with parasympathetic fibers
- - - - Presynaptic ⎱ Parasym-
—— Postsynaptic ⎰ pathetic
- - - - Presynaptic ⎱ Sympathetic
—— Postsynaptic ⎰
—— Visceral afferents running
with sympathetic fibers
- - - - Somatic motor
—— Somatic afferent

C

FIGURE 4.19 *Continued.*

nerves of the uterus are located in the
myometrium

- The **endometrium**—the inner mucous
coat—firmly adheres to the myometrium.
In the sexually mature female, much of
this layer is shed and renewed during the
menstrual cycle.

The *principal supports of the uterus* are the
pelvic fascia and the **urinary bladder** on which
the uterus normally rests. The cervix is the least
mobile part of the uterus because it is held in position by ligaments that are condensations of the
parietal pelvic fascia or endopelvic fascia, which
may also contain smooth muscle (see Fig. 4.26):

- *Transverse cervical (cardinal) ligaments*
extend from the cervix and lateral parts of
the fornix of the vagina to the lateral walls
of the pelvis
- *Uterosacral ligaments* pass superiorly and
slightly posteriorly from the sides of the
cervix to the middle of the sacrum; they
are palpable on rectal examination.

The **broad ligament of the uterus** is a double layer of peritoneum that extends from the
sides of the uterus to the lateral walls and floor
of the pelvis (Fig. 4.20*A*). The broad ligament

assists in keeping the uterus relatively centered in the pelvis, but mostly contains the
ovaries, uterine tubes, and related structures,
including the vasculature that serves them.
The two layers of the ligament are continuous
with each other at a free edge that surrounds
the uterine tube. Laterally the peritoneum of
the broad ligament is prolonged superiorly
over the ovarian vessels as the **suspensory ligament of ovary** (Fig. 4.20). The **ligament of
ovary** lies posterosuperiorly and the **round ligament of uterus** lies anteroinferiorly between
the layers of the broad ligament. The part of
the broad ligament by which the ovary sus-
pends is the **mesovarium** (Fig. 4.20*B*). The
part of the broad ligament forming the mesentery of the uterine tube is the **mesosalpinx.**
The major part of the broad ligament, or **mesometrium,** is below the mesosalpinx and
mesovarium.

Relations of Uterus (Fig. 4.20). Peritoneum
covers the uterus anteriorly and superiorly
(Fig. 4.11*B*), except for the vaginal part of the
cervix. The **peritoneum** is reflected anteriorly
from the uterus onto the bladder and posteriorly over the posterior part of the fornix of
the vagina onto the rectum. Anteriorly, the

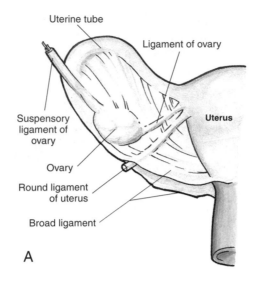

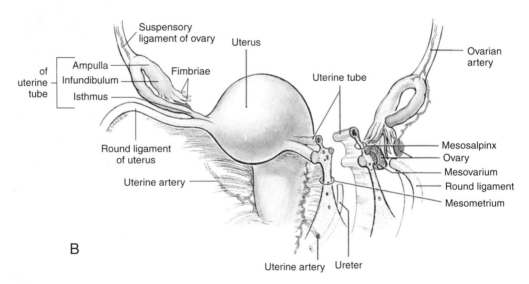

FIGURE 4.20   Uterus, uterine tubes, and broad ligament. A. Relationship of the broad ligament to the ovary and its ligaments, anterior view. **B.** Anterolateral view of sagittal sections showing the mesentery of the uterus (mesometrium), ovary (mesovarium), and uterine tube (mesosalpinx).

uterine fundus and upper body of the uterus are separated from the urinary bladder by the **vesicouterine pouch** (Fig. 4.17*B*) because the peritoneum is reflected from the uterus onto the posterior margin of the superior surface of the bladder; the inferior uterine body (isthmus) and cervix lie in direct contact with the bladder without intervening peritoneum. This allows uterine/cervical cancer to invade the urinary bladder. Posteriorly, the body and supravaginal part of the cervix are separated from the **sigmoid colon** by a layer of peritoneum and the peritoneal cavity and from the rectum by the **rectouterine pouch** (Fig. 4.17*B*). *Laterally, the uterine artery crosses the ureter superiorly, near the cervix,* in the root of the broad ligament (Fig. 4.20*B*).

Vasculature of Uterus. The blood supply derives mainly from the **uterine arteries** with an additional supply from the ovarian arteries (Fig. 4.18*A*, Table 4.4). The **uterine veins** run in the broad ligament, draining the **uterine venous plexus** formed on each side of the uterus and vagina (Fig. 4.18*B*). Veins from this plexus drain into the **internal iliac veins**. *The uterine lymphatic vessels follow three main routes* (Fig. 4.19*A*):

• Most vessels from the uterine fundus pass to the **lumbar lymph nodes,** but some vessels pass to the **external iliac lymph nodes** or run along the round ligament of the uterus to the **superficial inguinal lymph nodes.**

• Vessels from the uterine body pass within the broad ligament to the **external iliac lymph nodes.**

• Vessels from the uterine cervix pass to the **internal iliac and sacral lymph nodes.**

Innervation of Uterus. The nerves to the uterus derive from the **uterovaginal plexus** (Fig. 4.19, *B* and *C*), which travels with the uterine artery at the junction of the base of the peritoneal broad ligament and the supe-

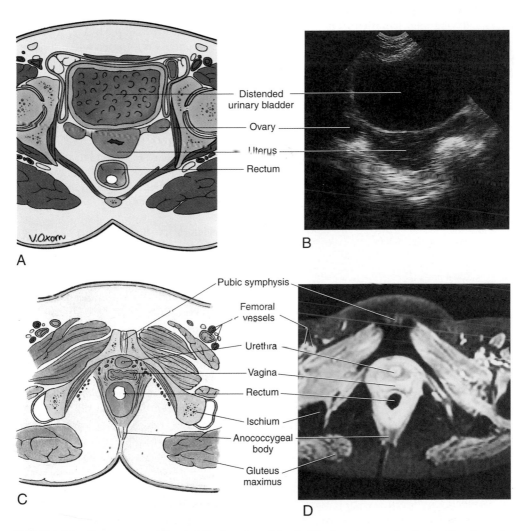

FIGURE 4.21   Transverse sections of the female pelvis. A. Drawing of an anatomical section through the urinary bladder, uterus, and rectum. **B.** Transverse ultrasound scan. **C.** Drawing of an anatomical section through the urethra, vagina, and rectum. **D.** Transverse magnetic resonance image (MRI).

rior part of the fascial transverse cervical ligament. The **uterovaginal plexus** is one of the
pelvic plexuses that extend to the pelvic viscera from the **inferior hypogastric plexus** (Fig.
4.19, *B* and *C*). Sympathetic, parasympathetic, and visceral afferent fibers pass
through this plexus. **Sympathetic innervation**
originates in the lower thoracic spinal cord
segments and passes through lumbar splanchnic nerves and the intermesenteric/hypogas-
tric series of plexuses. **Parasympathetic innervation** originates in the S2 through S4 spinal
cord segments and passes through the **pelvic
splanchnic nerves** to the inferior hypogas-
tric/uterovaginal plexus. Visceral afferent
fibers, carrying pain sensation from the uterine fundus, travel retrogradely with the sympathetic fibers to the lower thoracic/upper
lumbar spinal ganglia; those from the cervix
and upper vagina travel with the parasympathetic fibers to the sacral spinal ganglia.

HYSTERECTOMY

Hysterectomy (excision of the uterus) is performed
through the lower anterior abdominal wall or through the
vagina. Because the uterine artery crosses anterior to the
ureter near the lateral fornix of the vagina, the ureter is in
danger of being inadvertently clamped or severed when
the uterine artery is tied off during a hysterectomy. The
point of crossing of the artery and the ureter is approximately 2 cm superior to the ischial spine.

Caudal Epidural Block

A caudal epidural block must be administered in advance
of childbirth, which is not possible with a precipitous birth.
The anesthetic agent is administered using an in-dwelling
catheter in the *sacral canal* (see Chapter 5), enabling ad-
ministration of more anesthetic agent for a deeper or more
prolonged anesthesia if necessary. Within the sacral canal,
the anesthesia bathes the S2 through S4 spinal nerve roots,
including the pain fibers from the uterine cervix and upper
vagina, and the afferent fibers from the pudendal nerve.
Thus, the entire birth canal, pelvic floor, and majority of the
perineum are anesthetized but the lower limbs usually are
not affected. Since visceral afferent fibers from the uterine
fundus ascend to the upper lumbar spinal ganglia, they are
also not affected and sensations of uterine contraction are
still perceived. This is important to women selecting partic-
ipatory methods of childbirth.

Uterine Tubes

The uterine tubes extend from the uterine
horns and open into the peritoneal cavity near
the ovaries (Fig. 4.20). The uterine tubes lie in
the **mesosalpinx** formed by the free edges of
the broad ligament. Typically, the tubes extend
posterolaterally to the lateral pelvic walls
where they ascend and arch over the ovaries,
but ultrasound studies demonstrate that the
position of the tubes and ovaries is variable
(dynamic) in life, and right and left sides are
often asymmetrical. *Each uterine tube is divisible into four parts* (Fig. 4.20*B*):

- The **infundibulum** is the funnel-shaped
  distal end that opens into the peritoneal
  cavity through the **abdominal os** (ostium,
  opening). The fingerlike processes of the
  infundibulum—the **fimbriae**—spread over
  the medial surface of the ovary; one large
  ovarian fimbria is attached to the superior
  pole of the ovary.
- The **ampulla,** the widest and longest part,
  begins at the medial end of the
  infundibulum.
- The **isthmus,** the thick-walled part, enters
  the uterine horn.
- The **uterine part,** the short intramural
  segment that passes through the wall of
  the uterus and opens through the **uterine
  os** into the uterine cavity.

Vasculature of Uterine Tubes. The tubal
branches arise as anastomosing terminal
branches of the **uterine and ovarian arteries**
(Fig. 4.18*A*). The tubal veins drain into the
ovarian veins and **uterine venous plexus** (Fig.
4.18*B*). The lymphatic vessels drain to the
lumbar lymph nodes (Fig. 4.19*A*).

Innervation of Uterine Tubes. The nerve
supply derives partly from the **ovarian plexus**
and partly from the **uterine plexus** (Fig. 4.19,
B and *C*). Afferent fibers ascend through the
ovarian plexus and lumbar splanchnic nerves
to cell bodies in the T11 through L1 spinal
ganglia.

INFECTIONS OF FEMALE GENITAL TRACT

Because the female genital tract communicates with the
peritoneal cavity through the abdominal ostia, infections
of the vagina, uterus, and uterine tubes may result in peritonitis. Conversely, inflammation of the tube (*salpingitis*)
may result from infections that spread from the peritoneal

cavity. A major cause of infertility in women is blockage of the uterine tubes, often the result of infection that causes salpingitis.

Salpingography
Patency of the uterine tubes may be determined by *salpingography,* a radiographic procedure involving injection of a water-soluble radiopaque material into the uterus—*hysterosalpingography.* The material enters the uterine tubes, and if the tubes are patent, passes from the abdominal os into the peritoneal cavity.

Ligation of Uterine Tubes
Ligation of the uterine tubes is a surgical method of birth control. *Abdominal tubal ligation* is usually performed through a short suprapubic incision made just at the pubic hairline. *Laparoscopic tubal ligation* is done with a laparoscope that is similar to a small telescope with a powerful light. It is inserted through a small incision, usually near the umbilicus. Oocytes discharged from the ovaries that enter the tubes of these patients die and are soon absorbed.

Tubal Pregnancy
Occasionally a fertilized oocyte fails to reach the uterus and develops into an advanced embryo in the uterine tube. On the right side, the vermiform appendix often lies close to the ovary and uterine tube. This close relationship explains why a *ruptured tubal pregnancy* and the resulting peritonitis may be misdiagnosed as acute appendicitis. In both cases, the parietal peritoneum is inflamed in the same general area and the pain is referred to the right lower quadrant of the abdomen.

Ovaries

The almond-shaped ovaries are most commonly located close to the lateral pelvic walls suspended by the **mesovarium**—part of the broad ligament (Fig. 4.21*B*). The distal end of the ovary connects to the lateral wall of the pelvis by the **suspensory ligament of the ovary** (Fig. 4.20*A*). This ligament conveys the ovarian vessels, lymphatics, and nerves to and from the ovary, and constitutes the lateral part of the mesovarium. The ovary also attaches to the uterus by the **ligament of ovary** (ovarian ligament), which runs within the mesovarium. The ligament connects the proximal (uterine) end of the ovary to the lateral angle of the uterus, just inferior to the entrance of the uterine tube.

Vasculature of Ovaries. The ovarian arteries from the abdominal aorta descend along the posterior abdominal wall. At the pelvic brim, the **ovarian arteries** cross over the external iliac vessels and enter the suspensory ligaments (Figs. 4.18*A* and 4.20*B*). The ovarian artery sends branches through the mesovarium to the ovary and through the mesosalpinx to supply the uterine tube. The ovarian and tubal branches anastomose with ovarian and tubal branches of the uterine artery. Veins draining the ovary form a **pampiniform plexus of veins** near the ovary and uterine tube (Fig. 4.18*B*). The veins of the plexus merge to form a singular **ovarian vein,** which leaves the lesser pelvis with the ovarian artery. The right ovarian vein ascends to enter the *IVC;* the left ovarian vein drains into the *left renal vein.* The **lymphatic vessels** follow the ovarian blood vessels and join those from the uterine tubes and fundus of the uterus as they ascend to the **lumbar lymph nodes** (Fig. 4.19*A*).

Innervation of Ovaries. The nerves descend along the ovarian vessels from the **ovarian plexus**, which communicates with the uterine plexus (Fig. 4.19, *B* and *C*). The parasympathetic fibers in the plexus are derived from the **pelvic splanchnic nerves.** Afferent fibers from the ovary enter the spinal cord through T10 and T11 nerves.

RECTUM

The rectum is the part of the alimentary tract that is continuous proximally with the sigmoid colon and distally with the anal canal (Fig. 4.22*A*). The *rectosigmoid junction* lies at the level of S3 vertebra. The rectum follows the curve of the sacrum and coccyx, and ends anteroinferior to the tip of the coccyx where the rectum turns posteroinferiorly and becomes the **anal canal**. The dilated terminal part, the **ampulla of the rectum,** supports and retains the fecal mass before it is expelled during defecation. The rectum is S-shaped and has three flexures as it follows the sacrococcygeal curve (Fig. 4.22 *B*). Its terminal part bends sharply in a posterior direction—**anorectal flexure**—as it perforates the pelvic diaphragm to become the anal canal. The roughly 80° anorectal flexure (angle) is an important mechanism for fecal conti-

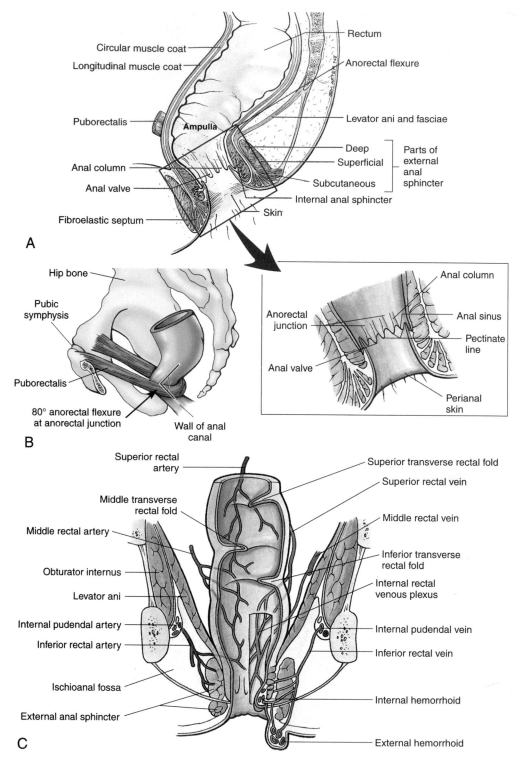

FIGURE 4.22   **Rectum and anal canal. A.** Median section showing the anal sphincters. Inset drawing of the anal canal. **B.** Puborectalis muscle. **C.** Coronal section showing arterial supply (right side) and venous drainage (left side) with hemorrhoids.

nence, being maintained during the resting state by the tonus of the puborectalis muscle (Fig. 4.22*B*) and by its active contraction during peristaltic contractions if defecation is not to occur. The relation of puborectalis during defecation results in straightening of the anorectal junction. At each of three concavities formed by lateral flexures of the rectum are **superior, middle, and inferior trectal folds** of the mucous and submucous coats overlying thickened parts of the circular muscle layer of the rectal wall (Fig. 4.22, *A* and *C*).

Peritoneum covers the anterior and lateral surfaces of the superior third of the rectum (Fig. 4.11), only the anterior surface of the middle third, and no surface of the inferior third because it is subperitoneal. *In males* the peritoneum reflects from the rectum to the posterior wall of the bladder where it forms the floor of the **rectovesical pouch.** *In females* the peritoneum reflects from the rectum to the posterior fornix of the vagina, where it forms the floor of the **rectouterine pouch.** In both sexes, lateral reflections of peritoneum from the upper one-third of the rectum form *pararectal fossae,* which permit the rectum to distend as it fills with feces.

The rectum rests posteriorly on the inferior three sacral vertebrae and the coccyx, anococcygeal ligament, median sacral vessels, and inferior ends of the sympathetic trunks and sacral plexuses. *In males* the rectum is related anteriorly to the fundus of the urinary bladder, terminal parts of the ureters, ductus deferentes, seminal glands, and prostate (Figs. 4.16 and 4.17). The *rectovesical septum* lies between the fundus of the bladder and the ampulla of the rectum and is closely associated with the seminal glands and prostate. *In females* the rectum is related anteriorly to the vagina (Figs. 4.8 and 4.20*C*) and is separated from its posterior fornix and the cervix by the **rectouterine pouch** (Fig. 4.11*B*). Inferior to this pouch, the weak rectovaginal septum separates the superior half of the posterior wall of the vagina from the rectum.

Vasculature of Rectum. The continuation of the inferior mesenteric artery, the **superior rectal artery,** supplies the proximal part of the rectum. The two **middle rectal arteries**—usually arising from the *inferior vesical* (male) *or uterine* (female) *arteries*—supply the middle and inferior parts of the rectum, and the **inferior rectal arteries**—arising from the internal pudendal arteries—supply the anorectal junction and anal canal (Fig. 4.22*C*). Blood from the rectum drains via superior, middle, and inferior **rectal veins.** Because the superior rectal vein drains into the portal venous system and the middle and inferior rectal veins drain into the systemic system, this communication is an important area of *portacaval anastomosis* (p. 180). The submucosal **rectal venous plexus** surrounds the rectum and communicates with the vesical venous plexus in males and the uterovaginal venous plexus in females. The rectal venous plexus consists of two parts, the **internal rectal venous plexus** just deep to the epithelium of the rectum and the external **rectal venous plexus** external to the muscular wall of the rectum.

- *Lymphatic vessels from the superior half of the rectum* ascend along the superior rectal vessels to the **pararectal lymph nodes** (Fig. 4.23*A*); lymph then passes to lymph nodes in the inferior part of the mesentery of the sigmoid colon and from them to the **inferior mesenteric** and **lumbar lymph nodes.**
- *Lymphatic vessels from the inferior half of the rectum* ascend with the middle rectal arteries and drain into the **internal iliac lymph nodes.**

Innervation of Rectum. The nerve supply to the rectum is from the sympathetic and parasympathetic systems (Fig. 4.23*B*). The rectum derives its sympathetic supply from the lumbar part of the sympathetic trunk and the **superior hypogastric plexus** through plexuses on the branches of the inferior mesenteric artery. The parasympathetic supply derives from the **pelvic splanchnic nerves.** Fibers pass from these nerves to the left and right **inferior hypogastric plexuses** to supply the rectum. Visceral afferent or sensory fibers also join these plexuses and reach the spinal cord through the pelvic splanchnic or **lumbar splanchnic nerves.**

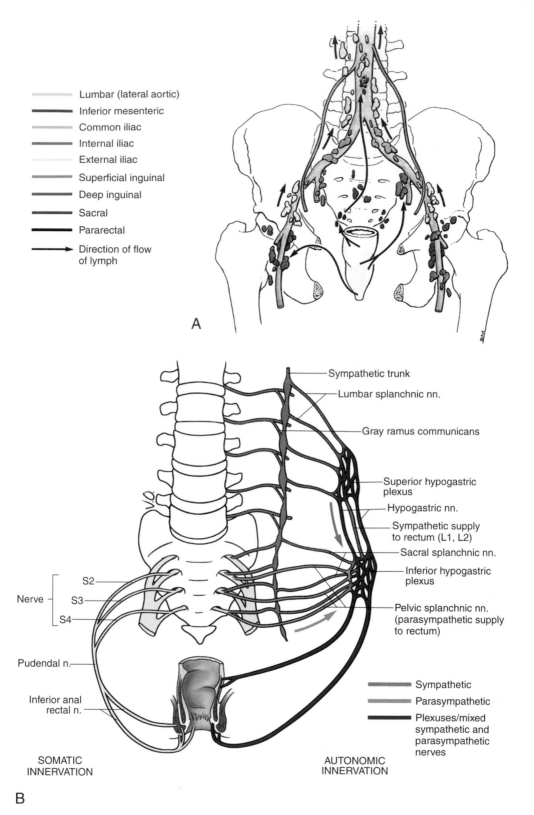

Lumbar (lateral aortic)
Inferior mesenteric
Common iliac
Internal iliac
External iliac
Superficial inguinal
Deep inguinal
Sacral
Pararectal
→ **Direction of flow of lymph**

A

Sympathetic trunk
Lumbar splanchnic nn.
Gray ramus communicans
Superior hypogastric plexus
Hypogastric nn.
Sympathetic supply to rectum (L1, L2)
Sacral splanchnic nn.
Inferior hypogastric plexus
Pelvic splanchnic nn. (parasympathetic supply to rectum)

Nerve {
S2
S3
S4
}

Pudendal n.

Inferior anal rectal n.

Sympathetic
Parasympathetic
Plexuses/mixed sympathetic and parasympathetic nerves

SOMATIC INNERVATION

AUTONOMIC INNERVATION

B

FIGURE 4.23   Rectum and anal canal. A. Lymphatic drainage. *Arrows,* lymph flow to lymph nodes.
B. Innervation. Anterior views. The splanchnic nerves and hypogastric plexuses are retracted laterally.

ANAL CANAL

The anal canal is the terminal part of the large intestine that extends from the upper aspect of the pelvic diaphragm to the anus. The anal canal begins where the rectal ampulla abruptly narrows at the level of the U-shaped sling formed by the puborectalis muscle (Fig. 4.22, *A* and *B*). The anal canal ends at the **anus,** the external outlet of the gastrointestinal tract. The anal canal, surrounded by **internal** and **external anal sphincters,** descends posteroinferi-orly between the **anococcygeal body** (liga-ment) and the **perineal body** (Fig. 4.24*B*). The anal canal is normally collapsed except during passage of feces. Both sphincters must relax before defecation can occur. The **external anal sphincter** is a large voluntary sphincter that forms a broad band on each side of the infe-rior two-thirds of the anal canal (Fig. 4.22). This sphincter blends superiorly with the pub-orectalis muscle. The sphincter is supplied mainly by S4 through the inferior anal (rectal) nerve (Fig. 4.23*B*). The **internal anal sphincter** is an involuntary sphincter surrounding the su-perior two-thirds of the anal canal. It is a thickening of the circular muscle layer of the intestine. The internal anal sphincter is inner-vated (caused to contract) by the sympathetic system. It is inhibited (loses its tonic contrac-

tion and is allowed to expand passively) by the parasympathetic system. The internal anal sphincter is tonically contracted most of the time to prevent leakage of fluid or flatus; how-ever, it relaxes in response to the pressure of feces or gas distending the rectal ampulla, re-quiring voluntary contraction of the puborec-talis and external anal sphincter if defecation is not to occur.

Interior of Anal Canal

The superior half of the mucous membrane of the anal canal is characterized by a series of lon-gitudinal ridges—**anal columns** (Fig. 4.22*A*). These columns contain the terminal branches of the superior rectal artery and vein. The **anorec-tal junction,** indicated by the superior ends of the anal columns, is where the rectum joins the anal canal. The inferior ends of these columns are joined by **anal valves.** Superior to the valves are small recesses—**anal sinuses.** When com-pressed by feces, the anal sinuses exude mucus that aids in evacuation of feces from the anal canal. The inferior comb-shaped limit of the anal valves forms an irregular line—the **pecti-nate line**—that indicates the junction of the su-perior part of the anal canal (derived from the hindgut) and the inferior part (derived from the proctodeum). The anal canal superior to the pectinate line differs from the part inferior to the pectinate line in its arterial supply, innerva-tion, and venous and lymphatic drainage. These differences result from their different embry-ological origins (Moore and Persaud, 1998).

Vasculature of Anal Canal

The **superior rectal artery** supplies the anal canal superior to the pectinate line (Fig. 4.22*C*). The two **inferior rectal arteries** supply the infe-rior part of the anal canal, as well as the sur-rounding muscles and perianal skin. The **mid-dle rectal arteries** assist with the blood supply to the anal canal by forming anastomoses with the superior and inferior rectal arteries. The **in-ternal rectal venous plexus** drains in both direc-tions from the level of the pectinate line. *Supe-rior to the pectinate line,* the internal rectal venous plexus drains chiefly into the **superior rectal vein**—a tributary of the inferior mesenteric vein—and the portal system (Fig. 4.22*C*). *Inferior to the pectinate line,* the internal rectal venous plexus drains into the **inferior rectal veins**—tributaries of the inferior caval venous system—around the margin of the external anal sphincter. The **middle rectal veins**—tributaries of the internal iliac veins (also caval tributaries)—mainly drain the muscularis externa of the rectal ampulla and form anastomoses with the superior and inferior rectal veins. *Superior to the pectinate line,* the lymphatic vessels drain into the **internal iliac lymph nodes** and through them into the common iliac and lumbar lymph nodes (Fig. 4.23*A*). *Inferior to the pectinate line* the lymphatic vessels drain into the **superficial inguinal lymph nodes.**

Innervation of Anal Canal

The nerve supply to the anal canal superior to the pectinate line is visceral innervation from the **inferior hypogastric plexus** (sympathetic and parasympathetic fibers [Fig. 4.23*B*]). The superior part of the anal canal is sensitive only to stretching. *The nerve supply of the anal canal inferior to the pectinate line* is somatic innervation from the **inferior anal (rectal) nerves,** branches of the pudendal nerve. Therefore, this part of the anal canal is sensitive to pain, touch, and temperature.

PERINEUM

The perineum refers to both an external surface area and a shallow "compartment" of the body. In the anatomical position, the perineum (external surface area) is the narrow region between the proximal parts of the thighs. However, when the lower limbs are abducted, the perineum is a diamond-shaped area extending from the mons pubis anteriorly, the medial surfaces (insides) of the thighs laterally, and the gluteal folds and upper end of the intergluteal (natal) cleft posteriorly (Fig. 4.24). Some obstetricians apply the term perineum to a more restricted region—the area between the vagina and anus. The perineal compartment lies inferior to the inferior pelvic aperture and is separated from

---

HEMORRHOIDS

Internal hemorrhoids ("piles") are prolapses of the *internal rectal venous plexus* (Fig. 4.22*C*). They are thought to result from a breakdown of the muscularis mucosae, a smooth muscle layer deep to the mucosa. Internal hemorrhoids tend to strangulate and ulcerate. *External hemorrhoids* are thromboses (blood clots) in the veins of the *external rectal venous plexus* and are covered by skin. Predisposing factors for hemorrhoids include pregnancy, chronic constipation, and any disorder that results in increased intra-abdominal pressure.

The anastomoses between the superior, middle, and inferior rectal veins form clinically important communications between the portal and systemic venous systems (p. 180). The superior rectal vein drains into the inferior mesenteric vein, whereas the middle and inferior rectal veins drain through the systemic system into the IVC. Any abnormal increase in pressure in the valveless portal system may cause enlargement of the superior rectal veins, causing an increase in blood flow in the internal rectal venous plexus, resulting in internal hemorrhoids. In *portal hypertension,* as in *hepatic cirrhosis,* the anastomotic veins in the anal canal and elsewhere become varicose. However, hemorrhoids occur most often in the absence of portal hypertension.

Because visceral afferent nerves supply the anal canal superior to the pectinate line, an incision or a needle insertion in this region is painless. However, *the anal canal inferior to the pectinate line is very sensitive* (e.g., to the prick of a hypodermic needle) because it is supplied by the *inferior anal (rectal) nerves* containing somatic sensory fibers.

---

the pelvic cavity by the pelvic diaphragm. *The osseofibrous structures marking the boundaries of the perineum (perineal compartment)* (Figs. 4.24 and 4.25) are the:

* Pubic symphysis—anteriorly
* Inferior pubic and ischial (ischiopubic) rami—anterolaterally
* Ischial tuberosities—laterally
* Sacrotuberous ligaments—posterolaterally
* Inferiormost sacrum and coccyx.

A transverse line joining the anterior ends of the ischial tuberosities divides the perineum into two triangles (Fig. 4.25):

* The **anal triangle,** containing the anus, is posterior to this line.
* The **urogenital (UG) triangle,** containing the root of the scrotum and penis in males and the external genitalia in females, is anterior to this line.

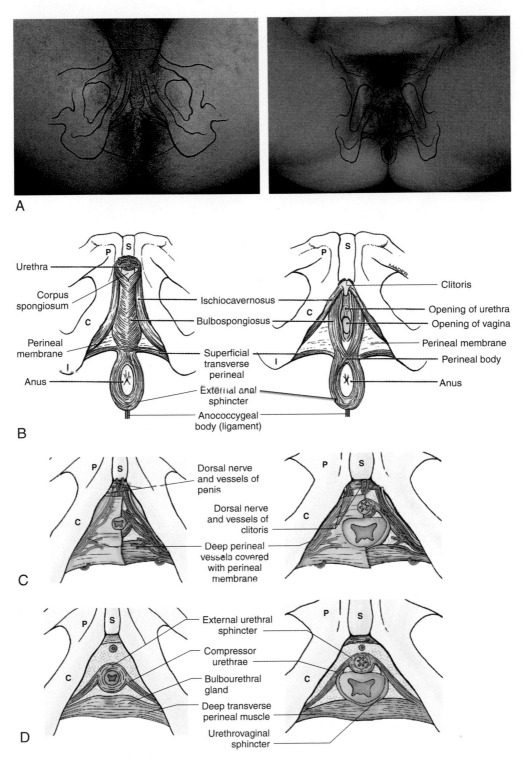

FIGURE 4.24   Perineum. A. Male (*left*) and female (*right*). **B.** Observe the boundaries of structures in the perineal compartment. *P,* body of pubis; *S,* pubic symphysis; *C,* conjoint ramus formed by inferior rami of ischium and pubis; *I,* ischial tuberosity. **C.** Perineal membrane and vessels. **D.** External urethral sphincter, urethrovaginal sphincter, and compressor urethrae.

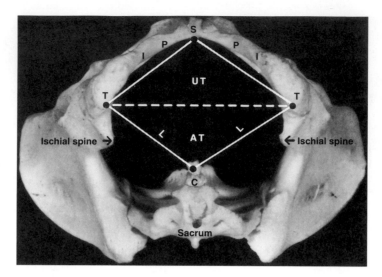

FIGURE 4.25 **Pelvic outlet of the female pelvis.** *UT,* urogenital triangle; *AT,* anal triangle; *S,* pubic symphysis; *P,* inferior pubic rami; *I,* ischial rami; *T,* ischial tuberosities; *C,* coccyx.

The **perineal membrane** (Fig. 4.24*B*), a thin sheet of tough deep fascia, stretches between the right and left sides of the pubic arch. Lying in the urogenital triangle, the perineal membrane covers the anterior part of the pelvic outlet. The perineal body is an irregular fibromuscular mass located in the median plane between the anal canal and the perineal membrane. It lies deep to the skin and subcutaneous tissue, posterior to the vestibule of the vagina or bulb of the penis, and anterior to the anus and anal canal. The perineal body attaches to the posterior border of the perineal membrane. It contains collagenous and elastic fibers and both skeletal and smooth muscle. The perineal body is variable in size and consistency, with relatively little fat deep to the overlying skin. *The perineal body is the site of convergence of several muscles* (Fig. 4.24):

- Bulbospongiosus
- External anal sphincter
- Superficial and deep transverse perineal muscles.

PELVIC AND PERINEAL FASCIA

The **pelvic fascia** is connective tissue that occupies all the space between the membranous peritoneum and the muscular pelvic walls and floor not occupied by pelvic organs. This "layer" is a continuation of the comparatively thin endoabdominal fascia that lies between the muscular abdominal walls and the peritoneum superiorly. Traditionally, the pelvic fascia has been described as having parietal and visceral components (Fig. 4.26). The **visceral pelvic fascia** (endopelvic fascia) surrounds the pelvic viscera and their nerves and vessels and binds them to each other and to the parietal pelvic fascia. The **parietal pelvic fascia** is a membranous layer of variable thickness that

---

DISRUPTION OF PERINEAL BODY

The perineal body is an especially important structure in women because it is the final support of the pelvic viscera. Stretching or tearing of this attachment for the perineal muscles can occur during childbirth, removing support from the inferior part of the posterior wall of the vagina. As a result, *prolapse of the vagina* through the vaginal orifice may occur.

Episiotomy

During vaginal surgery and labor, an *episiotomy*—surgical incision of the perineum and lower, posterior vaginal wall—is often made to enlarge the vaginal orifice and to prevent a jagged tear of the perineal muscles.

lines the internal (deep or pelvic) aspect of the muscles forming the walls and floor of the pelvis. The parietal pelvic fascia also forms part of the pelvic floor (superior and inferior fascia of the pelvic diaphragm), and is separated from the parietal peritoneum by extraperitoneal fat. The parietal pelvic fascia covers the pelvic surfaces of the **obturator internus, piriformis, coccygeus, sphincter urethrae,** and **levator ani muscles** (Fig. 4.26, *B, E,* and *F*). The name given to the fascia is derived from the muscle it encloses (e.g. obturator fascia). The parietal pelvic fascia attaches to the periosteum of the ilium just inferior to the pelvic brim. *In females* this fascia attaches to the posterior aspect of the body of the pubis, the bladder, cervix of the uterus, vagina, and rectum to form the pubovesical, cardinal (transverse cervical), and uterosacral ligaments. *In males* the parietal pelvic fascia is attached to the rectum, prostate, urinary bladder, and pubis. The fascia attached to the prostate and bladder forms the medial and lateral *pubovesical (puboprostatic) ligaments*.

The **hypogastric sheath** is a thick band of condensed pelvic fascia (Fig. 4.26, *B* and *E*). This fascial condensation gives passage to essentially all the vessels and nerves passing from the lateral wall of the pelvis to the pelvic viscera, along with the ureters and, in the male, the ductus deferens. As it extends medially from the lateral wall, the hypogastric sheath divides into three laminae ("leaflets" or "wings") that pass to or between the pelvic organs, conveying neurovascular structures and providing support. The three laminae of the hypogastric sheath, from anterior to posterior, are (Fig. 4.26, *B* and *E*):

*   The *lateral ligament of the bladder,* passing to the bladder, conveying the superior vesical arteries and veins
*   The *middle lamina in the male* forming the *rectovesical septum* between the posterior surface of the bladder and the prostate anteriorly and the rectum posteriorly. *In the female,* the middle lamina passes medially to the uterine cervix and vagina as the *cardinal (transverse cervical) ligament*—also known clinically as the *lateral cervical* or *Mackenrodt ligament.* In its uppermost portion, at the base of the broad ligament,

the uterine artery runs transversely toward the cervix while the ureters course immediately beneath them as they pass on each side of the cervix toward the bladder.
*   The posteriormost lamina passes to the rectum, conveying the middle rectal artery and veins.

The **retropubic space** (Fig. 4.26, *B* and *E*) is between the parietal pelvic fascia and the anterior surface of the urinary bladder. It contains loose connective tissue, fat, vessels, and nerves. The connective tissue and fat accommodate expansion of the urinary bladder as urine accumulates.

The **perineal fascia** consists of superficial and deep layers (Fig. 4.27). The **subcutaneous tissue** (superficial fascia) consists of a fatty superficial layer and a membranous (deep) layer (Colles fascia). *In females,* the fatty superficial layer continues anteriorly into the labia majora and from there into the mons pubis and the fatty superficial layer of the abdomen (Camper fascia). *In males,* the fatty superficial layer is greatly diminished in the urogenital triangle, being replaced altogether in the penis and scrotum with smooth (dartos) muscle. It is continuous between the scrotum and thighs with the subcutaneous tissue of the abdomen and posteriorly with a similar layer in the anal region. The **membranous layer** is attached posteriorly to the posterior margin of the perineal membrane and the perineal body. Laterally it is attached to the **fascia lata** (deep fascia) of the uppermost medial aspect of the thigh. Anteriorly, the membranous layer of superficial perineal fascia is continuous with the dartos muscle in the scrotum; however, on each side of and anterior to the scrotum, the membranous layer becomes continuous with the membranous layer of the abdomen. *In females,* the membranous layer of the abdomen (Scarpa fascia) passes superior to the fatty layer forming the labia majora and becomes continuous with the membranous layer of the subcutaneous fascia of the abdomen.

The *deep perineal fascia* (investing or Gallaudet fascia) intimately invests the ischiocavernosus, bulbospongiosus, and superficial transverse perineal muscles. It is also attached

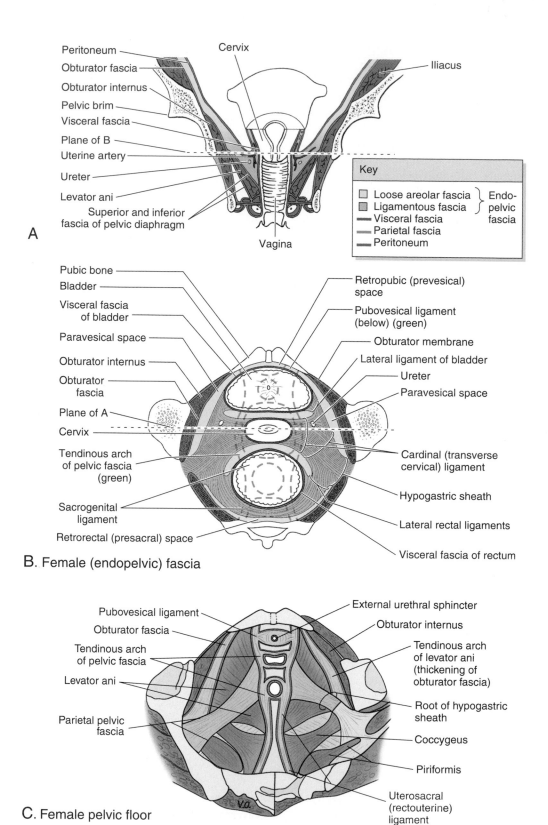

FIGURE 4.26 **Pelvic fascia: endopelvic fascia and fascial ligaments. A.** Coronal section of a female pelvis. **B.** Transverse section of a female pelvis at the level shown in (**A**). **C.** Floor of the female pelvis.

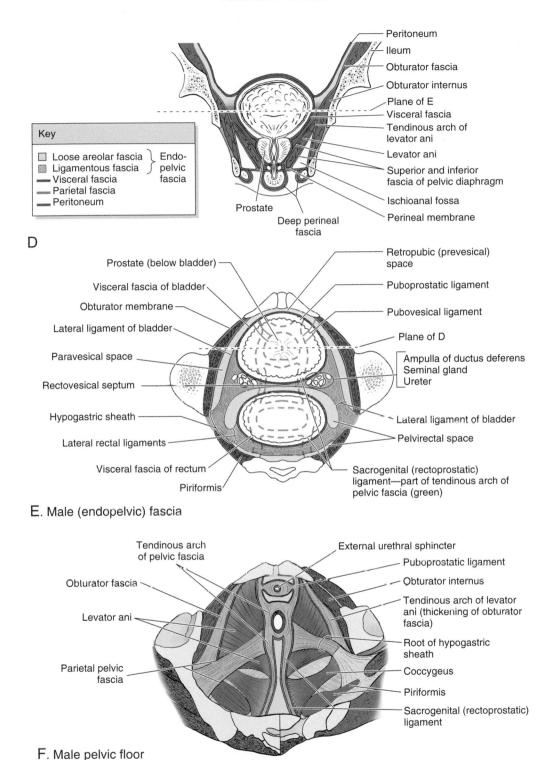

Key

- ☐ Loose areolar fascia ⎫ Endo-
- ☐ Ligamentous fascia ⎬ pelvic
- ▬ Visceral fascia ⎭ fascia
- ▬ Parietal fascia
- ▬ Peritoneum

Peritoneum
Ileum
Obturator fascia
Obturator internus
Plane of E
Visceral fascia
Tendinous arch of levator ani
Levator ani
Superior and inferior fascia of pelvic diaphragm
Ischioanal fossa
Perineal membrane

Prostate
Deep perineal fascia

D

Prostate (below bladder)
Visceral fascia of bladder
Obturator membrane
Lateral ligament of bladder
Paravesical space
Rectovesical septum
Hypogastric sheath
Lateral rectal ligaments
Visceral fascia of rectum
Piriformis

Retropubic (prevesical) space
Puboprostatic ligament
Pubovesical ligament
Plane of D
Ampulla of ductus deferens
Seminal gland
Ureter
Lateral ligament of bladder
Pelvirectal space
Sacrogenital (rectoprostatic) ligament—part of tendinous arch of pelvic fascia (green)

E. Male (endopelvic) fascia

Tendinous arch of pelvic fascia
Obturator fascia
Levator ani
Parietal pelvic fascia

External urethral sphincter
Puboprostatic ligament
Obturator internus
Tendinous arch of levator ani (thickening of obturator fascia)
Root of hypogastric sheath
Coccygeus
Piriformis
Sacrogenital (rectoprostatic) ligament

F. Male pelvic floor

FIGURE 4.26 *Continued.* **D.** Coronal section of a male pelvis at the level shown in (**E**). **E.** Transverse section of the male pelvis at the level shown in (**D**). **F.** Floor of the male pelvis.

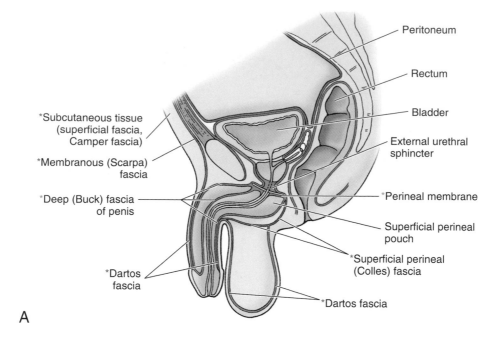

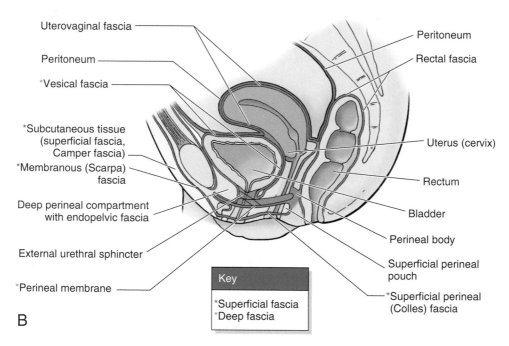

FIGURE 4.27   Fascia of the pelvis and perineum. A. Median section of a male pelvis. **B.** Median section of a female pelvis.

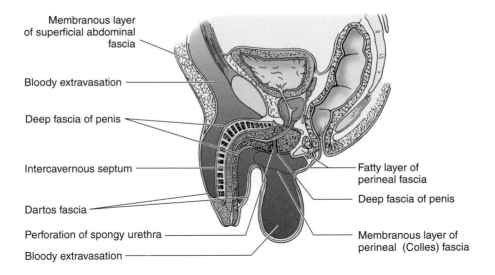

Membranous layer of superficial abdominal fascia

Bloody extravasation

Deep fascia of penis

Intercavernous septum

Dartos fascia

Perforation of spongy urethra

Bloody extravasation

Fatty layer of perineal fascia

Deep fascia of penis

Membranous layer of perineal (Colles) fascia

C

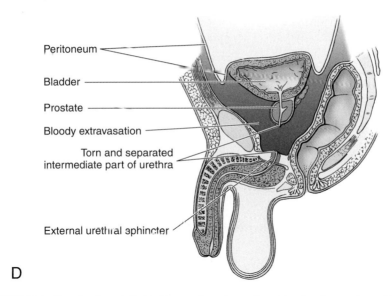

Peritoneum

Bladder

Prostate

Bloody extravasation

Torn and separated intermediate part of urethra

External urethral sphincter

D

FIGURE 4.27 *Continued.* **C.** Median section of a male pelvis showing rupture of the corpus spongiosum and spongy urethra. This results in urine passing from it (extravasation) into the superficial perineal pouch. **D.** Median section of a male pelvis showing rupture of the intermediate part of the urethra. Rupture of this part of the urethra results in extravasation of urine and blood into the deep perineal pouch.

laterally to the ischiopubic ramus superior to the attachment of the membranous layer of superficial perineal fascia. Anteriorly it is fused to the suspensory ligament of the penis and is continuous with the deep fascia covering the external oblique muscle of the abdomen and the rectus sheath. The deep perineal fascia is fused with the suspensory ligament of the clitoris in females and the deep fascia of the abdomen, as in males.

Superficial Perineal Pouch

The superficial perineal pouch (compartment) is a potential space between the membranous layer of superficial perineal fascia and the perineal membrane (Figs. 4.26 and 4.27).

In males the superficial perineal pouch contains the:

• Root (bulb and crura of the penis and muscles associated with it (ischiocavernosus and bulbospongiosus and their covering of deep perineal fascia)
• Proximal part of the spongy urethra
• Superficial transverse perineal muscles
• Branches of the internal pudendal vessels
• Branches of the pudendal nerves (perineal nerves).

In females the superficial perineal pouch contains the:

• Root (crura) of the clitoris and the muscle associated with it (ischiocavernosus)
• Bulbs of the vestibule and the surrounding muscle (bulbospongiosus)
• Superficial transverse perineal muscles
• Related vessels and nerves (branches of internal pudendal vessels, perineal nerves)
• Greater vestibular glands (p. 273).

Deep Perineal Pouch

The deep perineal pouch (space) is not an enclosed compartment; it is open superiorly. This pouch and the deep urogenital muscles are bounded below by the perineal membrane; however, the pouch extends superiorly as the anterior recesses of the ischioanal fossa (see Fig. 4.29).

In males the deep perineal pouch contains the:

• Intermediate part of the urethra
• External urethral sphincter muscle
• Bulbourethral glands
• Deep transverse perineal muscles
• Related vessels and nerves.

In females the deep perineal pouch contains the:

• Proximal part of the urethra
• External urethral sphincter muscle
• Deep transverse perineal muscles
• Related vessels and nerves.

Traditionally, a trilaminar *urogenital (UG) diaphragm* was described as the main constituent of the deep perineal pouch. The long-held concept of a flat, essentially two-dimensional UG diaphragm is erroneous (Wendell-Smith, 1995). According to this concept, the UG diaphragm consisted of the perineal membrane (inferior fascia of UG diaphragm) on the bottom and a "superior fascia of the UG diaphragm" on top, between which was a flat muscular sheet composed of a disclike sphincter urethra and the transversely oriented deep transverse perineal muscle. Only the descriptions of the perineal membrane and of the deep transverse perineal muscles of the male appear to be supported by evidence; the female deep transverse perineal muscles are mainly smooth muscle. *The strong perineal membrane, extending between the ischiopubic rami and separating the superficial and deep perineal pouches, is the final passive support of the pelvic viscera.* Immediately superior to the posterior half of the perineal membrane, the flat, sheetlike *deep transverse perineal muscle,* when developed, offers dynamic support for the pelvic viscera. As described by Oelrich (1980), however, the urethral sphincter is not a flat, planar structure, and the only "superior fascia" is the fascia of the external urethral sphincter.

The **external urethral sphincter** is more tube- and troughlike than disclike, and in the male only a part of the muscle forms a circular investment (a true sphincter) for the intermediate part of the urethra inferior to the prostate (Fig. 4.28*A*). Its larger, troughlike part extends vertically to the neck of the bladder, displacing the prostate and investing the prostatic urethra anteriorly and anterolaterally only. As the prostate develops from urethral glands, the muscle atrophies or is displaced by the prostate posteriorly and posterolaterally. Whether this part of the muscle compresses or dilates the prostatic urethra is a matter of some controversy.

In the female the external urethral sphincter is more properly a "urogenital sphincter," according to Oelrich (1983). Here too, he described a part forming a true anular sphincter around the urethra, but this having several additional parts extending from it (Fig. 4.28*B*): a superior part, extending to the

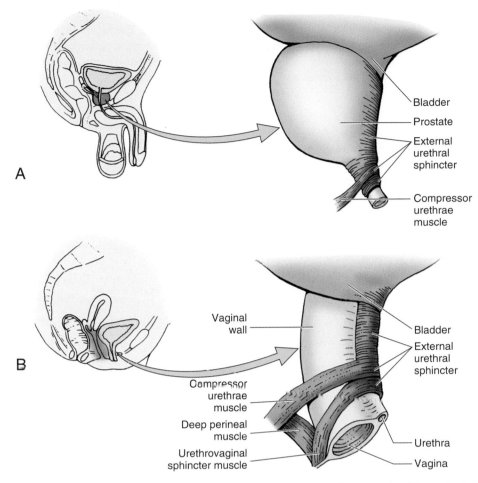

FIGURE 4.28 **Urethra. A.** External urethral sphincter and compressor urethrae muscle of the male. Lateral view. **B.** External urethral sphincter, compressor urethrae, and urethrovaginal sphincter muscles of the female. Lateral view.

neck of the bladder; a subdivision described as extending inferolaterally to the ischial ramus on each side (the **compressor urethrae muscle**); and yet another bandlike part, which encircles both the vagina and urethra (**urethrovaginal sphincter muscle**). In both the male and female, the musculature described, rather than lying in the plane of the deep perineal muscle, is actually oriented perpendicular to it.

PELVIC DIAPHRAGM

The pelvic diaphragm—consisting of the levator ani and coccygeus muscles, together with

RUPTURE OF URETHRA IN MALES AND EXTRAVASATION OF URINE

Rupture of the spongy urethra results in urine passing into the superficial perineal pouch (Fig. 4.27C). The attachments of the perineal fascia determine the direction of flow of the extravasated urine. Hence, urine and blood may pass into the loose connective tissue in the scrotum, around the penis, and superiorly into the fatty layer of subcutaneous connective tissue of the lower anterior abdominal wall. The urine cannot pass far into the thighs because the superficial perineal fascia blends with the fascia lata (deep fascia) enveloping the thigh muscles, just distal to the inguinal ligament. In addition, urine cannot pass posteriorly into the anal triangle because the superficial and deep layers of perineal fascia are continuous with each other at the posterior edge of the perineal membrane. Rupture of the intermediate part of the urethra results in extravasation of urine and blood into the deep perineal pouch (Fig. 4.27D).

the fascia above and below them—separates the pelvic cavity from the perineum (Fig. 4.29). *The pelvic diaphragm forms the funnel-shaped floor of the pelvic cavity and the inverted V-shaped roof of each ischioanal fossa.*

Ischioanal Fossae

The ischioanal fossae (formerly ischiorectal fossae) around the wall of the anal canal are large fascia-lined, wedge-shaped spaces between the skin of the anal region and the pelvic diaphragm (Fig. 4.29*B*). The apex of each fossa lies superi-orly where the levator ani muscle arises from the obturator fascia. The ischioanal fossae, wide inferiorly and narrow superiorly, are filled with fat and loose connective tissue. The two ischioanal fossae communicate by means of the deep postanal space over the **anococcygeal body** (ligament), a fibrous mass located between the anal canal and the tip of the coccyx (Fig. 4.29*B*).

Each ischioanal fossa is bounded:

- Laterally by the ischium and the inferior part of the obturator internus, covered with obturator fascia

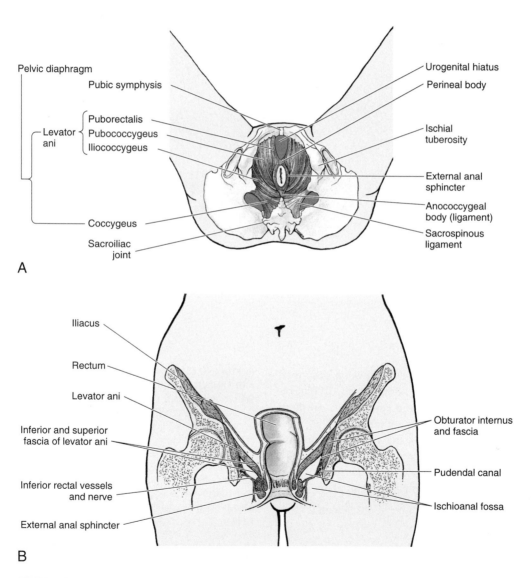

FIGURE 4.29   Pelvic diaphragm and ischioanal fossae. A. Inferior view of the pelvic diaphragm. **B.** Coronal section of the pelvis through the rectum, anal canal, and ischioanal fossae.

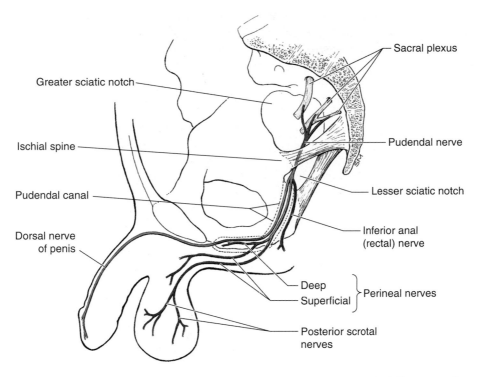

FIGURE 4.30   Diagram of the pudendal nerve in a male. The five regions in which it runs are shown in color. The perineal nerves in the female give rise to labial branches and the dorsal nerve of the clitoris.

- Medially by the anal canal to which the levator ani descends and which the external anal sphincter surrounds
- Posteriorly by the gluteus maximus
- Anteriorly by the external urethral sphincter and deep transverse perineal muscles and their fascia. These parts of the fossae, superior to the perineal membrane, are known as the *anterior recesses of the ischioanal fossae.*

The ischioanal fossae are traversed by tough, fibrous bands and filled with fat, forming the *fat bodies of the ischioanal fossae.* These fat bodies support the anal canal but are readily displaced to permit expansion of the anal canal during the passage of feces. The **pudendal canals** on the lateral walls of the ischioanal fossae contain the *internal pudendal vessels* and the **pudendal nerves** (Fig. 4.30). Posteriorly these vessels and the nerve give rise to the inferior rectal vessels and inferior anal (rectal) nerves, respectively, which cross the ischioanal fossae and become superficial as they supply the external anal

sphincter and the perianal skin. Two other cutaneous nerves, the perforating branch of S2 and S3 and the perineal branch of S4 nerve, also pass through the ischioanal fossae.

Pudendal Canal

The pudendal canal is a space within the obturator fascia (Figs. 4.29*B* and 4.30), which covers the medial aspect of the obturator internus muscle and lines the lateral wall of the ischioanal fossa. The pudendal canal begins at the posterior border of the ischioanal fossa and runs from the **lesser sciatic notch** adjacent to the ischial spine to the posterior edge of the perineal membrane. The internal pudendal artery and vein, the pudendal nerve, and the nerve to the obturator internus enter this canal at the lesser sciatic notch, inferior to the ischial spine. The **pudendal nerve** supplies most of the innervation to the perineum. The pudendal nerve supplies the skin, organs, and muscles of the perineum; it is therefore concerned with micturition, defecation, erection, ejaculation, and, in the female, parturition. Toward the distal end of the pudendal canal, the pudendal nerve splits, giving rise to the perineal nerves and continuing as the **dorsal nerve of penis or clitoris.** These nerves run anteriorly on each side of the internal pudendal artery. The **superficial perineal nerves** give scrotal or labial (cutaneous) branches, and the **deep perineal nerve** supplies the muscles of the deep and superficial perineal pouches, the skin of the vestibule of the vagina, and the mucosa of the inferiormost part of the vagina. The dorsal nerve of the penis or clitoris, a sensory nerve, runs through the deep perineal pouch to reach its area of supply. The **inferior anal (rectal) nerve** arises from the pudendal nerve at the entrance of the pudendal canal and crosses the ischioanal fossa to reach the anus. The inferior anal nerve supplies the external anal sphincter and perianal skin and communicates with the posterior scrotal or labial and perineal nerves. The **dorsal nerve of the penis or clitoris,** a sensory branch of the pudendal nerve, runs through the deep perineal pouch to reach its area of supply.

ISCHIOANAL ABSCESSES

The ischioanal fossae are occasionally the sites of infection that may result in the formation of *ischioanal abscesses*. These collections of pus are annoying and painful. Diagnostic signs of an ischioanal abscess are fullness and tenderness between the anus and ischial tuberosity. An ischioanal abscess may open spontaneously into the contralateral ischioanal fossa (horseshoe abscess), anal canal, rectum, or perianal skin.

MALE PERINEUM

The superficial structures of the male perineum (perineal area) are the penis and scrotum. The urethra in the bladder neck and the prostatic urethra, the first two parts of the male urethra, are described with the pelvis (p. 230). The **intermediate (membranous) part of the urethra** is the shortest and narrowest part of the urethra, except for the external urethral orifice. It begins at the apex of the prostate and ends at the bulb of the penis, where it is continuous with the spongy urethra (Fig. 4.13*A*). The intermediate part of the urethra traverses the deep perineal pouch, where it is surrounded by the external urethral sphincter and the perineal membrane.

Posterolateral to this part of the urethra are the small **bulbourethral glands** (Fig. 4.13) and their slender ducts, which open into the proximal part of the spongy urethra. The **spongy urethra,** the longest part, passes through the *bulb* and *corpus spongiosum* of the penis. It begins at the distal end of the intermediate part of the urethra and ends at the **external urethral orifice** (Figs. 4.31*D* and 4.32). There are minute openings of the ducts of mucus-secreting *urethral glands* into the spongy urethra. **Lymphatic vessels** from the intermediate part of the urethra drain mainly into the **internal iliac lymph nodes** (Fig. 4.33), whereas most vessels from the spongy urethra pass to the **deep inguinal lymph nodes,** but some vessels pass to the external iliac lymph nodes.

Penis

The penis is the male organ of copulation and the outlet for urine and semen. The penis consists of a **root, body,** and **glans penis** (Fig. 4.31*D*). It is composed of three cylindrical bodies of erectile cavernous tissue—the **corpora cavernosa** and the **corpus spongiosum**—each having a fibrous outer covering or capsule, the **tunica albuginea** (Fig. 4.31*B*). Superficial to this covering is the **deep fascia of the penis,** the continuation of the deep perineal fascia that forms a membranous covering for the corpora, binding them together. The corpus spongiosum contains the **spongy urethra.** The corpora cavernosa are fused with each other in the median plane, except posteriorly where they separate to form the **crura of the penis** (Figs. 4.31*A* and 4.32*B*). The **root of the penis** consists of the crura and bulb, surrounded by the **ischiocavernosus** and **bulbospongiosus muscles** (Figs. 4.24*B* and 4.31). The root is located in the superficial perineal pouch (Fig. 4.27*A*). The **crura** and **bulb of the penis** are the proximal ends of the corpora and contain erectile tissue. The **body of the penis** is the free part that is pendulous in the flaccid condition. Except for a few fibers of the bulbospongiosus near the root of the penis and the ischiocavernosus that embrace the crura, the penis has no muscles. Distally the corpus spongiosum of the penis expands to form the **glans penis** (Fig. 4.31). The margin of the glans projects beyond the ends of the corpora cavernosa to form the **corona of**

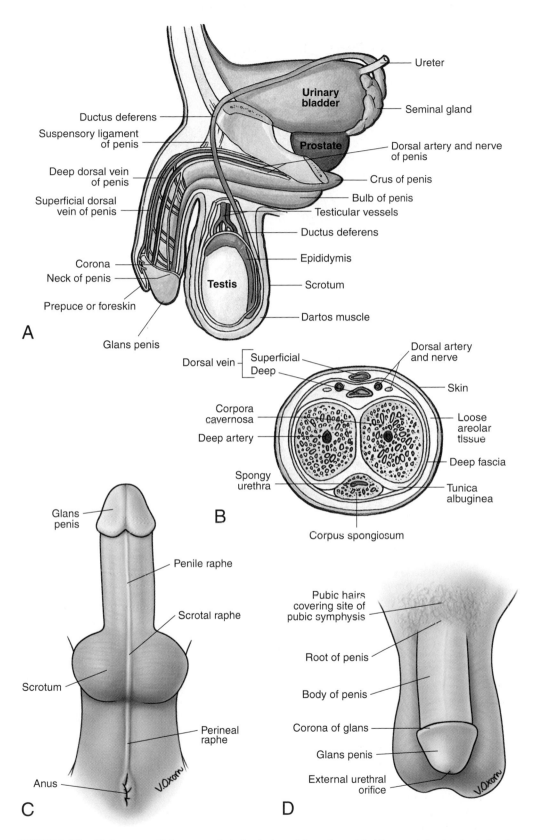

FIGURE 4.31 **Male urogenital organs. A.** Lateral view of the urinary bladder, prostate, seminal gland, and male genital organs. **B.** Transverse section through the body of the penis. **C.** Ventral aspect of penis and scrotum. The spongy urethra is deep to the penile raphe. **D.** Dorsum of penis.

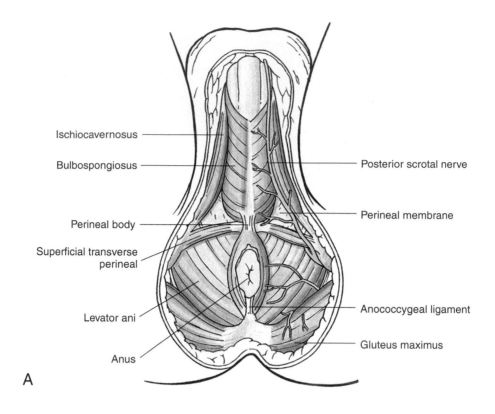

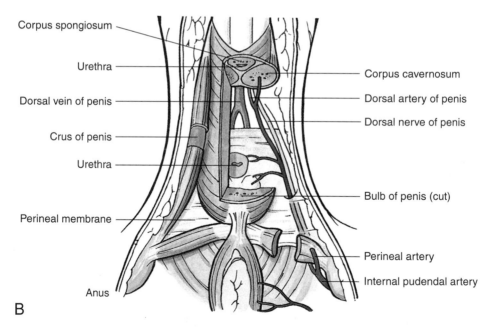

FIGURE 4.32 Dissections of the male perineum. A. Superficial dissection. **B.** Deep dissection.

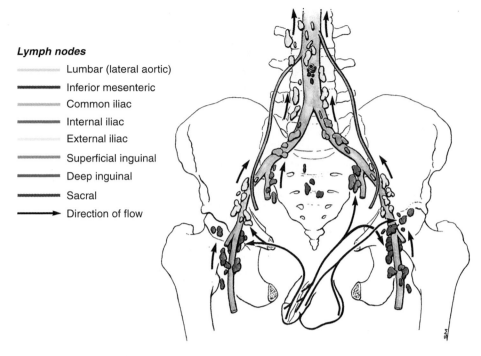

Lymph nodes

	Lumbar (lateral aortic)
	Inferior mesenteric
	Common iliac
	Internal iliac
	External iliac
	Superficial inguinal
	Deep inguinal
	Sacral
→	Direction of flow

FIGURE 4.33 **Lymphatic drainage of the penis and scrotum.** *Arrows,* lymph flow to lymph nodes.

the gland. The slitlike opening of the spongy urethra, the **external urethral orifice,** is located at or near the tip of the glans (Fig. 4.31). The skin and fascia of the penis are prolonged as a double layer of skin, the **prepuce** (foreskin), which covers the glans to a variable extent (Fig. 4.31*A*). The *fundiform ligament of the penis* is a band of elastic fibers of the subcutaneous tissue that arises from the pubic symphysis. It passes inferiorly and splits to form a sling that is attached to the deep fascia of the penis. The **suspensory ligament of the penis** is the deep fascia that firmly attaches the root of the penis to the pubic symphysis, pubic rami, and perineal membrane (Fig. 4.31*A*).

The **superficial perineal muscles** are the superficial transverse perineal, bulbospongiosus, and ischiocavernosus (Table 4.7). These muscles are in the superficial perineal pouch and are supplied by the perineal nerves.

Vasculature of Penis. The penis is supplied by branches of the **internal pudendal arteries** (Table 4.6).

- *Dorsal arteries* run in the interval between the corpora cavernosa on each side of the deep dorsal vein, supplying the fibrous tissue around the corpora and penile skin
- *Deep arteries* pierce the crura and run within the corpora cavernosa, supplying the erectile tissue in these structures
- The *artery of the bulb of the penis* supplies the posterior part of the corpus spongiosum and the bulbourethral gland.

Superficial and deep branches of the **external pudendal arteries** (Table 4.6) supply the penile skin, anastomosing with branches of the internal pudendal arteries. Blood from the cavernous spaces of the corpora is drained by a venous plexus that becomes the **deep dorsal vein of the penis** in the deep fascia (Fig. 4.31, *A* and *B*). This vein passes deep to the inferior pubic (arcuate) ligament and joins the **prostatic venous plexus** (Fig. 4.13*B*). Blood from the superficial coverings of the penis (skin and dartos fascia) drains into the **superficial dorsal vein,** which ends in the superficial external pudendal vein. Some blood also passes to the lat-

TABLE 4.6. ARTERIAL SUPPLY OF PERINEUM

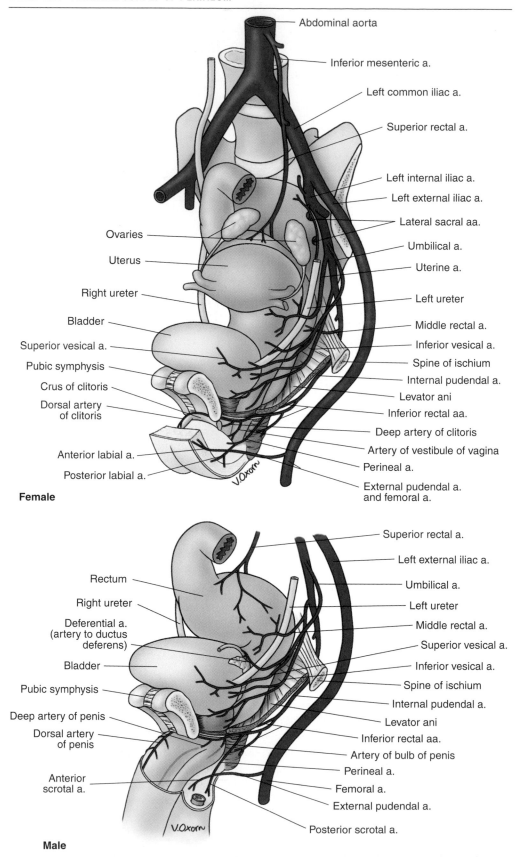

Abdominal aorta

Inferior mesenteric a.

Left common iliac a.

Superior rectal a.

Left internal iliac a.

Left external iliac a.

Lateral sacral aa.

Umbilical a.

Uterine a.

Ovaries

Uterus

Right ureter

Left ureter

Bladder

Middle rectal a.

Superior vesical a.

Inferior vesical a.

Pubic symphysis

Spine of ischium

Crus of clitoris

Internal pudendal a.

Dorsal artery of clitoris

Levator ani

Inferior rectal aa.

Deep artery of clitoris

Anterior labial a.

Artery of vestibule of vagina

Posterior labial a.

Perineal a.

External pudendal a. and femoral a.

Female

Superior rectal a.

Left external iliac a.

Rectum

Umbilical a.

Right ureter

Left ureter

Deferential a. (artery to ductus deferens)

Middle rectal a.

Superior vesical a.

Bladder

Inferior vesical a.

Pubic symphysis

Spine of ischium

Deep artery of penis

Internal pudendal a.

Dorsal artery of penis

Levator ani

Inferior rectal aa.

Artery of bulb of penis

Perineal a.

Anterior scrotal a.

Femoral a.

External pudendal a.

Posterior scrotal a.

V.Oxorn

Male

TABLE 4.6. *CONTINUED*

Artery	Origin	Course	Distribution
Internal pudendal	Internal iliac artery	Leaves pelvis through greater sciatic foramen; hooks around ischial spine and enters perineum by way of lesser sciatic foramen and passes to pudendal canal	Perineum and external genital organs
Inferior rectal	Internal pudendal artery	Leaves pudendal canal and crosses ischioanal fossa to anal canal	Distal portion of anal canal
Perineal	Internal pudendal artery	Leaves pudendal canal and enters superficial perineal space	Supplies superficial perineal muscles and scrotum
Posterior scrotal or labial	Terminal branches of perineal artery	Runs in subcutaneous tissue of posterior scrotum or labium majus	Skin of scrotum or labium majus
Artery of bulb of penis or vestibule	Internal pudendal artery	Pierces perineal membrane to reach bulb of penis or vestibule of vagina	Supplies bulb of penis or vestibule and bulbourethral gland (male) and greater vestibular gland (female)
Deep artery of penis or clitoris	Terminal branch of internal pudendal artery	Pierces perineal membrane to reach corpora cavernosa of penis or clitoris	Supplies erectile tissue of penis or clitoris
Dorsal artery of penis or clitoris	Terminal branch of internal pudendal artery	Pierces perineal membrane and passes through suspensory ligament of penis or clitoris to run on dorsum of penis or clitoris	Skin of penis and erectile tissue of penis or clitoris
External pudendal, superficial and deep branches	Femoral artery	Pass medially across the thigh to reach the scrotum of labia majora	External genitalia and superomedial part of the thigh

eral pudendal vein. The **superficial inguinal lymph nodes** receive most of the lymph from the penis (Fig. 4.33*C*).

Innervation of Penis. The nerves derive from the S2 through S4 segments of the spinal cord. The **dorsal nerve of the penis**—a terminal branch of the **pudendal nerve** (Fig. 4.30)—arises in the pudendal canal and passes anteriorly into the deep perineal pouch. It supplies the skin, glans, and spongy urethra. The penis is supplied with a variety of sensory nerve endings—especially the glans—and thus is highly sensitive. Branches of the *ilioinguinal nerve* supply the skin at the root of the penis.

Scrotum

The scrotum is a cutaneous fibromuscular sac for the testes and associated structures (Fig. 4.32*A*). It is situated posteroinferior to the penis and inferior to the pubic symphysis. The bilateral embryonic formation of the scrotum is indicated by the midline **scrotal raphe** (Fig. 4.31*C*), which is continuous on the ventral surface of the penis with the

ERECTION, EMISSION, AND EJACULATION

When a male is stimulated erotically, arteriovenous anastomoses—by which blood is normally able to bypass the "empty" potential spaces (sinuses) of the corpora cavernosa—are closed. The smooth muscle in the fibrous trabeculae and coiled arteries relaxes as a result of *parasympathetic stimulation* (S1 through S4 through the cavernous nerves from the prostatic nerve plexus). As a result the arteries straighten, enlarging their lumina and allowing blood to flow into and dilate the cavernous spaces in the corpora of the penis. The bulbospongiosus and ischiocavernosus muscles compress the venous plexuses at the periphery of the corpora cavernosa, impeding the return of venous blood. As a result the corpora become enlarged, rigid, and the penis erects. During **emission,** semen (sperms and glandular secretions) is delivered to the prostatic urethra through the ejaculatory ducts after peristalsis of the ductus deferentes and seminal glands. *Prostatic fluid* is added to the seminal fluid as the smooth muscle in the prostate contracts. During **ejaculation,** semen is expelled from the urethra through the external urethral orifice. *Ejaculation results from:*

- Closure of the urethral sphincter at the neck of the bladder—sympathetic (L1 and L2 nerves)
- Contraction of the prostatic and urethral muscles—a parasympathetic response (S2 through S4 nerves)
- Contraction of the bulbospongiosus muscles—pudendal nerves (S2 through S4).

After ejaculation, the penis gradually returns to a flaccid state, resulting from sympathetic stimulation that causes constriction of the smooth muscle in the coiled arteries. The bulbospongiosus and ischiocavernosus muscles relax, allowing more blood to flow into the veins. Blood is slowly drained from the cavernous spaces in the penile corpora into the deep dorsal vein.

penile raphe and posteriorly along the median line of the perineum as the **perineal raphe.** The contents of the scrotum (testes and epididymides) are described with the abdomen (see Chapter 2).

Vasculature of Scrotum. The anterior aspect of the scrotum is supplied by the **external pudendal arteries** (Table 4.6) and the posterior aspect is supplied by the **internal pudendal arteries.** The scrotum also receives branches from the testicular and cremasteric arteries. The **scrotal veins** accompany the arteries and join the external pudendal veins. **Lymphatic vessels** from the scrotum drain into the **superficial inguinal lymph nodes** (Fig. 4.33).

Innervation of Scrotum. The anterior aspect of the scrotum is supplied by the anterior scrotal nerves derived from the **ilioinguinal nerve,** and by the genital branch of the **genitofemoral nerve** (p. 194). The posterior aspect of the scrotum is supplied by **posterior scrotal nerves,** superficial branches of the perineal nerves (Fig. 4.30) and by the perineal branch of the *posterior femoral cutaneous nerve.*

FEMALE PERINEUM

The superficial structures of the female perineum (perineal area) are the clitoris, labia majora, and labia minora. *The female perineum is bounded by the:*

- Mons pubis
- Medial aspects (insides) of the thighs
- Gluteal folds
- The superior end of the intergluteal cleft—the cleft between the buttocks—where the tip of the coccyx is palpable.

Female External Genitalia

The female external genitalia—the **pudendum** or **vulva** (Fig. 4.34*A*)—include the:

- Mons pubis
- Labia majora
- Labia minora
- Clitoris
- Vestibule
- Greater vestibular glands.

The vulva serves:

- As sensory and erectile tissue for sexual arousal and intercourse
- To direct the flow of urine
- To prevent entry of foreign material into the urogenital tract
- As padding upon which the body weight rests when straddling, as when riding a bicycle.

Mons Pubis. The mons pubis is the rounded fatty prominence anterior to the pubic symphysis, pubic tubercle, and superior pubic rami. The amount of fat in the mons increases at puberty and decreases after menopause. After puberty the mons pubis is covered with coarse pubic hairs.

TABLE 4.7. MUSCLES OF PERINEUM

Muscle	Origin	Insertion	Innervation	Action(s)
External anal sphincter	Skin and fascia surrounding anus and coccyx via anococcygeal body	Perineal body	Inferior anal (rectal) nerve (Fig. 4.30)	Closes anal canal
Bulbospongiosus	Male: median raphe, ventral surface of bulb of penis, and perineal body	Male: corpora spongiosum and cavernosa and fascia of bulb of penis		Male: compresses bulb of penis and assists in erection of penis
	Female: perineal body	Female: fascia of corpus cavernosa		Females: reduces lumen of vagina and assists in erection of clitoris
Ischiocavernosus	Ischial ramus and tuberosity	Crus of penis or clitoris	Deep branch of perineal nerve, a branch of pudendal nerve (Fig. 4.30)	Maintains erection of penis or clitoris by compression of outflow veins
Superficial transverse perineal	Ischial ramus and tuberosity	Perineal body		Supports perineal body
Deep transverse perineal	Inner aspect of ischiopubic ramus	Median raphe, perineal body, and external anal sphincter		Fixes perineal body
External urethral sphincter	Inferior pubic ramus and ischial tuberosity	Surrounds urethra; in females some fibers also enclose vagina		Compresses urethra; also compresses vagina in females

Labia Majora. The labia majora are prominent folds of skin that bound the *pudendal cleft*—the slit between the labia majora—and indirectly provide protection for the urethral and vaginal orifices. Each labium majus—largely filled with subcutaneous fat containing smooth muscle—passes inferoposteriorly from the mons pubis toward the anus. The external aspects of the labia in the adult are covered with pigmented skin containing many sebaceous glands and are covered with crisp pubic hair. The internal aspects of the labia are smooth, pink, and hairless.

Labia Minora. The labia minora are folds of fat-free, hairless skin. They are enclosed in the pudendal cleft within the labia majora. They have a core of spongy connective tissue containing erectile tissue and many small blood vessels. Although the internal surface of each labium minus consists of thin moist skin, it has the typical pink color of a mucous membrane and contains many sensory nerve endings.

Vestibule. The vestibule is the space or cavity between the labia minora that contains the openings of the urethra, vagina, and ducts of the greater and lesser vestibular glands (Fig. 4.34, *A* and *D*). The **external urethral orifice** is located posteroinferior to the glans clitoris and anterior to the vaginal orifice. On each side of the external urethral orifice are the openings of the ducts of the *paraurethral glands*. The size and appearance of the **vaginal orifice** vary with

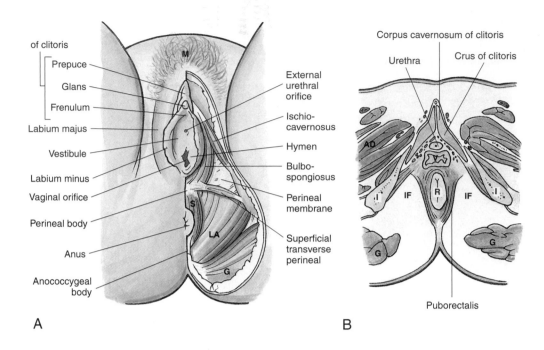

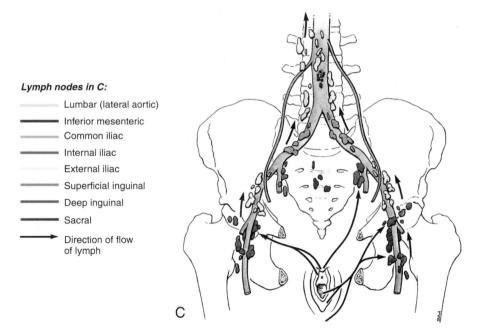

FIGURE 4.34   Female perineum. A. Left side has been dissected to show muscles. *M,* mons pubis; *S,* external anal sphincter; *LA,* levator ani; *G,* gluteus maximus. **B.** Transverse section of the female perineum. *AD,* adductor muscles of thigh; *V,* vagina; *I,* ischium; *IF,* ischioanal fossa; *R,* rectum; *G,* gluteus maximus. **C.** Lymphatic drainage of the vulva (external genitalia). *Arrows,* lymph flow to lymph nodes.

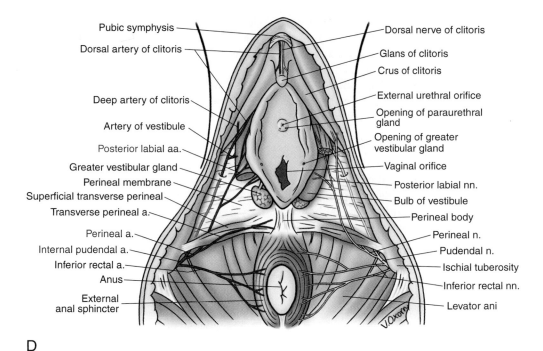

Pubic symphysis
Dorsal artery of clitoris
Deep artery of clitoris
Artery of vestibule
Posterior labial aa.
Greater vestibular gland
Perineal membrane
Superficial transverse perineal
Transverse perineal a.
Perineal a.
Internal pudendal a.
Inferior rectal a.
Anus
External anal sphincter

Dorsal nerve of clitoris
Glans of clitoris
Crus of clitoris
External urethral orifice
Opening of paraurethral gland
Opening of greater vestibular gland
Vaginal orifice
Posterior labial nn.
Bulb of vestibule
Perineal body
Perineal n.
Pudendal n.
Ischial tuberosity
Inferior rectal nn.
Levator ani

D

FIGURE 4.34 *Continued.* **D.** Blood supply and innervation.

the condition of the **hymen,** a thin fold of mucous membrane surrounding the vaginal orifice. The hymen at first covers the orifice and after its rupture, surrounds it (Fig. 4.34*A*).

Bulbs of Vestibule. The bulbs of the vestibule are paired *masses of elongated erectile tissue* that lie along the sides of the vaginal orifice under cover of the bulbospongiosus muscles (Fig. 4.34*D*). The bulbs are homologous with the bulb of the penis and the corpus spongiosum.

Vestibular Glands. The **greater vestibular glands** are on each side of the vestibule, posterolateral to the vaginal orifice (Fig. 4.34*D*). The glands are round or oval and are partly overlapped posteriorly by the bulbs of the vestibule and both are enclosed by the bulbospongiosus muscle. The slender ducts of these glands pass deep to the bulbs and open into the vestibule on each side of the vaginal orifice. These glands secrete mucus into the vestibule during sexual arousal. The **lesser vestibular glands** are smaller glands on each side of the vestibule that open into it between the urethral and vaginal orifices. These glands

secrete mucus into the vestibule, which moistens the labia and vestibule.

Clitoris. The clitoris is an erectile organ located where the labia minora meet anteriorly. The clitoris consists of a *root* and a *body,* which are composed of two **crura,** two **corpora cavernosa,** and a **glans** (Fig. 4.34, *A* and *D*). The anteriormost parts of the labia minora pass anterior to the clitoris and form the **prepuce of the clitoris** (Fig. 4.34*A*). A more posterior or deeper part of the labia minora passes posterior to the clitoris and forms the **frenulum of the clitoris** (Fig. 4.34*A*). The clitoris enlarges upon tactile stimulation and is highly sensitive. The glans clitoris is the most highly innervated part of the clitoris.

Vasculature of Vulva. The arterial supply to the vulva is from the **external pudendal arteries** (Table 4.6) and one internal pudendal artery on each side. The **internal pudendal artery** supplies the skin, sex organs, and perineal muscles. The labial arteries are branches of the internal pudendal artery, as are those of the clitoris (Fig. 4.34*D*). The labial veins are tributaries of the

internal pudendal veins and companion veins (L. venae comitantes). Venous engorgement during the excitement phase of sexual response causes an increase in the size and consistency of the clitoris and the bulbs of the vestibule. The vulva contains a rich network of **lymphatic vessels** that pass laterally to the **superficial inguinal lymph nodes** (Fig. 4.34C).

Innervation of Vulva. The nerves to the vulva are the anterior labial nerves (branches of the **ilioinguinal nerve**); the genital branch of the **genitofemoral nerve**; the perineal branch of the **femoral cutaneous nerve of thigh**, and **posterior labial nerves**—branches of the **perineal nerves** (Fig. 4.34D). *Parasympathetic stimulation produces:*

- Increased vaginal secretion
- Erection of the clitoris
- Engorgement of erectile tissue in the bulbs of the vestibule

Perineal Fascia and Muscles

The *superficial perineal fascia* (Fig. 4.30B) consists of a more superficial fatty layer and a deeper membranous layer of subcutaneous connective tissue (Colles fascia). These layers are continuous in the labia majora. The deep layer of fascia attaches medially to the pubic symphysis and laterally to the body of the pubis. The **superficial perineal muscles** (Fig. 4.34A) include the:

- Superficial transverse perineal
- Ischiocavernosus
- Bulbospongiosus.

The slender, **superficial transverse perineal muscle** (L. transversus perinei superficialis) passes in the base of the superficial perineal pouch from the ischial ramus to the perineal body. The **ischiocavernosus,** another slender muscle, attaches to the ischial ramus and partially surrounds the crus of the clitoris (Fig. 4.34, *A* and *B*). The **bulbospongiosus,** a thin wide muscle, is separated from its contralateral partner by the vagina. It arises from the perineal body, passes around the vagina, and inserts into the clitoris. In its course it covers the bulb of the vestibule and the greater vestibular

gland. Acting together, the bulbospongiosus muscles constrict the vagina weakly (Table 4.7).

The **perineal body** is a fibromuscular structure that supports the posterior wall of the vagina and is the center of a musculofibrous "cross-member" that *forms the final dynamic support of the pelvic viscera* (Fig. 4.34A). The perineal body lies between the inferior part of the vagina and the anal canal and is held in position by the attachment of the perineal and levator ani muscles, the other parts of the "cross-member."

DILATION OF URETHRA
The female urethra is very distensible because it contains considerable elastic tissue, as well as smooth muscle. It can easily dilate without injury to it; consequently, the passage of catheters or cystoscopes in females is much easier than it is in males.

Inflammation of Greater Vestibular Glands
The greater vestibular glands (Bartholin glands) are usually not palpable, except when infected. *Bartholinitis*—inflammation of the greater vestibular glands—may result from a number of pathogenic organisms. Infected glands may enlarge to a diameter of 4 to 5 cm and impinge on the wall of the rectum.

Pudendal and Ilioinguinal Nerve Blocks
To relieve the pain experienced during childbirth, *pudendal nerve block anesthesia* may be performed by injecting a local anesthetic agent into the tissues surrounding the pudendal nerve. The injection may be made where the pudendal nerve crosses the lateral aspect of the sacrospinous ligament, near its attachment to the ischial spine. Although a pudendal nerve block anaesthetizes most of the perineum, it does not abolish sensation from the anterior part of the perineum that is innervated by the ilioinguinal nerve. To abolish pain from the anterior part of the perineum, an *ilioinguinal nerve block* is performed. The *posterior cutaneous nerve of the thigh* must also be blocked to provide thorough anesthesia.

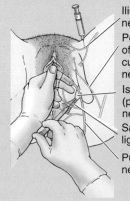

Ilioinguinal nerve block site

Perineal branch of posterior cutaneous nerve of thigh

Ischial spine (pudendal nerve block site)

Sacrospinous ligament

Pudendal nerve

5 Back

*T*he back—*the posterior aspect of the trunk inferior to the neck and superior to the gluteal region* (buttocks)—is the region of the body to which the head, neck, and limbs are attached. Because of their close association with the trunk, the back of the neck and the posterior and deep cervical muscles and vertebra are described in this chapter. The back consists of skin, subcutaneous tissue—a layer of loose irregular connective tissue consisting of fatty tissue containing cutaneous nerves and vessels—deep fascia, muscles and their vessels and nerves, ligaments, vertebral column, ribs (in thoracic region), spinal cord and meninges (membranes covering spinal cord), and various nerves and vessels.

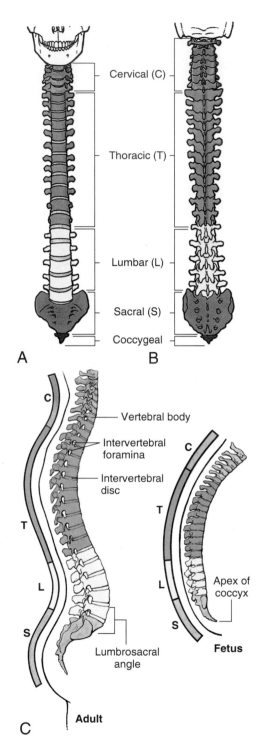

FIGURE 5.1 Vertebral column and curvatures.
A. Anterior view. **B.** Posterior view. **C.** Curvatures of
the vertebral column of the adult and fetus, lateral
view. *C,* cervical; *T,* thoracic; *L,* lumbar; *S,* sacral.

VERTEBRAL COLUMN

The vertebral column (spine, backbone)—
extending from the cranium (skull) to the
apex (tip) of the coccyx—*forms the skeleton
of the neck* and back and the main part of the
axial skeleton (bones of cranium, vertebral
column, ribs, and sternum). *The vertebral
column:*

- Protects the spinal cord and spinal
  nerves
- Supports the weight of the body
- Provides a partly rigid and flexible axis for
  the body and a pivot for the head
- Plays an important role in posture and
  locomotion—movement from one place to
  another.

The adult vertebral column typically consists of 33 vertebrae arranged in five regions:
7 cervical, 12 thoracic, 5 lumbar, 5 sacral, and
4 coccygeal (Fig. 5.1). The **lumbosacral angle**
occurs at the junction of the lumbar region of
the vertebral column and sacrum. *Motion occurs between only 24 vertebrae:* 7 cervical, 12
thoracic, and 5 lumbar. The sacral vertebrae
are fused in adults to form the **sacrum,** and
the four coccygeal vertebrae are fused to form
the **coccyx.** The vertebrae gradually become
larger as the vertebral column descends to the
sacrum and then tapers toward the apex of
the coccyx. These structural differences are
related to the fact that the successive vertebrae bear increasing amounts of the body's
weight as the column descends. The vertebral
column is flexible because it consists of small
bones—the **vertebrae**—that are separated by
intervertebral (IV) discs. The cervical, thoracic, and lumbar vertebrae articulate at synovial joints that facilitate and control the vertebral column's flexibility. The vertebral
bodies contribute approximately three
fourths of the height of the vertebral column
and the IV discs of fibrocartilage contribute
approximately one fourth. The shape and
strength of the vertebrae and IV discs, ligaments, and muscles provide stability to the
vertebral column.

CURVATURES OF VERTEBRAL COLUMN

The vertebral column in adults has four curvatures: cervical, thoracic, lumbar, and sacral (Fig. 5.1*C*). The curvatures provide a flexible support (shock-absorbing resilience) for the body. The thoracic and sacral curvatures are concave anteriorly, whereas the cervical and lumbar curvatures are concave posteriorly. The thoracic and sacral curvatures are **primary curvatures** that develop during the fetal period. Primary curvatures are caused by differences in height between the anterior and posterior parts of the vertebrae. The cervical and lumbar curvatures are **secondary curvatures** that begin to appear in the cervical region during the fetal period but do not become obvious until infancy. Secondary curvatures are caused mainly by differences in thickness between the anterior and posterior parts of the IV discs. The **cervical curvature** becomes prominent when an infant begins to hold its head erect. The **lumbar curvature** becomes obvious when an infant begins to walk and assumes the upright posture. This curvature—generally more pronounced in females—ends at the **lumbosacral angle** formed at the junction of L5 vertebra with the sacrum. The **sacral curvature** also differs in males and females; it is sharper in females.

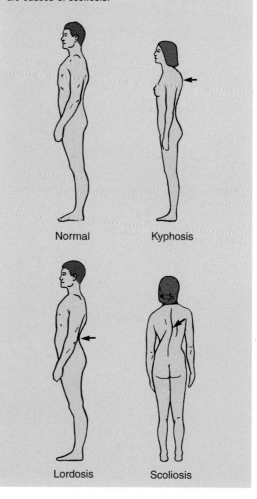

Normal   Kyphosis

Lordosis   Scoliosis

STRUCTURE AND FUNCTION OF VERTEBRAE

Vertebrae vary in size and other characteristics from one region of the vertebral column to another and to a lesser degree within each region. *A typical vertebrae consists of a vertebral body, vertebral arch, and seven processes* (Fig. 5.2). The **vertebral body**—the anterior, more massive part of the vertebra—gives strength to the vertebral column and supports body weight. The vertebral bodies, especially from T4 inferiorly, become progressively larger to bear the progressively greater body weight. The **vertebral arch**—posterior to the vertebral body—is formed by right and left pedicles and laminae. The **pedicles** are short, stout processes that join the vertebral arch to the vertebral body. The pedicles project posteriorly to meet two broad, flat plates of bone—the **laminae.** The vertebral arch and the posterior surface of the vertebral body form the walls of the **vertebral foramen**—the aperture in each vertebra. The succession of vertebral foramina in the articulated column forms the **vertebral canal,** which contains the spinal cord, meninges (protective membranes), fat, spinal nerve roots, and vessels. The indentations formed by the projection of the body and articular processes above and below the pedicles are **vertebral notches** (Fig. 5.2*B*). The superior and inferior vertebral notches of adjacent vertebrae contribute to

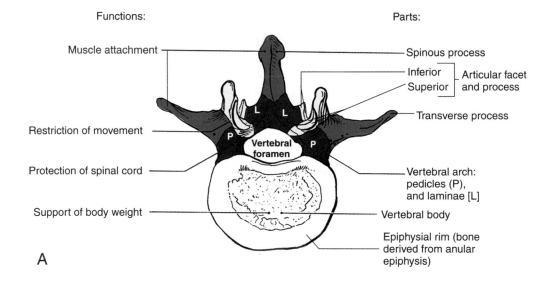

Functions:

Muscle attachment

Restriction of movement

Protection of spinal cord

Support of body weight

Parts:

Spinous process

Inferior / Superior — Articular facet and process

Transverse process

Vertebral arch: pedicles (P), and laminae [L]

Vertebral body

Epiphysial rim (bone derived from anular epiphysis)

Vertebral foramen

A

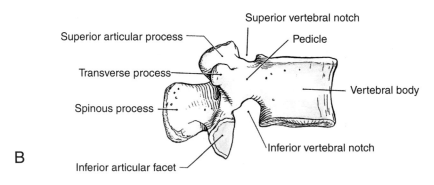

Superior articular process

Transverse process

Spinous process

Superior vertebral notch

Pedicle

Vertebral body

Inferior vertebral notch

Inferior articular facet

B

FIGURE 5.2   Parts and functions of typical vertebra. A. Superior view. **B.** Lateral view.

the formation of the **IV foramina,** which give passage to spinal nerve roots and accompanying vessels, and contain the spinal ganglia (dorsal root ganglia).

Seven processes arise from the vertebral arch of a typical vertebra:

- The **spinous process** projects posteriorly from the vertebral arch at the junction of the laminae and overlaps the vertebra below.
- Two **transverse processes** project posterolaterally from the junctions of the pedicles and laminae.
- **Four articular processes**—two superior and two inferior—also arise from the junctions of the pedicles and laminae. Each articular process has an **articular facet** covered, in life, with articular cartilage.

The spinous and two transverse processes project from the vertebral arch and afford attachments for deep back muscles and form levers that help the muscles to move the vertebrae. The articular processes are in apposition with corresponding processes of vertebrae superior and inferior to them. Their function is to restrict movements in certain directions or at least to determine which movements may be permitted. The interlocking of the articular processes also prevents the vertebrae from slipping anteriorly. The direction of the **articular facets** on the articular processes determines the direction of movement allowed in any particular region.

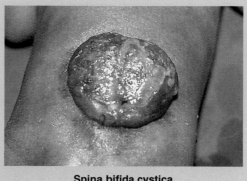

Spina bifida cystica

REGIONAL CHARACTERISTICS OF VERTEBRAE

The features of "typical" vertebrae demonstrate characteristic modifications specific to each region of the vertebral column; for example, cervical vertebrae are characterized by the presence of foramina in their transverse processes (Table 5.1). In addition, some individual vertebrae have distinguishing characteristics; *C7 vertebra, for example, has a long spinous process that forms a prominence under the skin,* especially when the neck is flexed. The main regional characteristics of vertebrae are summarized in Tables 5.1 to 5.4.

JOINTS OF VERTEBRAL COLUMN

The joints of the vertebral column include the joints of *vertebral bodies, joints of vertebral arches, craniovertebral joints, costovertebral joints* (Chapter 2), and *sacroiliac joints* (Chapter 4).

Joints of Vertebral Bodies

The joints of the vertebral bodies are *secondary cartilaginous joints* (symphyses) designed for weight-bearing and strength. The articulating surfaces of adjacent vertebrae are connected by IV discs and ligaments (Fig. 5.3). The **IV discs,** interposed between the bodies of adjacent vertebrae, provide strong attachments between the vertebral bodies. *Each IV disc consists of:*

- An anulus fibrosus—the outer fibrous part
- A nucleus pulposus—the gelatinous central mass.

SPINA BIFIDA

The common congenital anomaly of the vertebral column is *spina bifida occulta,* in which the laminae of L5 and/or S1 fail to develop normally and fuse. This bony defect, present in up to 24% of people, is concealed by skin but its location is often indicated by a tuft of hair. Most people with spina bifida occulta have no back problems. In severe types of the anomaly, such as **spina bifida cystica,** one or more vertebral arches may almost completely fail to develop (Moore and Persaud, 1998). Spina bifida cystica is associated with herniation of the meninges (*meningocele*) and/or the spinal cord (*meningomyelocele*). Usually, neurological symptoms are present in severe cases of meningomyelocele (e.g., paralysis of limbs and disturbances in bladder and bowel control).

TABLE 5.1. CERVICAL VERTEBRAE

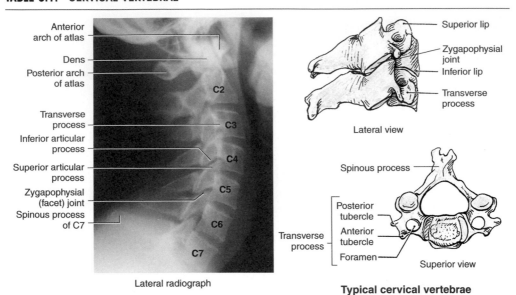

Lateral radiograph

Lateral view

Typical cervical vertebrae

Superior view

Cervical vertebrae (C1–C7) form skeleton of neck. They are typical vertebrae except for C1 and C2.

Part	Distinctive Characteristics
Body	Small and wider from side to side than anteroposteriorly; superior surface is concave and inferior surface is convex
Vertebral foramen	Large and triangular
Transverse processes	Transverse foramina (L. foramina transversarium); small or absent in C7; vertebral arteries and accompanying venous and sympathetic plexuses pass through foramina, except C7, which transmits only small accessory vertebral veins; anterior and posterior tubercles
Articular processes	Superior facets directed superoposteriorly; inferior facets directed inferoanteriorly
Spinous process	C3–C5 short and bifid (split in two parts); process of C6 is long but that of C7 is longer (C7 is called the vertebra prominens)

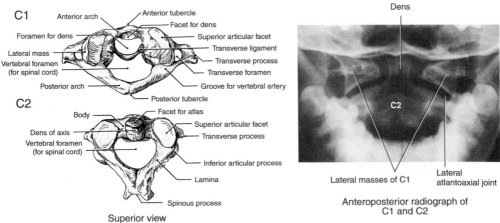

Superior view

Anteroposterior radiograph of C1 and C2

C1 and C2 vertebrae are atypical. The ringlike C1 vertebra, the atlas, is somewhat kidney-shaped when viewed from above or below. Its concave superior articular facets receive the occipital condyles. C1 has no spinous process or body and consists of two lateral masses connected by anterior and posterior arches. C1 carries the cranium and rotates on C2's large flat superior articular facets. C2 vertebra, the axis, is the strongest cervical vertebra. Its distinguishing feature is the dens, which projects superiorly from its body.

TABLE 5.2.   THORACIC VERTEBRAE

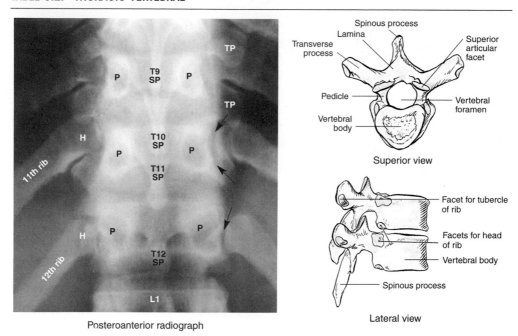

Posteroanterior radiograph

Superior view

Lateral view

Thoracic vertebrae (T1–T12) form posterior part of skeleton of thorax and articulate with ribs. Space between vertebral bodies is site of intervertebral disc. *P,* pedicle; *arrows,* costovertebral joints.

Part	Distinctive Characteristics
Body	Heart-shaped; has one or two facets for articulation with head of a rib *(H)*
Vertebral foramen	Circular and smaller than in cervical and lumbar regions
Transverse process *(TP)*	Long and strong and extends posterolaterally; length diminishes from T1–T12 (T1–T10 have facets for articulation with tubercle of a rib)
Articular processes	Superior facets directed posteriorly and slightly laterally; inferior facets directed anteriorly and slightly medially
Spinous process *(SP)*	Long and slopes posteroinferiorly; tip extends to level of vertebral body below

There is no IV disc between C1 (atlas) and C2 (axis) vertebrae. The most inferior functional disc is between L5 and S1 vertebrae. The discs vary in thickness in different regions; they are thickest in the lumbar region and thinnest in the superior thoracic region. The discs are thicker anteriorly in the cervical and lumbar regions and more uniform in thickness in the thoracic region.

The **anulus fibrosus** is a ring consisting of concentric lamellae of fibrocartilage forming the circumference of the IV disc (Fig. 5.3). The anuli insert into the smooth, rounded rims (epiphysial "rings") on the articular surfaces of the vertebral bodies (Fig. 5.2A).

The lamellae of the anuli fibrosi are thinner and less numerous posteriorly than they are anteriorly or laterally. The **nucleus pulposus**—the central core of the IV disc—is more cartilaginous than fibrous and is normally highly elastic in young people. The nucleus pulposus is located more posteriorly than centrally and

TABLE 5.3. LUMBAR VERTEBRAE

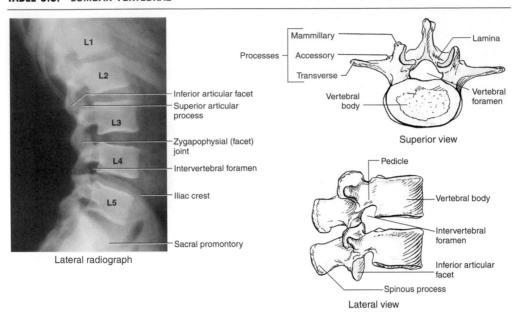

Lateral radiograph

L1
L2
L3
L4
L5

Inferior articular facet
Superior articular process
Zygapophysial (facet) joint
Intervertebral foramen
Iliac crest
Sacral promontory

Processes — Mammillary / Accessory / Transverse
Lamina
Vertebral body
Vertebral foramen

Superior view

Pedicle
Vertebral body
Intervertebral foramen
Inferior articular facet
Spinous process

Lateral view

Lumbar vertebrae (L1–L5) are larger and heavier than in other regions. Space between vertebral bodies is site of intervertebral disc

Part	Distinctive Characteristics
Body	Massive; kidney-shaped when viewed from above or below
Vertebral foramen	Triangular; larger than in thoracic region and smaller than in cervical region
Transverse processes	Long and slender; accessory process on posterior surface of base of each process
Articular processes	Superior facets directed posteromedially (or medially); inferior facets directed anterolaterally (or laterally); mammillary process on posterior surface of each superior articular process
Spinous process	Short and sturdy

has a high water content that is maximal at birth and decreases with advancing age. It acts like a shock absorber for axial forces and like a semifluid ball-bearing during flexion, extension, rotation, and lateral flexion of the vertebral column. *The nucleus pulposus is avascular.* It receives its nourishment by diffusion from blood vessels at the periphery of the anulus fibrosus and vertebral body.

The **anterior longitudinal ligament** (Fig. 5.3*A*) is a strong, broad fibrous band that covers and connects the anterolateral aspects of the vertebral bodies and IV discs. The ligament extends from the pelvic surface of the sacrum to the anterior tubercle of C1 vertebra (atlas) and the occipital bone anterior to the foramen magnum. *The anterior longitudinal ligament maintains stability of the intervertebral joints and helps prevent hyperextension of the vertebral column.*

The **posterior longitudinal ligament** is a much narrower, somewhat weaker band than

TABLE 5.4. SACRUM AND COCCYX

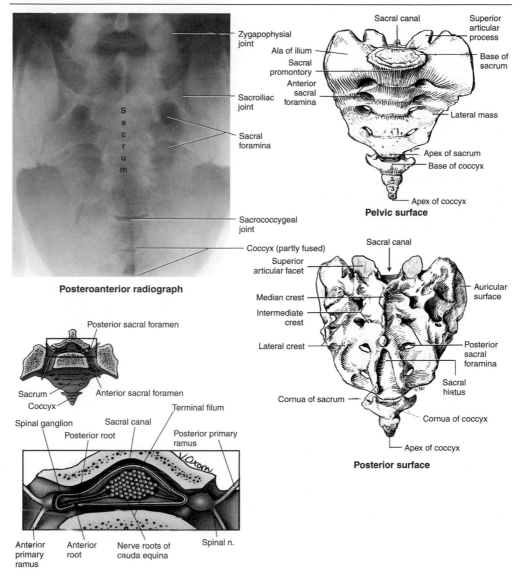

Posteroanterior radiograph

Pelvic surface

Posterior surface

The large, wedge-shaped **sacrum** in adults is composed of five fused sacral vertebrae. The sacrum provides strength and stability to the pelvis and transmits body weight to the pelvic girdle through the **sacroiliac joints**. The base of the sacrum is formed by the superior surface of S1 vertebra. Its superior articular processes articulate with the inferior articular processes of L5 vertebra. The projecting anterior edge of the body of the first sacral vertebra is the **sacral promontory**.

On the pelvic and dorsal surfaces are four pairs of sacral foramina for the exit of the rami of the first four sacral nerves and the accompanying vessels. The pelvic surface of the sacrum is smooth and concave. The four transverse lines indicate where fusion of the sacral vertebrae occurred. The posterior surface of the sacrum is rough and convex. The fused spinous processes form the **median sacral crest**. The inverted U-shaped **sacral hiatus** results from the absence of the laminae and spinous processes of S4 and S5 vertebrae. The hiatus leads into the sacral canal, the inferior end of the vertebral canal. The **sacral cornua** (L. horns), representing the inferior articular processes of S5 vertebra, project inferiorly on each side of the sacral hiatus and are a helpful guide to its location. The lateral surface of the sacrum has an ear-shaped articular surface that participates in the sacroiliac joint.

The vertebrae of the tapering **coccyx** are remnants of the skeleton of the embryonic tail-like caudal eminence. The vertebrae are reduced in size and have no pedicles, laminae, or spinous processes. The distal three vertebrae fuse during middle life to form the coccyx, a beaklike bone that articulates with the sacrum.

Surface Anatomy of Vertebral Column

The tips of the spinous processes of some cervical and all thoracic and lumbar vertebrae are palpable and often visible when the vertebral column is flexed. In the photograph, the *large arrow* indicates the prominent C7 spinous process and the *small arrow* indicates the T2 spinous process. The short bifid spinous processes of C3 through C5 vertebrae may be felt in the *nuchal (neck) groove* between the neck muscles, but they are not easy to palpate because they lie deep to the surface. There is a slight depression posterior to the arch of the atlas (C1 vertebra) because it has no spinous process. C6, C7, and T1 are palpated easily when the neck is fully flexed. In the anatomi-cal position, there is a furrow over the spinous processes of the lower thoracic and lumbar vertebrae. The spinous processes of lumbar vertebrae are large and easy to observe and palpate. A plane transecting the highest points of the iliac crests usually passes through the L4 spinous process and the L4/L5 IV disc. The transverse processes of C1, C6, and C7 vertebrae are also palpable. Those of C1 can be palpated by deep pressure posteroinferior to the tips of the mastoid processes of the temporal bones (bony prominences posterior to the ears). The transverse processes of other vertebrae are covered with thick muscles and are felt only with difficulty.

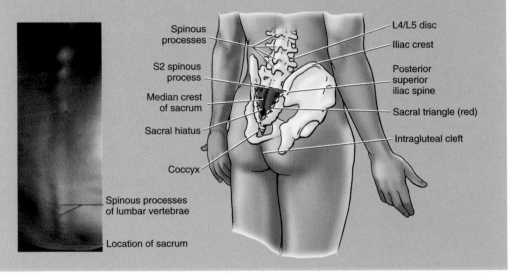

Spinous processes
S2 spinous process
Median crest of sacrum
Sacral hiatus
Coccyx
Spinous processes of lumbar vertebrae
Location of sacrum
L4/L5 disc
Iliac crest
Posterior superior iliac spine
Sacral triangle (red)
Intragluteal cleft

DISLOCATION OF VERTEBRAE

The bodies of cervical vertebrae can be dislocated in neck injuries with less force than is required to fracture them. Because of the large vertebral canal in the cervical region, slight dislocation can occur without damaging the spinal cord. When a cervical vertebra is severely dislocated, it injures the spinal cord. However, the vertebra may self-reduce ("slip back into place") so that a radiograph or magnetic resonance image (MRI) may not indicate that the cord has been injured.

The transition from the relatively inflexible thoracic region to the much more mobile lumbar region occurs abruptly. Consequently, T11 or T12 are the most commonly fractured noncervical vertebrae (i.e., a "broken back" versus a "broken neck"). *Fractures of the interarticular parts of the vertebral laminae of L1 (spondylolysis) may result in forward displacement of L5 vertebral body relative to the sacrum (S1 vertebra—spondylolisthesis).* The posterior fragment, consisting of most of the vertebral arch, remains in normal relation to the sacrum, but the anterior fragment and the L5 vertebral body may move anteriorly. It is the anterior displacement of most of the vertebral column that constitutes spondylolisthesis. *Spondylolisthesis at the L5/S1 articulation* may result in pressure on the spinal nerves, causing back and lower limb pain.

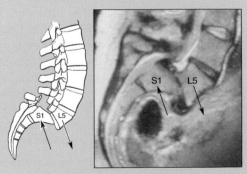

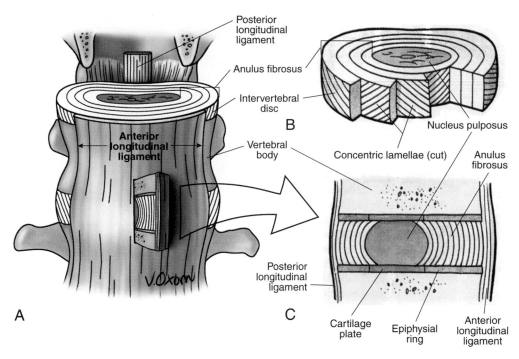

FIGURE 5.3   Intervertebral (IV) discs and longitudinal ligaments. A. Anterior view. **B.** Transverse section of IV disc showing concentric lamellae of anulus fibrosus. **C.** Sagittal section of IV disc.

the anterior longitudinal ligament. The posterior longitudinal ligament runs within the vertebral canal along the posterior aspect of the vertebral bodies. It is attached to the IV discs and the posterior edges of the vertebral bodies from C2 (axis) to the sacrum. *The posterior longitudinal ligament helps prevent hyperflexion of the vertebral column and posterior protrusion of the IV discs.* It is well provided with nociceptive (pain) nerve endings.

Uncovertebral "joints" (of Luschka) are between the uncinate (hooklike) processes of C3 through C6 vertebrae and the bevelled surfaces of the vertebral bodies superior to them (Fig. 5.4). The "joints" (fissures) are at the lateral and posterolateral margins of the IV discs. These jointlike structures are covered with cartilage and contain a capsule filled with fluid. They are considered to be synovial joints by some; others consider them to be degenerative spaces in the discs that are filled with extracellular fluid. *The uncovertebral "joints" are frequent sites of spur formation (projecting processes of bone) that may cause neck pain.*

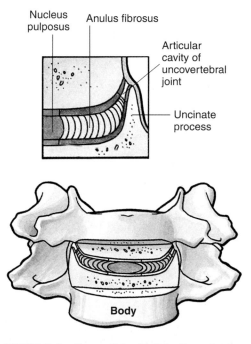

FIGURE 5.4   Uncovertebral joints. These joints are at the posterolateral margin of the cervical IV discs.

HERNIATION OF IV DISCS

With increasing age, the anuli fibrosi begin to undergo degenerative changes, apparently from wear and tear. Consequently an anulus, usually in the lumbar region, may protrude (herniate). In older people, the nuclei pulposi lose their turgor (fullness) and become thinner because of dehydration and degeneration. The age changes in the IV discs account in part for the slight loss in height that occurs during old age. Decrease in the height of an IV disc also results in narrowing of the IV foramina, which may cause compression of spinal nerves or nerve roots. If degeneration of the posterior longitudinal ligament and wearing of the anulus fibrosus has occurred, the nucleus pulposus may herniate into the vertebral canal and compress the spinal cord or nerve roots of spinal nerves in the cauda equina. *Disc protrusions* (herniations, "slipped discs") usually occur posterolaterally where the anulus is relatively thin and poorly supported by the posterior or anterior longitudinal ligaments. The *localized back pain* of a herniated disc results from pressure on the longitudinal ligaments and periphery of the anulus fibrosus and from local inflammation resulting from chemical irritation by substances from the ruptured nucleus pulposus. Chronic pain resulting from the spinal nerve roots being compressed by the herniated disc is referred to the area (dermatome) supplied by that nerve. *Approximately 95% of lumbar disc protrusions occur at the L4/L5 or L5/S1 levels.* Symptom-producing IV disc protrusions occur in the cervical region almost as often as in the lumbar region. As degenerative changes occur, the cervical IV discs thin out and the uncinate processes approach the beveled inferior surfaces of the cervical vertebrae superiorly. This results in encroachment of the IV foramina, pressure on the nerve roots, and neck pain. Cervical disc problems—associated with injuries—may also occur in young persons.

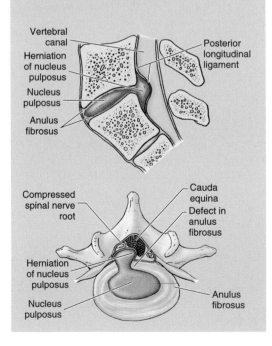

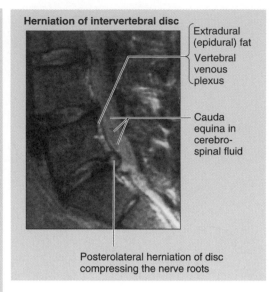

Herniation of intervertebral disc

Extradural (epidural) fat

Vertebral venous plexus

Cauda equina in cerebro-spinal fluid

Posterolateral herniation of disc compressing the nerve roots

Vertebral canal
Herniation of nucleus pulposus
Nucleus pulposus
Anulus fibrosus
Posterior longitudinal ligament

Compressed spinal nerve root
Herniation of nucleus pulposus
Nucleus pulposus
Cauda equina
Defect in anulus fibrosus
Anulus fibrosus

Joints of Vertebral Arches

The joints of the vertebral arches are the **zygapophysial joints** (facet joints). These articulations are plane synovial joints between the superior and inferior articular processes (L. zygapophyses) of adjacent vertebrae. Each joint is surrounded by a thin, loose **articular capsule,** which is attached to the margins of the articular facets of the articular processes of adjacent vertebrae (Fig. 5.5, *B* and *C*). Accessory ligaments unite the laminae, transverse processes, and spinous processes and help to stabilize the joints. *The zygapophysial joints permit gliding movements between the vertebrae;* the shape and disposition of the articular surfaces determine the type of movement possible. The zygapophysial joints are innervated by articular branches that arise from the medial branches of the posterior primary rami of spinal nerves (Fig. 5.6).

Accessory Ligaments of Intervertebral Joints

The laminae of adjacent vertebral arches are joined by broad, yellow elastic fibrous tissue—the **ligamenta flava** (L. flavus, yellow)—that extend almost vertically from the lamina above to the lamina below (Fig. 5.5*A*). The ligaments bind the laminae of the adjoining vertebrae together, forming part of the posterior wall of the vertebral canal. The ligamenta flava resist separation of the vertebral laminae, thereby arresting abrupt flexion of the

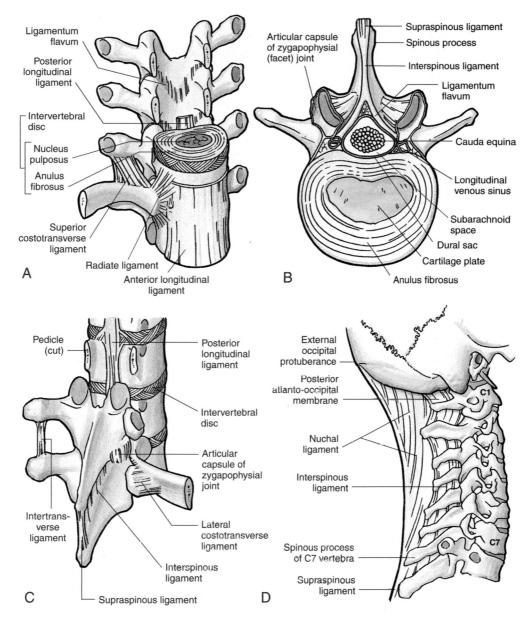

FIGURE 5.5 **Joints and ligaments of the vertebral column. A.** Anterior view. Pedicles of upper vertebrae have been sawn through and their bodies have been removed. A rib and its costovertebral joint and associated ligaments are illustrated also. **B.** Transverse section of an IV disc and associated ligaments. The nucleus pulposus has been removed to show the hyaline cartilage plate covering the superior surface of the vertebral body. **C.** Dorsolateral view. The vertebral arch of the upper vertebra has been removed. **D.** Lateral view. Ligaments of the cervical region.

vertebral column and usually preventing injury to the IV discs. The strong elastic ligamenta flava help to preserve the normal curvatures of the vertebral column and assist with straightening of the column after flexing. Adjacent spinous processes are united by weak **interspinous ligaments** and strong cordlike **supraspinous ligaments** (Fig. 5.5, *B* and *C*). The latter ligament merges superiorly with the **nuchal ligament** (L. ligamentum nuchae), the strong median ligament of the neck (*nucha* refers to back of neck). The nuchal ligament—composed of thickened fibroelastic tissue—attaches to the external occipital protuberance and the posterior border of the foramen magnum to the spinous processes of the cervical vertebrae. Because of the shortness of the C3 through C5 spinous processes, the nuchal ligament substitutes for bone in providing muscular attachments. The **intertransverse ligaments** (Fig. 5.5*C*), connecting adjacent transverse processes, consist

of scattered fibers in the cervical region and fibrous cords in the thoracic region. In the lumbar region they are thin and membranous.

Craniovertebral Joints
The craniovertebral joints include the:

- Atlanto-occipital joint—between the atlas (C1 vertebra) and the occipital bone of the cranium
- Atlantoaxial joints—between C1 and C2 vertebrae.

Atlanto—a Greek prefix—refers to the atlas. *These suboccipital articulations are synovial joints that have no IV discs.* Their design allows a wider range of movement than in the rest of the vertebral column.

Atlanto-occipital Joints. These articulations between the lateral masses of C1 (atlas) and the occipital condyles (Fig. 5.7*C*) permit nodding of the head, such as the neck flexion and extension

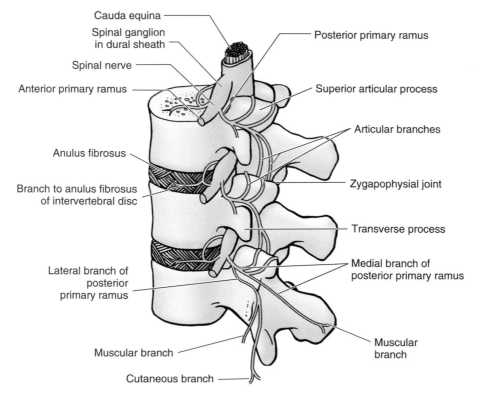

FIGURE 5.6   Nerves of vertebral joints. The posterior primary ramus arises from the spinal nerve outside the IV foramen and divides into medial and lateral branches, which supply the zygapophysial joints.

Labels on figure: Cauda equina; Spinal ganglion in dural sheath; Spinal nerve; Anterior primary ramus; Anulus fibrosus; Branch to anulus fibrosus of intervertebral disc; Lateral branch of posterior primary ramus; Muscular branch; Cutaneous branch; Posterior primary ramus; Superior articular process; Articular branches; Zygapophysial joint; Transverse process; Medial branch of posterior primary ramus; Muscular branch

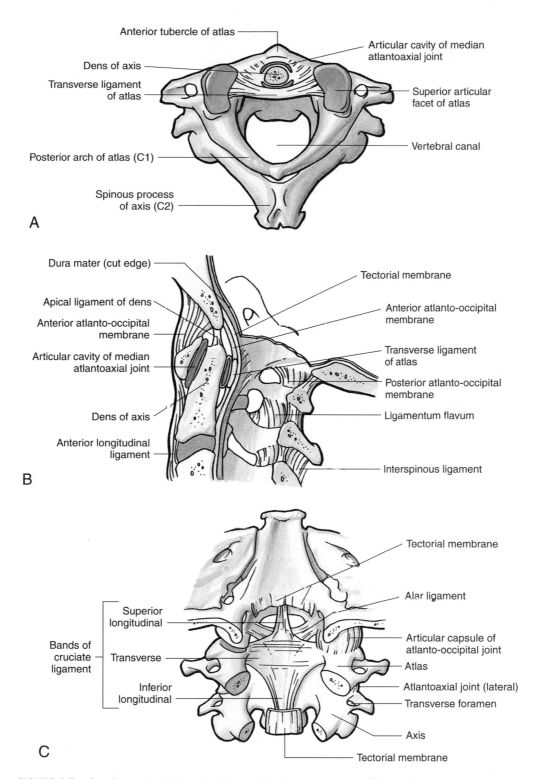

FIGURE 5.7 Craniovertebral joints. A. Atlantoaxial joint, superior view. Observe the large vertebral foramen of atlas (C1 vertebra), which is divided into two foramina by the transverse ligament. The larger posterior foramen is for the spinal cord, and the smaller anterior foramen is for the dens of the axis (C2 vertebra). **B.** Median section showing the ligaments and joints. **C.** Posterior view. Observe the bow-shaped transverse ligament of atlas that, by addition of superior and inferior bands, becomes the cross-shaped cruciate ligament.

occurring when indicating approval—the "yes" movement. The main movement is flexion, with a little lateral bending and rotation. These joints also permit sideways tilting of the head. The *atlanto-occipital joints are synovial joints of the condyloid type* and have thin, loose articular capsules composed of fibrous capsules lined by synovial membranes. The cranium and C1 are also connected by anterior and posterior **atlanto-occipital membranes,** which extend from the anterior and posterior arches of C1 to the anterior and posterior margins of the foramen magnum (Fig. 5.7*B*). The anterior and posterior atlanto-occipital membranes prevent excessive movement of the atlanto-occipital joints.

Atlantoaxial Joints. There are three atlantoaxial articulations (Fig. 5.7*A*):

- Two lateral atlantoaxial joints between the lateral masses of C1 and C2 vertebrae
- One median atlantoaxial joint between the dens of C2 and the anterior arch and transverse ligament of the atlas.

The **transverse ligament of the atlas** is a strong band extending between the tubercles on the medial aspects of the lateral masses of C1 vertebrae. It holds the dens of C2 against the anterior arch of C1, forming the posterior wall of a socket for the dens. Vertically oriented superior and inferior **longitudinal bands** pass from the transverse ligament to the occipital bone superiorly and to the body of C2 inferiorly. Together, the transverse ligament and the longitudinal bands form the **cruciate ligament** (formerly the cruciform ligament), so named because of its resemblance to a cross (Fig. 5.7*C*).

The **alar ligaments** extend from the sides of the dens to the lateral margins of the foramen magnum. These short, rounded cords—just smaller than a pencil—attach the cranium to C1 vertebra and check rotation (side-to-side movements) of the head when it is turned.

The **tectorial membrane** is the strong superior continuation of the posterior longitudinal ligament across the central atlantoaxial joint through the foramen magnum to the central floor of the cranial cavity. It runs from the body of C2 vertebra to the internal surface of the occipital bone and covers the alar and transverse ligaments (Fig. 5.7, *B* and *C*).

Movement (mainly rotation) at all three atlantoaxial joints permits the head to be turned from side to side, as occurs when rotating the head to indicate disapproval (the "no" movement). During this movement, the cranium and C1 vertebra rotate on C2 vertebra as a unit. *Excessive rotation of the atlantoaxial joints is prevented by the alar ligaments.* During rotation of the head, the dens of C2 is the axis or pivot that is held in a socket or collar formed by the anterior arch of the atlas and the transverse ligament of the atlas. The articulation of the dens of C2 with C1 (central atlantoaxial joint) is described as a pivot joint, whereas the C1/C2 zygapophysial joints (lateral atlantoaxial joints) are gliding-type synovial joints.

RUPTURE OF TRANSVERSE LIGAMENT OF ATLAS
When the transverse ligament ruptures or is weakened by disease, the dens is set free, resulting in *atlantoaxial subluxation*—incomplete dislocation of the atlantoaxial joint. When complete dislocation occurs, the dens may be driven into the upper cervical region of the spinal cord, causing *quadriplegia* (paralysis of all four limbs), or into the medulla of the brainstem, causing death.

Rupture of Alar Ligaments
The alar ligaments are weaker than the transverse ligament of the atlas. Consequently, combined flexion and rotation of the head may tear one or both alar ligaments. Rupture of an alar ligament results in an increase of approximately 30% in the range of movement to the opposite side.

MOVEMENTS OF VERTEBRAL COLUMN

The following movements of the vertebral column are possible (Fig. 5.8): flexion, extension, lateral bending, and rotation (torsion). The range of movement of the vertebral column varies according to the region and the individual. The mobility of the column results primarily from the compressibility and elasticity of the IV discs. *The range of movement of the vertebral column is limited by the:*

- Thickness, elasticity, and compressibility of IV discs
- Shape and orientation of zygapophysial joints

- Tension of articular capsules of the above joints
- Resistance of back muscles and ligaments (such as the ligamenta flava and the posterior longitudinal ligament).

The back muscles producing movements of the vertebral column are discussed subsequently; however, the movements are not produced exclusively by the back muscles. They are assisted by gravity and the action of the anterolateral abdominal muscles (see Chapter 3). Movements between adjacent vertebrae take place on the resilient nuclei pulposi of the IV discs and at the zygapophysial joints. The orientation of the latter joints permits some movements and restricts others. In the thoracic region, for example, the slightly oblique orientation of the zygapophysial joints allows some rotation and lateral bending but prevents flexion of the vertebral column. Although movements between adjacent vertebrae are relatively small, especially in the thoracic region, the summation of all of the small movements produces a considerable range of movement of the vertebral column as a whole (e.g., when bending to touch the toes).

Movements of the vertebral column are freer in the cervical and lumbar regions than elsewhere. Flexion, extension, lateral bending, and rotation of the neck are especially free because the:

- IV discs, although thin relative to most other discs, are thick relative to the small size of the vertebral bodies at this level

- Articular surfaces of the zygapophysial joints are relatively large and the joint planes are almost horizontal
- Articular capsules of the zygapophysial joints are loose
- Neck is slender (with less surrounding soft tissue bulk).

The sagittally oriented joint planes of the lumbar region are conducive to flexion and extension. *Extension of the vertebral column is most marked in the lumbar region* and usually is more extensive than flexion; however, the interlocking articular processes here prevent rotation. The lumbar region, like the cervical region, has large IV discs (the largest ones occur here) relative to the size of the vertebral bodies. *Lateral bending of the vertebral column is greatest in the cervical and lumbar regions.* The thoracic region, in contrast, has IV discs that are thin relative to the size of the vertebral bodies. Relative stability is also conferred on this part of the vertebral column through its connection to the sternum by the ribs and costal cartilages. The joint planes here lie on an arc that is centered on the vertebral body, permitting rotation in the thoracic region. This rotation of the upper trunk, in combination with the rotation permitted in the cervical region and that at the atlantoaxial joints, enables the torsion of the axial skeleton that occurs as one looks back over the shoulder. *Flexion is almost nonexistent in the thoracic region, and lateral bending is severely restricted.*

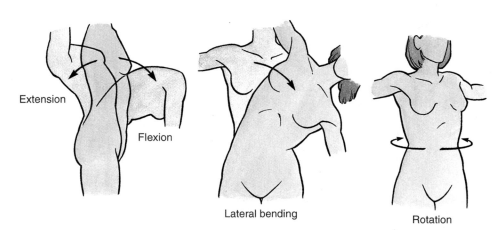

FIGURE 5.8 Movements of the vertebral column.

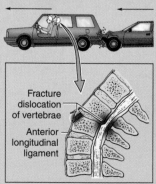
VASCULATURE OF VERTEBRAL COLUMN

Spinal arteries supplying the vertebrae (Fig. 5.9*A*) are branches of the:

- Vertebral and ascending cervical arteries in the neck
- Posterior intercostal arteries in the thoracic region
- Subcostal and lumbar arteries in the abdomen
- Iliolumbar and lateral and medial sacral arteries in the pelvis.

Spinal arteries enter the IV foramina and divide mostly into terminal arteries distributed to the posterior and anterior roots of the spinal nerves and their coverings. Some **radicular arteries** continue as irregularly spaced **segmental medullary arteries** that anastomose with the longitudinal arteries that supply the spinal cord (p. 308).

Spinal veins form venous plexuses along the vertebral column both inside (**internal vertebral venous plexus**) and outside (**external vertebral venous plexus**) the vertebral canal (Fig. 5.9, *B* and *C*). The large, wide, tortuous **basivertebral veins** are in the substance of the vertebral bodies. They emerge from foramina on the surfaces of the vertebral bodies (mostly the posterior aspect) and drain into the external and especially the internal vertebral venous plexuses. The **intervertebral veins** accompany the spinal nerves through the IV foramina. These veins drain blood from the spinal cord and vertebral venous plexuses.

MUSCLES OF BACK

Most body weight is anterior to the vertebral column, especially in obese people; consequently, the many strong muscles attached to the spinous and transverse processes of vertebrae are necessary to support and move the vertebral column. *There are three groups of muscles in the back:*

- The superficial and intermediate groups include *extrinsic back muscles* that produce and control limb and respiratory movements, respectively.

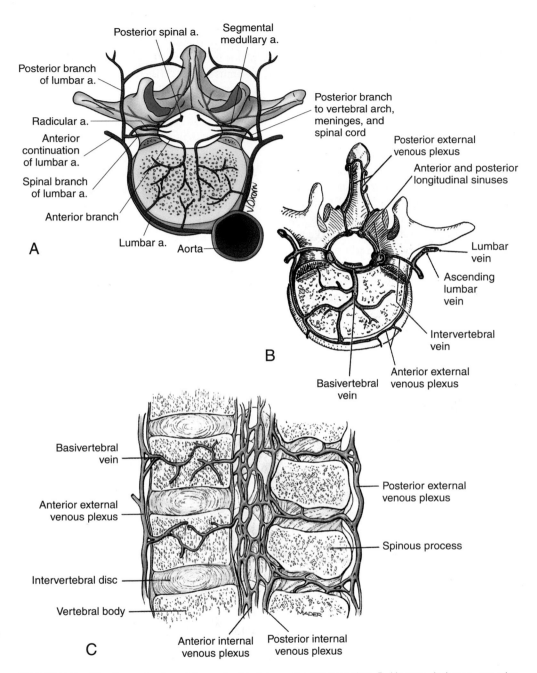

FIGURE 5.9 **Blood supply of vertebrae. A.** Arterial supply, superior view. **B.** Venous drainage, superior view. **C.** Vertebral venous plexuses, median section.

- The deep group includes the true or *intrinsic back muscles* that specifically act on the vertebral column, producing movements and maintaining posture.

SUPERFICIAL OR EXTRINSIC BACK MUSCLES

The *superficial extrinsic back muscles* (trapezius, latissimus dorsi, levator scapulae, and rhomboids) connect the upper limbs to the trunk and control limb movements (see Chapter 7).These muscles, although located in the back region, for the most part receive their nerve supply from the anterior rami of cervical nerves and act on the upper limb. The trapezius receives its motor fibers from a cranial nerve, the accessory nerve (CN XI). The *intermediate extrinsic back muscles* (serratus posterior) are superficial respiratory muscles and are described with muscles of the thoracic wall in Chapter 2.

DEEP OR INTRINSIC BACK MUSCLES

The deep (true) or intrinsic back muscles are innervated by the posterior rami of spinal nerves and act to maintain posture and control movements of the vertebral column (Fig. 5.10). These muscles—extending from the pelvis to the cranium—are enclosed by fascia that attaches medially to the nuchal ligament, the tips of the spinous processes, the supraspinous ligament, and the median crest of the sacrum. The fascia attaches laterally to the cervical and lumbar transverse processes and to the angles of the ribs. The thoracic and lumbar parts of the fascia constitute the **thoracolumbar fascia** (Fig. 5.11). The posterior aponeuroses of the transverse abdominal and internal oblique muscles split into two strong sheets—the middle and posterior layers of the thoracolumbar fascia—which enclose the deep muscles of the back. The anterior layer of thoracolumbar fascia is the deep fascia of the quadratus lumborum (quadratus lumborum fascia). The deep back muscles are grouped according to their relationship to the surface (Table 5.5).

Superficial Layer of Intrinsic Back Muscles

The **splenius muscles** (splenii)—thick and flat—lie on the lateral and posterior aspects of the neck, covering the vertical intrinsic muscles obliquely, somewhat like a bandage, which explains their name (L. splenion, bandage). The splenius muscles arise from the midline and extend superolaterally to the cervical vertebrae (*splenius cervicus*) and cranium (*splenius capitis*). These muscles cover and hold the deep neck muscles in position (Fig. 5.10, Table 5.5).

Intermediate Layer of Intrinsic Back Muscles

The **erector spinae muscles** (sacrospinalis) lie in a groove on each side of the vertebral column (Fig. 5.10). The *massive erector spinae— the chief extensor of the vertebral column— divides into three muscle columns:*

- Iliocostalis—lateral column
- Longissimus—intermediate column
- Spinalis—medial column.

Each column is divided regionally into three parts according to its superior attachments (e.g., iliocostalis lumborum, iliocostalis thoracis, and iliocostalis cervicis). The common origin of the three erector spinae columns is through a broad tendon that attaches inferiorly to the posterior part of the iliac crest, the posterior aspect of the sacrum, the sacroiliac ligaments, and the sacral and inferior lumbar spinous processes. Although the muscle columns are generally identified as isolated muscles, each column is actually composed of many overlapping shorter fibers—a design that provides stability, localized action, and segmental vascular and neural supply. Clinically, this design clearly demonstrates the localization of symptoms that occur with injury (e.g., strains). The attachments, nerve supply, and actions of the erector spinae are described in Table 5.5.

Deep Layer of Intrinsic Back Muscles

Deep to the erector spinae muscles is an obliquely disposed group of muscles—the **transversospinal muscle group** (L. transversospinalis)—comprised of the semispinalis, multifidus, and rotatores. *These muscles originate from transverse processes of vertebrae and pass to spinous processes of more superior vertebrae.* They occupy the "gutter" between the collective transverse and spinous processes (Fig. 5.10, *B* and *C*).

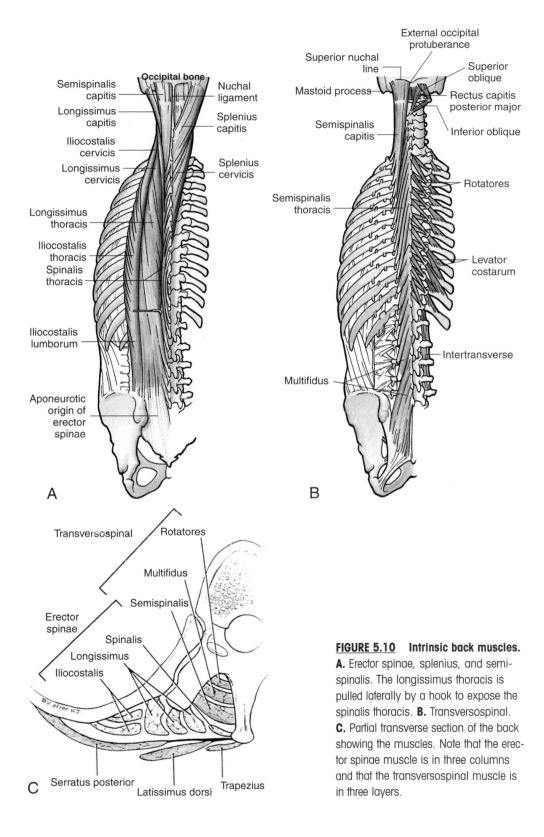

A. Semispinalis capitis, Longissimus capitis, Iliocostalis cervicis, Longissimus cervicis, Longissimus thoracis, Iliocostalis thoracis, Spinalis thoracis, Iliocostalis lumborum, Aponeurotic origin of erector spinae, Occipital bone, Nuchal ligament, Splenius capitis, Splenius cervicis

B. Superior nuchal line, Mastoid process, Semispinalis capitis, Semispinalis thoracis, Multifidus, External occipital protuberance, Superior oblique, Rectus capitis posterior major, Inferior oblique, Rotatores, Levator costarum, Intertransverse

C. Transversospinal, Rotatores, Multifidus, Semispinalis, Erector spinae, Spinalis, Longissimus, Iliocostalis, Serratus posterior, Latissimus dorsi, Trapezius

FIGURE 5.10 **Intrinsic back muscles.** **A.** Erector spinae, splenius, and semispinalis. The longissimus thoracis is pulled laterally by a hook to expose the spinalis thoracis. **B.** Transversospinal. **C.** Partial transverse section of the back showing the muscles. Note that the erector spinae muscle is in three columns and that the transversospinal muscle is in three layers.

TABLE 5.5. DEEP OR INTRINSIC BACK MUSCLES

Muscles	Origin	Insertion	Nerve Supply[a]	Main Action(s)
Superficial layer				
Splenius	*Splenius capitis*: inferior part of nuchal ligament (Fig. 5.5D), spinous processes (SPs) of C7–T3 or T4 vertebrae, and supraspinous ligament	*Splenius capitis*: fibers run superolaterally to mastoid process of temporal bone and inferior to lateral third of superior nuchal line of occipital bone		*Bilaterally*: extend head *Unilaterally*: laterally bend (flex) and rotate face to same side
	Splenius cervicis: SPs of T3–T6 vertebrae	*Splenius cervicis*: posterior tubercles of transverse processes (TVPs) of C1–C3 or C4 vertebrae		*Bilaterally*: extend neck *Unilaterally*: laterally bend and rotate neck toward same side
Intermediate layer				
Erector spinae	*Common origin*: posterior sacrum, iliac crest, sacrotuberous ligament, dorsal sacroiliac ligament, SPs of TVPs T11–L5 vertebrae, and supraspinous ligament. Additional sites of origin are outlined below.	*Iliocostalis: lumborum, thoracis, and cervicis*: fibers run superiorly to angles of lower ribs and cervical TVPs *Longissimus: thoracis, cervicis, and capitis*: fibers run superiorly to ribs between tubercles and angles, to TVPs in thoracic and cervical regions, and to mastoid process of temporal bone *Spinalis: thoracis, cervicis, and capitis*: fibers run superiorly to SPs in the upper thoracic region and to cranium	Posterior rami of spinal nerves	
Parts of erector spinae:				
1. Iliocostalis:				
Lumborum	Common origin of erector spinae	Angles of lower 6–12 ribs		Extend and laterally bend vertebral column
Thoracis	Angles of 6–12 ribs	Angles of ribs 1–6, TVPs of C7 vertebrae		
Cervicis	Angles of 3–6 ribs	Posterior tubercles of TVPs of C4–C6 vertebrae		

Muscle	Origin	Insertion	Innervation	Action
2. Longissimus:				
Thoracis	Common origin of erector spinae, also TVPs and accessory processes of L1–L5 vertebrae, and middle layer of thoracolumbar fascia	TVPs of T1–T12 vertebrae between tubercules and angles of lower 9–10 ribs		Extend and laterally bend vertebral column
Cervicis	TVPs of T1–T5 vertebrae	TVPs and articular processes of C2–C6 vertebrae		Extend head
Capitis	TVPs of T1–T5 vertebrae and articular processes of C4–C7 vertebrae	Mastoid process of temporal bone		
3. Spinalis:				
Thoracis	SPs of T11–L2 vertebrae	SPs of T1–T4 vertebrae, sometimes down to T8 SP of C2 vertebrae; occasionally SPs of C3 and C4 vertebrae		Extend vertebral column
Cervicis (often absent)	Inferior part of nuchal ligament, SPs of C7–T2 vertebrae			Extend head
Capitis (blends with semispinalis capitis)	Articular processes of C4–C6 vertebrae TVPs of C7–T6 (T7) vertebrae	Occipit (back of head) between superior and inferior nuchal lines of occipital bone	Posterior rami of spinal nerves	
Deep layer				
Transversospinal:	Transverse processes (TVPs):	Spinous processes (SPs):		
	Semispinalis arises from TVPs of C4–T12 vertebrae	Semispinalis thoracis, cervicis, and capitis; fibers run superomedially to occipital bone and SPs in thoracic and cervical regions, spanning 4–6 segments		Extend head and thoracic and cervical regions of vertebral column and rotate them contralaterally
	Multifidus arises from sacrum and ilium, TVPs of T1–T3, and articular processes of C4–C7 vertebrae	Multifidus: fibers pass superomedially to SPs of vertebrae above, spanning 2–4 segments		Stabilizes vertebrae during local movements of vertebral column
	Rotatores arise from TVPs of vertebrae; are best developed in thoracic region	Rotatores: pass superomedially to attach to junction of lamina and TVP, or SP of vertebra above their origin, spanning 1–2 segments		Stabilize vertebrae and assist with local extension and rotary movements of vertebral column; may function as organs of proprioception

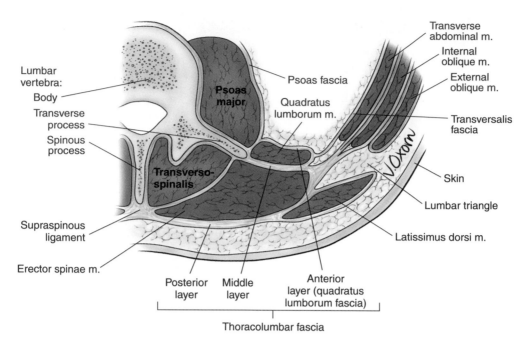

FIGURE 5.11   Muscles and fascia of the back. Transverse section of lower part.

- The semispinalis is superficial; spans four to six segments
- The multifidus is deeper; spans two to four segments
- The rotatores are deepest; span one to two segments.

The **semispinalis,** as its name indicates, arises from approximately half the vertebral column ("spine"). It is divided into three parts according to the vertebral level of their superior attachments: semispinalis capitis, semispinalis cervicis, and semispinalis thoracis. **Semispinalis capitis** is responsible for the longitudinal bulges at the back of the neck near the median plane (Fig. 5.10). It ascends from the cervical and thoracic transverse processes to the occipital bone. **Semispinalis thoracis and cervicis** pass superomedially from the transverse processes to the thoracic and cervical spinous processes of more superior vertebrae.

The **multifidus** consists of short, triangular muscular bundles that are thickest in the lumbar region. Each muscular bundle passes obliquely superiorly and medially and attaches along the whole length of the spinous process of the adjacent superior vertebra.

The **rotatores** or rotator muscles—best developed in the thoracic region—are the deepest of the three layers of transversospinal muscles (Fig. 5.10, *A* and *C*). They arise from the transverse process of one vertebra and insert into the root of the spinous processes of the next one or two vertebrae superiorly.

The *interspinal* (L. interspinales), *intertransverse* (L. intertransversarii), and elevators of ribs (L. levatores costarum) are the smallest of the deep back muscles. The interspinal and intertransverse muscles connect spinous and transverse processes, respectively.

Muscles Producing Movements of Intervertebral Joints

The principal muscles producing movements of the cervical, thoracic, and lumbar IV joints are summarized in Table 5.6. Structures limiting movement of the vertebral column are summarized in Table 5.7. Smaller muscles generally have higher densities of *muscle spindles* (sensors of proprioception—the sense of one's position—that are interdigitated among the muscle's fibers) than do large muscles. It has been presumed that this is because small muscles are

TABLE 5.6. PRINCIPAL MUSCLES PRODUCING MOVEMENTS OF INTERVERTEBRAL JOINTS

A. Cervical Region

Flexion	Extension	Lateral Bending	Rotation

Bilateral action of
  Longus coli
  Scalene
  Sternocleidomastoid
	Bilateral action of
	  Splenius capitis
	  Semispinalis capitis
	  and cervicis
		Unilateral action of
		  Iliocostalis cervicis
		  Longissimus capitis and cervicis
		  Splenius capitis and cervicis
			Unilateral action of
			  Rotatores
			  Semispinalis capitis and
			   cervicis
			  Multifidus
			  Splenius cervicis

B. Thoracic and Lumbar Regions

Flexion	Extension	Lateral Bending	Rotation

Bilateral action of
  Rectus abdominus
  Psoas major
  Gravity
	Bilateral action of
	  Erector spinae
	  Multifidus
	  Semispinalis
	   thoracis
		Unilateral action of
		  Iliocostalis thoracis and
		   lumborum
		  Longissimus thoracis
		  Multifidus
		  External and internal oblique
		  Quadratus lumborum
			Unilateral action of
			  Rotatores
			  Multifidus
			  External oblique
			   acting synchronously
			   with opposite internal
			   oblique
			  Semispinalis thoracis

TABLE 5.7. STRUCTURES LIMITING MOVEMENT OF VERTEBRAL COLUMN

A. Cervical Region

Movement	Limiting Structures
Flexion	• Ligaments: posterior atlantoaxial, posterior longitudinal, flavum, tectorial membrane • Posterior neck muscles • Anulus fibrosus (tension posteriorly)
Extension	• Ligaments: anterior longitudinal, anterior atlantoaxial • Anterior neck muscles • Anulus fibrosus (tension anteriorly) • Spinous processes (contact between adjacent spinous processes)
Lateral Bending	• Ligaments: alar ligament tension limits movement to contralateral side • Anulus fibrosus (tension laterally) • Zygapophysial (facet) joints
Rotation	• Ligaments: alar ligament tension limits movement to ipsilateral side • Anulus fibrosus

B. Thoracic and Lumbar Regions

Movement	Limiting Structures
Flexion	• Ligaments: supraspinous, interspinous, flavum • Capsules of zygapophysial (facet) joints • Extensor muscles • Vertebral bodies (apposition anteriorly) • Intervertebral disc (compression anteriorly) • Anulus fibrosus (tension posteriorly)
Extension	• Ligaments: anterior longitudinal • Capsules of zygapophysial joints • Abdominal muscles • Spinous processes (contact between adjacent processes) • Anulus fibrosus (tension anteriorly) • Intervertebral discs (compression posteriorly)
Lateral Bending	• Ligaments: contralateral side • Contralateral muscles that laterally bend trunk • Contact between iliac crest and thorax • Anulus fibrosus (tension of contralateral fibers) • Intervertebral disc (compression ipsilaterally)
Rotation	• Ligaments: costovertebral • Ipsilateral external oblique, contralateral internal oblique • Articular facets (apposition) • Anulus fibrosus

Modified from Clarkson M. *Musculoskeletal assessment. Joint Range of Motion and Muscle Strength*, 2nd ed. Baltimore: Lippincott Williams & Wilkins, 2000.

used for the most precise movements, such as fine postural movements or manipulation, and therefore require more proprioceptive feedback. The movements described for small muscles are assumed from the location of their attachments, the direction of the muscle fibers, and from activity measured by *electromyography* as movements are performed (p. 24). Muscles such as the rotatores, however, are so small and are placed in positions of such relatively poor mechanical advantage that their ability to produce the movements described is somewhat questionable. Furthermore, such small muscles often are redundant to other larger muscles having superior mechanical advantage. Hence, it has been proposed that the smaller muscles of small-large muscle pairs function more as "kinesiological monitors"—organs of proprioception—and that the larger muscles are the producers of motion.

BACK STRAINS

Back strain is a common back problem that usually results from extreme movements of the vertebral column, such as extension or rotation. *Back strain refers to some stretching or microscopic tearing of muscle fibers and/or ligaments of the back.* The muscles usually involved are those producing movements of the lumbar IV joints, especially the erector spinae. If the weight is not properly balanced on the vertebral column, strain is exerted on the muscles. This is undoubtedly a common cause of low back pain. As a protective mechanism, the back muscles go into spasm following an injury or in response to inflammation of structures such as ligaments.

SUBOCCIPITAL AND DEEP NECK MUSCLES

The **suboccipital region**—upper back of neck—is the triangular area (*suboccipital triangle*) inferior to the occipital region of the head, including the posterior aspects of C1 and C2 vertebrae. The **suboccipital triangle** lies deep to the trapezius and semispinalis capitis muscles (Fig. 5.12). The four small muscles in the suboccipital region, rectus capitis posterior major and minor and superior and inferior oblique, are innervated by the posterior ramus of C1, the **suboccipital nerve.** These muscles are mainly postural muscles, but they act on the head—directly or indirectly—as indicated by "capitis" in their name.

- *Rectus capitis posterior major* arises from the spinous process of C2 vertebra and inserts into the lateral part of the **inferior nuchal line** of the occipital bone.

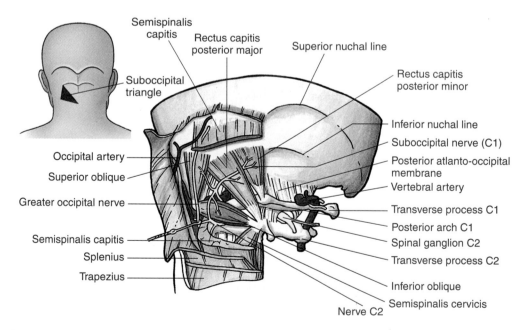

FIGURE 5.12   Suboccipital region and deep neck muscles. This drawing of a dissection shows muscles, nerves, and arteries.

- *Rectus capitis posterior minor* arises from the posterior tubercle on the posterior arch of C1 vertebra and inserts into the medial third of the inferior nuchal line.
- *Inferior oblique of head* (obliquus capitis inferior) arises from the spinous process of C2 vertebra and inserts into the transverse process of C1 vertebra. The name of this muscle is somewhat misleading; it is the only "capitis" muscle that has no attachment to the cranium.
- *Superior oblique of head* (obliquus capitis superior) arises from the transverse process of C1 and inserts into the occipital bone between the superior and inferior nuchal lines.

The actions of the suboccipital group of muscles is to extend the head on C1 and rotate the head and C1 on C2 vertebrae (Fig. 5.10). *The boundaries and contents of the suboccipital triangle are:*

- Superomedially—rectus capitis posterior major
- Superolaterally—superior oblique
- Inferolaterally—inferior oblique

- Floor—posterior atlanto-occipital membrane and posterior arch of C1
- Roof—semispinalis capitis
- Contents—*vertebral artery* and *suboccipital nerve* (C1).

The principal muscles producing movements of the craniovertebral joints are summarized in Tables 5.8 and 5.9, and the nerve supply of the muscles in the suboccipital triangle, back of the neck, and back are summarized in Table 5.10.

ISCHEMIA (REDUCED BLOOD SUPPLY) OF BRAINSTEM
The winding course of the vertebral arteries through the suboccipital triangle becomes clinically significant when blood flow through them is reduced, as occurs with *arteriosclerosis*. Under these conditions, prolonged turning of the head—as occurs when backing up a motor vehicle—may cause dizziness and other symptoms from interference with the blood supply to the brainstem.

SPINAL CORD AND MENINGES

The spinal cord, spinal meninges, and related structures are in the **vertebral canal** (Fig. 5.13)

TABLE 5.8. PRINCIPAL MUSCLES PRODUCING MOVEMENTS OF ATLANTO-OCCIPITAL JOINTS

Flexion	Extension	Lateral Bending
Longus capitis	Rectus capitis posterior major and minor	Sternocleidomastoid
Rectus capitis anterior	Superior oblique of head	Superior and inferior oblique of head
Anterior fibers of sternocleidomastoid	Semispinalis capitis	Rectus capitis lateralis (Table 9.5)
	Splenius capitis	Longissimus capitis
	Longissimus capitis	Splenius capitis
	Trapezius	

TABLE 5.9. PRINCIPAL MUSCLES PRODUCING ROTATION AT ATLANTOAXIAL JOINTS[a]

Ipsilateral[b]	Contralateral
Inferior oblique of head	Sternocleidomastoid
Rectus capitis posterior, major and minor	Semispinalis capitis
Longissimus capitis	
Splenius capitis	

[a]Rotation is the specialized movement at these joints. Movement of one joint involves the other.
[b]Same side to which head is rotated.

TABLE 5.10.   NERVE SUPPLY OF SUBOCCIPITAL TRIANGLE, BACK, AND BACK OF NECK

Nerve	Origin	Course	Distribution
Suboccipital	Posterior ramus C1 nerve	Runs between cranium and first cervical vertebra to reach suboccipital triangle	Muscles of suboccipital triangle
Greater occipital	Posterior ramus C1 nerve	Emerges inferior to inferior oblique and ascends to back of scalp	Skin over neck and occipital bone
Lesser occipital	Anterior ramus of C2 nerve and sometimes C3 nerve	Pass directly to skin	Skin of neck and scalp
Posterior rami	Spinal nerves	Pass segmentally to muscles and skin	Intrinsic muscles of back and overlying skin adjacent to vertebral column

The **spinal cord,** the major reflex center and conduction pathway between the body and the brain, is a cylindrical structure that is slightly flattened anteriorly and posteriorly. It is protected by the vertebrae and their associated ligaments and muscles, the spinal meninges, and the cerebrospinal fluid (CSF). *The spinal cord begins as a continuation of the medulla oblongata,* the caudal part of the brainstem. In the newborn, the inferior end of the spinal cord usually is opposite the IV disc between L2 and L3 vertebrae. *In adults, the spinal cord usually ends opposite the IV disc between L1 and L2 vertebrae*; however, it may terminate as high as T12 or as low as L3. Thus, the spinal cord occupies only the superior two thirds of the **vertebral canal**. *The spinal cord is enlarged in two regions for innervation of the limbs:*

* The **cervical enlargement** extends from C4 through T1 segments of the spinal cord, and most of the anterior rami of the spinal nerves arising from it form the *brachial plexus of nerves* that innervates the upper limbs (Chapter 7).
* The **lumbosacral enlargement** extends from T11 through L1 segments of the spinal cord, and the anterior rami of the spinal nerves arising from it contribute to the *lumbar and sacral plexuses of nerves* that innervate the lower limbs (Chapter 6). The spinal nerve roots arising from the lumbosacral enlargement and medullary

cone form the **cauda equina**—the bundle of spinal nerve roots running through the *lumbar cistern* (subarachnoid space).

STRUCTURE OF SPINAL NERVES

Thirty-one pairs of spinal nerves are attached to the spinal cord—8 cervical, 12 thoracic, 5 lumbar, 5 sacral, and 1 coccygeal (Fig. 5.13A). Multiple rootlets emerge from the posterior and anterior surfaces of the spinal cord and converge to form posterior and anterior **roots of the spinal nerves** (Fig. 5.14A). The part of the spinal cord from which the rootlets of one pair of roots emerge is a **segment of the spinal cord**. The posterior roots of the spinal nerves contain afferent (or sensory) fibers from skin, subcutaneous and deep tissues, and, often, viscera. The anterior roots of spinal nerves contain efferent (or motor) fibers to skeletal muscle and many contain presynaptic autonomic fibers. The cell bodies of somatic axons contributing to the ventral roots are in the **anterior horns of gray substance** (matter) of the spinal cord (Fig. 5.14B), whereas the cell bodies of axons making up the posterior roots are outside the spinal cord in the **spinal ganglia** (posterior root ganglia) at the distal ends of the posterior roots. The posterior and anterior nerve roots unite at their points of exit from the vertebral canal to form a **spinal nerve.** The

1st cervical nerves lack posterior roots in 50% of people, and the coccygeal nerve (Co1) may be absent. Each spinal nerve divides almost immediately into a **posterior primary ramus** and **anterior primary ramus** (Fig. 5.14*A*). The posterior rami supply the skin and deep muscles of the back; the anterior rami supply the limbs and the rest of the trunk.

In adults, the spinal cord is shorter than the vertebral column; hence, there is a progressive obliquity of the spinal nerve roots as the cord descends (Fig. 5.13). Because of the increasing distance between the spinal cord segments and the corresponding vertebrae, the length of the nerve roots increases progressively as the inferior end of the vertebral column is approached. The lumbar and sacral nerve rootlets are the longest. They descend until they reach the IV foramina of exit in the lumbar and sacral regions of the vertebral column,

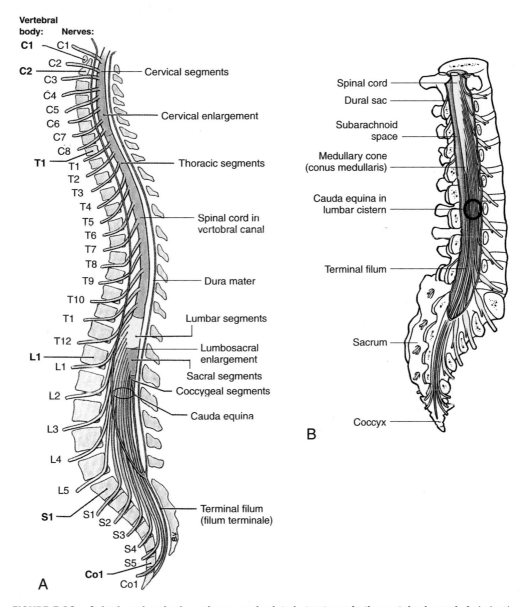

FIGURE 5.13 **Spinal cord, spinal meninges, and related structures in the vertebral canal. A.** Lateral view. **B.** Posterolateral view. These drawings illustrate the relation of the spinal cord segments and spinal nerves to the adult vertebral column.

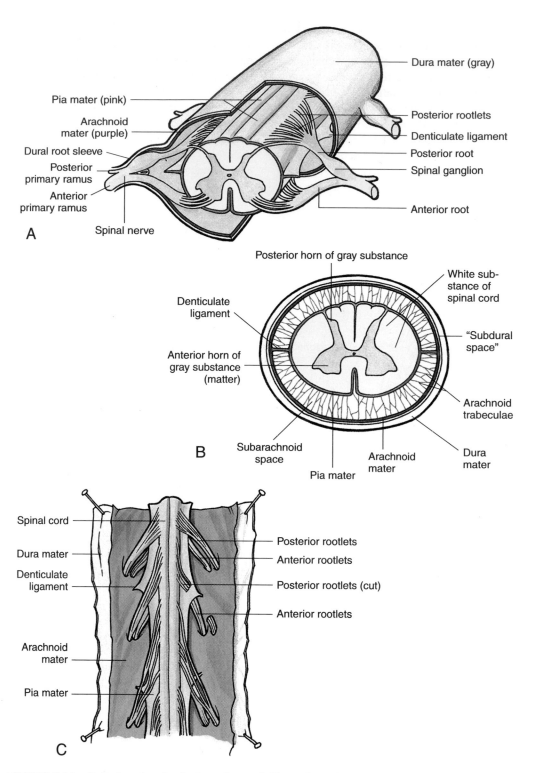

FIGURE 5.14　Spinal cord and spinal meninges. A. Three-dimensional drawing of the spinal cord and meninges. **B.** Transverse section of the spinal cord and meninges. **C.** The meninges have been cut and spread out. The pia mater (*pink*) covers the spinal cord and projects laterally as the denticulate ligament.

respectively. The bundle of spinal nerve roots in the **lumbar cistern** (subarachnoid space) within the vertebral canal caudal to the termination of the spinal cord resembles a horse's tail, hence its name—**cauda equina** (L. horse tail). The inferior end of the spinal cord has a conical shape and tapers into the **medullary cone** (L. conus medullaris). From its inferior end, the **terminal filum** (L. filum terminale) descends among the spinal nerve roots in the cauda equina. The terminal filum is the vestigial remnant of the caudal part of the spinal cord that was in the tail-like caudal eminence of the embryo. It consists primarily of pia mater but its proximal end also includes vestiges of neural tissue, connective tissue, and neuroglial tissue. The terminal filum takes on layers of arachnoid and dura mater as it penetrates the inferior end of the dural sac and passes through the **sacral hiatus** to attach ultimately to the dorsum of the coccyx (p. 307). The terminal filum serves as an anchor for the end of the **dural sac**—the continuation of the dura inferior to the medullary cone.

COMPRESSION OF LUMBAR SPINAL NERVE ROOTS

The lumbar spinal nerves increase in size from above downward, whereas the IV foramina decrease in diameter. Consequently, the L5 spinal nerve roots are the thickest and their foramina, the narrowest. This increases the chance that these nerve roots will be compressed if herniation of the nucleus pulposus of an IV disc occurs (p. 286).

SPINAL MENINGES AND CEREBROSPINAL FLUID

Collectively, the dura mater (dura), arachnoid mater (arachnoid), and pia mater (pia) surrounding the spinal cord form the **spinal meninges.** These membranes and CSF surround, support, and protect the spinal cord and the spinal nerve roots, including those in the cauda equina (p. 307).

The **spinal dura mater,** composed of tough, fibrous, and elastic tissue, is the outermost covering membrane of the spinal cord (Fig. 5.14). The spinal dura is separated from the vertebrae by the **extradural (epidural) space** (Table 5.11). The dura forms the **dural sac,** a long tubular sheath within the vertebral canal (Fig. 5.14*B*). The dural sac adheres to the margin of the foramen magnum of the cranium, where it is continuous with the cranial dura mater. The dural sac is pierced by the spinal nerves and is anchored inferiorly to the coccyx by the **terminal filum.** The spinal dura extends into the IV foramina and along the posterior and anterior nerve roots distal to the spinal ganglia to form **dural root sleeves** (Fig. 5.14*A*). These sleeves adhere to the periosteum lining the IV foramina and end by blending with the epineurium of the spinal nerves.

The **arachnoid mater**—a delicate, avascular membrane composed of fibrous and elastic tissue—lines the dural sac and the dural root sleeves and encloses the CSF-filled subarachnoid space containing the spinal cord, spinal nerve roots, and spinal ganglia (Fig. 5.14, *B* and *C*). *The arachnoid is not attached to the dura but is held against the inner surface of the dura by the pressure of the CSF.* In a lumbar spinal puncture, the needle traverses the dura and arachnoid simultaneously (p. 307). Their apposition is the dura-arachnoid surface, often erroneously referred to as the "subdural space." *No such space exists normally.* Bleeding into this artifactual space creates a *subdural hematoma* in the pathological space. In the cadaver—because of the absence of CSF—the arachnoid falls away from the internal surface of the dura and lies loosely on the spinal cord. The arachnoid is separated from the pia mater on the surface of the spinal cord by the **subarachnoid space** containing CSF (Table 5.10). Delicate strands of connective tissue, the **arachnoid trabeculae,** span the subarachnoid space connecting the arachnoid and pia (Fig. 5.14*B*).

The **pia mater**—the innermost covering membrane of the spinal cord—consists of flattened cells with long, equally flattened processes that closely follow all the surface features of the spinal cord (Fig. 5.14, *B* and *C*). The pia also covers the roots of the spinal nerves and spinal blood vessels. Inferior to the medullary cone, the pia continues as the terminal filum.

The spinal cord is suspended in the dural sac by the saw-toothed **denticulate ligament**

TABLE 5.11.   SPACES ASSOCIATED WITH SPINAL MENINGES

Space	Location	Contents
Extradural (epidural)	Between wall of vertebral canal and dura mater	Fat, loose connective tissue, internal venous plexuses, and distal to L2 vertebra, the roots of spinal nerves
Subdural[a]	Between dura and arachnoid mater	Capillary layer of serous fluid
Subarachnoid	Between arachnoid and pia mater	CSF, arachnoid trabeculae, spinal arteries, and veins

[a]Recent evidence indicates that the subdural space is a creation of a cleft in this area as the result of tissue damage Haines (2002).

on each side (L. denticulus, a small tooth). These ligaments are lateral extensions from the lateral surface of the pia midway between the posterior and anterior nerve roots. Twenty to twenty-two of these processes—shaped much like shark's teeth—attach to the internal surface of the dural sac. The uppermost part of the denticulate ligament attaches to the occipital dura immediately inside the foramen magnum. The lowermost part of the denticulate ligament passes between T12 and L1 nerve roots.

Subarachnoid Space

The subarachnoid space lies between the arachnoid and pia and is filled with CSF (Figs. 5.13B and 5.14B, Table 5.11). The enlargement of the space in the dural sac, caudal to the medullary cone, is the **lumbar cistern** containing the **cauda equina**.

LUMBAR SPINAL PUNCTURE

To obtain a sample of CSF from the lumbar cistern, a *lumbar puncture needle*—fitted with a stylet—is inserted into the subarachnoid space. Lumbar spinal puncture (spinal tap) is performed with the patient leaning forward or lying on the side with the back flexed. Flexion of the vertebral column facilitates insertion of the needle by stretching the ligamenta flava and spreading the laminae and spinous processes apart. Under aseptic conditions, the needle is inserted in the midline between the spinous processes of L3 and L4 (or L4 and L5) vertebrae. At these levels in adults, there is little danger of damaging the spinal cord.

Epidural Block

An anaesthetic agent can be injected into the extradural (epidural) space using the position described for lumbar spinal puncture. The anesthetic has a direct effect on the spinal nerve roots of the cauda equina after they exit from the dural sac. The patient loses sensation inferior to the level of the block. An anesthetic agent can also be injected through the sacral hiatus into the extradural space in the sacral canal—a *caudal epidural block*. The agent spreads superiorly and acts on the spinal nerves (*caudal analgesia*). The distance the agent ascends (and hence the number of nerves affected) depends on the amount injected and on the position assumed by the patient.

Laminectomy

Laminectomy is a surgical procedure that exposes the spinal cord. The laminae of several vertebrae are removed to relieve pressure on neural structures from bony fragments, protruding discs, tumors, hematomas, and other lesions.

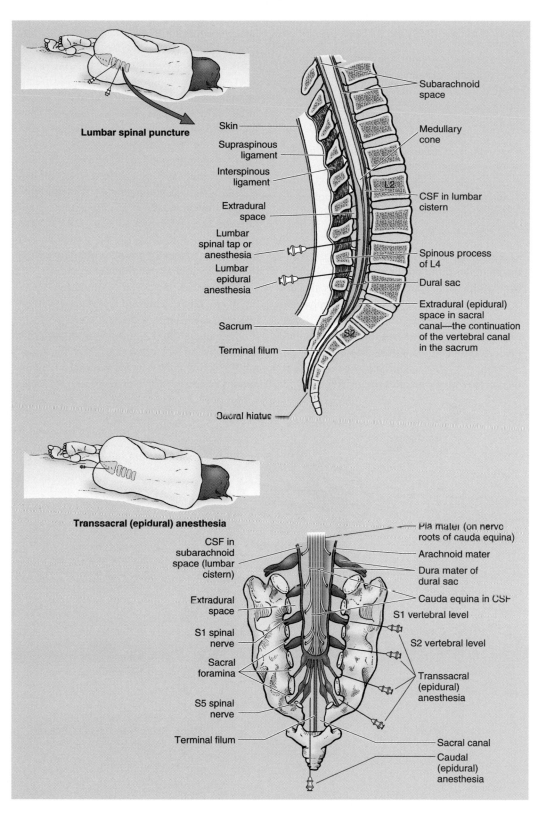

Lumbar spinal puncture

Skin

Supraspinous ligament

Interspinous ligament

Extradural space

Lumbar spinal tap or anesthesia

Lumbar epidural anesthesia

Sacrum

Terminal filum

Sacral hiatus

Subarachnoid space

Medullary cone

L2

CSF in lumbar cistern

Spinous process of L4

Dural sac

Extradural (epidural) space in sacral canal—the continuation of the vertebral canal in the sacrum

S2

Transsacral (epidural) anesthesia

CSF in subarachnoid space (lumbar cistern)

Extradural space

S1 spinal nerve

Sacral foramina

S5 spinal nerve

Terminal filum

Pia mater (on nerve roots of cauda equina)

Arachnoid mater

Dura mater of dural sac

Cauda equina in CSF

S1 vertebral level

S2 vertebral level

Transsacral (epidural) anesthesia

Sacral canal

Caudal (epidural) anesthesia

VASCULATURE OF SPINAL CORD

The arteries supplying the spinal cord arise from branches of the vertebral, ascending cervical, deep cervical, intercostal, lumbar, and lateral sacral arteries (Fig. 5.15). *Three longitudinal arteries supply the spinal cord:*

- An *anterior spinal artery,* formed by union of branches of vertebral arteries
- *Paired posterior spinal arteries,* each of which is a branch of either the vertebral artery or the posteroinferior cerebellar artery.

The spinal arteries run longitudinally from the medulla of the brainstem to the medullary cone of the spinal cord. By themselves, the anterior and posterior spinal arteries supply only the short superior part of the spinal cord. Most proximal spinal nerves and roots are accompanied by **radicular arteries,** *which do not reach the posterior, anterior, or spinal arteries.* **Segmental medullary arteries** occur irregularly in place of radicular arteries—*they are really just larger vessels that pass all the way to the spinal arteries.* The segmental medullary arteries are derived from spinal branches of the ascending cervical, deep cervical, vertebral, posterior intercostal, and lumbar arteries. The medullary segmental arteries enter the vertebral canal through the IV foramina and are located chiefly where the need for a good blood supply to the spinal cord is greatest—the cervical and lumbosacral enlargements. The **anterior (great) radicular artery** (of Adamkiewicz) reinforces the circulation to two thirds of the spinal cord, including the lumbosacral enlargement. It usually arises on the left at low thoracic or upper lumbar levels.

The anterior and posterior **spinal veins** (Fig. 5.9, *B* and *C*) are arranged longitudinally; they communicate freely with each other and are drained by up to 12 anterior and posterior medullary and radicular veins. The veins draining the spinal cord join the **internal vertebral venous plexuses** in the extradural space. The

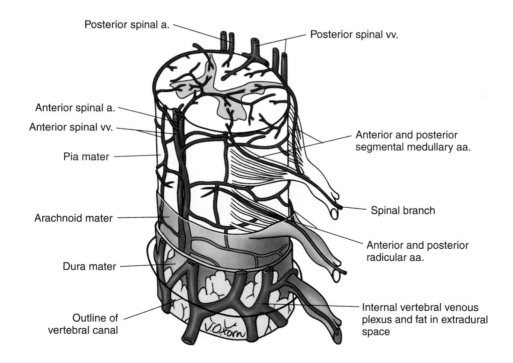

A

FIGURE 5.15   Vasculature of the spinal cord. A. Arterial supply and venous drainage of the spinal cord.

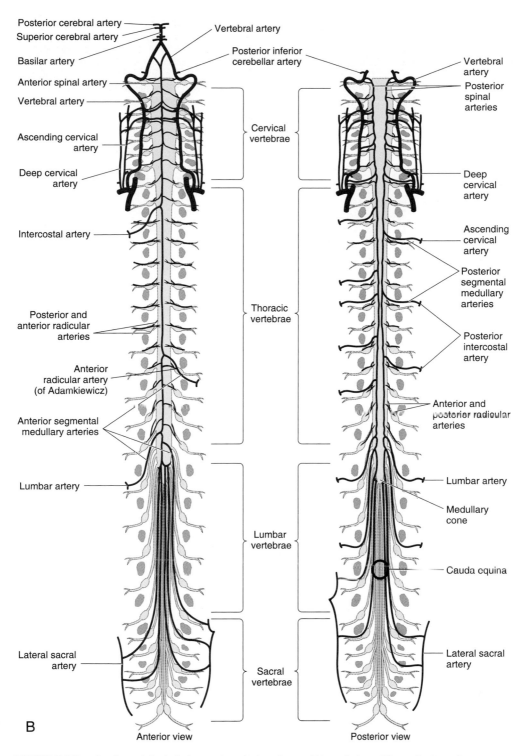

FIGURE 5.15 *Continued.* **B.** Anterior and posterior views of the arteries of the spinal cord.

internal vertebral venous plexus is continuous laterally through all IV foramina and superiorly through the foramen magnum to communicate with dural venous sinuses and vertebral veins in the cranium (see Chapter 8). The internal vertebral plexus also communicates with the external vertebral venous plexus on the external surface of the vertebrae.

ISCHEMIA OF SPINAL CORD

The segmental reinforcements of blood supply from the segmental medullary arteries are important in supplying the anterior and posterior spinal arteries. Fractures, dislocations, and fracture-dislocations may interfere with the blood supply to the spinal cord from the spinal and medullary arteries. *Deficiency of blood supply (ischemia) of the spinal cord affects its function and can lead to muscle weakness and paralysis.* The spinal cord may also suffer circulatory impairment if the segmental medullary arteries, particularly the *anterior radicular artery* (of Adamkiewicz), are narrowed by *obstructive arterial disease.*

Sometimes the aorta is purposely occluded ("cross-clamped") during surgery. Patients undergoing such surgeries, and those suffering ruptured aneurysms of the aorta or occlusion of the anterior radicular artery, may lose all sensation and voluntary movement inferior to the level of impaired blood supply to the spinal cord (*paraplegia*) secondary to death of neurons in the part of the spinal cord supplied by the anterior spinal artery.

When systemic blood pressure drops severely for 3 to 6 minutes, blood flow from the medullary segmental arteries to the anterior spinal artery supplying the midthoracic region of the spinal cord may be reduced or stopped. These patients may also lose sensation and voluntary movement in the areas supplied by the affected level of the spinal cord.

Alternative Circulation Pathways

The *vertebral venous plexuses* are important because blood may return from the pelvis or abdomen through these plexuses and reach the heart via the SVC when the IVC is obstructed. These veins also can provide a route for metastasis of cancer cells to the vertebrae or the brain from an abdominal or pelvic tumor (e.g., prostate cancer).

MEDICAL IMAGING OF BACK

Radiographical examination of the vertebral column usually requires both anteroposterior and lateral views (Fig. 5.16). Conventional radiographs are excellent for high-contrast struc-

tures such as bone. The advent of *digital radiography* allows improved contrast resolution.

Computed tomography (CT) differentiates between the white and gray substance of the brain and spinal cord. CT improves the radiological assessment of fractures of the vertebral column, particularly in determining the degree of compression of the spinal cord. The very

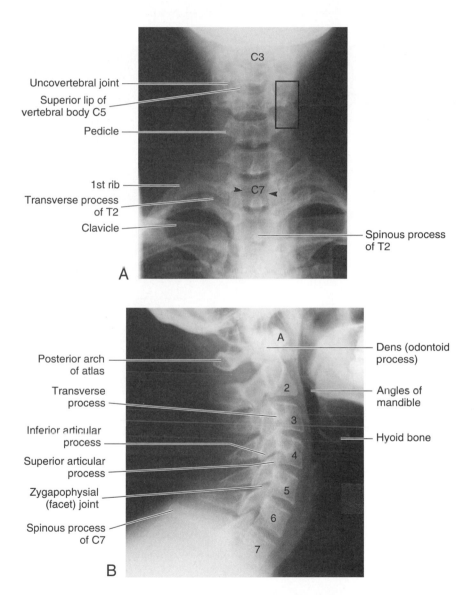

FIGURE 5.16 **Radiographs of cervical region of vertebral column. A.** Anteroposterior (AP) view. The *arrowheads* indicate the margins of the column of air (*black*) in the trachea. The *boxed area* outlines the column of articular processes and the overlapping transverse processes. **B.** Lateral view. Observe that the anterior arch of the atlas (*A*) is in a plane that is anterior to the curved line joining the anterior borders of the bodies of the vertebrae. The vertebral bodies of C2 through C7 are numbered. Observe also the long spinous process (C7)—vertebra prominens. (Courtesy of Dr. J. Heslin, Toronto, Ontario, Canada.)

dense vertebrae attenuate much of the x-ray beam and therefore appear white on the scans (Fig. 5.17). The IV discs have a higher density than the surrounding adipose tissue in the extradural (epidural) space and the CSF in the subarachnoid space. Herniations of the IV discs are therefore recognizable in CT images.

Magnetic resonance imaging (MRI), like CT, is a computer-assisted imaging procedure, but x-rays are not used as with CT. MRI produces extremely good images of the vertebral column, spinal cord, and CSF (Fig. 5.18). MRI clearly demonstrates the components of IV discs and shows their relationship to the vertebral bodies and longitudinal ligaments. Herniations of the nucleus pulposus and its relationship to the spinal nerve roots also are well defined (see p. 286).

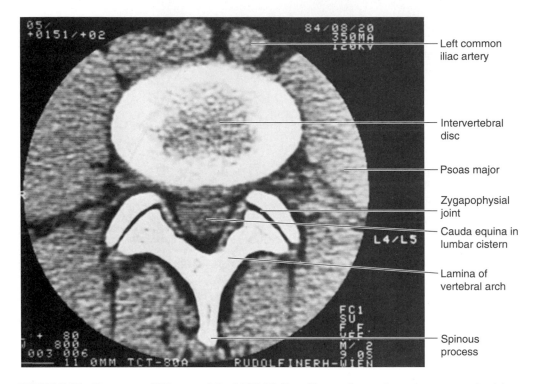

FIGURE 5.17   Transverse CT image of the L4/L5 IV disc. Observe the cauda equina, zygapophysial joints, and vertebral arch.

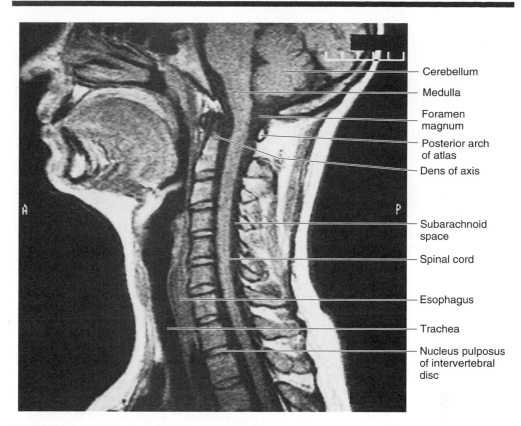

FIGURE 5.18   Midsagittal MRI of the lower head and neck. Observe the cerebellum, medulla, spinal cord, and cervical region of the vertebral column.

6 Lower Limb

*T*he lower limb (extremity) is specialized to support body weight and locomotion and for maintaining equilibrium. The lower limbs are connected to the trunk by the **pelvic girdle,** a bony ring formed by the two hip bones—joined at the **pubic symphysis** (L. symphysis pubis)—and the sacrum. *The lower limb has four parts* (Fig. 6.1):

- **Hip** (*blue*), containing the **hip bone** and *hip joint,* which connects the skeleton of the limb to the vertebral column
- **Thigh** (*purple*), containing the **femur,** which connects the hip and knee; the **patella** covers the anterior surface of the knee

- **Leg** (*pink*), the part between the knee and ankle containing the **tibia** (shin bone) and **fibula** (calf bone), which connects the knee and ankle; *the fibula does not articulate with the femur*
- **Foot** (*orange*), the distal part of the leg containing the *tarsus* (which connects the ankle and foot), *metatarsus,* and *phalanges* (toe bones).

BONES OF LOWER LIMB

Body weight is transferred from the vertebral column to the pelvic girdle and from the pelvic girdle through the hip joints to the femurs. Weight is then transferred to the tibias at the knee joints and to the feet at the ankle joints.

HIP BONE

The hip bone forms the bony connection between the trunk and lower limb. Each mature hip bone is formed by the fusion of three bones: *ilium, ischium,* and *pubis* (Figs. 6.2 and 6.3). At puberty these bones are still separated by a **triradiate cartilage.** The cartilage disappears and the bones begin to fuse at 15 to 17 years of age; little or no trace of their lines of fusion is visible between the 20th and 25th years.

The **ilium**—the superior and largest part of the hip bone—forms the superior part of the **acetabulum** (Fig. 6.3), the cuplike cavity (socket) on the lateral aspect of the hip bone for articulation with the head of the femur. The ilium consists of a **body,** which joins the pubis and ischium to the acetabulum, and an **ala** (wing), which is bordered superiorly by the **iliac crest.** The **ischium** forms the posteroinferior part of the acetabulum and hip bone. The ischium consists of a **body,** where it joins the ilium and superior ramus of the pubis to form the acetabulum. The **ramus of ischium** joins the inferior ramus of the pubis to form the **ischiopubic ramus** (Fig. 6.3*B*). The **pubis** forms the anterior part of the acetabulum and the anteromedial part of the hip bone. The pubis has a **body** that articulates with its fellow at the pubic symphysis. It also has two **rami,** superior and inferior.

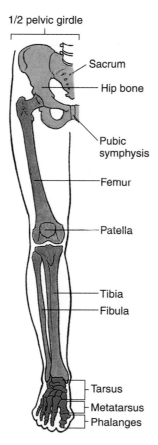

1/2 pelvic girdle

- Sacrum
- Hip bone
- Pubic symphysis
- Femur
- Patella
- Tibia
- Fibula
- Tarsus
- Metatarsus
- Phalanges

FIGURE 6.1 **Regions and bones of the lower limb.** Anterior view. Regions: Hip (*blue*), thigh (*purple*), leg (*pink*), and foot (*orange*).

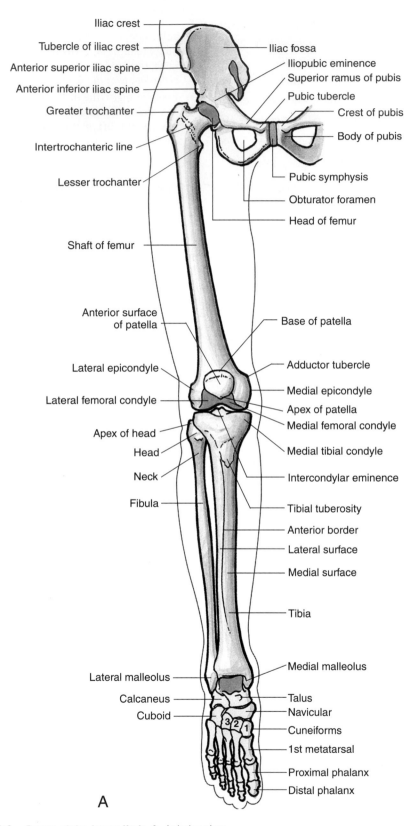

Iliac crest

Tubercle of iliac crest

Anterior superior iliac spine

Anterior inferior iliac spine

Greater trochanter

Intertrochanteric line

Lesser trochanter

Shaft of femur

Anterior surface of patella

Lateral epicondyle

Lateral femoral condyle

Apex of head

Head

Neck

Fibula

Lateral malleolus

Calcaneus

Cuboid

Iliac fossa

Iliopubic eminence

Superior ramus of pubis

Pubic tubercle

Crest of pubis

Body of pubis

Pubic symphysis

Obturator foramen

Head of femur

Base of patella

Adductor tubercle

Medial epicondyle

Apex of patella

Medial femoral condyle

Medial tibial condyle

Intercondylar eminence

Tibial tuberosity

Anterior border

Lateral surface

Medial surface

Tibia

Medial malleolus

Talus

Navicular

Cuneiforms

1st metatarsal

Proximal phalanx

Distal phalanx

A

FIGURE 6.2   **Bones of the lower limb. A.** Anterior view.

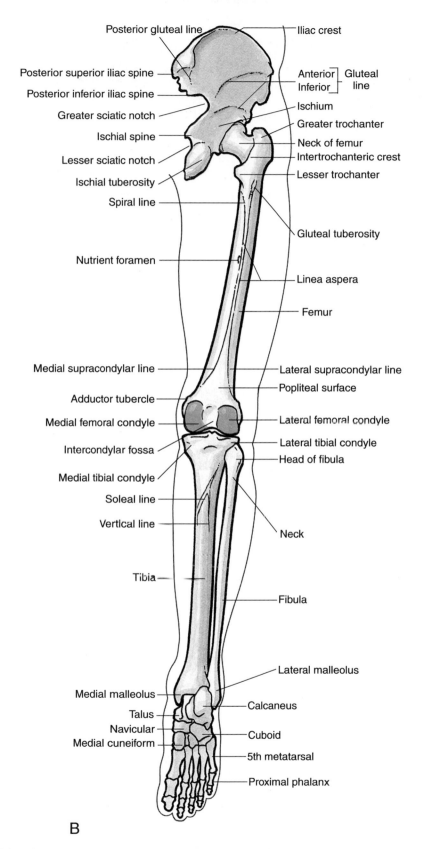

Posterior gluteal line

Iliac crest

Posterior superior iliac spine

Anterior · Gluteal
Inferior · line

Posterior inferior iliac spine

Ischium

Greater sciatic notch

Greater trochanter

Ischial spine

Neck of femur

Lesser sciatic notch

Intertrochanteric crest

Ischial tuberosity

Lesser trochanter

Spiral line

Gluteal tuberosity

Nutrient foramen

Linea aspera

Femur

Medial supracondylar line

Lateral supracondylar line

Adductor tubercle

Popliteal surface

Medial femoral condyle

Lateral femoral condyle

Intercondylar fossa

Lateral tibial condyle

Medial tibial condyle

Head of fibula

Soleal line

Vertical line

Neck

Tibia

Fibula

Lateral malleolus

Medial malleolus

Calcaneus

Talus

Navicular

Cuboid

Medial cuneiform

5th metatarsal

Proximal phalanx

B

FIGURE 6.2 *Continued.* **B.** Posterior view.

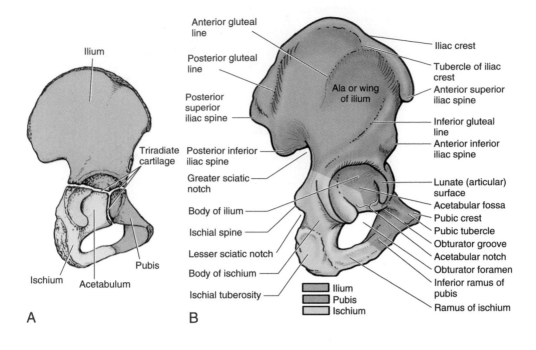

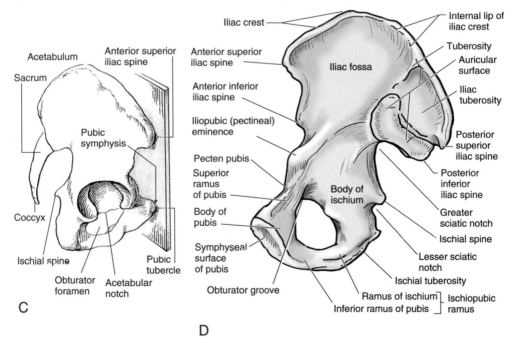

FIGURE 6.3 **Hip bone. A.** Parts of the hip bone of a 13-year-old. Lateral view. **B.** Right hip bone of an adult in the anatomical position. Lateral aspect. **C.** Alignment of the hip bone in the anatomical position. Lateral view. In the anatomical position shown here, the anterior superior iliac spine and the anterior aspect of the pubis lie in the same vertical plane. **D.** Right hip bone of an adult in the anatomical position.

To place the hip bone in the anatomical position, place it so that the acetabulum faces laterally and slightly anteriorly (Fig. 6.3*C*). *When the hip bone is in the anatomical position, the:*

- Anterior superior iliac spine and anterosuperior aspect of the pubis lie in the same vertical plane
- Ischial spine and superior end of the pubic symphysis are approximately in the same horizontal plane
- Symphyseal surface of the pubis is vertical, parallel, and close to the median plane
- Internal aspect of the body of the pubis faces almost directly superiorly
- Acetabulum faces inferolaterally, with the acetabular notch directed inferiorly
- Obturator foramen lies inferomedial to the acetabulum.

FRACTURES OF HIP BONE
Fracture of the hip bone often results from a violent injury such as occurs in a major vehicular accident. Anteroposterior compression of the hip bones fractures the pubic rami. Lateral compression of the pelvis may fracture the acetabula, as may falls on the feet (e.g., from a roof) when the limbs are extended.

FEMUR

The femur—the longest and heaviest bone in the body—transmits body weight from the hip bone to the tibia when a person is standing. The femur consists of a shaft (body) and proximal and distal ends (Fig. 6.2). The **femoral shaft** is slightly bowed anteriorly. Most of the shaft is smoothly rounded, except for a prominent double-edge ridge on its posterior aspect—the **linea aspera**—that diverges inferiorly. The proximal end of the femur consists of a head, neck, and two trochanters (greater and lesser). The femoral **head** projects superomedially and slightly anteriorly when articulating with the acetabulum. The femoral head is attached to the femoral shaft by the **neck** of the femur at an angle (115–140°, averaging 126°) to the long axis of the bone; the angle varies with age and sex. The angle is more acute in females because of the increased breadth of the lesser pelvis and the greater obliquity of the femoral shaft. Although this architecture allows greater mobility

of the femur at the hip joint, it imposes considerable strain on the neck of the femur. Where the neck joins the shaft are two large, blunt elevations—the trochanters. The conical **lesser trochanter** with its rounded tip extends medially from the posteromedial part of the junction of the femoral neck and shaft (Fig. 6.2*A*). The **greater trochanter** is a large, laterally placed mass that projects superomedially where the neck joins the shaft. The **intertrochanteric line** is a roughened ridge running from the greater to the lesser trochanter. A similar but smoother ridge, the **intertrochanteric crest,** joins the trochanters posteriorly (Fig. 6.2*B*). The distal end of the femur ends in two spirally curved **femoral condyles** (medial and lateral). *The femoral condyles articulate with the tibial condyles to form the knee joint.*

FEMORAL FRACTURES
Fractures of the femoral neck are fairly common, especially in persons with osteoporosis (reduction in quantity of bone). These fractures often interrupt the blood supply to the femoral head, resulting in bone degeneration. Fractures between the greater and lesser trochanters (*intertrochanteric fractures*) or through the trochanters (*pertrochanteric fractures*) are common in persons older than 60 years. The femoral shaft is large and strong; however, a violent direct injury, such as may be sustained in an automobile accident, may fracture it.

Coxa Vara and Coxa Valga
The *angle of inclination* that the long axis of the femoral neck makes with the shaft (**A**) varies with age, sex, and

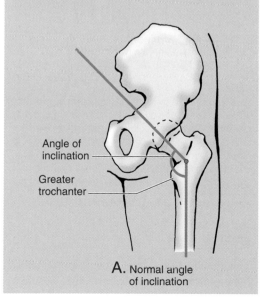

Angle of inclination

Greater trochanter

A. Normal angle of inclination

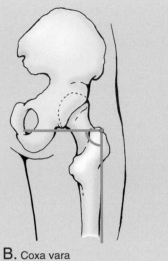

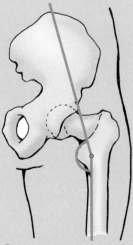

B. Coxa vara
(abnormally decreased
angle of inclination)

C. Coxa valga
(abnormally increased
angle of inclination)

Continued
development of the femur (e.g., consequent to a congenital defect in ossification of the femoral neck). It also may change with any pathological process that weakens the neck of the femur (e.g., rickets). When the angle of inclination is decreased, the condition is *coxa vara* (**B**); when it is increased it is *coxa valga* (**C**). Coxa vara causes a mild shortening of the lower limb and limits passive abduction of the hip.

PATELLA

The patella (knee cap) is a large *sesamoid bone*—formed intratendinously after birth an-

terior to the knee joint (Fig. 6.2*A*). This triangular-shaped bone articulates with the patellar surface of the femur. The subcutaneous **anterior surface of patella** is convex; the thick **base** (superior border) slopes inferoanteriorly; the two lateral and medial **borders** converge inferiorly to form the pointed **apex,** and the **articular surface** (posterior surface) has a smooth, oval articular area that is divided into articular facets by a *vertical ridge* (p. 385).

TIBIA

The large, weight-bearing **tibia** articulates with the femoral condyles superiorly, the talus inferiorly, and, laterally, with the fibula at its proximal and distal ends (Figs. 6.2 and 6.4). The **nutrient foramen** of the tibia, the largest in the skeleton, is located on the posterior aspect of the proximal third of the bone. The *nutrient canal* runs a long inferior course in the bone before it opens into the medullary (marrow) cavity. The distal end of the tibia is smaller than the proximal end and has facets for articulation with the fibula and talus. The **medial malleolus** is an inferiorly directed projection from the medial side of the distal end of the tibia.

FIBULA

The slender **fibula** lies posterolateral to the tibia and serves mainly for muscle attachment (Figs. 6.2 and 6.4). At its distal end, the fibula enlarges to form the **lateral malleolus,** which is more prominent and more posteriorly placed than the medial malleolus and extends approximately 1 cm further distally. *The fibula is not directly involved in weight-bearing;* however, its lateral malleolus helps hold the talus in its socket. The shafts of the tibia and fibula are connected by an **interosseous membrane** throughout most of their lengths.

PATELLAR FRACTURES
A direct blow on the patella may fracture it in two or more fragments. *Transverse patellar fractures* may result from a blow to the knee or from sudden contraction of the quadriceps muscle (p. 333), for example, when

one slips and attempts to prevent a backward fall. The proximal fragment of the patella is pulled superiorly with the quadriceps tendon and the distal fragment remains with the patellar ligament.

Tibial and Fibular Fractures

The tibia is the most common long bone to be fractured and is the most frequent site of a *compound fracture—* one in which the skin is perforated and blood vessels are torn (**A**). *Fracture of the tibia through the nutrient canal predisposes to nonunion of the bone fragments,* resulting from damage to the nutrient artery. The tibial shaft is sub- cutaneous and unprotected anteromedially throughout its course (**B**). It is narrowest (and weakest) at the junction of its inferior and middle thirds. *Fractures of the fibula commonly occur just proximal to the lateral malleolus* and often are associated with fracture-dislocations of the ankle joint (**C**). When a person slips, forcing the foot into an excessively inverted position, the ankle ligaments tear, forcibly tilting the talus against the lateral malleolus and shearing it off.

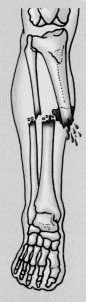

A. Compound (open) fracture with external bleeding

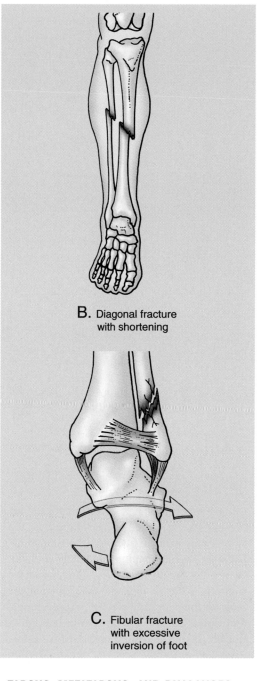

B. Diagonal fracture with shortening

C. Fibular fracture with excessive inversion of foot

Bone Grafts

The fibula is a common source of bone for grafting. Even after a piece of the fibular shaft has been removed, walk- ing, running, and jumping can be normal. The perios- teum and nutrient artery are generally removed with the piece of bone so that the graft will remain alive and grow when transplanted to another site. The transplanted piece of fibula, secured in its new site, eventually restores the blood supply of the bone to which it is now attached. Healing proceeds as if merely a fracture were at each of its ends.

TARSUS, METATARSUS, AND PHALANGES

The **bones of the foot** comprise the tarsus, metatarsus, and phalanges (Figs. 6.2 and 6.5).

Tarsus

The tarsus consists of seven bones: calcaneus, talus, cuboid, navicular, and three cunei-

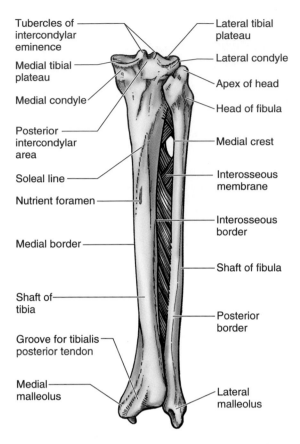

FIGURE 6.4   Bones of the leg. Posterior view of the tibia and fibula connected by the interosseous membrane.

forms. Only the talus articulates with the leg bones. The **calcaneus** (heel bone) is the largest and strongest bone in the foot. It articulates with the talus superiorly and the cuboid anteriorly (Fig. 6.5*A*). The calcaneus transmits most of the body weight from the talus to the ground. The **talar shelf** (L. sustentaculum tali)—projecting from the superior border of the medial surface of the calcaneus—supports the head of the talus (Fig. 6.5*B*). The lateral surface of the calcaneus has an oblique ridge (Fig. 6.5*C*)—the **fibular trochlea** (peroneal trochlea). The posterior part of the calcaneus has a prominence—**calcaneal tuberosity** (L. tuber, calcanei)—which has medial, lateral, and anterior tubercles (Fig. 6.5*B*). The **talus** (ankle bone) has a *head, neck,* and *body* (Fig. 6.5*C*). The talus rests on the anterior two thirds of the calca-

neus. The superior surface of the body of the talus—the **trochlea** (pulley)—bears the weight of the body transmitted from the tibia and articulates with the distal ends of the tibia and fibula. The head of the talus articulates anteriorly with the navicular. The rounded **talar head** rests partially on the **talar shelf** of the calcaneus (Fig. 6.5, *B* and *E*). The **navicular** (L. little ship), a flattened, boat-shaped bone, is located between the talar head and the cuneiforms. The medial surface of the navicular projects inferiorly as the **navicular tuberosity.** If the tuberosity is too prominent, it may press against the medial part of the shoe and cause foot pain. The **cuboid** is the most lateral bone in the distal row of the tarsus. Anterior to the **tuberosity of cuboid** (Fig. 6.5*B*), on the lateral and plantar surfaces of the bone, is a *groove for the*

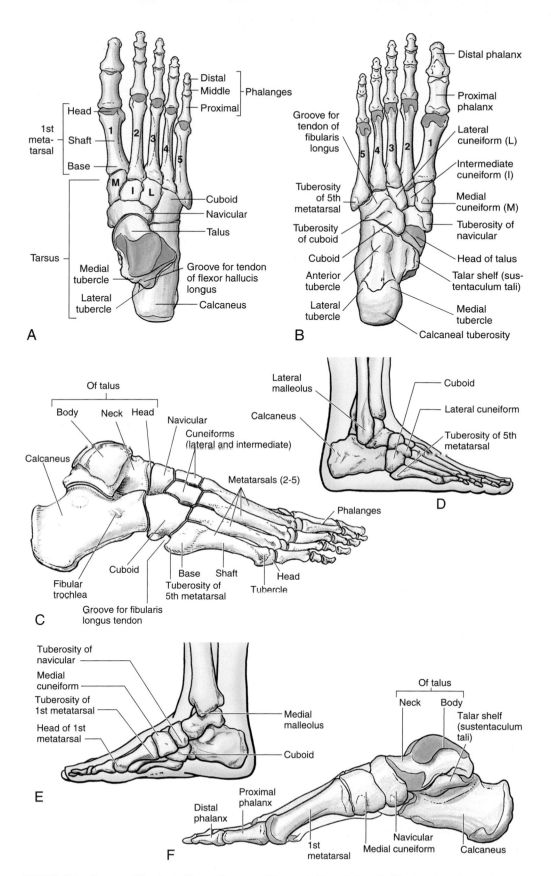

FIGURE 6.5 **Bones of the foot.** *Blue,* articular cartilages. **A.** Dorsal view. **B.** Plantar view. **C** and **D.** Lateral views. **E** and **F.** Medial views.

tendon of the fibularis longus muscle (Fig. 6.5, *B* and *C*). There are three **cuneiform bones:** medial (1st), intermediate (2nd), and lateral (3rd). Each cuneiform (L. wedge-shaped) articulates with the navicular posteriorly and the base of the appropriate metatarsal anteriorly. In addition, the lateral cuneiform articulates with the cuboid.

Metatarsus

The metatarsus consists of five bones (metatarsals), which connect the tarsus and phalanges. They are numbered from the medial side of the foot (Fig. 6.5, *B* and *C*). The 1st metatarsal is shorter and stouter than the others. The 2nd metatarsal is the longest. Each bone consists of a **base** (proximally), a **shaft** (body), and a **head** (distally). The bases of the metatarsals articulate with the cuneiform and cuboid bones and the heads articulate with the proximal phalanges. *The base of the 5th metatarsal* has a large **tuberosity** (Fig. 6.5C) that projects over the lateral margin of the cuboid.

Phalanges

There are 14 phalanges: the 1st digit (great toe) has two phalanges (proximal and distal); the other four digits have three each—proximal, middle, and distal (Fig. 6.5, *A* and *B*). Each phalanx consists of a **base** (proximally), a **shaft** (body), and a **head** (distally). The phalanges of the 1st digit are short, broad, and strong.

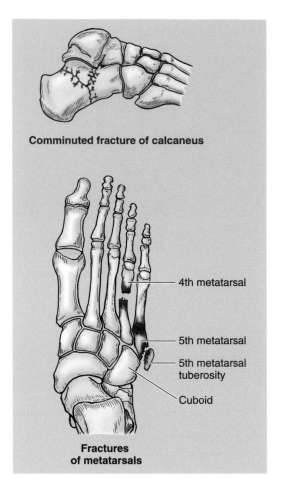

Comminuted fracture of calcaneus

4th metatarsal

5th metatarsal

5th metatarsal tuberosity

Cuboid

Fractures of metatarsals

FRACTURES OF FOOT BONES

Fractures of the calcaneus occur in persons who fall on their heels (e.g., from a ladder). Usually this bone breaks into several fragments (*comminuted fracture*) that disrupt the subtalar joint where the talus articulates with the calcaneus (p. 398). *Fractures of the talar neck* may occur during severe dorsiflexion of the ankle (e.g., when a person is pressing extremely hard on the brake pedal of a car during a head-on collision). *Fractures of the metatarsals and phalanges* usually occur when a heavy object falls on the foot or when the foot is run over by a wheel bearing heavy weight. Metatarsal fractures are also common in dancers, especially female ballet dancers using the demipointe technique. The "dancer's fracture" usually occurs when she/he loses balance, putting the full body weight on the metatarsal and fracturing the bone.

FASCIA, VESSELS, AND NERVES OF LOWER LIMB

The **fascia of the lower limb** consists of superficial and deep layers (Fig. 6.6). Together, they form an enveloping sheath for the limb that binds structures together. The superficial layer of **subcutaneous tissue** (superficial fascia) lies deep to the skin and consists of loose connective tissue that contains cutaneous nerves, a variable amount of fat, superficial veins, lymphatic vessels, and lymph nodes. The connective tissue fibers blend with those in the dermis of the skin so that no distinct plane of cleavage is detectable. The subcutaneous tissue of the hip and thigh is continuous with that of the inferior part of the anterolateral abdominal wall and buttock. At the knee the subcutaneous tissue loses its fat

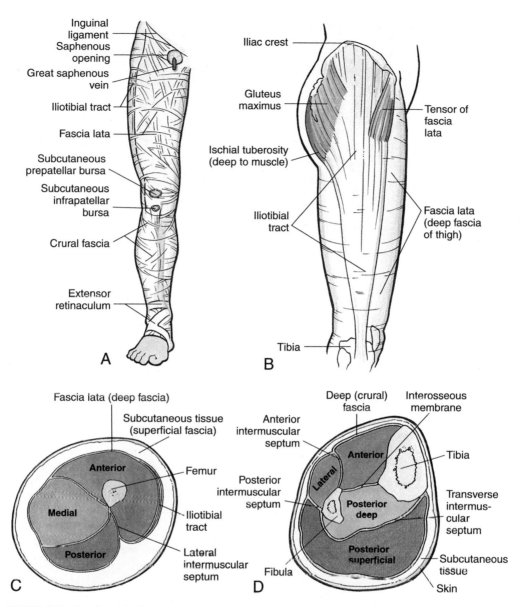

FIGURE 6.6 **Fascia of the lower limb. A.** Anterior view of deep fascia. **B.** Lateral view of the hip and thigh, especially to show the iliotibial tract of the fascia lata (deep fascia of thigh). **C.** Transverse section of the thigh showing its fascial compartments. **D.** Transverse section of the leg showing its fascial compartments.

and blends with the deep fascia, but fat is present in the subcutaneous tissue of the leg.

The **deep fascia,** a dense layer of connective tissue between the subcutaneous tissue and the muscles, invests the lower limb like an elastic stocking. It forms fibrous septa that separate muscles from one another and invest

them (Fig. 6.6, *C* and *D*). *The deep fascia of the thigh is called* **fascia lata** (L. broad fascia) and the *deep fascia of the leg,* **crural fascia** (L. crus, leg). *The fascia lata attaches:*

- Superiorly to the inguinal ligament, pubic arch, body of pubis, and pubic tubercle

Surface Anatomy of Lower Limb Bones

When your hands are on your hips, they rest on the **iliac crests,** the curved superior borders of the alae (wings) of the ilium. The anterior third of the crest is easily palpated because it is subcutaneous. The highest point of the crest is at the level of the IV disc between L4 and L5 vertebrae. Clinically, this level is used as a landmark for inserting a needle when performing a lumbar puncture to obtain cerebrospinal fluid (p. 306). The iliac crest ends anteriorly at the rounded **anterior superior iliac spine,** which is easy to palpate, especially in thin persons, because it is subcutaneous and often visible. **The ischial tuberosity** is easily palpated in the inferior part of the buttock when the thigh is flexed. It bears body weight when sitting. The thick gluteus maximus and fat obscure the tuberosity when the thigh is extended. The **gluteal fold,** a prominent skin fold containing fat, coincides with the inferior border of the gluteus maximus.

The **greater trochanter of the femur** is easily palpable on the lateral side of the hip approximately 10 cm inferior to the iliac crest. Because it lies close to the skin, the greater trochanter causes discomfort when you lie on your side on a hard surface. In the anatomical position, a line joining the tips of the greater

trochanters normally passes through the centers of the femoral heads and pubic tubercles. The **shaft of the femur** usually is not palpable because it is covered with large muscles. The **femoral condyles** are subcutaneous and easily palpated when the knee is flexed or extended. The patellar surface of the femur is where the **patella** (kneecap) slides during flexion and extension of the leg. The lateral and medial margins of the patellar surface can be palpated when the leg is flexed. The **adductor tubercle,** a small prominence of bone, may be felt at the superior part of the medial femoral condyle.

The **tibial tuberosity,** an oval elevation on the anterior surface of the tibia, is palpable approximately 5 cm distal (inferior) to the apex of the patella. *The subcutaneous anteromedial surface of the entire tibia is also easy to palate.* The skin covering it is freely movable. The prominence at the ankle, the **medial malleolus,** is also subcutaneous and its inferior end is blunt. The medial and lateral **tibial condyles** can be palpated anteriorly at the sides of the **patellar ligament** (p. 333), especially when the knee is flexed. The **head of fibula** can be palpated easily at the level of the superior part of the tibial tuberosity because its knoblike head is subcutaneous at the posterolateral aspect of the knee

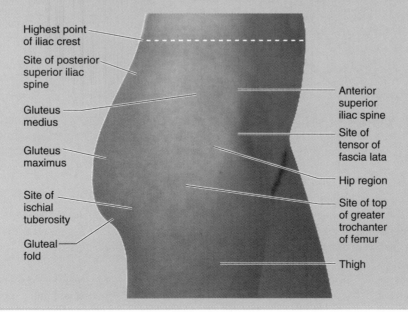

Highest point of iliac crest

Site of posterior superior iliac spine

Gluteus medius

Gluteus maximus

Site of ischial tuberosity

Gluteal fold

Anterior superior iliac spine

Site of tensor of fascia lata

Hip region

Site of top of greater trochanter of femur

Thigh

Continued

(p. 370). The **neck of fibula** can be palpated just distal to the fibular head. Only the distal part (¼ to ⅓) of the shaft of the fibula is subcutaneous. Palpate your **lateral malleolus,** noting that it is subcutaneous and that its inferior end is sharp. Observe that the tip of the lateral malleolus extends farther (about 1 cm) distally and more posteriorly than does the tip of the **medial malleolus**—the prominence on the medial side of the ankle (**A**).

The **talar head** is palpable anteromedial to the proximal part of the lateral malleolus when the foot is inverted and anterior to the medial malleolus when the foot is everted. Eversion of the foot makes the talar head more prominent as it moves away from the navicular. The talar head occupies the space between the talar shelf and the navicular tuberosity. When the foot is plantarflexed, the superior surface of the **talar body** can be palpated on the anterior aspect of the ankle, anterior to the inferior end of the tibia. The posterior, medial, and lateral surfaces of the **calcaneus** can be palpated easily. The weight-bearing **medial tubercle of calcaneus** on the plantar surface of the foot is broad and large but is not usually easily palpable (**B**). The **fibular trochlea** (Fig. 6.5*C*), a lateral extension of the calcaneus, may be detectable as a small tubercle on the lateral aspect of the calcaneus, anteroinferior to the tip of the lateral malleolus. The **navicular tuberosity** is easily seen and palpated on the medial aspect of the foot, inferoanterior to the tip of the **medial malleolus**. Usually, palpation of bony prominences on the plantar surface of the foot is difficult because of the thick skin, fascia, and pads of fat. The cuboid and cuneiforms are difficult to identify individually by palpation. The **cuboid** can be felt somewhat indistinctly on the lateral aspect of the foot, posterior to the base of the 5th metatarsal. The **medial cuneiform** can be indistinctly palpated between the tuberosity of the navicular and the base of the 1st metatarsal.

The **head of 1st metatarsal** forms a prominence on the medial aspect of the foot. The medial and lateral **sesamoids** inferior to the head of this metatarsal can be felt to slide when the 1st digit is moved passively. The **tuberosity of 5th metatarsal** forms a prominent landmark on the lateral aspect of the foot and can be palpated easily at the midpoint of the lateral border of the foot. The shafts of the **metatarsals** and **phalanges** can be felt on the dorsum of the foot between the extensor tendons (p. 370).

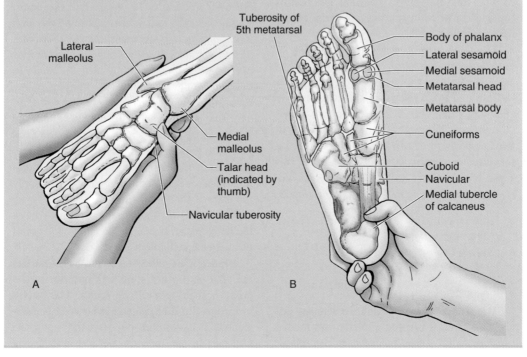

Lateral malleolus

Tuberosity of 5th metatarsal

Medial malleolus

Talar head (indicated by thumb)

Navicular tuberosity

Body of phalanx
Lateral sesamoid
Medial sesamoid
Metatarsal head
Metatarsal body
Cuneiforms
Cuboid
Navicular
Medial tubercle of calcaneus

A

B

- Laterally and posteriorly to the iliac crest
- Posteriorly to the sacrum, coccyx, sacrotuberous ligament, and ischial tuberosity.

The **fascia lata** attaches distally to the subcutaneous bone around the knee and is continuous with the crural fascia. The fascia lata is extremely strong laterally because it encloses large thick muscles, especially where it is thickened to form the **iliotibial tract** (Fig. 6.6B). This broad strip of fibers is also the aponeurosis of the **tensor of fascia lata** (L. tensor fasciae latae) and **gluteus maximus muscles.** The distal end of the straplike iliotibial tract attaches to the tubercle on the anterolateral aspect of the lateral condyle of the tibia (Gerdy tubercle). The **saphenous opening** in the fascia lata is a deficiency in the deep fascia inferior to the medial part of the inguinal ligament and inferolateral to the pubic tubercle (Fig. 6.6A). The sievelike *cribriform fascia* (fibrofatty tissue), derived from the subcutaneous connective tissue, occupies the saphenous opening. The **great saphenous vein** passes through the saphenous opening and cribriform fascia to enter the femoral vein. Some efferent lymphatic vessels from the superficial inguinal lymph nodes also pass through the saphenous opening and cribriform fascia to enter the deep inguinal lymph nodes (see Fig. 6.8A).

The thigh muscles are within three fascial compartments—anterior, medial, and posterior—the walls of which are formed by the fascia lata and three fascial **intermuscular septa** (Fig. 6.6C) that arise from the internal aspect of the fascia lata and are attached deeply to the linea aspera of the femur. The **lateral intermuscular septum** is strong; the other two septa are relatively weak. *The intermuscular septa divide the thigh into three compartments:*

- *Anterior compartment* (hip flexion/knee extension)
- *Posterior compartment* (hip extension/knee flexion)
- *Medial compartment* (hip adduction).

The **crural fascia**—continuous with the fascia lata—attaches to the anterior and medial borders of the tibia, where it is continuous with its periosteum (Fig. 6.6B). The crural fascia is thick in the proximal part of the anterior aspect of the leg, where it forms part of the proximal attachments of the underlying muscles. Although thin in the distal part of the leg, the crural fascia is thickened where it forms the **extensor retinaculum** (Fig. 6.6A). Anterior and posterior intermuscular septa pass from the deep surface of the crural fascia and attach to the corresponding margins of the fibula. *The interosseous membrane and the crural intermuscular septa divide the leg into three compartments* (Fig. 6.6D):

- Anterior (dorsiflexor) compartment
- Lateral (fibular or everter) compartment
- Posterior (plantarflexor) compartment.

The **transverse intermuscular septum** divides the plantarflexor muscles in the posterior compartment into superficial and deep groups.

CUTANEOUS INNERVATION OF LOWER LIMB

The area of skin supplied by cutaneous branches from a single spinal nerve is a **dermatome** (Fig. 6.7A). The dermatomes L1 through L5 extend as a series of bands from the posterior midline of the trunk into the limbs, passing laterally and inferiorly around the limb to its anterior and medial aspects. Dermatomes S1 and S2 pass inferiorly along the posterior aspect of the limb, separating near the ankle to pass to the lateral and medial margins of the foot. *Adjacent dermatomes overlap considerably*; that is, each segmental nerve overlaps the territories of its neighbors, except at the **axial line**—the line of junction of dermatomes supplied from discontinuous spinal levels. Cutaneous nerves in the subcutaneous tissue supply the skin of the lower limb (Fig. 6.7B). These nerves, except for some in the proximal part of the limb, are branches of the lumbar and sacral plexuses (see Chapters 4 and 5).

Branches of subcostal nerve (T12) supply the skin of the hip and thigh anterior to the greater trochanter of the femur. The lateral branch of the **iliohypogastric nerve** (L1, occasionally T12) supplies skin over the superolateral part of the buttock. Several branches of

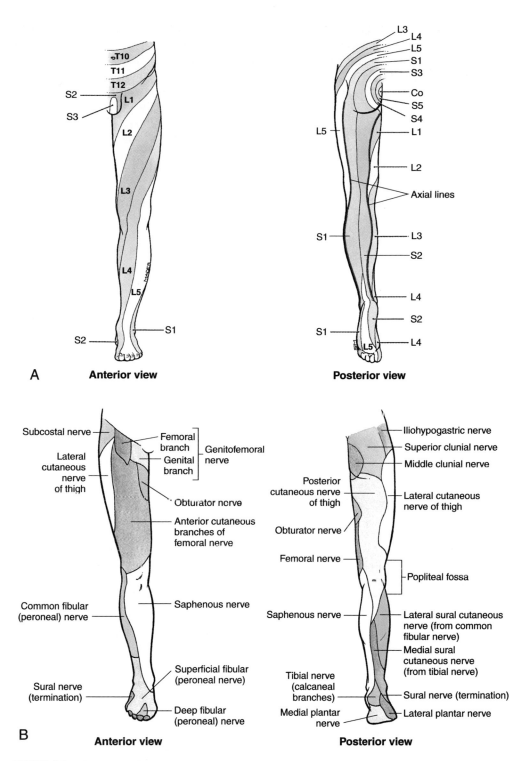

A   **Anterior view**   **Posterior view**

B   **Anterior view**   **Posterior view**

FIGURE 6.7   **Cutaneous innervation of the lower limb. A.** Anterior and posterior views of the lower limb showing dermatomes (areas of distribution of each spinal nerve to skin). **B.** Similar views showing the distribution of peripheral cutaneous nerves, usually containing fibers from more than one spinal nerve.

330   Essential Clinical Anatomy

the **ilioinguinal nerve** (L1, occasionally T12) supply skin over the proximal anteromedial part of the thigh. The femoral branch of the **genitofemoral nerve** (L2 and L3) supplies skin just inferior to the middle part of the inguinal ligament. The **lateral cutaneous nerve of thigh** (lateral femoral cutaneous nerve)—L2 and L3—passes deep to the inguinal ligament just medial to the anterior superior iliac spine. Anterior branches become superficial approximately 10 cm distal to the inguinal ligament to supply skin on the lateral and anterior parts of the thigh. A posterior branch passes posteriorly across the lateral and posterior surfaces of the thigh to supply skin from the level of the greater trochanter to the middle of the area just proximal to the knee. The **anterior cutaneous branches of femoral nerve** (Fig. 6.7*B*) arise in the femoral triangle (p. 341) and pierce the fascia lata to supply skin on the me-

dial and anterior aspects of the thigh. The **posterior cutaneous nerve of thigh** (posterior femoral cutaneous nerve)—S2 and S3—supplies skin on the posterior aspect of the thigh and over the posterior aspect of the knee (popliteal fossa). The **saphenous nerve** (longest branch of the femoral nerve) supplies skin on the medial side of the leg and foot. The **sural nerve** (formed by union of the medial sural cutaneous branch of the tibial nerve and the fibular communicating branch of the common fibular nerve) supplies skin on the posterior and lateral aspects of the leg and on the lateral side of the foot. The **common fibular (peroneal) nerve** supplies skin on the lateral part of the posterior aspect of the leg through its branch, the **lateral sural cutaneous nerve**. The **superficial fibular (peroneal) nerve** supplies skin on the distal third of the anterior surface of the leg and dorsum of the foot. The

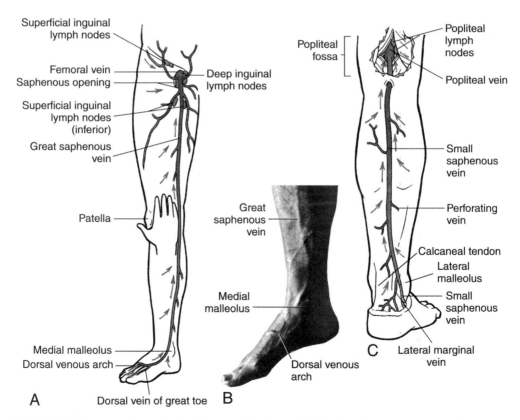

FIGURE 6.8 Venous and lymphatic drainage of the lower limb. A. Great saphenous vein and superficial lymphatic drainage. Anterolateral view. The *green arrows* indicate superficial lymphatic drainage to the inguinal nodes. **B.** Photograph showing the course of the great saphenous vein. Medial view. **C.** Small saphenous vein and superficial lymphatic drainage (*green arrows*) to the popliteal lymph nodes, posterior view.

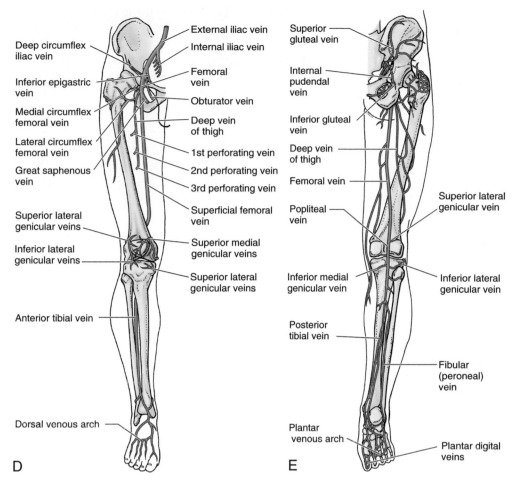

Deep circumflex iliac vein
Inferior epigastric vein
Medial circumflex femoral vein
Lateral circumflex femoral vein
Great saphenous vein
Superior lateral genicular veins
Inferior lateral genicular veins
Anterior tibial vein
Dorsal venous arch

External iliac vein
Internal iliac vein
Femoral vein
Obturator vein
Deep vein of thigh
1st perforating vein
2nd perforating vein
3rd perforating vein
Superficial femoral vein
Superior medial genicular veins
Superior lateral genicular veins

D

Superior gluteal vein
Internal pudendal vein
Inferior gluteal vein
Deep vein of thigh
Femoral vein
Popliteal vein
Inferior medial genicular vein
Posterior tibial vein
Plantar venous arch

Superior lateral genicular vein
Inferior lateral genicular vein
Fibular (peroneal) vein
Plantar digital veins

E

FIGURE 6.8 *Continued.* **D.** Deep venous drainage. Anterior view. **E.** Deep venous drainage. Posterior view.

deep fibular (peroneal) nerve supplies skin of the 1st interdigital cleft of the dorsum of the foot and adjacent sides of the dorsal aspects of the 1st and 2nd toes. The **medial plantar nerve** supplies skin on the medial side of the sole of the foot and the adjacent sides of the plantar aspect of the first three toes. The **lateral plantar nerve** supplies skin on the sole of the foot and toes lateral to a line splitting the 4th toe. **Calcaneal branches** (from tibial and sural nerves) supply skin of the heel (Fig. 6.7*B*).

VENOUS DRAINAGE OF LOWER LIMB

The lower limb has superficial and deep veins; the superficial veins are in the subcutaneous tissue, and the deep veins are deep to (be-

neath) the deep fascia, accompanying all major arteries. Superficial and deep veins have valves, but they are more numerous in deep veins. The two major **superficial veins** are the great and small saphenous veins (Fig. 6.8).

The **great saphenous vein** is formed by the union of the **dorsal vein of great toe** and the **dorsal venous arch** of the foot. *The great saphenous vein* (Fig. 6.8*A*):

- Ascends anterior to the *medial malleolus*
- Passes posterior to the *medial femoral condyle*
- Anastomoses freely with the *small saphenous vein*
- Traverses the *saphenous opening* in the fascia lata
- Empties into the *femoral vein.*

The **small saphenous vein** arises on the lateral side of the foot from the union of the dorsal vein of the small toe with the dorsal venous arch. *The small saphenous vein* (Fig. 6.8C):

- Ascends posterior to the *lateral malleolus* as a continuation of the **lateral marginal vein**
- Passes along the lateral border of the *calcaneal tendon*
- Inclines to the midline and penetrates the deep fascia
- Ascends between the heads of the *gastrocnemius muscle*
- Empties into the **popliteal vein** in the popliteal fossa.

Perforating veins penetrate the deep fascia close to their origin from the superficial veins (Fig. 6.8C). They *contain valves* that, when functioning normally, allow blood to flow only from the superficial veins to the deep veins. The perforating veins pass through the deep fascia at an oblique angle so that when muscles contract and pressure increases inside the deep fascia, the perforating veins are compressed. This also prevents blood from flowing from the deep to the superficial veins. This pattern of venous blood flow—from superficial to deep—is the route followed by most blood from the lower limb. It is important for proper venous return from the limb because it enables muscular contractions to propel blood toward the heart against the pull of gravity—*musculovenous pump* (p. 29).

The **deep veins** in the lower limb accompany all the major arteries and their branches. Instead of occurring as a single vein in the limbs, the deep veins usually occur as paired, frequently interconnecting **companion veins** (L. venae comitantes) that flank the artery they accompany. They are contained within a vascular sheath with the artery, whose pulsations also help to compress and move blood in the veins (Fig. 6.8, *D* and *E*).

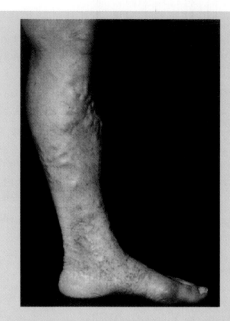

Varicose Veins

Saphenous Vein Grafts
Vein grafts obtained by surgically harvesting parts of the great saphenous vein are used to bypass obstructions in blood vessels (e.g., an occlusion of a coronary artery or its branches). When part of the vein is used as a bypass, it is reversed so that the valves do not obstruct blood flow.

LYMPHATIC DRAINAGE OF LOWER LIMB

The lower limb has superficial and deep lymphatic vessels. For the main part, the **superficial lymphatic vessels** accompany the saphenous veins and their tributaries. The lymphatic vessels accompanying the great saphenous vein enter the **superficial inguinal lymph nodes** (Fig. 6.8A). Most lymph from these nodes passes to the **external iliac lymph nodes**; some lymph passes via the **deep inguinal lymph nodes.** The lymphatic vessels accompanying the small saphenous vein enter the **popliteal lymph nodes,** which surround the popliteal vein in the fat of the popliteal fossa (Fig. 6.8C). The **deep lymphatic vessels** of the leg accompany deep veins and enter the **popliteal lymph nodes.** Most lymph from these nodes ascends through deep lymphatic vessels of the thigh to the **deep inguinal lymph nodes** (Fig. 6.8A). These nodes lie beneath the deep fascia on the medial aspect of the femoral vein. Lymph from the deep nodes passes to the **external iliac lymph nodes** (p. 352).

INCOMPETENT VALVES
When the valves of the perforating veins are incompetent (dilated so that their cusps do not close), contractions of the calf muscles, which normally propel the blood deeply, cause a reverse flow of blood. As a result, the superficial veins become enlarged and tortuous—*varicose veins.*

ORGANIZATION OF THIGH MUSCLES

The thigh muscles are organized into three compartments by **intermuscular septa** that pass between the muscles from the fascia lata to the femur (Fig. 6.6C). The compartments—*anterior, medial,* and *posterior*—are named on the basis of their location.

ANTERIOR THIGH MUSCLES

The anterior thigh muscles—**hip flexors and knee extensors**—are in the *anterior compartment of the thigh.* For attachments, nerve supply, and main actions of these muscles, see Figures 6.9 and 6.10 and Table 6.1. The **anterior thigh muscles** are:

- **Pectineus:** a flat quadrangular muscle, located in the anterior part of the superomedial aspect of the thigh, that *adducts and flexes the thigh* and assists with medial rotation of the thigh.
- **Iliopsoas** (*chief flexor of the thigh*)**:** formed by the merger of two muscles, the psoas major and iliacus. The fleshy parts of the two muscles lie in the abdomen, merging as they enter the thigh by passing deep to the inguinal ligament and attaching to the lesser trochanter of the femur.
- **Tensor of fascia lata** (L. tensor fasciae latae)**:** a fusiform muscle that lies on the lateral side of the hip, enclosed between two layers of fascia lata. *The tensor of fascia lata is primarily a flexor of the thigh;* however, it generally does not act independently. To produce flexion it acts in concert with the iliopsoas. *The tensor of* fascia lata also tenses the fascia lata and iliotibial tract, thereby helping to support the femur on the tibia when standing.

- **Sartorius:** this long, ribbonlike muscle is the most superficial muscle in the anterior thigh; it passes obliquely (lateral to medial) across the superoanterior part of the thigh and acts across both the hip and knee joints.
- **Quadriceps femoris** (L. four-headed femoral muscle)**:** the *great extensor of the leg* forms the main bulk of the anterior thigh muscles. The quadriceps covers almost all the anterior aspect and sides of the femur. **The quadriceps has four parts:**

  - **Rectus femoris**—located on the anterior aspect of the thigh; this part of the muscle also crosses and helps the iliopsoas flex the hip joint
  - **Vastus lateralis**—located on the lateral aspect of the thigh
  - **Vastus intermedius**—located deep to the rectus femoris between the vastus medialis and vastus lateralis
  - **Vastus medialis**—located on the medial aspect of the thigh.

The tendons of the four parts of the quadriceps unite to form the **quadriceps tendon** (Fig. 6.9B), a broad band that attaches to the patella. The **patellar ligament**—the continuation of the quadriceps tendon—attaches the patella to the **tibial tuberosity.** The patella increases the power of the already strong quadriceps femoris by holding the quadriceps tendon away from the distal end of the femur. This improves the tendon's angle to the tibial tuberosity and increases its leverage. A small, flat muscle, the **articular muscle of knee** (L. articularis genus), a derivative of the vastus intermedius (Fig. 6.9F), attaches superiorly to the inferior part of the anterior aspect of the femur and inferiorly to the synovial capsule of the knee joint and the wall of the suprapatellar bursa. The articular muscle of the knee pulls the synovial capsule superiorly during extension of the leg so that it will not be caught between the patella and femur within the knee joint.

MEDIAL THIGH MUSCLES

The medial thigh muscles—**adductor group**—are in the medial compartment of the thigh

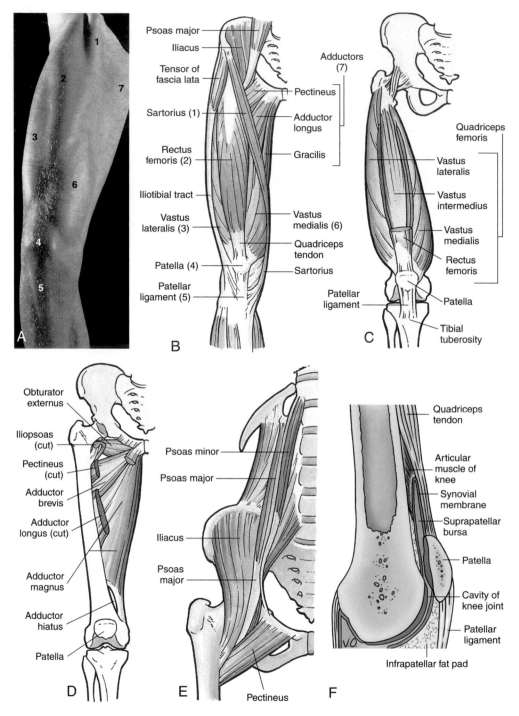

FIGURE 6.9 **Anterior and medial thigh muscles. A–E**. Anterior views. **F**. Medial view. **A**. Surface anatomy **B**. Muscles. Numbers in **A** refer to structures labelled in **B**. **C**. Quadriceps femoris; most of the rectus femoris has been removed to show the vastus intermedius. **D**. Deep dissection of the medial compartment of the thigh. **E**. Iliopsoas (psoas major and iliacus) and pectineus. **F**. Articular muscle of the knee (L. articularis genus).

TESTING QUADRICEPS FUNCTION

The quadriceps femoris is tested with the person in the prone position and the knee partly flexed. The person extends the knee against resistance. If the quadriceps is functioning normally, it can be seen and felt easily; if it is paralyzed, the person cannot extend the leg against resistance. A person with *paralysis of the quadriceps* may press on the distal end of the thigh during walking to prevent flexion of the knee joint.

Patellar Tendon Reflex

Tapping the patellar ligament with a reflex hammer normally elicits the patellar reflex (knee jerk). This reflex is tested by having the person sit with the legs dangling. A firm strike on the patellar ligament with a reflex hammer usually causes the leg to extend. If the reflex is normal, a hand on the patient's quadriceps should feel the muscle contract. This reflex tests the L2 through L4 nerves. Tapping the patellar ligament activates muscle spindles in the quadriceps; afferent impulses from these spindles travel in the femoral nerve to the spinal cord. From here, efferent impulses are transmitted via motor fibers in the femoral nerve to the quadriceps, resulting in a jerklike contraction of the muscle and extension of the leg at the knee joint. *Diminution or absence of the patellar tendon reflex* may result from any lesion that interrupts the innervation of the quadriceps muscle (e.g., peripheral nerve disease).

Chondromalacia Patellae

Chondromalacia patellae ("runner's knee") is a common knee problem for runners and jumpers (e.g., in basketball). The soreness and aching around and/or deep to the patella results from *quadriceps imbalance*. This condition may be caused by a blow to the patella or from extreme flexion of the knee joint (e.g., during squatting and jumping).

Genu Valgum and Genu Varum

The femur is set obliquely, creating an angle with the tibia at the knee (**A**). A medial angulation of the leg in relation to the thigh (**B**) is a deformity called *genu varum* (bowleg) that causes unequal weight distribution. All the pressure is taken by the inside of the knee joint, which results in *arthrosis*—destruction of knee cartilage. Because of the exaggerated knee angle in genu varum, the patella tends to move laterally when the leg is extended. This movement is increased by the pull of the vastus lateralis. A lateral angulation of the leg (**C**) in relation to the thigh (exaggeration of knee angle) is *genu valgum* (knock-knee).

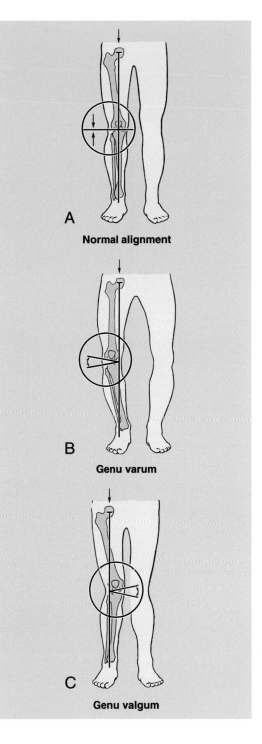

A Normal alignment

B Genu varum

C Genu valgum

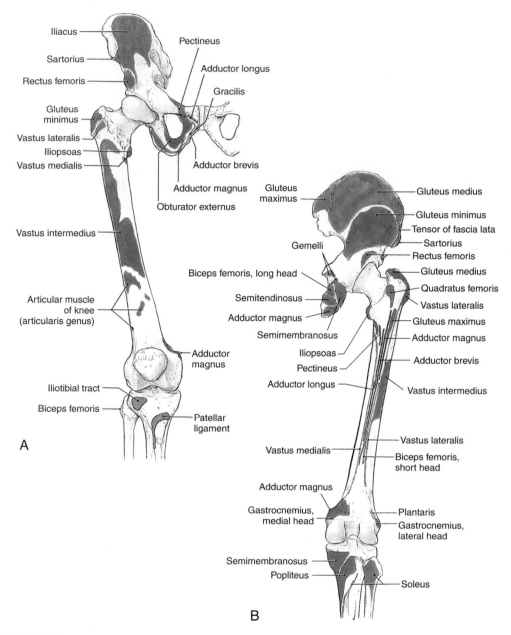

FIGURE 6.10   Attachments of muscles to the bones of the lower limb. A. Anterior view. **B.** Posterior view. *Proximal attachments* are shown in salmon color and distal attachments are shown in blue.

(Fig. 6.9, *B* and *D,* Table 6.2). *The adductor group consists of:*

- **Adductor longus:** most anterior muscle in the group
- **Adductor brevis:** lies deep to the pectineus and adductor longus muscles

- **Adductor magnus:** largest adductor muscle—composed of adductor and "hamstring" parts; the parts differ in their attachments, nerve supply, and main actions
- **Gracilis:** a long, straplike muscle lying along the medial side of the thigh and

TABLE 6.1. ANTERIOR THIGH MUSCLES

Muscle	Proximal Attachment	Distal Attachment	Innervation[a]	Main Action(s)
Pectineus	Superior ramus of pubis	Pectineal line of femur, just inferior to lesser trochanter	Femoral nerve (**L2** and L3); may receive a branch from obturator nerve	Adducts and flexes thigh; assists with medial rotation of thigh
Iliopsoas				
Psoas major	Sides of T12-L5 vertebrae and discs between them; transverse processes of all lumbar vertebrae	Lesser trochanter of femur	Anterior rami of lumbar nerves (**L1**, **L2**, and L3)	Acting jointly in flexing thigh at hip joint and in stabilizing this joint[b]
Iliacus	Iliac crest, iliac fossa, ala of sacrum, and anterior sacroiliac ligaments	Tendon of psoas major, lesser trochanter, and femur distal to it	Femoral nerve (**L2** and L3)	
Tensor of fascia lata (L. tensor fasciae latae)	Anterior superior iliac spine and anterior part of iliac crest	Iliotibial tract that attaches to lateral condyle of tibia	Superior gluteal (L4 and L5)	Abducts, medially rotates, and flexes thigh; helps to keep knee extended; steadies trunk on thigh
Sartorius	Anterior superior iliac spine and superior part of notch inferior to it	Superior part of medial surface of tibia	Femoral nerve (L2 and L3)	Flexes, abducts, and laterally rotates thigh at hip joint; flexes leg at knee joint[c]
Quadriceps femoris				
Rectus femoris	Anterior inferior iliac spine and ilium superior to acetabulum	Base of patella and by patellar ligament to tibial "tuberosity"[d]	Femoral nerve (L2, **L3,** and **L4**)	Extends leg at knee joint; rectus femoris also steadies hip joint and helps iliopsoas to flex thigh
Vastus lateralis	Greater trochanter and lateral lip of linea aspera of femur			
Vastus medialis	Intertrochanteric line and medial lip of linea aspera of femur			
Vastus intermedius	Anterior and lateral surfaces of shaft of femur			

[a]Numbers indicate spinal cord segmental innervation of nerves [e.g., **L1, L2,** and L3 indicate that nerves supplying psoas major are derived from first three lumbar segments of the spinal cord; boldface type (**L1, L2**) indicates main segmental innervation]. Damage to one or more of these spinal cord segments or to motor nerve roots arising from them results in paralysis of the muscles concerned.

[b]Psoas major is also a postural muscle that helps control deviation of trunk and is active during standing.

[c]Four actions of sartorius (L. sartor, tailor) produce the once common crosslegged sitting position used by tailors—hence the name.

TABLE 6.2.   MEDIAL THIGH MUSCLES

Muscle	Proximal Attachment	Distal Attachment[a]	Innervation[b]	Main Action(s)
Adductor longus	Body of pubis inferior to pubic crest	Middle third of linea aspera of femur	Obturator nerve, (L2, **L3,** and L4)	Adducts thigh
Adductor brevis	Body and inferior ramus of pubis	Pectineal line and proximal part of linea aspera of femur		Adducts thigh and to some extent flexes it
Adductor magnus	*Adductor part:* inferior ramus of pubis, ramus of ischium *Hamstring part:* ischial tuberosity	*Adductor part:* gluteal tuberosity, linea aspera, medial supracondylar line *Hamstring part:* adductor tubercle of femur	*Adductor part:* obturator nerve (L2, **L3,** and **L4**) *Hamstring part:* tibial part of sciatic nerve (**L4**)	Adducts thigh; its adductor part also flexes thigh, and its hamstring part extends it
Gracilis	Body and inferior ramus of pubis	Superior part of medial surface of tibia	Obturator nerve (**L2** and L3)	Adducts thigh, flexes leg, and helps rotate it medially
Obturator externus	Margins of obturator foramen and obturator membrane	Trochanteric fossa of femur	Obturator nerve (L3 and **L4**)	Laterally rotates thigh; steadies head of femur in acetabulum

Collectively, the first four muscles listed are the adductors of the thigh, but their actions are more complex (e.g., they act as flexors of the hip joint during flexion of the knee joint and are active during walking).
[a]See Figure 6.10 for muscle attachments.
[b]See Table 6.1 for explanation of segmental innervation.

knee; it is the only adductor muscle to cross and act at the knee joint as well as the hip joint

- **Obturator externus:** a deeply placed fan-shaped muscle in the superomedial part of the thigh.

An opening between the aponeurotic attachment of the adductor part of the adductor magnus and the tendon of the "hamstring" part—the **adductor hiatus** (Fig. 6.9D)—leads from the anterior compartment of the thigh into the popliteal fossa. *The main action of the adductor group of muscles is to adduct the thigh* (e.g., when pressed together while riding a horse). Three adductors (longus, brevis, and magnus) are used in all movements in which the thighs are ad-

ducted. They also aid in returning the rotated thigh to the neutral position and are important stabilizing muscles during flexion and extension of the thigh.

The **obturator artery**—a branch of the *internal iliac artery* (Table 6.3)—distributes largely outside the pelvis. It runs inferoanteriorly, passing through the **obturator foramen** to enter the medial compartment of the thigh. Its anterior branch supplies the obturator externus, pectineus, adductors of thigh, and gracilis. Its posterior branch gives off an acetabular branch that supplies the head of the femur.

The **obturator nerve** (L2–L4)—the principal nerve of the lumbar plexus—arises from anterior branches of L2 through L4 nerves and descends along the medial border of the psoas

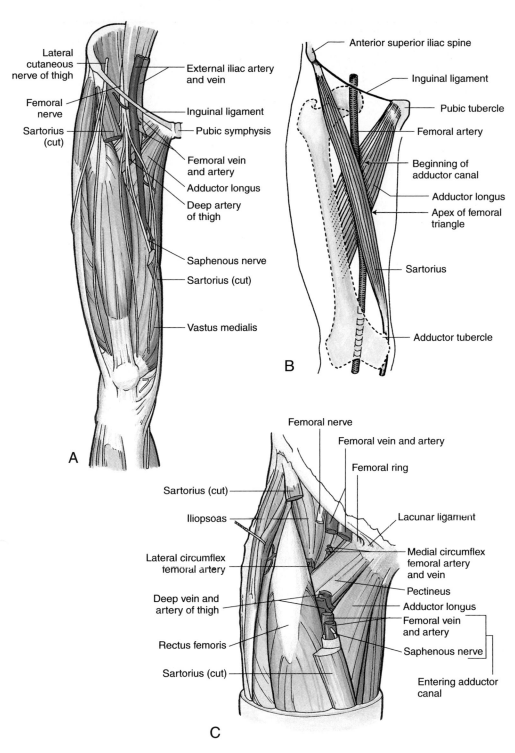

FIGURE 6.11 **Relations of the femoral triangle.** Anterior views. **A.** Dissection of the femoral triangle containing muscles, the femoral nerve, and vessels. **B.** Adductor (subsartorial) canal. **C.** Deep dissection showing the floor of the femoral triangle.

TABLE 6.3. ARTERIAL SUPPLY TO THIGH AND GLUTEAL REGION

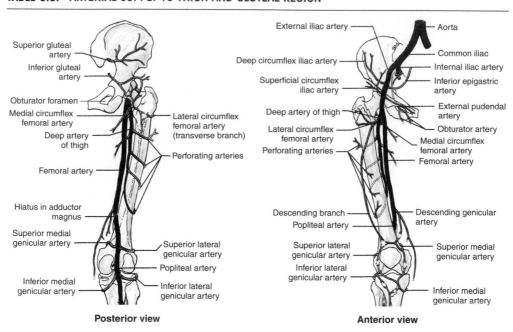

Posterior view   **Anterior view**

Artery	Origin	Course	Distribution
Femoral	Continuation of external iliac artery distal to inguinal ligament	Descends through femoral triangle, enters adductor canal, and ends at adductor hiatus; becomes popliteal artery	Supplies anterior and anteromedial surfaces of thigh
Deep artery of thigh	Femoral artery about 4 cm distal to inguinal ligament	Passes inferiorly, deep to adductor longus	Perforating branches pass through adductor magnus to posterior and lateral compartments of thigh
Lateral circumflex femoral	Deep artery of thigh; may arise from femoral artery	Passes laterally deep to sartorius and rectus femoris and divides into three branches	Ascending branch supplies anterior part of gluteal region; transverse branch winds around femur; descending branch descends to knee and joins genicular anastomoses
Medial circumflex femoral	Deep artery of thigh or may arise from femoral artery	Passes medially and posteriorly between pectineus and iliopsoas, enters gluteal region, and divides into two branches	Supplies most blood to head and neck of femur; transverse branch takes part in cruciate anastomosis of thigh; ascending branch joins inferior gluteal artery

Continued

TABLE 6.3. *CONTINUED*

Artery	Origin	Course	Distribution
Obturator	Internal iliac artery	Passes through obturator foramen, enters medial compartment of thigh, and divides into anterior and posterior branches	Anterior branch supplies obturator externus, pectineus, adductors of thigh, and gracilis; posterior branch supplies muscles attached to ischial tuberosity
Superior gluteal		Enters gluteal region through greater sciatic foramen, superior to piriformis, and divides into superficial and deep branches; anastomoses with inferior gluteal and medial circumflex femoral arteries	*Superficial branch:* gluteus maximus *Deep branch:* runs between gluteus medius and minimus and supplies them and tensor of fascia lata
Inferior gluteal		Enters gluteal region through greater sciatic foramen, inferior to piriformis, and descends on medial side of sciatic nerve; anastomoses with superior gluteal artery and participates in cruciate anastomosis of thigh, involving first perforating artery of deep femoral and medial and lateral circumflex femoral arteries	Supplies gluteus maximus, obturator internus, quadratus femoris, and superior parts of hamstrings
Internal pudendal		Enters gluteal region through greater sciatic foramen and descends posterior to ischial spine (see Fig 6.16); enters perineum through lesser sciatic foramen	Supplies external genitalia and muscles in the perineal region; does not supply gluteal region

muscle (see Chapter 3). It enters the thigh through the obturator foramen and divides into anterior and posterior branches. The anterior branch supplies the adductor longus, adductor brevis, gracilis, and pectineus; the posterior branch supplies the obturator externus and adductor magnus.

GROIN PULL
The terms "pulled groin" and "groin injury" refer to a strain, stretching, and some tearing of the proximal attachments of the anteromedial thigh muscles. The injury usually involves the flexor and adductor muscles. Groin pulls usually occur in sports that require quick starts, such as hockey, baseball, and short distance racing.

Transplantation of Gracilis
Because the gracilis is a relatively weak member of the adductor group, it can be removed without noticeable loss of its actions on the leg. Hence, surgeons often transplant the gracilis, or part of it, with its nerve and blood vessels to replace a damaged muscle in the hand, for example. Once transplanted, the muscle soon produces good digital flexion and extension. The gracilis may also be used to replace the anal sphincters.

Femoral Triangle
The femoral triangle—*a junctional region between the trunk and lower limb*—is a triangular fascial space in the anterosuperior third of the thigh (Fig. 6.11). *It appears as a depression inferior to the inguinal ligament* when the thigh is

flexed, abducted, and laterally rotated. *The femoral triangle is bounded:*

- Superiorly by the *inguinal ligament*
- Medially by the *adductor longus*
- Laterally by the *sartorius.*

The *base of the femoral triangle* is formed by the *inguinal ligament.* The *apex of the triangle* is where the lateral border of the sartorius crosses the medial border of the adductor longus. The muscular *floor of the femoral triangle* is formed from lateral to medial by the iliopsoas and pectineus. The *roof of the femoral triangle* is formed by fascia lata, cribriform fascia, subcutaneous tissue, and skin. *The contents of the femoral triangle, from lateral to medial, are the:*

- Femoral nerve and its branches
- Femoral sheath and its contents
- Femoral artery and several of its branches
- Femoral vein and its proximal tributaries, such as the great saphenous vein and deep veins of the thigh (Fig. 6.8*D*).

The femoral triangle is bisected by the femoral artery and vein, which, respectively, leave and enter the adductor canal at its apex (Fig. 6.11*C*). The **adductor canal** is a space in the middle third of the thigh between the vastus medialis and adductor muscles.

Femoral Nerve. The femoral nerve (L2 through L4)—*the largest branch of the lumbar plexus*—forms within the psoas major in the abdomen and descends posterolaterally through the pelvis to the midpoint of the inguinal ligament (Fig. 6.11*A*). It then passes deep to this ligament and *enters the femoral triangle lateral to the femoral vessels.* After entering the triangle, the femoral nerve divides into several terminal branches supplying the anterior thigh muscles. It also sends articular branches to the hip and knee joints and provides cutaneous branches to the anteromedial thigh (Fig. 6.7*B*). The terminal branch of the femoral nerve—the **saphenous nerve**—descends through the femoral triangle, lateral to the **femoral sheath** containing the femoral vessels. *The saphenous nerve*

accompanies the femoral artery and vein through the adductor canal (Fig. 6.11*A*). It then becomes superficial by passing between the sartorius and gracilis when the femoral vessels transverse the adductor hiatus. The saphenous nerve runs anteroinferiorly to supply the skin and fascia on the anteromedial aspects of the knee, leg, and foot.

Femoral Sheath. A *funnel-shaped, fascial tube,* the femoral sheath extends 3 to 4 cm inferior to the inguinal ligament and encloses proximal parts of the femoral vessels and femoral canal (Fig. 6.12). *The femoral sheath does not enclose the femoral nerve.* The sheath is formed by an inferior prolongation of the transversalis and iliopsoas fascia of the abdomen deep to the inguinal ligament (see Chapter 3). The femoral sheath ends by becoming continuous with the tunica adventitia—loose connective tissue covering—of the femoral vessels. The medial wall of the femoral sheath is pierced by the great saphenous vein and lymphatic vessels. *The femoral sheath allows the femoral artery and vein to glide deep to the inguinal ligament during movements of the hip joint.* The femoral sheath is subdivided into three compartments by vertical septa derived from extraperitoneal connective tissue of the abdomen. **The compartments of the femoral sheath are the:**

- *Lateral compartment for the femoral artery*
- *Intermediate compartment for the femoral vein*
- *Medial compartment, which is the femoral canal.*

The **femoral canal**—the smallest of the three femoral sheath compartments—is the short conical medial compartment of the sheath that lies between the medial edge of the femoral sheath and the femoral vein. The small (1 cm wide) *base or opening of the femoral canal*—its proximal or abdominal end—is directed superiorly and, although oval shaped, is called the **femoral ring** (Figs. 6.11*C* and 6.12). **The femoral canal:**

- Extends distally to the level of the proximal edge of the **saphenous opening**

- Allows the femoral vein to expand when venous return from the lower limb is increased or backs up, as when holding one's breath
- Is a main pathway for lymphatic vessels from the lower limb (inguinal nodes) to the abdomen (external iliac nodes)
- Contains loose connective tissue, fat, and sometimes a deep inguinal lymph node (Cloquet node).

The boundaries of the femoral ring are:

- Laterally, a partition between the femoral canal and femoral vein
- Posteriorly, superior ramus of the pubis covered by the pectineus and its fascia
- Medially, the **lacunar ligament**

- Anteriorly, the medial part of the inguinal ligament.

Femoral Artery. The femoral artery—*the chief artery to the lower limb*—is the continuation of the external iliac artery (Fig. 6.11*A*, Table 6.3). *The femoral artery:*

- Begins at the inguinal ligament, passing midway between the anterior superior iliac spine and the pubic symphysis
- Enters the femoral triangle deep to the midpoint of the inguinal ligament, *lateral to the femoral vein*
- Lies posterior to the fascia lata and descends on adjacent borders of the iliopsoas and pectineus, forming the floor of the femoral triangle

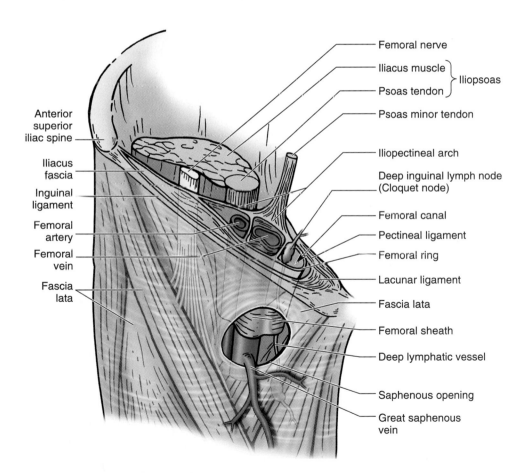

FIGURE 6.12 **Femoral sheath and contents.** Superior end of the anterior aspect of the thigh. The femoral nerve is external and lateral to the sheath.

- Bisects the femoral triangle and exits at its apex to *enter the adductor canal,* deep to sartorius
- Exits the adductor canal by passing through the *adductor hiatus* and becoming the *popliteal artery.*

The **deep artery of thigh** (L. profunda femoris)—the largest branch of the femoral artery and *the chief artery to the thigh*—arises in the femoral triangle (Fig. 6.11*A,* Table 6.3). It passes deeply in the thigh as it descends so that it lies posterior to the femoral artery and vein on the medial side of the femur. The deep artery of the thigh leaves the femoral triangle between the pectineus and adductor longus and descends posterior to the latter muscle, giving off perforating arteries that supply the adductor magnus, hamstring, and vastus lateralis muscles. The **circumflex femoral arteries** are usually branches of the deep artery of the thigh, but they may arise directly from the femoral artery. They encircle the thigh, anastomose with each other and other arteries, and supply the thigh muscles and the proximal end of the femur. The **medial circumflex femoral artery** *supplies most of the blood to the head and neck of the femur.* It passes deeply between the iliopsoas and pectineus to reach the posterior part of the thigh. The **lateral circumflex femoral artery** passes laterally, deep to the sartorius and rectus femoris (Fig. 6.11*C*), and between the branches of the femoral nerve. Here it divides into branches that supply the head of femur and the muscles on the lateral side of the thigh.

The **obturator artery** (Table 6.3) helps the deep artery of thigh supply the adductor muscles. Arising either from the internal iliac artery or as an *accessory or aberrant obturator artery* from the inferior epigastric artery, the obturator artery passes through the *obturator foramen,* enters the thigh, and divides into anterior and posterior branches, which straddle the adductor brevis muscle. The posterior branch gives off an *acetabular branch* that supplies the femoral head.

The **femoral vein** (Fig. 6.11*A*) is *the continuation of the popliteal vein proximal to the adductor hiatus.* As it ascends through the adductor canal, the femoral vein lies posterolateral and then posterior to the femoral artery (Fig. 6.11*C*). The femoral vein enters the femoral sheath lateral to the femoral canal and ends posterior to the inguinal ligament (Fig. 6.12), where it *becomes the external iliac vein.* In the inferior part of the femoral triangle, the femoral vein receives the deep vein of thigh, great saphenous vein, and other tributaries. The **deep vein of thigh,** formed by the union of three or four perforating veins, enters the femoral vein inferior to the inguinal ligament and inferior to the termination of the great saphenous vein.

FEMORAL PULSE AND CANNULATION OF FEMORAL ARTERY

The pulse of the femoral artery is usually palpable just inferior to the midpoint of the inguinal ligament (Fig. 6.12). Normally the pulse is strong; however, if the lumina of the common or external iliac arteries are partially occluded, the pulse may be diminished. The femoral artery may be compressed here to control arterial bleeding following lower limb trauma. The femoral artery is easily exposed and cannulated at the base of the femoral triangle (e.g., for cardioangiography—radiography of the heart and great vessels following introduction of contrast material). For *left cardiac angiography,* a long slender catheter is inserted percutaneously into the femoral artery and passed superiorly in the aorta to the openings of the coronary arteries (see Chapter 2).

Cannulation of Femoral Vein

The femoral vein usually is not palpable but its position can be located by feeling the pulsations of the femoral artery, which lies just lateral to it (Fig. 6.12). In thin people the femoral vein is surprisingly close to the surface and may be mistaken for the great saphenous vein. *It is therefore important to know that the femoral vein has no tributaries at this level except for the great saphenous vein* that joins it approximately 3 cm inferior to the inguinal ligament. To secure blood samples and take pressure recordings from the right chambers of the right side of the heart and/or from the pulmonary artery, or for *right cardiac angiography,* a long slender catheter is inserted into the femoral vein as it passes through the femoral triangle. Under fluoroscopic control, the catheter is passed through the external and common iliac veins and IVC into the right atrium of the heart (see Chapter 2).

Femoral Hernia

The femoral ring is a weak area in the lower anterior abdominal wall (Fig. 6.12) *that is the site of a femoral hernia,* a protrusion of abdominal viscera (often a loop of small intestine) through the femoral ring into the femoral canal. A femoral hernia is more common in women than in men. The hernial sac compresses the contents of the femoral canal and distends its wall. Initially, the hernia is relatively small because it is contained within the femoral canal, but it can enlarge by passing through the *saphenous opening* into the subcutaneous tissue of the thigh. *Strangulation of a femoral hernia* may occur and interfere with the blood supply to the herniated intestine, and this vascular impairment may result in tissue necrosis.

Adductor Canal

The adductor (subsartorial) canal—approximately 15 cm in length—*is a narrow fascial tunnel in the thigh* (Fig. 6.11, *B* and *C*). Located deep to the middle third of the sartorius, it provides an intermuscular passage through which the femoral vessels pass to reach the *popliteal fossa* and become *popliteal vessels*. The adductor canal begins where the sartorius crosses over the adductor longus and ends at the *adductor hiatus* (Fig. 6.11*B*). *The contents of the adductor canal are the:*

- Femoral artery and vein
- Saphenous nerve
- Nerve to vastus medialis.

   The adductor canal is bounded:

- Anteriorly and laterally by the vastus medialis
- Posteriorly by the adductors longus and magnus
- Medially by the sartorius.

GLUTEAL REGION

The gluteal region lies posterior to the pelvis between the iliac crest and the inferior border of the gluteus maximus muscles (Fig. 6.13). The **intergluteal cleft** (clunial or natal cleft) separates the buttocks from each other. The **gluteal muscles**—maximus, medius, and minimus—form the bulk of the buttocks. The **gluteal sulcus** lies inferior to the **gluteal fold,** which covers the inferior border of the gluteus maximus when the thigh is extended. The **gluteal sulcus** indicates the inferior boundary of the buttock and the superior boundary of the thigh.

GLUTEAL LIGAMENTS

The parts of the bony pelvis—hip bones, sacrum, and coccyx—are bound together by dense ligaments (Fig. 6.14). The **sacrotuberous** and **sacrospinous ligaments** convert the sciatic notches in the hip bones into the greater and lesser sciatic foramina. The **greater sciatic foramen** is the passageway for structures entering or leaving the pelvis. It is helpful to think of this foramen as the "door" through which all lower limb arteries and nerves leave the pelvis and enter the gluteal region. The **lesser sciatic foramen** is a passageway for structures entering or leaving the perineum.

GLUTEAL MUSCLES

The gluteal muscles (Fig. 6.15 and 6.16) consist of:

- Three large glutei (maximus, medius, and minimus), which are *mainly extensors, abductors, and medial rotators of the thigh.*

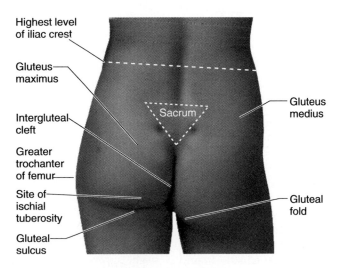

Highest level of iliac crest

Gluteus maximus

Intergluteal cleft

Greater trochanter of femur

Site of ischial tuberosity

Gluteal sulcus

Sacrum

Gluteus medius

Gluteal fold

FIGURE 6.13 **Surface anatomy of the gluteal region.** Posterior view.

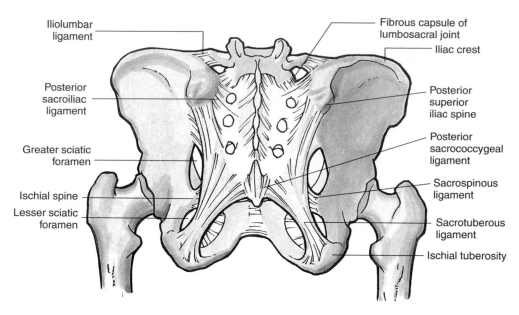

FIGURE 6.14   Lumbar and pelvic ligaments. Posterior view.

- A deeper group of smaller muscles (piriformis, obturator internus, gemelli, and quadratus femoris), which are covered by the inferior half of the gluteus maximus and are the *lateral rotators of the thigh*. They also stabilize the hip joint by steadying the head of the femur in the acetabulum.

For the attachments, nerve supply, and main actions of the gluteal muscles, see Table 6.4.

Three *gluteal bursae*—membranous sacs containing a capillary layer of synovial fluid—separate the gluteus maximus from adjacent structures. The bursae are located in the subcutaneous tissue in areas subject to friction, for example, between a muscle and a bony prominence. The usual bursae associated with the gluteus maximus are:

- The **trochanteric bursae** separate superior fibers of the gluteus maximus from the greater trochanter of the femur.
- The **ischial bursa** separates the inferior part of the gluteus maximus from the ischial tuberosity.
- The **gluteofemoral bursa** separates the iliotibial tract—the fibrous reinforcement of the fascia lata into which most fibers of the gluteus maximus insert (Fig. 6.16*B*)—from

the superior part of the proximal attachment of the vastus lateralis, a thigh muscle.

TROCHANTERIC AND ISCHIAL BURSITIS
Diffuse deep pain in the gluteal and lateral thigh regions, especially during stair climbing or rising from a seated position, may be caused by *trochanteric bursitis*, characterized by tenderness over the greater trochanter of the femur. Inflammation of the ischial bursa—*ischial bursitis*—may result from excessive friction (e.g., when cycling for a long period).

GLUTEAL NERVES

Several nerves arise from the *sacral plexus* and either supply the gluteal region—such as the superior and inferior gluteal nerves—or pass through it to supply the perineum and thigh (e.g., the pudendal and sciatic nerves, respectively). Table 6.5 describes the origin and distribution of the gluteal nerves. The skin of the gluteal region is richly innervated by superficial gluteal nerves, the *clunial nerves* (L. clunes, buttocks). The superior, middle, and inferior **clunial nerves** supply skin over the buttock (Fig. 6.5*B*). The **deep gluteal nerves** are the sciatic, posterior cutaneous nerve of the thigh, superior gluteal and inferior gluteal

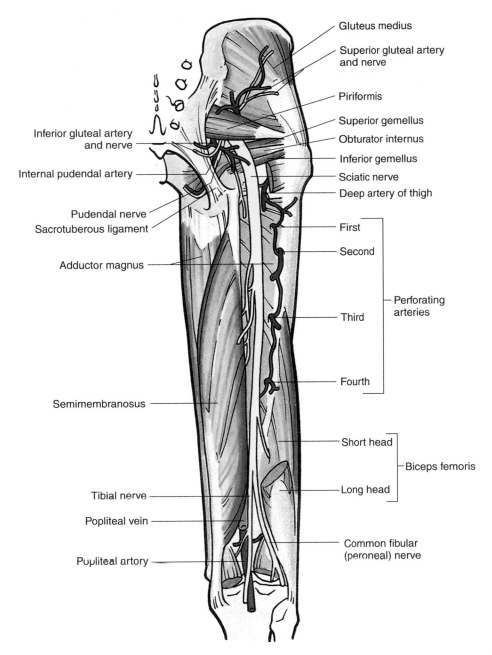

FIGURE 6.15 **Gluteal and posterior thigh muscles.** Dissection showing the relation of vessels and nerves to these muscles.

nerves, nerve to the quadratus femoris, puden-dal nerve, and nerve to the obturator internus (Table 6.5). All these nerves are branches of the sacral plexus and leave the pelvis through the greater sciatic foramen (Fig. 6.14). Except for the superior gluteal nerve, they all emerge inferior to the piriformis muscle (Fig. 6.15). The pudendal nerve supplies no structures in the gluteal region; it supplies structures in the perineum (Chapter 4).

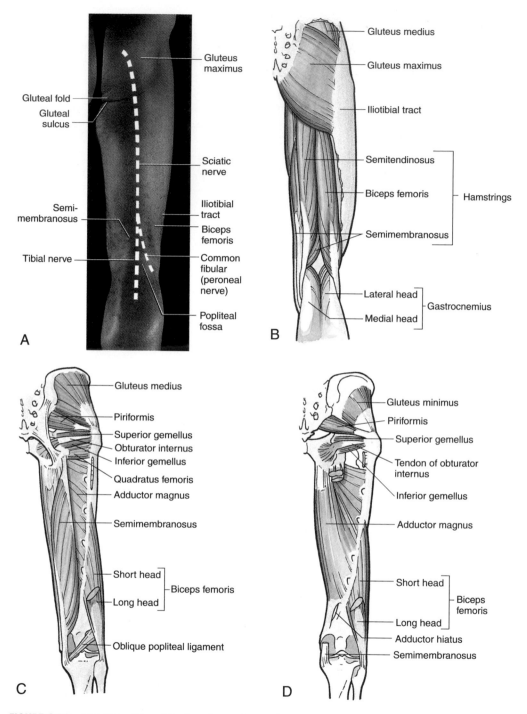

FIGURE 6.16 Muscles of the gluteal region and posterior aspect of the thigh. A. Surface anatomy.
B. Superficial dissection of the gluteus maximus and hamstrings. **C.** Deeper dissection showing the gluteus medius, lateral rotators of the hip joint, semimembranosus, and the short head of the biceps femoris. **D.** Still deeper dissection showing the gluteus minimus and adductor magnus.

TABLE 6.4.   MUSCLES OF GLUTEAL REGION

Muscle	Proximal Attachment	Distal Attachment[a]	Innervation[b]	Main Action(s)
Gluteus maximus	Ilium posterior to posterior gluteal line, dorsal surface of sacrum and coccyx, and sacrotuberous ligament	Most fibers end in iliotibial tract that inserts into lateral condyle of tibia; some fibers insert on gluteal tuberosity of femur	Inferior gluteal nerve (L5, **S1**, and **S2**)	Extends thigh and assists in its lateral rotation; steadies thigh and assists in rising from sitting position
Gluteus medius	External surface of ilium between anterior and posterior gluteal lines	Lateral surface of greater trochanter of femur	Superior gluteal nerve (**L5** and S1)	Abduct and medially rotate thigh; keeps pelvis level when opposite leg is raised
Gluteus minimus	External surface of ilium between anterior and inferior gluteal lines	Anterior surface of greater trochanter of femur		
Piriformis	Anterior surface of sacrum and sacrotuberous ligament	Superior border of greater trochanter of femur	Branches of anterior rami of **S1** and S2	Laterally rotate, extended thigh and abduct flexed thigh; steady femoral head in acetabulum
Obturator internus	Pelvic surface of obturator membrane and surrounding bones	Medial surface of greater trochanter of femur[c]	Nerve to obturator internus (L5 and **S1**)	
Gemelli, superior and inferior	Superior, ischial spine; inferior, ischial tuberosity		Superior gemellus: same nerve supply as obturator internus. Inferior gemellus: same nerve supply as quadratus femoris	
Quadratus femoris	Lateral border of ischial tuberosity	Quadrate tubercle on intertrochanteric crest of femur and inferior to it	Nerve to quadratus femoris (L5 and S1)	Laterally rotates thigh[d]; steadies femoral head in acetabulum

[a]See Figures 6.10 and 6.16 for muscle attachments.
[b]See Table 6.1 for explanation of segmental innervation.
[c]Gemelli muscles blend with tendon of obturator internus muscle as it attaches to greater trochanter of femur.
[d]There are six lateral rotators of the thigh: piriformis, obturator internus, gemelli (superior and inferior), quadratus femoris, and obturator externus. These muscles also stabilize the hip joint.

GLUTEAL ARTERIES

The gluteal arteries arise, directly or indirectly, from the **internal iliac arteries** (Fig. 6.17A, Table 6.3). The major gluteal branches of the internal iliac artery are the:

- Superior gluteal artery
- Inferior gluteal artery
- Internal pudendal artery.

The **superior** and **inferior gluteal arteries** leave the pelvis through the greater sciatic foramen and pass superior and inferior to the piriformis, respectively. The **internal pudendal artery** passes through the gluteal region but does not supply any structures in the buttock.

TABLE 6.5.   NERVES OF GLUTEAL REGION

Nerve	Origin	Course	Distribution[a] in Gluteal Region
Clunial (superior, middle, and inferior)	Superior: posterior rami of L1–L3 nerves Middle: posterior rami of S1–S3 nerves Inferior: posterior cutaneous nerve of thigh (anterior rami of S2–S3)	Superior nerves cross iliac crest; middle nerves exit through posterior sacral foramina and enter gluteal region; inferior nerves curve around inferior border of gluteal maximus	Supplies skin of gluteal region (buttocks) as far as greater trochanter
Sciatic	Sacral plexus (L4–S3)	Leaves pelvis through greater sciatic foramen inferior to piriformis and enters gluteal region	Supplies no muscles in gluteal region
Posterior cutaneous nerve of thigh	Sacral plexus (S1–S3)	Leaves pelvis through greater sciatic foramen inferior to piriformis, runs deep to gluteus maximus, and emerges from its inferior border	Supplies skin of buttock through inferior clunial branches and skin over posterior aspect of thigh and calf; lateral perineum, upper medial thigh via perineal branch
Superior gluteal	Anterior rami of L4–S1 nerves	Leaves pelvis through greater sciatic foramen superior to piriformis and runs between gluteus medius and minimus	Innervates gluteus medius, gluteus minimus, and tensor of fascia lata
Inferior gluteal	Anterior rami of L5–S2 nerves	Leaves pelvis through greater sciatic foramen inferior to piriformis and divides into several branches	Supplies gluteus maximus
Nerve to quadratus femoris	Anterior rami of L4, L5, and S1 nerves	Leaves pelvis through greater sciatic foramen deep to sciatic nerve	Innervates hip joint, inferior gemellus, and quadratus femoris
Pudendal	Anterior rami of S2–S4 nerves	Enters gluteal region through greater sciatic foramen inferior to piriformis; descends posterior to sacrospinous ligament; enters perineum through lesser sciatic foramen	Supplies most innervation to the perineum; supplies no structures in gluteal region
Nerve to obturator internus	Anterior rami of L5, S1, and S2 nerves	Enters gluteal region through greater sciatic foramen inferior to piriformis; descends posterior to ischial spine; enters lesser sciatic foramen and passes to obturator internus	Supplies superior gemellus and obturator internus

[a]See Fig. 6.7B for cutaneous innervation of lower limb.

INJURY TO SUPERIOR GLUTEAL NERVE

Section of the superior gluteal nerve results in a character-istic motor loss, resulting in weakened abduction of the thigh by the gluteus medius, a disabling *gluteus medius limp,* and a *gluteal (waddling or Trendelenburg) gait,* a compensatory list of the body to the weakened gluteal side. The compensation occurs to put the center of gravity over the supporting lower limb. Medial rotation of the thigh is also severely impaired. When a person is asked to stand on one leg, the gluteus medius normally con-tracts as soon as the contralateral foot leaves the floor, preventing tipping of the pelvis on the unsupported side (**A**). When a person with paralysis of the superior gluteal nerve is asked to stand on one leg, the pelvis de-scends on the unsupported side (**B**), indicating that the gluteus medius on the contralateral (supported) side is weak or nonfunctional. This observation is a positive *Trendelenburg test.* When the pelvis descends on the unsupported side, the lower limb becomes, in effect, "too long" and does not clear the ground when the foot is brought forward in the "swing through" phase of walking. To compensate, the individual leans away from the unsupported side, raising the pelvis to allow

adequate room for the foot to come forward. This results in a characteristic "waddling gait." Another way to com-pensate is to lift the foot higher as it is brought for-ward—resulting in the so-called "steppage gait"—the same gait adopted in the presence of "foot-drop" from common fibular nerve paralysis (p. 360).

Injury to Sciatic Nerve

Injury to the sciatic nerve may occur in wounds of the but-tock (e.g., gunshot wounds). With respect to the sciatic nerve, the buttock has a side of safety (its lateral side) and a side of danger (its medial side). Wounds or sur-gery on the medial side may injure the sciatic nerve and its branches to muscles in the posterior aspect of the thigh (Fig. 6.16). Paralysis of these muscles results in impairment of thigh extension and leg flexion.

Intragluteal Injections

The gluteal region is a common site for intramuscular in-jection of drugs because the gluteal muscles are thick and large, providing a large area for venous absorption of drugs. Injections can be made safely only into the super-olateral part of the buttock (green area in drawing).

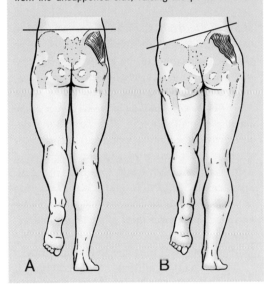

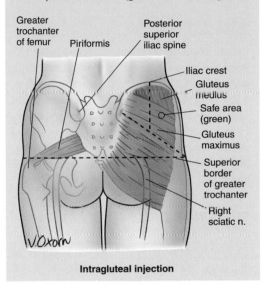

Intragluteal injection

GLUTEAL VEINS

The gluteal veins—tributaries of the **internal iliac veins**—drain blood from the gluteal re-gion (Fig. 6.17*B*). The **superior** and **inferior gluteal veins** accompany the corresponding ar-teries through the greater sciatic foramen, su-perior and inferior to the piriformis, respec-tively. They communicate with tributaries of the femoral vein, thereby providing an alter-nate route for the return of blood from the lower limb if the femoral vein is occluded or

has to be ligated. The **internal pudendal veins** accompany the internal pudendal arteries and join to form a single vein that enters the inter-nal iliac vein. The pudendal veins drain blood from the perineum (see Chapter 4).

HEMATOMA OF BUTTOCK

Trauma to the buttock usually results from a hard fall (e.g., during figure skating). Because of the large gluteal veins between the gluteus maximus and medius, severe trauma often results in the formation of a large *hematoma* that re-sults in *ecchymosis*—a purplish patch caused by extrava-sation of blood into the subcutaneous tissue and skin.

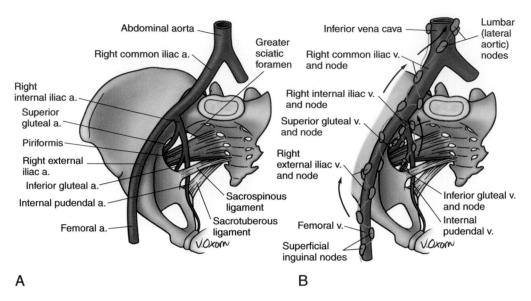

FIGURE 6.17   Vasculature of the gluteal region. A. Arteries. **B.** Veins and lymphatics.

GLUTEAL LYMPHATICS

Lymph from deep tissues of the buttocks follows the gluteal vessels to the **gluteal lymph nodes** (Fig. 6.17*B*) and from them to the internal, external, and common **iliac lymph nodes** and from them to the **lumbar lymph nodes.** Lymph from superficial tissues of the gluteal region enters the **superficial inguinal nodes.** Most superficial inguinal nodes send efferent lymphatic vessels to the **external iliac nodes.**

POSTERIOR THIGH MUSCLES

The three muscles in the posterior aspect of the thigh are the **hamstrings** (Figs. 6.15 and 6.16, Table 6.6):

- Semitendinosus
- Semimembranosus
- Biceps femoris (long head).

The hamstrings span the hip and knee joints, arise from the ischial tuberosity deep to the gluteus maximus, and are innervated by the tibial division of the sciatic nerve. *The hamstrings are extensors of the thigh* and *flexors of the leg, especially during walking.* Both actions cannot be performed fully at the same time. A fully flexed knee shortens the hamstrings so they cannot further contract to extend the thigh. Similarly, a fully extended hip shortens the hamstrings so they cannot act on the knee. When the thighs

and legs are fixed, the hamstrings can help to extend the trunk. For the attachments, nerve supply, and actions of the hamstrings, see Figures 6.10*B,* 6.15, 6.16, and Table 6.6.

The **sciatic nerve**—the largest nerve in the body—is *the continuation of the main part of the sacral plexus* (Table 6.5). The sciatic nerve descends from the gluteal region into the posterior thigh, where it lies on the adductor magnus and is crossed posteriorly by the long head of the biceps femoris (Figs. 6.16 and 6.18). *The sciatic nerve divides into the tibial and common fibular nerves in the inferior third of the thigh.* The sciatic nerve supplies articular branches to the hip joint and muscular branches to the hamstrings.

The **deep artery of thigh**—the largest branch of the femoral artery and *the chief artery of the thigh*—passes deeply in the femoral triangle to lie posterior to the femoral artery and vein on the medial side of the thigh. It descends in the medial compartment of the thigh deep to the adductor longus muscle, giving off **perforating arteries** (Figs. 6.15 and 6.18, Table 6.3), which pierce the adductor magnus to enter the posterior compartment and supply the hamstrings.

PULLED HAMSTRINGS

Pulled hamstrings are common in persons who run and/or kick (e.g., in quick-start sports such as baseball and soccer). The violent muscular exertion required to accelerate tears part of the proximal attachments of the hamstrings to the ischial tuberosity. Hamstring injuries may result from inadequate warming up before competition.

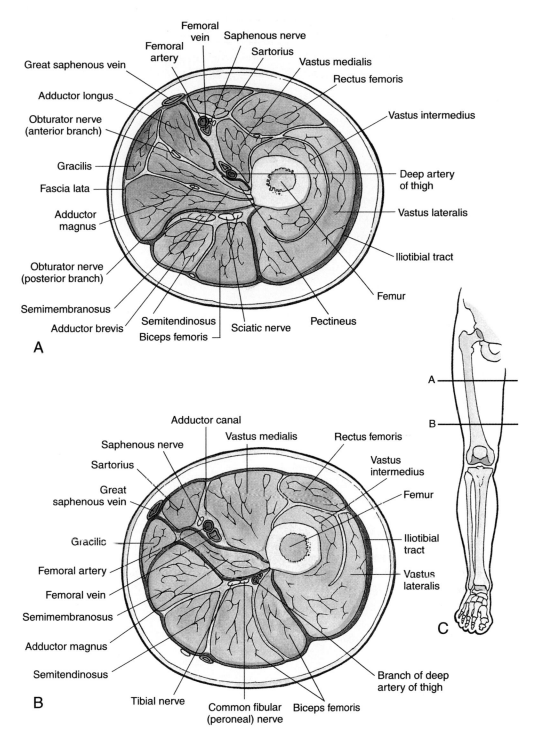

FIGURE 6.18 **Transverse sections of the thigh. A** and **B.** Muscles, vessels, and nerves. **C.** Orientation drawing showing the level of sections **A** and **B.**

TABLE 6.6. POSTERIOR THIGH MUSCLES

Muscle[a]	Proximal Attachment[b]	Distal Attachment	Innervation[c]	Main Action(s)
Semitendinosus	Ischial tuberosity	Medial surface of superior part of tibia	Tibial division of sciatic nerve (**L5, S1,** and S2)	Extend thigh; flex leg and rotate it medially; when thigh and leg are flexed, they can extend trunk
Semimembranosus		Posterior part of medial condyle of tibia		
Biceps femoris	*Long head:* ischial tuberosity *Short head:* linea aspera and lateral supracondylar line of femur	Lateral side of head of fibula; tendon is split at this site by fibular collateral ligament of knee	*Long head:* tibial division of sciatic nerve (L5, **S1,** and S2) *Short head:* common fibular (peroneal) division of sciatic nerve (L5, **S1,** and S2)	Flexes leg and rotates it laterally; extends thigh (e.g., when starting to walk)

[a]Collectively these three muscles are known as hamstrings (Figs. 6.15 and 6.16).
[b]See Figure 6.10 for muscle attachments.
[c]See Table 6.1 for explanation of segmental innervation.

POPLITEAL FOSSA

The popliteal fossa is the diamond-shaped space posterior to the knee (Fig. 6.19). All important vessels and nerves from the thigh to the leg pass through this fossa.

The popliteal fossa is formed:

- *Superolaterally* by the biceps femoris (superolateral border)
- *Superomedially* by the semimembranosus, lateral to which is the semitendinosus (*superomedial border)*
- *Inferolaterally* and *inferomedially* by the lateral and medial heads of the gastrocnemius, respectively (*inferolateral and inferomedial borders)*
- *Posteriorly* by skin, subcutaneous tissue, and popliteal fascia (*roof of the fossa*)
- *Anteriorly* by the popliteal surface of the femur, fibrous capsule of the knee joint (including the oblique popliteal ligament), and fascia over the popliteus, which together form the *floor of the popliteal fossa* (see Fig. 6.23, *C* and *D*).

The contents of the popliteal fossa (Fig. 6.19B) include the:

- Small saphenous vein
- Popliteal artery and vein and genicular branches
- Tibial and common fibular nerves
- Posterior cutaneous nerve of the thigh (p. 329)
- Popliteal lymph nodes and lymphatic vessels (p. 330).

FASCIA OF POPLITEAL FOSSA

The subcutaneous tissue overlying the fossa contains fat, the small saphenous vein (although it may penetrate the deep fascia at a more inferior level), and three cutaneous nerves: the terminal branch(es) of the *posterior cutaneous nerve of the thigh* and the *medial and lateral sural cutaneous nerves.* The **popliteal fascia** is a strong sheet of deep fascia that forms a protective covering for neurovascular structures passing from the thigh through the popliteal fossa to

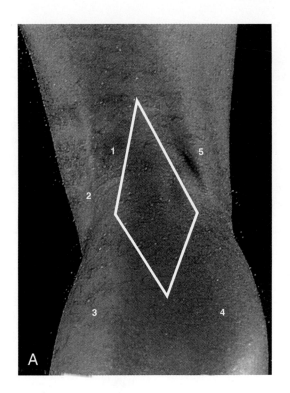

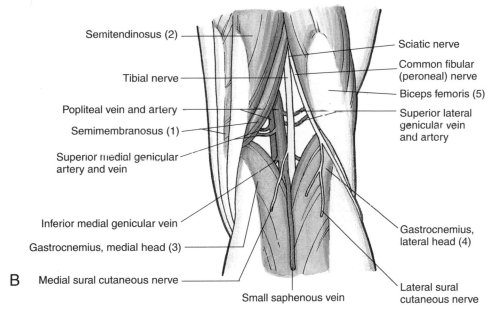

Semitendinosus (2)

Tibial nerve

Popliteal vein and artery

Semimembranosus (1)

Superior medial genicular artery and vein

Inferior medial genicular vein

Gastrocnemius, medial head (3)

Medial sural cutaneous nerve

Sciatic nerve

Common fibular (peroneal) nerve

Biceps femoris (5)

Superior lateral genicular vein and artery

Gastrocnemius, lateral head (4)

Lateral sural cutaneous nerve

Small saphenous vein

FIGURE 6.19 **Popliteal fossa.** Posterior views of the right fossa. **A.** Surface anatomy. *Numbers* refer to structures in **B.** The diamond-shaped gap in the muscles overlying the fossa is outlined. **B.** Dissection of the popliteal fossa showing its boundaries and contents.

the leg. The popliteal fascia is continuous with the fascia lata superiorly and crural fascia inferiorly. When the leg is extended, the popliteal fascia stretches and the semimembranosus moves laterally, providing further protection to the contents of the fossa.

BLOOD VESSELS IN POPLITEAL FOSSA

The **popliteal artery**—the *continuation of the femoral artery*—begins when the femoral artery passes through the **adductor hiatus** (Fig. 6.15, Table 6.7). The popliteal artery passes through the popliteal fossa and ends at the inferior border of the popliteus by dividing into the **anterior** and **posterior tibial arteries** (see Fig. 6.24). The deepest structure in the popliteal fossa, the popliteal artery, runs close to the articular capsule of the knee joint. Five genicular branches of the popliteal artery supply the articular capsule and knee ligaments. The **genicular arteries** are the lateral superior, medial superior, middle, lateral inferior, and medial inferior genicu-

TABLE 6.7.   ARTERIAL SUPPLY TO LEG

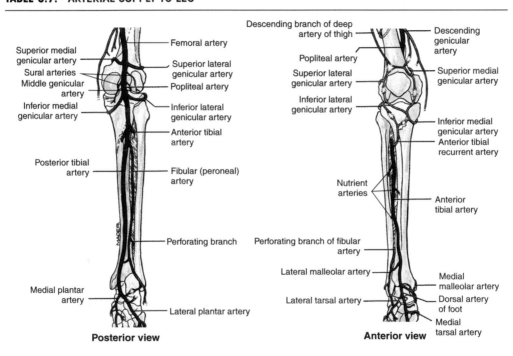

Posterior view

Anterior view

Artery	Origin	Course	Distribution
Popliteal	Continuation of femoral artery at adductor hiatus in adductor magnus	Passes through popliteal fossa to leg; ends at lower border of popliteus muscle by dividing into anterior and posterior tibial arteries	Superior, middle, and inferior genicular arteries to both lateral and medial aspects of knee
Anterior tibial	Popliteal artery	Passes into anterior compartment through gap in superior part of interosseous membrane and descends on this membrane between tibialis anterior and extensor digitorum longus	Anterior compartment of leg

TABLE 6.7. *CONTINUED*

Artery	Origin	Course	Distribution
Posterior tibial	Popliteal artery	Passes through posterior compartment of leg and terminates distal to flexor retinaculum by dividing into medial and lateral plantar arteries	Posterior and lateral compartments of leg; circumflex fibular branch joins anastomoses around knee; nutrient artery passes to tibia
Fibular (peroneal)	Posterior tibial artery	Descends in posterior compartment adjacent to posterior intermuscular septum	Posterior compartment of leg: perforating branches supply lateral compartment of leg
Superior genicular arteries (medial and lateral)	Popliteal artery	Curve around proximal aspect of femoral condyles to the knee anteriorly	Knee joint as part of genicular anastomosis
Inferior genicular arteries (medial and lateral)	Popliteal artery	Pass anterior to medial and lateral heads of gastrocnemius to the anterior aspect of the knee	Knee joint as part of genicular anastomosis
Middle genicular artery	Popliteal artery	Pierces oblique popliteal ligament (Fig. 6.16)	Cruciate ligaments and synovial membrane of knee joint
Sural arteries	Popliteal artery	Arise in popliteal fossa and pass to muscles	Gastrocnemius, plantaris, and proximal soleus

Observe the **genicular anastomosis**—the arterial network of genicular arteries around the patella and femoral and tibial condyles.

lar arteries (Fig. 6.19*B*, Table 6.7). These arteries participate in the formation of the **genicular anastomosis** (L. genu, knee), *a network of genicular arteries around the knee*. The muscular branches of the popliteal artery supply the hamstring, gastrocnemius, soleus, and plantaris muscles. The superior muscular branches of the popliteal artery have clinically important anastomoses with the terminal part of the deep artery of thigh and gluteal arteries (Table 6.3).

The **popliteal vein** is formed at the distal border of the popliteus (Fig. 6.19*B*). Throughout its course, the popliteal vein is close to the popliteal artery and lies superficial to and in the same fibrous sheath as the artery. *The popliteal vein ends at the adductor hiatus where it becomes the femoral vein* (Fig. 6.16*D*). The **small saphenous vein** passes from the posterior aspect of the lateral malleolus to the popliteal fossa, where it pierces the deep popliteal fascia and enters the popliteal vein.

POPLITEAL PULSE

Because the popliteal artery is deep in the popliteal fossa, it may be difficult to feel the *popliteal pulse*. Palpation of this pulse is commonly performed by placing the patient in the prone position with the knee flexed to relax the popliteal fascia and hamstrings. The pulsations are best felt in the inferior part of the fossa. Weakening or loss of the popliteal pulse is a sign of femoral artery obstruction.

Popliteal Aneurysm

A *popliteal aneurysm* (dilation of the popliteal artery) usually causes edema (swelling) and pain in the popliteal fossa. If the femoral artery has to be ligated, blood can bypass the occlusion via the genicular anastomosis and reach the popliteal artery distal to the ligation.

NERVES IN POPLITEAL FOSSA

The **sciatic nerve** usually ends at the superior angle of the popliteal fossa by dividing into the tibial and common fibular nerves (Fig. 6.19*B*, Table 6.8). The **tibial nerve**—the medial, larger terminal branch of the sciatic nerve—*is the most superficial of the three main central components of the popliteal fossa* (i.e., nerve, vein, and artery); however, it is deep and in a protected position (Fig. 6.20). *The tibial nerve bisects the fossa as it passes from its superior to its inferior angle.* While in the fossa, the tibial nerve gives branches to the soleus, gastrocnemius, plantaris, and popliteus muscles. A **medial sural cutaneous nerve** also derives from the tibial nerve, which joins the **lateral sural cutaneous nerve** at a highly variable level to form the **sural nerve.** This nerve supplies the lateral side of the leg and ankle. The **common fibu-**

lar nerve (Figs. 6.20, *A* and *B* and 6.21*B*)—the lateral, smaller terminal branch of the sciatic nerve—begins at the superior angle of the popliteal fossa and follows closely the medial border of the biceps femoris and its tendon along the superolateral boundary of the popliteal fossa. The common fibular nerve leaves the fossa by passing superficial to the lateral head of the gastrocnemius and then passes over the posterior aspect of the head of the fibula. *The common fibular nerve winds around the fibular neck, where it is vulnerable to injury.* Here it divides into its terminal branches, the superficial and deep fibular nerves.

TABLE 6.8.   NERVES OF LEG

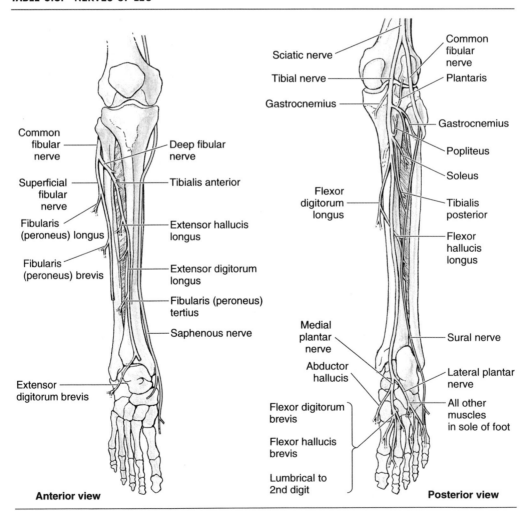

Anterior view   **Posterior view**

TABLE 6.8. *CONTINUED*

Nerve	Origin	Course	Distribution in Leg
Saphenous	Femoral nerve	Descends with femoral vessels through femoral triangle and adductor canal and then descends with great saphenous vein	Supplies skin on medial side of leg and foot
Sural	Usually arises from both tibial and common fibular nerves	Descends between heads of gastrocnemius and becomes superficial at the middle of the leg; descends with small saphenous vein and passes inferior to the lateral malleolus to the lateral side of foot	Supplies skin on posterior and lateral aspects of leg and lateral side of foot
Tibial ⎤ Sciatic nerve		Forms as sciatic bifurcates at apex of popliteal fossa; descends through popliteal fossa and lies on popliteus; runs inferiorly on the tibialis posterior with the posterior tibial vessels; terminates beneath the flexor retinaculum by dividing into the medial and lateral plantar nerves	Supplies posterior muscles of leg and knee joint
Common fibular ⎦		Forms as sciatic bifurcates at apex of popliteal fossa and follows medial border of biceps femoris and its tendon; passes over posterior aspect of head of fibula and then winds around neck of fibula deep to fibularis longus, where it divides into deep and superficial fibular nerves	Supplies skin on lateral part of posterior aspect of leg via its branch, the lateral sural cutaneous nerve; also supplies knee joint via its articular branch
Superficial fibular ⎤ Common fibular nerve		Arises between fibularis longus and neck of fibula and descends in lateral compartment of the leg; pierces deep fascia at distal third of leg to become subcutaneous	Supplies fibularis longus and brevis and skin on distal third of anterior surface of leg and dorsum of foot
Deep fibular ⎦		Arises between fibularis longus and neck of fibula; passes through extensor digitorum longus and descends on interosseous membrane; crosses distal end of tibia and enters dorsum of foot	Supplies anterior muscles of leg, dorsum of foot, and skin of first interdigital cleft; sends articular branches to joints it crosses (Fig. 6.7B)

LEG

The leg contains the tibia and fibula, bones that connect the knee and ankle. The **tibia,** the weight-bearing bone, is larger and stronger than the **fibula.** The leg bones are connected by the **interosseous membrane** (Fig. 6.20*A*). *The leg is divided into three compartments*—anterior, lateral, and posterior—by the anterior and posterior **intermuscular septa** and the interosseous membrane (Fig. 6.20*B*).

ANTERIOR COMPARTMENT OF LEG

The anterior compartment—the *extensor compartment of leg*—is located anterior to the interosseous membrane, between the lateral surface of the tibial shaft and the anterior intermuscular septum. The anterior compartment is bounded anteriorly by crural fascia and skin. *The four muscles in the anterior compartment* (Figs. 6.20 and 6.21) *are:*

- Tibialis anterior
- Extensor digitorum longus
- Extensor hallucis longus
- Fibularis tertius.

These muscles are mainly dorsiflexors of the ankle joint and extensors of the toes. For their attachments, nerve supply, and main actions, see Table 6.9.

The **superior extensor retinaculum** is a strong, broad band of deep fascia (Fig. 6.21*A*), passing from the fibula to the tibia, proximal to the malleoli. It binds down the muscle tendons in the anterior compartment, preventing them from bowstringing anteriorly during dorsiflexion of the ankle joint. The **inferior extensor retinaculum,** a Y-shaped band of deep fascia, attaches laterally to the anterosuperior surface of the calcaneus. It forms a strong loop around the tendons of the fibularis tertius and extensor digitorum longus muscles.

The **deep fibular nerve** (Fig. 6.21*B*, Table 6.8)—*the nerve in the anterior compartment*—is one of the two terminal branches of the common fibular nerve. The deep fibular nerve arises between the fibularis longus muscle and the fibular neck, and after entering the compartment, accompanies the anterior tibial artery. The **anterior tibial artery** (Fig. 6.21*B*, Table 6.7)—*the artery in the anterior compartment*—supplies structures in the anterior compartment. The smaller terminal branch of the popliteal artery, the anterior tibial artery begins at the inferior border of the popliteus. It passes anteriorly through a gap in the superior part of the interosseous membrane and descends on the anterior surface of this membrane between the tibialis anterior and extensor digitorum longus. It ends at the ankle joint, midway between the malleoli (Fig. 6.21*B*), where it becomes the **dorsal artery of foot** (L. arteria dorsalis pedis).

INJURY TO COMMON FIBULAR NERVE

Because of its superficial position at the knee, *the common fibular nerve is the most commonly injured nerve in the lower limb,* mainly because it winds superficially around the neck of the fibula. This nerve may be severed during fracture of the fibular neck or severely stretched when the knee joint is injured or dislocated. *Severance of the common fibular nerve results in paralysis of all muscles in the anterior and lateral compartments of the leg* (Table 6.9). The loss of eversion of the foot and dorsiflexion of the ankle causes **foot-drop**—the foot passively plantarflexes and inverts, causing the toes to drag on the floor when walking. The person compensates by developing a high stepping ("steppage") gait, raising the foot as high as is necessary to keep the toes from hitting the ground. In addition, the foot slaps down when the heel is planted, producing a distinctive "clop." There also is a variable loss of sensation on the anterolateral aspect of the leg and dorsum of the foot.

Anterior Tibialis Strain

Anterior tibialis strain (shin splints)—edema and pain in the area of the distal third of the tibia—is a painful condition of the anterior compartment of the leg that follows vigorous and/or lengthy exercise. The anterior tibial muscles swell from sudden overuse and the edema and muscle-tendon inflammation reduce blood flow to the muscles. The swollen muscles are painful and tender to pressure.

LATERAL COMPARTMENT OF LEG

The lateral compartment is bounded by the lateral surface of the fibula, the anterior and posterior intermuscular septa, and the crural fascia (Figs. 6.20 and 6.22). The lateral compartment contains two muscles: the fibularis longus and brevis. See Table 6.9 for their attachments, nerve supply, and main actions.

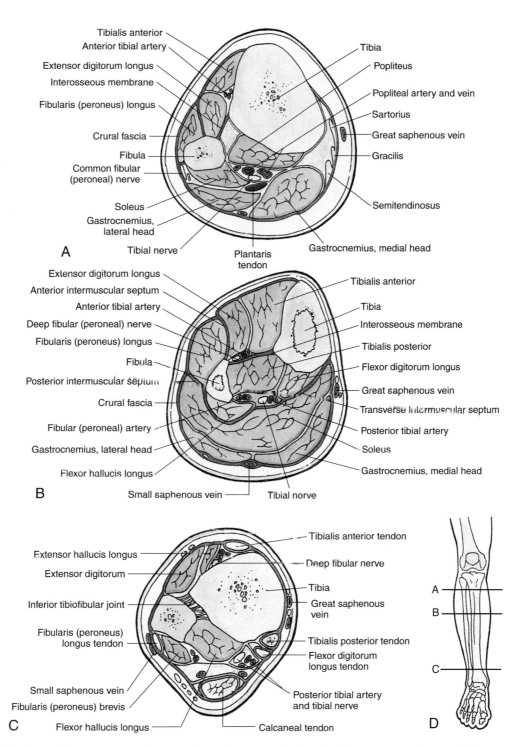

FIGURE 6.20 **Bones, muscles, vessels, and nerves of the leg. A–C.** Transverse sections of the leg. **D.** Orientation drawing showing the level of sections.

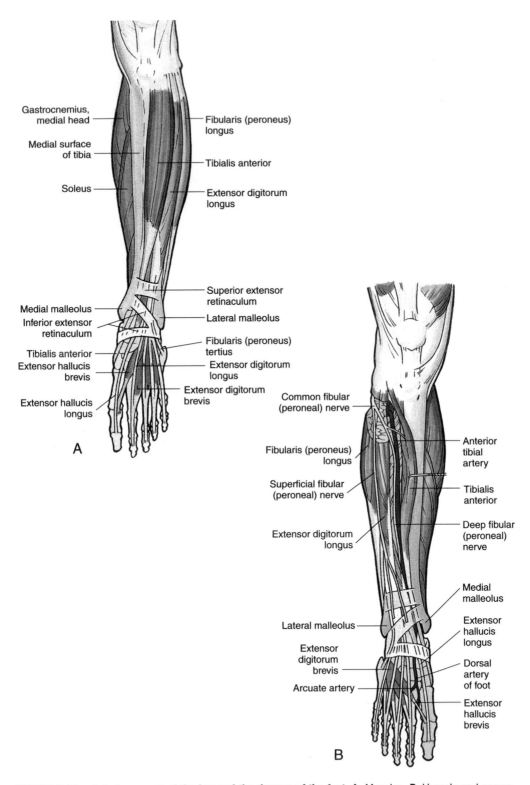

A

FIGURE 6.21   **Anterior aspect of the leg and the dorsum of the foot. A.** Muscles. **B.** Vessels and nerves. Muscles are separated to display these structures.

TABLE 6.9. MUSCLES OF ANTERIOR AND LATERAL LEG

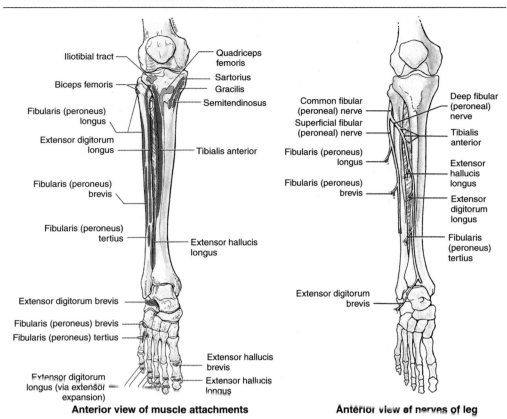

Anterior view of muscle attachments

Anterior view of nerves of leg

Muscle	Proximal Attachment	Distal Attachment	Innervation	Main Action(s)
Anterior compartment				
Tibialis anterior	Lateral condyle and superior half of lateral surface of tibia and interosseous membrane	Medial and inferior surfaces of medial cuneiform and base of 1st metatarsal	Deep fibular (peroneal) nerve (**L4** and L5)	Dorsiflexes ankle and inverts foot
Extensor hallucis longus	Middle part of anterior surface of fibula and interosseous membrane	Dorsal aspect of base of distal phalanx of great toe (hallux)	Deep fibular (peroneal) nerve (L5 and S1)	Extends great toe and dorsiflexes ankle
Extensor digitorum longus	Lateral condyle of tibia and superior three fourths of anterior surface of interosseous membrane	Middle and distal phalanges of lateral four digits		Extends lateral four digits and dorsiflexes ankle
Fibularis (peroneus) tertius	Inferior third of anterior surface of fibula and interosseous membrane	Dorsum of base of 5th metatarsal		Dorsiflexes ankle and aids in eversion of foot
Lateral compartment				
Fibularis (peroneus) longus	Head and superior two thirds of lateral surface of fibula	Base of 1st metatarsal and medial cuneiform	Superficial fibular (peroneal) nerve (**L5, S1,** and S2)	Evert foot and weakly plantarflex ankle
Fibularis (peroneus) brevis	Inferior two thirds of lateral surface of fibula	Dorsal surface of tuberosity on lateral side of base of 5th metatarsal		

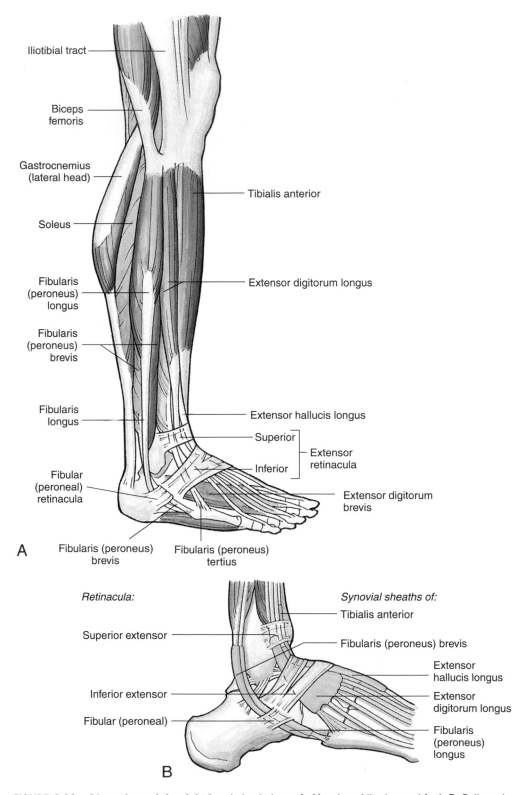

Iliotibial tract

Biceps
femoris

Gastrocnemius
(lateral head)

Soleus

Fibularis
(peroneus)
longus

Fibularis
(peroneus)
brevis

Fibularis
longus

Fibular
(peroneal)
retinacula

Tibialis anterior

Extensor digitorum longus

Extensor hallucis longus

Superior
Inferior
} Extensor
retinacula

Extensor digitorum
brevis

A

Fibularis (peroneus)
brevis

Fibularis (peroneus)
tertius

Retinacula:

Superior extensor

Inferior extensor

Fibular (peroneal)

Synovial sheaths of:
Tibialis anterior

Fibularis (peroneus) brevis

Extensor
hallucis longus

Extensor
digitorum longus

Fibularis
(peroneus)
longus

B

FIGURE 6.22 **Dissections of the right leg.** Lateral views. **A.** Muscles of the leg and foot. **B.** Retinacula
and synovial sheaths of the tendons (*blue*) at the ankle.

The **superficial fibular nerve**—*the nerve in the lateral compartment*—is the other terminal branch of the common fibular nerve (Table 6.8). It supplies skin on the distal part of the anterior surface of the leg and nearly all the dorsum of the foot. *The lateral compartment of the leg does not have an artery.* The muscles are supplied by perforating branches of the **anterior tibial artery** and inferiorly by perforating branches of the **fibular artery** (Table 6.7).

POSTERIOR COMPARTMENT OF LEG

The posterior compartment is the largest of the three leg compartments. The *calf muscles* in the compartment are divided into superficial and deep groups by the **transverse intermuscular septum** (Fig. 6.20*B*). The tibial nerve and posterior tibial vessels supply both divisions of the posterior compartment and run between the superficial and deep groups of muscle, just deep to the transverse intermuscular septum.

Superficial Muscle Group

The superficial muscle group—*gastrocnemius, soleus,* and *plantaris*—forms a powerful muscular mass in the calf (Fig. 6.23). For attachments, nerve supply, and main actions of these muscles, see Table 6.10. The two-headed **gastrocnemius** and the **soleus** form the large three-headed **triceps surae** (L. sura, calf). This muscle has a common tendon—the **calcaneal tendon** (L. tendo calcaneus, Achilles tendon)—which attaches to the calcaneus. A *superficial calcaneal bursa* lies between the skin and calcaneal tendon, and a *deep calcaneal bursa* (*retrocalcaneal bursa*) is located between the tendon and calcaneus. *The triceps surae plantarflexes the ankle joint, raising the heel against the resistance of the body's weight* (e.g., by "standing on toes").

INFLAMMATION AND RUPTURE OF CALCANEAL TENDON
Inflammation, strain, and rupture of the calcaneal tendon often occur during running and quick-start sports (e.g., squash). *Rupture of the calcaneal tendon* results in abrupt calf pain. Persons with this injury cannot use the limb, and a lump appears in the calf owing to shortening of the triceps surae. After complete rupture of the tendon, the foot can be dorsiflexed to a greater extent than normal, but the person cannot easily plantarflex the foot.

Calcaneal Tendon Reflex
The *ankle reflex* is elicited by striking the tendon briskly with a reflex hammer. This tendon reflex tests the S1 and S2 nerve roots. If the S1 nerve root is cut or compressed, the ankle reflex is virtually absent.

Gastrocnemius Strain
Gastrocnemius strain ("tennis leg") is a painful calf injury resulting from partial tearing of the medial belly of the gastrocnemius at or near its musculotendinous junction. It is caused by overstretching the muscle by concomitant full extension of the knee and dorsiflexion of the ankle joint.

Calcaneal Bursitis
Calcaneal bursitis—*inflammation and swelling of the deep calcaneal bursa*—is fairly common in persons competing in long-distance running, basketball, and tennis. It is caused by excessive friction on the bursa as the calcaneal tendon continuously slides over it.

Deep Muscle Group

Four muscles comprise the deep muscle group (Figs. 6.23 and 6.24):

- Popliteus
- Flexor digitorum longus
- Flexor hallucis longus
- Tibialis posterior.

For attachments, nerve supply, and main actions of these muscles, see Table 6.10. The **popliteus**—a thin, triangular muscle in the floor of the popliteal fossa (Fig. 6.23, *C* and *D*)—acts on the knee joint, whereas the other muscles act on the ankle and foot joints. The **flexor digitorum longus** is smaller than the flexor hallucis longus, even though it moves four digits. It passes diagonally into the sole of the foot, superficial to the tendon of the flexor hallucis longus, and divides into four tendons, which pass to the distal phalanges of the lateral four toes. The **flexor hallucis longus** is the powerful "push-off" muscle during walking, running, and jumping. It provides much of the spring to the step. The **tibialis posterior,** the deepest muscle in the group, lies between the flexor digitorum longus and the flexor hallucis longus in the same plane as the tibia and fibula.

The **tibial nerve** (L4, L5, and S1 through S3)—the larger of the two terminal branches of the **sciatic nerve** (Fig. 6.24)—leaves the popliteal fossa between the heads of the gas-

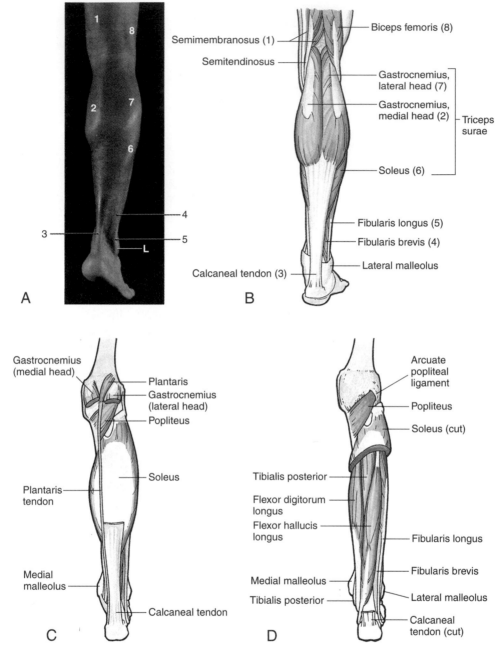

FIGURE 6.23   Muscles of the posterior thigh and leg. A. Surface anatomy. *Numbers* refer to the muscles labelled in **B.** *L,* lateral malleolus. **B.** Superficial muscles. **C.** Soleus, popliteus, and plantaris. **D.** Deep muscles.

trocnemius. *The tibial nerve supplies all muscles in the posterior compartment of the leg* (Table 6.10). Posteroinferior to the medial malleolus, *the tibial nerve divides into the medial* and *lateral plantar nerves.* A branch of the

tibial nerve, the *medial sural cutaneous nerve* unites with the communicating branch of the common fibular nerve to form the **sural nerve** (Table 6.8). This nerve supplies the skin of the lateral and posterior part of the inferior third

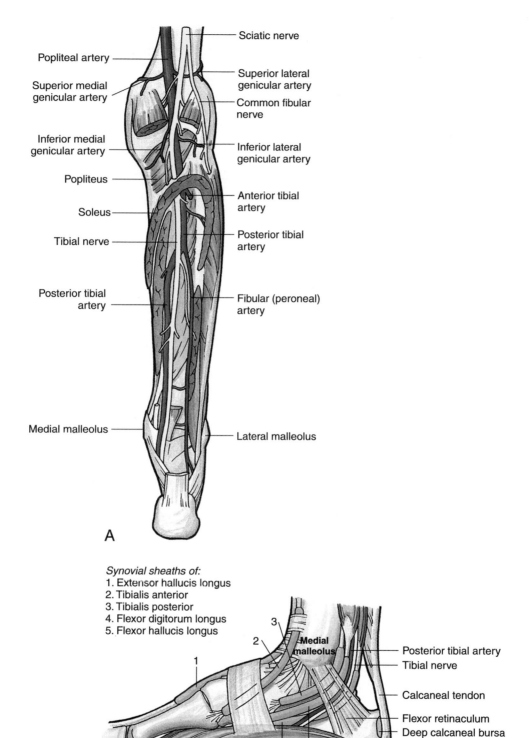

FIGURE 6.24 **Posterior leg and foot. A.** Deep dissection. Most of the soleus is cut away. **B.** Retinacula and synovial sheaths of the tendons at the ankle. Medial view.

TABLE 6.10.   MUSCLES OF POSTERIOR LEG

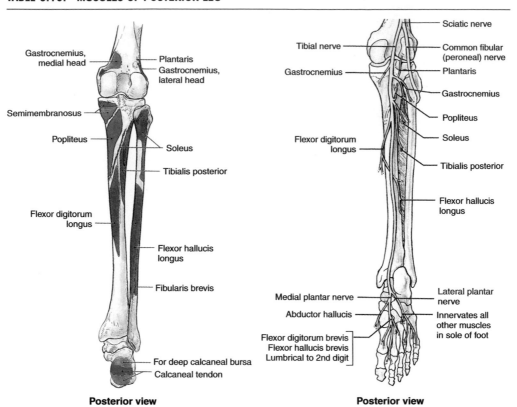

Posterior view   **Posterior view**

Muscle	Proximal Attachment	Distal Attachment	Innervation	Main Action(s)
Superficial muscle group				
Gastrocnemius	*Lateral head:* lateral aspect of lateral condyle of femur *Medial head:* popliteal surface of femur, superior to medial condyle	Posterior surface of calcaneus via calcaneal tendon (tendo calcaneus)	Tibial nerve (S1 and S2)	Plantarflexes ankle, raises heel during walking, and flexes leg at knee joint
Soleus	Posterior aspect of head of fibula, superior fourth of posterior surface of fibula, soleal line and medial border of tibia			Plantarflexes ankle and steadies leg on foot
Plantaris	Inferior end of lateral supracondylar line of femur and oblique popliteal ligament			Weakly assists gastrocnemius in plantarflexing ankle and flexing knee

Continued

TABLE 6.10. *CONTINUED*

Muscle	Proximal Attachment	Distal Attachment	Innervation	Main Actions
Deep muscle group				
Popliteus	Lateral surface of lateral condyle of femur and lateral meniscus	Posterior surface of tibia, superior to soleal line	Tibial nerve (L4, L5, and S1)	Weakly flexes knee and unlocks it
Flexor hallucis longus	Inferior two thirds of posterior surface of fibula and inferior part of interosseous membrane	Base of distal phalanx of great toe (hallux)	Tibial nerve (**S2** and S3)	Flexes great toe at all joints and plantarflexes ankle; supports medial longitudinal arch of foot
Flexor digitorum longus	Medial part of posterior surface of tibia inferior to soleal line, and by a broad tendon to fibula	Bases of distal phalanges of lateral four digits		Flexes lateral four digits and plantarflexes ankle; supports longitudinal arches of foot
Tibialis posterior	Interosseous membrane, posterior surface of tibia inferior to soleal line, and posterior surface of fibula	Tuberosity of navicular, cuneiform, and cuboid and bases of 2nd, 3rd, and 4th metatarsals	Tibial nerve (L4 and L5)	Plantarflexes ankle and inverts foot

of the leg and the lateral side of the foot. Articular branches of the tibial nerve supply the knee joint and medial calcaneal branches supply the skin of the heel.

INJURY TO TIBIAL NERVE

The tibial nerve is not commonly injured; however, the nerve may be injured by deep lacerations or wounds in the popliteal fossa. *Severance of the tibial nerve produces paralysis of the flexor muscles in the leg and the intrinsic muscles in the sole of the foot.* Persons with a tibial nerve injury cannot plantarflex their ankle or flex their toes. Loss of sensation also occurs on the sole of foot.

The **posterior tibial artery** (Fig. 6.24, Table 6.7), the larger terminal branch of the popliteal artery, **provides the main blood supply to the foot.** It begins at the distal border of

the popliteus and passes deep to the proximal attachment of the soleus. After giving off the **fibular artery,** its largest branch, the posterior tibial artery passes inferomedially on the posterior surface of the tibialis posterior. During its descent, it is accompanied by the tibial nerve and veins. The posterior tibial artery runs posterior to the medial malleolus. Deep to the flexor retinaculum and the origin of the abductor hallucis, the posterior tibial artery divides into *medial* and *lateral plantar arteries.* The **fibular artery**—*the largest branch of the posterior tibial artery*—begins inferior to the distal border of the popliteus (Fig. 6.24*A*). It passes obliquely toward the fibula and then descends along its medial side, usually within the flexor hallucis longus. The fibular artery gives muscular branches to the popliteus and

Surface Anatomy of Leg

The **tibialis anterior** lies superficially and is easily palpable just lateral to the anterior border of the tibia. As the foot is inverted and dorsiflexed, the large **tendon of tibialis anterior** (*6*) can be seen and palpated as it runs distally and medially over the anterior surface of the ankle joint to the medial side of the foot. The *pulse of the dorsal artery of the foot* (dorsalis pedis pulse) can be palpated lateral to the tendon of the tibialis anterior. If the great toe (1st digit) is dorsiflexed, the tendon of the **extensor hallucis longus** (*4*) can be palpated just lateral to the tendon of tibialis anterior. Also observe the **tendons of extensor hallucis brevis** (*1*) and extensor digitorum brevis (*5*). As the other toes are dorsiflexed, the **tendons of extensor digitorum longus** (*3*) can be palpated lateral to the extensor hallucis longus and fol-lowed to the four lateral digits. The **tendon of fibularis tertius** (*2*)—part of the extensor digitorum longus—may also be visible. The **fibularis longus** is subcutaneous throughout its course. The tendons of this muscle and the fibularis brevis are palpable when the foot is everted as they pass around the posterior aspect of the lateral malleolus. The **calcaneal tendon** can be followed easily to its attachment to the posterior part of the calcaneus. The **heads of gastrocnemius** are easily recognizable in the calf. The **soleus** can be palpated deep to and at the sides of the superior part of the calcaneal tendon. The soleus and gastrocnemius are easier to palpate when the foot is plantarflexed and when standing on the toes.

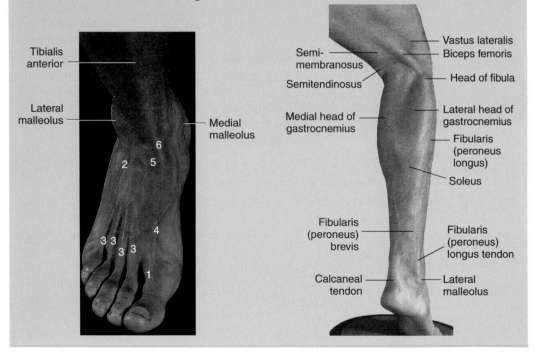

other muscles in the posterior and lateral compartments of the leg. It also supplies a **nutrient artery of the fibula.** The fibular artery usually pierces the interosseous membrane and passes to the dorsum of the foot. The **circumflex fibular artery** usually arises from the posterior tibial artery distal to the knee and passes laterally over the neck of the fibula to join the *genicular anastomosis.* The **nutrient artery of tibia** arises from the posterior tibial artery near its origin. The *calcaneal branches* of the **posterior tibial artery** supply the heel. A *malleolar branch* joins the network of vessels on the medial malleolus.

FOOT

The foot, distal to the leg, supports the weight of the body and has an important role in locomotion. The **foot** comprises the ankle, heel, metatarsus, sole, dorsum of foot, and toes. The **ankle** refers to the region of the ankle joint. The **skeleton of the foot** consists of 7 tarsal bones, 5 metatarsals, and 14 phalanges (Fig. 6.25). *The foot and its bones are divided into three parts:*

- *Hindfoot*—talus and calcaneus
- *Midfoot*—navicular, cuboid, and cuneiforms
- *Forefoot*—metatarsals and phalanges.

DEEP FASCIA OF FOOT

The deep fascia is thin on the dorsum of the foot, where it is continuous with the **inferior extensor retinaculum** (Fig. 6.21*A*). Over the lateral and posterior aspects, the deep fascia

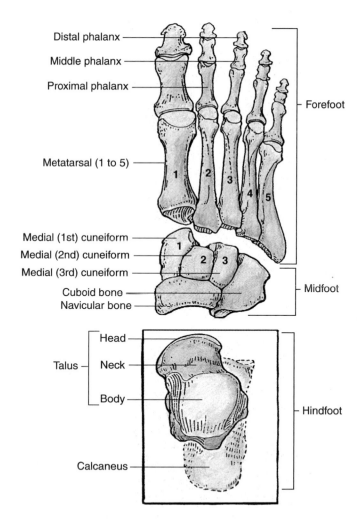

Distal phalanx
Middle phalanx
Proximal phalanx
Forefoot
Metatarsal (1 to 5)
1 2 3 4 5
Medial (1st) cuneiform
Medial (2nd) cuneiform
Medial (3rd) cuneiform
1 2 3
Cuboid bone
Navicular bone
Midfoot
Head
Talus — Neck
Body
Hindfoot
Calcaneus

FIGURE 6.25   Parts of the foot. Dorsal view.

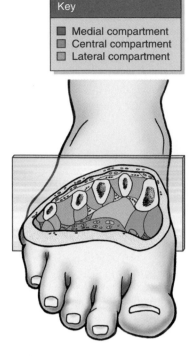

Key

■ Medial compartment
□ Central compartment
□ Lateral compartment

FIGURE 6.26   Compartments of the foot. Transverse section.

- **Central compartment**—containing the flexor digitorum brevis, flexor digitorum longus, quadratus plantae, lumbricals, proximal part of tendon flexor hallucis longus, and lateral plantar nerve and vessels
- **Lateral compartment**—containing the abductor and flexor digiti minimi brevis.

The muscles, nerves, and vessels in the sole are described according to these compartments; however, the muscles are more easily dissected in layers than by compartments.

PLANTAR FASCIITIS

Straining and inflammation of the plantar aponeurosis may result from running and high-impact aerobics, especially when inappropriate footwear such as old shoes are worn. Plantar fasciitis causes pain on the plantar surface of the heel and on the medial aspect of the foot. Point tenderness is located at the proximal attachment of the plantar aponeurosis to the medial tubercle of the calcaneus and on the medial surface of the bone. The pain increases with passive dorsiflexion of the great toe. If a *calcaneal spur* (bony process) protrudes from the medial calcaneal tubercle, the plantar fasciitis may produce the "heel spur syndrome." Usually a bursa develops at the end of the spur, which may become inflamed and tender.

---

of the foot is continuous with the **plantar fascia**—deep fascia of the sole—which has a thick central part—the **plantar aponeurosis**—and weaker medial and lateral parts (see Fig. 6.27A). The plantar fascia:

- Holds parts of the foot together
- Helps protect the plantar surface of the foot from injury
- Helps support the longitudinal arches of the foot—especially its plantar aponeurosis component.

The **plantar aponeurosis** arises posteriorly from the calcaneus and divides into five bands that split to enclose the digital tendons that attach to the margins of the fibrous digital sheaths and the sesamoid bones of the great toe. From the margins of the aponeurosis, vertical septa extend deeply to form *three compartments of the sole of the foot* (Fig. 6.26):

- **Medial compartment**—containing the abductor hallucis, flexor hallucis brevis, and medial plantar nerve and vessels

MUSCLES OF FOOT

The four muscular layers in the sole of the foot (Fig. 6.27) help maintain the arches of the foot and enable one to stand on uneven ground. The muscles are of little importance individually because fine control of the individual toes is not important to most people. In Table 6.11, note that the:

- **P**lantar interossei **ad**duct (**Pad**) and arise from a single metatarsal
- **D**orsal interossei **ab**duct (**Dab**) and arise from two metatarsals.

The *muscles on the dorsum of the foot* are the *extensor digitorum brevis* and *extensor hallucis brevis* (Fig. 6.21). These muscles form a fleshy mass on the lateral part of the dorsum of the foot. The **extensor digitorum brevis** extends digits 2 to 4 at the metatarsophalangeal joints, and the extensor hallucis brevis extends the great toe. The **extensor hallucis brevis** is part of the extensor digitorum brevis. Its small fleshy belly may be felt

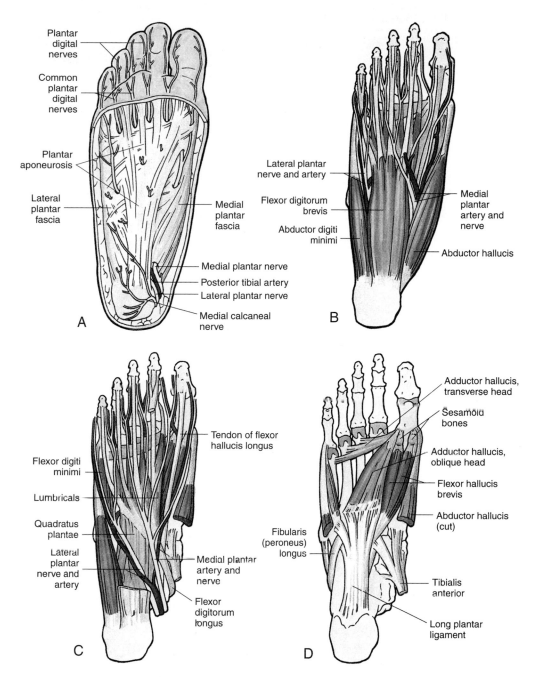

FIGURE 6.27 **Layers of plantar muscles. A.** Superficial dissection of the plantar aponeurosis. **B.** First layer. **C.** Second layer. **D.** Third layer. The fourth layer is not shown but is described in Table 6.11.

TABLE 6.11. MUSCLES IN SOLE OF FOOT

Muscle	Proximal Attachment	Distal Attachment	Innervation	Main Action(s)
First layer				
Abductor hallucis	Medial tubercle of tuberosity of calcaneus, flexor retinaculum, and plantar aponeurosis	Medial side of base of proximal phalanx of 1st digit	Medial plantar nerve (S2 and **S3**)	Abducts and flexes 1st digit (great toe, hallux)
Flexor digitorum brevis	Medial tubercle of tuberosity of calcaneus, plantar aponeurosis, and intermuscular septa	Both sides of middle phalanges of lateral four digits		Flexes lateral four digits
Abductor digiti minimi	Medial and lateral tubercles of tuberosity of calcaneus, plantar aponeurosis, and intermuscular septa	Lateral side of base of proximal phalanx of 5th digit	Lateral plantar nerve (S2 and **S3**)	Abducts and flexes 5th digit
Second layer				
Quadratus plantae	Medial surface and lateral margin of plantar surface of calcaneus	Posterolateral margin of tendon of flexor digitorum longus	Lateral plantar nerve (S2 and **S3**)	Assists flexor digitorum longus in flexing lateral four digits
Lumbricals	Tendons of flexor digitorum longus	Medial aspect of expansion over lateral four digits	*Medial one:* medial plantar nerve (S2 and **S3**) *Lateral three:* lateral plantar nerve (S2 and **S3**)	Flex proximal phalanges and extend middle and distal phalanges of lateral four digits
Third layer				
Flexor hallucis brevis	Plantar surfaces of cuboid and lateral cuneiforms	Both sides of base of proximal phalanx of 1st digit	Medial plantar nerve (S2 and **S3**)	Flexes proximal phalanx of 1st digit
Adductor hallucis	*Oblique head:* bases of metatarsals 2–4 *Transverse head:* plantar ligaments of metatarsophalangeal joints	Tendons of both heads attach to lateral side of base of proximal phalanx of 1st digit	Deep branch of lateral plantar nerve (S2 and **S3**)	Adducts 1st digit; assists in maintaining transverse arch of foot
Flexor digiti minimi brevis	Base of 5th metatarsal	Base of proximal phalanx of 5th digit	Superficial branch of lateral plantar nerve (S2 and **S3**)	Flexes proximal phalanx of 5th digit, thereby assisting with its flexion

Continued

TABLE 6.11. *CONTINUED*

Muscle	Proximal Attachment	Distal Attachment	Innervation	Main Action(s)
Fourth layer				
Plantar interossei (three muscles)	Bases and medial sides of metatarsals 3–5	Medial sides of bases of proximal phalanges of 3rd to 5th digits	Lateral plantar nerve (S2 and **S3**)	Adduct digits (2–4) and flex metatarsophalangeal joints
Dorsal interossei (four muscles)	Adjacent sides of metatarsals 1–5	*First:* medial side of proximal phalanx of 2nd digit *Second to fourth:* lateral sides of 2nd to 4th digits		Abduct digits (2–4) and flex metatarsophalangeal joints

when the toes are extended. Both muscles on the dorsum of the foot help the long extensors to extend the toes.

NERVES OF FOOT

The **tibial nerve** divides posterior to the medial malleolus into the **medial** and **lateral plantar nerves** (Fig. 6.27*C*, see Table 6.13). These nerves supply the intrinsic muscles of the foot except for the extensor digitorum brevis and extensor hallucis brevis, which are supplied by the **deep fibular nerve.** *The cutaneous innervation of the foot is supplied by the:*

- *Saphenous nerve*—medial side of the foot as far as the head of the 1st metatarsal
- *Superficial and deep fibular nerves*—dorsum of the foot
- *Medial and lateral plantar nerves*—sole of the foot
- *Sural nerve*—lateral aspect of the foot, including part of the heel
- *Calcaneal branches of the tibial and sural nerves*—heel.

ARTERIES OF FOOT

The arteries of the foot are terminal branches of the **anterior** and **posterior tibial arteries** (Table 6.12)—the dorsal and plantar arteries, respectively. The **dorsal artery of foot**—the *major source of blood supply to the toes*—is the direct continuation of the anterior tibial artery.

TABLE 6.12. ARTERIAL SUPPLY TO FOOT

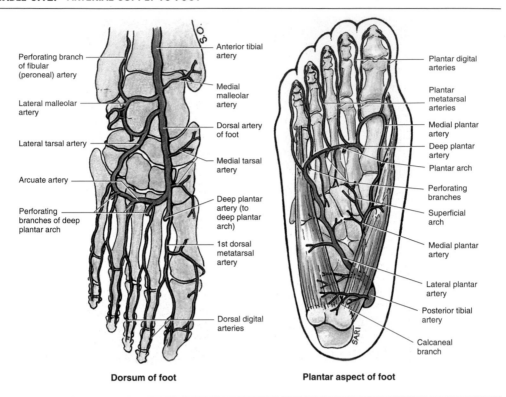

Dorsum of foot   **Plantar aspect of foot**

Artery	Origin	Course and Distribution
Dorsum of Foot		
Dorsal artery of foot (L. dorsalis pedis)	Continuation of anterior tibial artery distal to inferior extensor retinaculum	Descends anteromedially to 1st interosseous space and divides into plantar and arcuate arteries
Lateral tarsal artery		Runs an arched course laterally beneath extensor digitorum brevis to anastomose with branches of arcuate artery
Arcuate artery	Dorsal artery of foot	Runs laterally from 1st interosseous space across bases of lateral four metatarsals, deep to extensor tendons
Deep plantar artery		Passes to sole of foot and joins plantar arch
Metatarsal arteries:		
1st	Deep plantar artery	Run between metatarsals to clefts of toes where each vessel divides into two dorsal digital arteries. Also connected to plantar arch and plantar metatarsal arteries by perforating arteries.
2nd to 4th	Arcuate artery	
Dorsal digital arteries	Metatarsal arteries	Pass to sides of adjoining toes

Continued

TABLE 6.12. *CONTINUED*

Artery	Origin	Course and Distribution
Sole of Foot		
Medial plantar artery	Posterior tibial artery	Runs deep to abductor hallucis and then between it and flexor digitorum brevis
Lateral plantar artery		Runs anterolaterally deep to abductor hallucis and flexor digitorum brevis and then arches medially to form deep plantar arch
Deep plantar arch	Continuation of lateral plantar artery	Begins opposite base of 5th metatarsal and is completed medially by deep plantar artery
Perforating arteries (three)	Deep plantar arch	Pass to dorsum of foot
Plantar metatarsal arteries (four)		
Plantar digital arteries	Plantar metatarsal arteries	Supply toes

The **dorsal artery of foot** begins midway between the malleoli (at the ankle joint) and runs anteromedially, deep to the inferior extensor retinaculum between the extensor hallucis longus and extensor digitorum longus tendons on the dorsum of the foot. The dorsal artery gives off the **lateral tarsal artery** and then passes distally to the 1st interosseous space, where it divides into a **deep plantar artery** and an **arcuate artery** (Table 6.12). The arcuate artery gives off the 2nd, 3rd, and 4th dorsal **metatarsal arteries,** which run to the clefts of the toes, where each of them divides into two **dorsal digital arteries.** The deep plantar artery gives rise to the **1st dorsal metatarsal artery** and then joins the **plantar arch.**

DORSALIS PEDIS PULSE

The *dorsalis pedis pulse*—pulse of dorsal artery of foot or dorsalis pedis artery—is evaluated during a physical examination of the peripheral vascular system. Dorsalis pedis pulses may be palpated with the feet slightly dorsiflexed. The pulses usually are easy to palpate because the arteries are subcutaneous. Some healthy adults—and even children—have *congenitally nonpalpable dorsalis pedis pulses.* In these cases, the dorsal artery is replaced by an enlarged perforating fibular artery. A *diminished or absent dorsalis pedis pulse usually suggests vascular insufficiency resulting from arterial disease. Five "P signs" of acute occlusion are· pain, pallor, paresthesia (tingling), paralysis, and pulselessness.*

There are two neurovascular planes in the sole of the foot:

- A superficial one between the 1st and 2nd muscular layers
- A deep one between the 3rd and 4th muscular layers.

The **lateral plantar artery** and **nerve** course laterally between the muscles of the 1st and 2nd layers of plantar muscles (Fig. 6.27*B*). Their deep branches course medially between the muscles of the 3rd and 4th layers. The **arteries of the sole of foot** derive from the **posterior tibial artery**, which divides deep to the abductor hallucis to form the **medial** and **lateral plantar arteries**. They run parallel to the similarly named nerves. The **deep plantar arch** begins opposite the base of the 5th metatarsal as the continuation of the *lateral plantar artery*, coursing between the 3rd and 4th muscle layers. The arch is completed medially by union with the *medial plantar artery*, a branch of the dorsal ar-

TABLE 6.13. NERVES OF FOOT

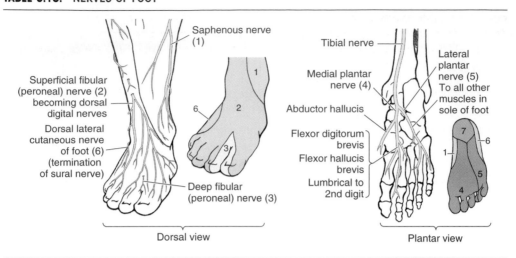

Dorsal view   Plantar view

Nerve	Origin	Course	Distribution in Foot
Saphenous (1)	Femoral nerve	Arises in femoral triangle and descends through thigh and leg; accompanies great saphenous vein anterior to medial malleolus and ends on medial side of foot	Supplies skin on medial side of foot as far anteriorly as head of 1st metatarsal
Superficial fibular (2)	Common fibular (peroneal) nerve	Pierces deep fascia in distal third of leg to become cutaneous and send branches to foot and digits	Supplies skin on dorsum of foot and all digits, except lateral side of 5th and adjoining sides of the 1st and 2nd digits
Deep fibular (3)		Passes deep to extensor retinaculum to enter dorsum of foot	Supplies extensor digitorum brevis and skin on contiguous sides of 1st and 2nd digits
Medial plantar (4)	Larger terminal branch of tibial nerve	Passes distally in foot between abductor hallucis and flexor digitorum brevis and divides into muscular and cutaneous branches	Supplies skin on medial side of sole of foot and sides of first three digits; also supplies abductor hallucis, flexor digitorum brevis, flexor hallucis brevis, and 1st lumbrical nerve
Lateral plantar (5)	Smaller terminal branch of tibial nerve	Passes laterally in foot between quadratus plantae and flexor digitorum brevis muscles and divides into superficial and deep branches	Supplies quadratus plantae, abductor digiti minimi, and flexor digiti minimi brevis; deep branch supplies plantar and dorsal interossei, lateral three lumbricals, and adductor hallucis; supplies skin on sole lateral to a line splitting 4th digit
Sural (6)	Usually arises from both tibial and common fibular nerves	Passes inferior to the lateral malleolus to lateral side of foot	Lateral aspect of foot
Calcaneal branches (7)	Tibial and sural nerves	Pass from distal part of posterior aspect of leg to skin on heel	Skin of heel

tery of the foot. As it crosses the foot, the deep plantar arch gives off four **plantar metatarsal arteries**, and three **perforating arteries** that pass to the dorsum of the foot, and many branches to the skin, fascia, and muscles in the sole of the foot (Table 6.12). These arteries join with the superficial branches of the medial and lateral plantar arteries to form the plantar digital arteries, supplying the adjacent digits.

WOUNDS OF SOLE OF FOOT

Wounds of the sole of the foot involving the plantar arch and its branches usually result in severe bleeding. Ligature of the arch is difficult because of its depth and the structures surrounding it.

VENOUS DRAINAGE OF FOOT

Dorsal digital veins running along the dorsum of each toe are continuous with the **dorsal metatarsal veins,** which join to form the **dorsal venous arch** in the subcutaneous tissue (p. 331). The dorsal arch communicates with the **plantar venous arch.** Veins converge toward the dorsal arch, which flows mainly toward the medial aspect of the foot to form the **great saphenous vein;** however, some veins flow laterally to form the **small saphenous vein.** The superficial veins of the sole unite to form a *plantar venous network* draining mainly into the **plantar venous network.** The deep veins of the sole begin as **plantar digital veins** on the plantar aspects of the digits. These veins communicate with the **dorsal digital veins** through perforating veins. Most blood from the foot returns through the deep veins that accompany the arteries.

LYMPHATIC DRAINAGE OF FOOT

The lymphatics of the foot begin in *subcutaneous plexuses* (p. 332). The collecting vessels consist of superficial and deep lymphatic vessels that follow the veins. Superficial lymphatic vessels are most numerous in the sole. They leave the foot medially along the *great saphenous vein* and laterally along the *small saphenous vein.* The vessels converging on the great saphenous vein accompany it to the inferior group of **superficial inguinal lymph nodes,** located along the termination of the great saphenous vein (p. 330). The superficial in-

guinal nodes drain in turn, mainly into the **external iliac lymph nodes** (Fig. 6.17*B*), but some nodes drain first into the deep inguinal nodes.

JOINTS OF LOWER LIMB

The joints of the lower limb include the joints of the pelvic girdle, lumbosacral joints, sacroiliac joints, and pubic symphysis, which are discussed in Chapter 4. The remaining joints of the lower limb are the hip joint, knee joint, tibiofibular joints, ankle joint, and foot joints.

HIP JOINT

The hip joint forms the connection between the lower limb and pelvic girdle. *It is a strong and stable multiaxial ball-and-socket type of synovial joint*—the femoral head is the ball and the acetabulum is the socket (Fig. 6.28). The hip joint is designed for stability as well as for a wide range of movement. During standing, the entire weight of the upper body is transmitted through the hip bones to the heads and necks of the femurs. The hip joint is mechanically most stable when a person is bearing weight—when carrying a heavy object, for example.

Articular Surfaces

The head of the femur articulates with the cuplike acetabulum of the hip bone. Because the depth of the acetabulum is increased by the fibrocartilaginous **acetabular labrum** (L. lip) and the **transverse acetabular ligament** (bridging the *acetabular notch*), more than half of the head fits within the acetabulum (Figs. 6.28 and 6.29). The acetabular labrum and transverse ligament "grasp" the femoral head. The head is covered with **articular cartilage,** except for the fovea (pit) for the ligament of the femoral head. The central and inferior part of the acetabulum, the **acetabular fossa** (Fig. 6.29), is thin, nonarticular, and often translucent.

Articular Capsule

The **fibrous part of the articular capsule** (fibrous capsule) permits free movement of the

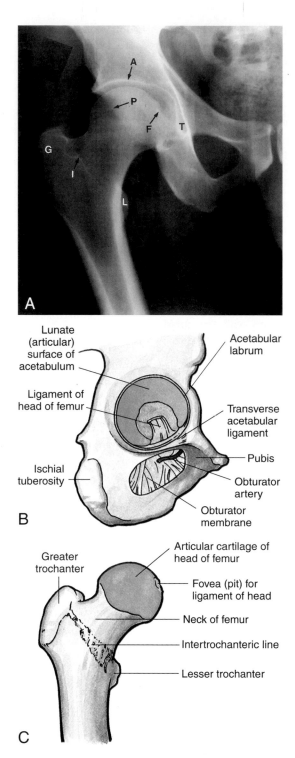

FIGURE 6.28   Articular surfaces of the hip joint. A. Radiograph. *A,* roof; *P,* posterior rim of the acetabulum; *F,* fovea (pit) for the ligament of the femoral head; *T,* "teardrop" appearance caused by superimposition of structures at the inferior margin of the acetabulum; *G,* greater trochanter; *I,* intertrochanteric crest; *L,* lesser trochanter. **B.** Hip bone and associated structures. Lateral view. **C.** Proximal femur. Anterior view.

joint. *The strong fibrous capsule* (Figs. 6.28 and 6.29):

- Attaches proximally to the *acetabulum* and transverse acetabular ligament
- Attaches distally to the *neck of the femur*
- Attaches anteriorly to the *intertrochanteric line* and the root of the greater trochanter
- Crosses to the femoral neck posteriorly— proximal to the *intertrochanteric crest*— but is not attached to it.

Most capsular fibers take a spiral course from the hip bone to the intertrochanteric line, with some deep fibers winding circularly around the neck, forming an **orbicular zone** (Fig. 6.29). These fibers form a collar that constricts the capsule and helps draw (screw) the femoral head tightly into the acetabulum during extension. Thick parts of the fibrous capsule form the ligaments of the hip joint (Fig. 6.30), which pass in a spiral fashion from the pelvis to the femur.

The **ligaments of the hip joint** are as follows:

- The fibrous capsule is reinforced anteriorly by the strong Y-shaped **iliofemoral ligament,** which attaches to the anterior inferior iliac spine and acetabular rim proximally and the intertrochanteric line distally. *The iliofemoral ligament prevents hyperextension of the hip joint during standing by screwing the femoral head into the acetabulum.*

- The fibrous capsule is reinforced inferiorly and anteriorly by the **pubofemoral ligament** that arises from the obturator crest of the pubic bone and passes laterally and inferiorly to merge with the fibrous capsule of the hip joint. This ligament blends with the medial part of the iliofemoral ligament and tightens during extension and abduction of the hip joint. *The pubofemoral ligament prevents overabduction of the hip joint.*

- The fibrous capsule is reinforced posteriorly by the **ischiofemoral ligament,** which arises from the ischial part of the acetabular rim and spirals superolaterally to the neck of the femur, medial to the base of the greater trochanter. *The ischiofemoral ligament, like the iliofemoral ligament, tends to screw the femoral head medially into the acetabulum, preventing hyperextension of the hip joint.*

The **synovial membrane of hip joint** (Fig. 6.29) lines the fibrous capsule and covers the:

- Neck of the femur between the attachment of the fibrous capsule and the edge of the articular cartilage of the head. Part of the deep portion of the synovial membrane forms **retinacular folds,** which reflect superiorly along the femoral neck as longitudinal bands. The folds contain retinacular blood vessels (branches of the medial [and a few from the lateral] femoral circumflex artery) that supply the head and neck of the femur.

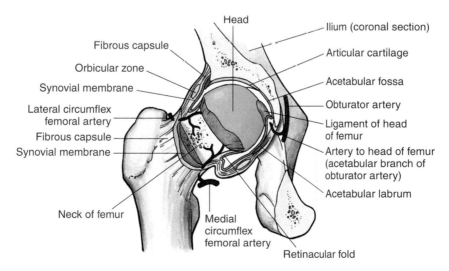

FIGURE 6.29   Blood supply of the head and neck of the femur. Anterior view. A section of bone has been removed from the femoral neck.

- Nonarticular area of the acetabulum, providing a covering for the ligament of the head of the femur.

A *synovial protrusion* beyond the free posterior margin of the fibrous capsule onto the femoral neck forms a *bursa for the obturator externus tendon*. The **ligament of head of femur** (Figs. 6.28 and 6.29) is weak and of little importance in strengthening the hip joint. Its wide end attaches to the margins of the acetabular notch and the transverse acetabular ligament; its narrow end attaches to the fovea (pit) in the femoral head. Usually the ligament contains a small **artery to head of femur.**

Hip Movements

Hip movements are flexion-extension, abduction-adduction, medial-lateral rotation, and

circumduction. Movements of the trunk at the hip joints are also important, such as those occurring when a person lifts the trunk from the supine position during sit-ups, for example. The degree of **flexion and extension** of the hip joint depends on the position of the knee. If the knee is flexed relaxing the hamstrings, the thigh can be more easily moved toward the anterior abdominal wall. Not all this movement occurs at the hip joint; some results from flexion of the vertebral column. **Abduction** of the hip joint is usually somewhat freer than adduction. **Rotation** of the hip joint can be carried through approximately one sixth of a circle when the thigh is extended and more when it is flexed. Lateral rotation is much more powerful than medial rotation. Muscles producing movements of the hip joint are illustrated in Figure 6.31. Structures limiting movement of the hip joint are summarized in Table 6.14.

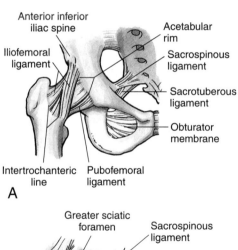
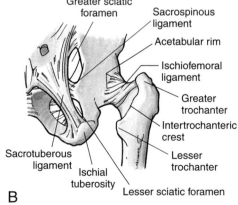

FIGURE 6.30   Ligaments of the pelvis and hip joint. A. Anterior view. **B.** Posterior view.

Blood Supply

The arteries supplying the hip joint (Fig. 6.29) *are the:*

- Medial and lateral **circumflex femoral arteries**—usually branches of the *deep artery of thigh* but occasionally branches of the femoral artery; the main blood supply is from the circumflex femoral arteries (especially the *medial circumflex femoral artery*) that travel in the retinacular folds.
- **Artery to head of femur,** a branch of the obturator artery.

Nerve Supply

The nerve supply of the hip joint is from the:

- *Femoral nerve* or its muscular branches (anteriorly)
- *Accessory obturator nerve,* if present (anteriorly)
- *Obturator nerve*—anterior division (inferiorly)
- *Superior gluteal nerve* (superiorly and posteriorly)
- *Nerve to quadratus femoris* (posteriorly).

Functional groups of muscles
acting at hip joint

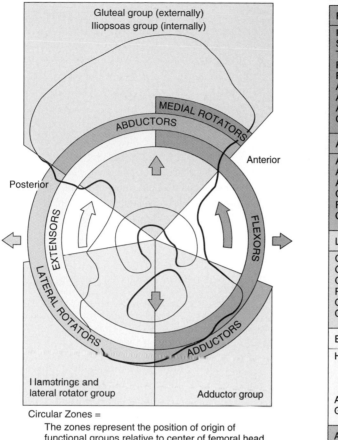

Flexors		
Iliopsoas		
Sartorius		
Tensor of fascia lata		
Rectus femoris		
Pectineus		
Adductor longus		
Adductor brevis		
Adductor magnus/anterior part		
Gracilis		
Adductors		
Adductor longus		
Adductor brevis		
Adductor magnus		
Gracilis		
Pectineus		
Obturator externus		
Lateral rotators		
Obturator externus		
Obturator internus		
Gemelli		
Piriformis		
Quadratus femoris		
Gluteus maximus		
Extensors		
Hamstrings:		
Semitendinosus		
Semimembranosus		
Long head, biceps femoris		
Adductor magnus/posterior part		
Gluteus maximus		
Abductors		
Gluteus medius		
Gluteus minimus		
Tensor of fascia lata		
Medial rotators		
Gluteus medius ⎫		
Gluteus minimus ⎬ Anterior parts		
Tensor of fascia lata ⎭		

Circular Zones =
The zones represent the position of origin of functional groups relative to center of femoral head in acetabulum (point of rotation). Pull is applied on the femur (femoral trochanters or shaft) from these positions.

Colored Arrows =
The arrows show the direction of rotation of femoral head caused by activity of functional groups.

FIGURE 6.31   Diagrammatic lateral view of the hip joint. Illustration shows the relative positions of muscles producing movements of the joint and the direction of the movement.

FRACTURE OF FEMORAL NECK
Fracture of the femoral neck often disrupts the blood supply to the femoral head. The medial circumflex femoral artery is clinically important because it supplies most of the blood to the head and neck of the femur. Its retinacular branches often are torn when the femoral neck is fractured or the hip joint is dislocated. In some cases the blood supplied to the femoral head through the artery in the ligament of the head may be the only blood received by the proximal fragment of the femoral head. If the blood vessels are ruptured, the fragment of bone may receive no blood or an inadequate amount and undergo *aseptic necrosis.*

Dislocation of Hip Joint
Acquired dislocation of the hip joint is uncommon because this articulation is so strong and stable. Nevertheless, dislocation may occur during an automobile accident, for example, when the hip is flexed, adducted, and medially

TABLE 6.14. STRUCTURES LIMITING MOVEMENTS OF HIP JOINT

Movement	Limiting Structures
Flexion	Soft tissue apposition Tension of articular capsule posteriorly Tension of gluteus maximus
Extension	Ligaments: iliofemoral, ischiofemoral, and pubofemoral Tension of iliopsoas
Abduction	Ligaments: pubofemoral, ischiofemoral, and inferior band of iliofemoral Tension of hip adductors
Adduction	Soft tissue apposition (thighs) Tension of iliotibial band, superior articular capsule, superior band of iliofemoral ligament, and hip abductors (especially when contralateral hip joint is abducted or flexed)
Internal rotation	Ligaments: ischiofemoral and posterior articular capsule Tension of external rotators of hip joint
External rotation	Ligaments: iliofemoral, pubofemoral, and anterior articular capsule Tension of medial rotators of hip joint

Modified from Clarkson HM: *Musculoskeletal Assessment. Joint Range of Motion and Manual of Muscle Strength,* 2nd ed. Baltimore: Lippincott Williams & Wilkins 2000.

Continued

rotated—often the position of the lower limb when a person is in a car. Posterior dislocations are most common. The fibrous capsule ruptures inferiorly and posteriorly, allowing the femoral head to pass through the tear in the capsule and over the posterior margin of the acetabulum onto the lateral surface of the ilium, shortening and medially rotating the affected limb.

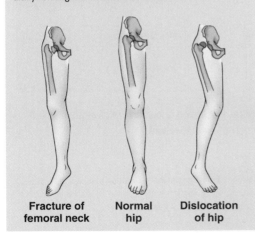

Fracture of femoral neck   Normal hip   Dislocation of hip

KNEE JOINT

The knee is primarily a *hinge type of synovial joint* allowing flexion and extension; however, the hinge movements are combined with gliding and rolling and with rotation about a vertical axis. Although the knee joint is well constructed, its function is commonly impaired when it is hyperextended (e.g., in body contact sports such as hockey).

Articular Surfaces

The articular surfaces of the knee joint are characterized by their large size and their complicated and incongruent shapes (Fig. 6.32). The femur slants medially at the knee, whereas the tibia is almost vertical. *The knee joint consists of three articulations:*

- Lateral and medial articulations between the femoral and tibial condyles
- Intermediate articulation between the patella and femur.

The stability of the knee joint (Fig. 6.33) *depends on the:*

- Strength and actions of surrounding muscles and their tendons
- Ligaments connecting the femur and tibia.

Of these supports, the muscles are most important; therefore, many sport injuries are preventable through appropriate conditioning and training. *The most important muscle in stabilizing the knee joint is the large quadriceps femoris,* particularly inferior fibers of the vastus medialis and lateralis.

Articular Capsule

The articular capsule of the knee joint is thin and is deficient in some areas. The strong fibrous part of the articular capsule—the **fibrous capsule** (Fig. 6.33*A*)—attaches to the femur superiorly, just proximal to the articular margins of the condyles and also to the **intercondylar fossa** posteriorly (Fig. 6.32*B*). The fibrous capsule is deficient on the lateral condyle to allow the popliteus tendon to pass out of the joint to attach to the tibia. Inferiorly, the fibrous capsule attaches to the articular margin of the tibia, except where the popliteus tendon crosses the bone. The

patella and **patellar ligament** serve as a capsule anteriorly (Fig. 6.33*A*). The extensive **synovial membrane** lines the internal aspect of the fibrous capsule and attaches to the periphery of the patella and the edges of the **menisci.** The synovial membrane reflects from the posterior aspect of the joint onto the **cruciate ligaments.** The reflection of the membrane between the tibia and patella covers the **infrapatellar fat pad.** The synovial membrane covering the fat pad and cruciate ligaments excludes them from the joint cavity (Fig. 6.33*A*). The knee joint cavity extends superior to the patella and deep to the quadriceps muscle as the **suprapatellar bursa.**

Ligaments

The fibrous capsule of the knee joint is strengthened by five extracapsular ligaments (Fig. 6.33):

* Patellar ligament
* Fibular collateral ligament

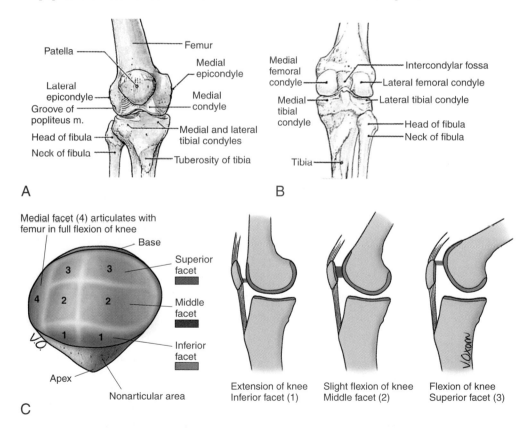

FIGURE 6.32   Bones of the right knee joint. A. Anterior view. **B.** Posterior view. **C.** Patella. Posterior view. Position of the patella during knee movements.

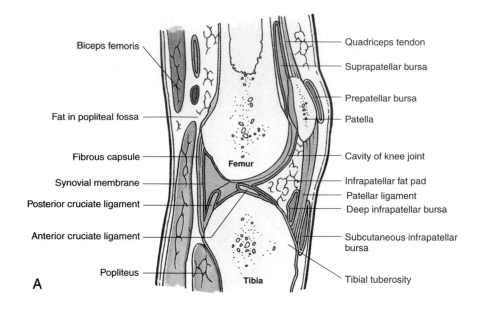

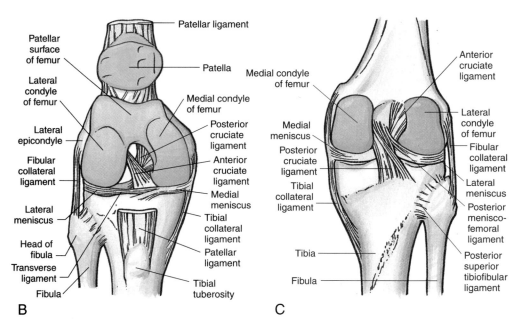

FIGURE 6.33 **Relations and ligaments of the knee joint. A.** Sagittal section. **B.** Anterior view. **C.** Posterior view.

- Tibial collateral ligament
- Oblique popliteal ligament
- Arcuate popliteal ligament.

The **patellar ligament,** the distal part of the quadriceps tendon, is a strong, thick fibrous band passing from the apex and adjoining mar-

gins of the patella to the **tibial tuberosity.** The **fibular collateral ligament,** rounded and cordlike, is strong. It extends inferiorly from the **lateral epicondyle of femur** to the lateral surface of the head of the fibula (Fig. 6.33, *B* and *C*). *The tendon of the popliteus passes deep to the fibular collateral ligament, separating it from* *the lateral meniscus.* The tendon of the biceps femoris is also split into two parts by this ligament. The **tibial collateral ligament** is a strong flat band that extends from the **medial epicondyle of femur** to the medial condyle and superior part of the medial surface of the tibia. *At its midpoint, the deep fibers of the tibial collateral ligament are firmly attached to the medial meniscus.* The **oblique popliteal ligament** (Fig. 6.16*C*) is a reflected expansion of the tendon of the semimembranosus that strengthens the fibrous capsule posteriorly. It arises posterior to the medial tibial condyle and passes superolaterally to attach to the central part of the posterior aspect of the fibrous capsule. The **arcuate popliteal ligament** (Fig. 6.23*D*) strengthens the fibrous capsule posteriorly. It arises from the posterior aspect of the fibular head, passes superomedially over the tendon of the popliteus, and spreads over the posterior surface of the knee joint.

The *intra-articular ligaments* within the knee joint consist of the *cruciate ligaments* and *menisci* (semilunar cartilages). The popliteus tendon is also intra-articular during part of its course. The **cruciate ligaments** (L. crux, a cross) *join the femur and tibia,* criss-crossing within the articular capsule of the joint but outside the synovial joint cavity (Figs. 6.33 and 6.34). The cruciate ligaments cross each other obliquely like the letter X, providing stability to the joint. The **anterior cruciate ligament** (ACL), the weaker of the two cruciate ligaments, arises from the anterior intercondylar area of the tibia, just posterior to the attachment of the medial meniscus. It extends superiorly, posteriorly, and laterally to attach to the posterior part of the medial side of the lateral condyle of the femur. The **ACL** has a relatively poor blood supply. It is slack when the knee is flexed and taut when it is fully extended, preventing posterior displacement of the femur on the tibia and hyperextension of the knee joint. When the joint is flexed at a right angle, the tibia cannot be pulled anteriorly because it is held by the ACL. The **posterior cruciate ligament** (PCL), the stronger of the two cruciate ligaments, arises from the posterior intercondylar area of the tibia. The **PCL** passes superiorly and anteriorly on the medial side of

the ACL to attach to the anterior part of the lateral surface of the medial condyle of the femur (Fig. 6.33*B*). The PCL tightens during flexion of the knee joint, preventing anterior displacement of the femur on the tibia or posterior displacement of the tibia on the femur. The PCL also helps prevent hyperflexion of the knee joint. In the weight-bearing flexed knee, the PCL is the main stabilizing factor for the femur (e.g., when walking downhill).

The **menisci of knee joint** are crescentic plates of fibrocartilage on the articular surface of the tibia that provide increased congruity for the articulating surface of the femoral condyles, which may act as shock absorbers (Fig. 6.35). The menisci are thicker at their external margins and taper to thin, unattached

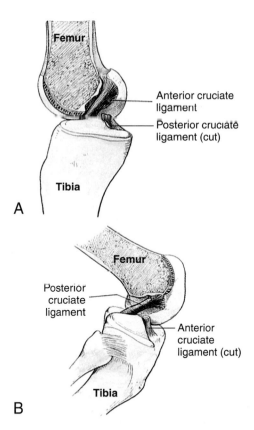

FIGURE 6.34 Cruciate ligaments of the knee joint. In each drawing, the femur has been sectioned longitudinally and the near half has been removed with the proximal part of the corresponding cruciate ligament. **A.** Anterior cruciate ligament. **B.** Posterior cruciate ligament.

edges in the interior of the joint. Wedge-shaped in transverse section, the menisci are firmly attached at their ends to the intercondylar area of the tibia. Their external margins attach to the fibrous capsule of the knee joint. The *coronary ligaments* are capsular fibers that attach the margins of the menisci to the tibial condyles. A slender fibrous band, the **transverse ligament of knee,** joins the anterior edges of the menisci (Fig. 6.35A), allowing them to move together during knee movements. The **medial meniscus** is C-shaped and broader posteriorly than anteriorly. Its ante-

rior end attaches to the anterior intercondylar area of the tibia, anterior to the attachment of the ACL. Its posterior end attaches to the posterior intercondylar area, anterior to the attachment of the PCL. *The medial meniscus firmly adheres to the deep surface of the tibial collateral ligament.* The **lateral meniscus** is nearly circular and is smaller and more freely movable than the medial meniscus. The tendon of the popliteus separates the lateral meniscus from the fibular collateral ligament. A strong tendinous slip, the **posterior meniscofemoral ligament,** joins the lateral meniscus to the PCL and the medial femoral condyle (Fig. 6.33C).

Knee Movements

Flexion and extension are the main knee movements; some rotation occurs when the knee is flexed. When the leg is fully extended with the foot on the ground, the knee "locks" because of medial rotation of the femur on the tibia. This position makes the lower limb a solid column and more adapted for weight-bearing. When the knee is "locked," the thigh and leg muscles can relax briefly without making the knee joint too unstable. To "unlock" the knee the popliteus contracts, rotating the femur laterally so that flexion of the knee can occur. The structures limiting movement of the knee are summarized in Table 6.15. *The main movements of the knee joint and the muscles producing them are:*

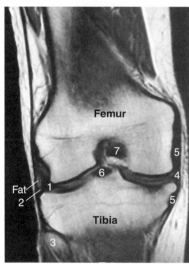

- *Flexion*—principally by the hamstrings but also by the gastrocnemius—movement is limited by contact between the calf and thigh
- *Rotation*—increasingly possible as the knee is flexed toward 60°
- *Medial rotation*—popliteus, semitendinosus, and slightly by semimembranosus—movement is checked by the cruciate ligaments
- *Lateral rotation*—biceps femoris—movement is checked as the collateral ligaments become taut
- *Extension*—principally by quadriceps—movement is limited as the cruciate and collateral ligaments become taut.

FIGURE 6.35 Cruciate ligaments and menisci of the knee joint. A. Superior view of the tibial plateau. The patella and quadriceps tendon are transected and the patellar fragment and patellar ligament are reflected anteriorly. **B.** Coronal MRI of the right knee. The numbers on the MRI refer to structures labelled in **A.**

KNEE JOINT INJURIES

Knee joint injuries are common because the knee is a mobile weight-bearing joint and its stability depends almost entirely on its associated ligaments and muscles. The knee joint is a main joint for sports that involve running, jumping, kicking, and changing directions. To perform these activities, the knee joint must be mobile; however, this mobility makes it susceptible to injuries. *The most common knee injuries in contact sports are ligament sprains,* which occur when the foot is fixed (e.g., in the ground). If a force is applied against the knee when the foot cannot move, ligament injuries may occur. The tibial and fibular collateral ligaments normally prevent disruption of the sides of the knee joint. They are tightly stretched when the leg is extended and thus usually prevent rotation of the tibia laterally or the femur medially.

Because the collateral ligaments are slack during flexion of the leg, they permit some rotation of the tibia on the femur in this position.

The firm attachment of the tibial collateral ligament to the medial meniscus is of considerable clinical significance because tearing of the tibial collateral ligament frequently results in concomitant tearing of the medial meniscus. The damage is frequently caused by a blow to the lateral side of the knee. Injury to the medial meniscus results from a twisting strain that is applied to the knee joint when it is flexed. Because the meniscus is firmly adherent to the tibial collateral ligament, twisting strains of this ligament may tear and/or detach the medial meniscus from the fibrous capsule. This injury is common in athletes who twist their flexed knees while running (e.g., in football and soccer). The ACL may tear when the tibial collateral ligament ruptures. First, the tibial collateral ligament ruptures, opening the joint on the medial side and possibly tearing the medial meniscus and ACL. Severe force directed anteriorly with the knee semiflexed may also tear the ACL, resulting in the "unhappy triad" of knee injuries (**A**). **ACL rupture,** one of the most common knee injuries in skiing accidents, for example, allows the tibia to slide anteriorly from the femur—*the anterior drawer sign* (**B**). Although strong, **PCL rupture** may occur when a person lands on the tibial tuberosity with the knee flexed (e.g., when falling on the floor in basketball). PCL ruptures usually occur in conjunction with tibial or fibular ligament tears.

These injuries also can occur in head-on collisions when seatbelts are not worn and the proximal end of the tibia strikes the dashboard. PCL ruptures allow the tibia to slide posteriorly from the femur—*the posterior drawer sign* (**C**).

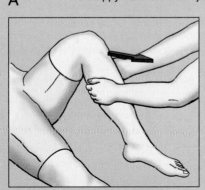

Anterior cruciate ligament (torn)

Tibial collateral ligament (torn)

Medial meniscus (torn)

A "Unhappy triad" of knee injuries

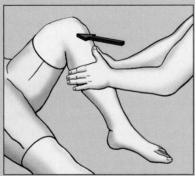

B. Anterior drawer sign (ACL)

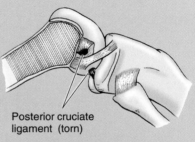

Half of bone is removed to show ligaments

Anterior cruciate ligament (torn)

The anterior cruciate ligament (**ACL**) prevents the femur from sliding posteriorly on the tibia and hyperextension of the knee and limits medial rotation of the femur when the foot is on the ground, and the leg is flexed.

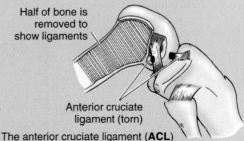

Posterior cruciate ligament (torn)

The posterior cruciate ligament (**PCL**) prevents the femur from sliding anteriorly on the tibia, particularly when the knee is flexed.

C. Posterior drawer sign (PCL)

TABLE 6.15. STRUCTURES LIMITING MOVEMENTS OF KNEE JOINT

Movement	Limiting Structures
Flexion (femoropatellar and femorotibial)	Soft tissue apposition posteriorly Tension of vastus lateralis, medialis, and intermedius Tension of rectus femoris (especially with hip joint extended)
Extension (femoropatellar and femorotibial)	*Ligaments:* anterior and posterior cruciates, fibular and tibial collateral, posterior articular capsule, and oblique popliteal ligament
Internal rotation (femorotibial with knee flexed)	*Ligaments:* anterior and posterior cruciates
External rotation (femorotibial with knee flexed)	*Ligaments:* fibular and tibial collateral

Modified from Clarkson HM: *Musculoskeletal Assessment. Joint Range of Motion and Manual of Muscle Strength,* 2nd ed. Baltimore: Lippincott Williams & Wilkins 2000.

Bursae Around Knee

Many bursae are located around the knee joint (Table 6.16) because most tendons run parallel to the bones and pull lengthwise across the joint during knee movements. Subcutaneous bursae—**prepatellar and infrapatellar bursae**—are also at the convex surface of the joint because the skin must be able to move freely during knee movements. *Four bursae communicate with the synovial cavity of the knee joint: suprapatellar bursa, popliteus bursa, anserine bursa,* and *gastrocnemius bursa* (Table 6.16).

Bursitis in Knee Region

The suprapatellar bursa communicates with the knee joint cavity; consequently, abrasions or penetrating wounds (e.g., a stab wound) superior to the patella may result in *suprapatellar bursitis* caused by bacteria entering the bursa from the torn skin. The infection may spread to the knee joint. *Prepatellar bursitis* is usually a friction bursitis caused by friction between the skin and patella. If the inflammation is chronic, the bursa becomes distended with fluid and forms a swelling ("housemaid's knee") anterior to the knee. *Subcutaneous infrapatellar bursitis* results from excessive friction between the skin and tibial tuberosity; the edema occurs over the proximal end of the tibia. *Deep infrapatellar bursitis* results in edema between the patellar ligament and tibia, superior to the tibial tuberosity.

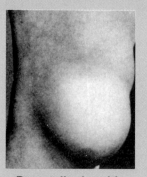

Prepatellar bursitis

Arteries and Nerves

The **arteries supplying the knee joint** are genicular branches of the femoral, popliteal, and anterior and posterior recurrent branches of the anterior tibial recurrent and circumflex fibular arteries, which form the **genicular anastomosis** around the knee joint (Table 6.7). The middle genicular branches of the popliteal artery penetrate the fibrous capsule of the joint and supply the cruciate ligaments, synovial membrane, and peripheral margins of the menisci. The **nerves of the knee joint** are branches of the obturator, femoral, tibial, and common fibular nerves (Table. 6.8).

TIBIOFIBULAR JOINTS

The tibia and fibula are connected by two joints: the proximal tibiofibular joint and the distal tibiofibular joint. In addition, an **interosseous membrane** joins the shafts of the bones (Fig. 6.36). Movement at the proximal joint is impossible without movement at the distal one. The **proximal tibiofibular joint** is a plane type of synovial joint between the fibular head and the lateral tibial condyle. The flat facet on the fibular head articulates with

TABLE 6.16. BURSAE AROUND KNEE

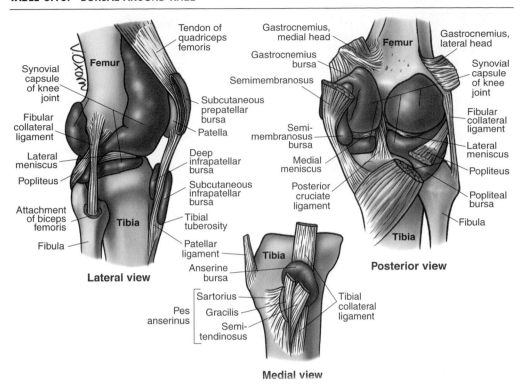

Bursae	Locations	Comments
Suprapatellar	Between femur and tendon of quadriceps femoris	Held in position by articular muscle of knee; communicates freely with synovial cavity of knee joint
Popliteus	Between tendon of popliteus and lateral condyle of tibia	Opens into synovial cavity of knee joint, inferior to lateral meniscus
Anserine	Separates tendons of sartorius, gracilis, and semitendinosus from tibia and tibial collateral ligament	Area where tendons of these muscles attach to tibia resembles the foot of a goose (L. pes, foot; L. anser, goose)
Gastrocnemius	Lies deep to proximal attachment of tendon of medial head of gastrocnemius	This bursa is an extension of synovial cavity of knee joint
Semimembranosus	Located between medial head of gastrocnemius and semimembranosus tendon	Related to the distal attachment of semimembranosus
Subcutaneous prepatellar	Lies between skin and anterior surface of patella	Allows free movement of skin over patella during movements of leg
Subcutaneous infrapatellar	Located between skin and tibial tuberosity	Helps knee to withstand pressure when kneeling
Deep infrapatellar	Lies between patellar ligament and anterior surface of tibia	Separated from knee joint by infrapatellar fatpad

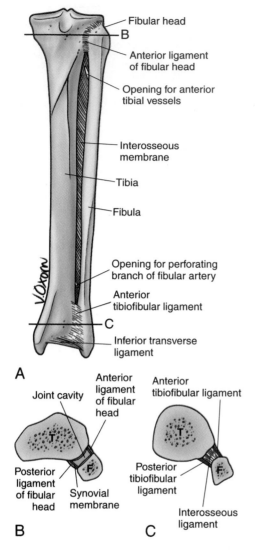

A

B

C

FIGURE 6.36 **Tibiofibular joints. A.** Anterior view. **B.** Proximal tibiofibular joint. Transverse section. **C.** Distal tibiofibular joint. Transverse section. *F,* fibula; *T,* tibia.

a similar facet located posterolaterally on the lateral tibial condyle. The *fibrous capsule* surrounds the joint and attaches to the margins of the articular surfaces of the fibula and tibia. The fibrous capsule is strengthened by **anterior** and **posterior ligaments of fibular head.** The *synovial membrane* lines the fibrous capsule. *Slight gliding movements of the proximal tibiofibular joint* occur during dorsiflexion and plantarflexion of the foot. The **arteries of proximal tibiofibular joint** are

from the inferior lateral genicular and anterior tibial recurrent arteries (Table 6.7). The **nerves of proximal tibiofibular joint** are from the common fibular nerve and the nerve to the popliteus.

The **distal tibiofibular joint** is a fibrous joint (syndesmosis). The integrity of this articulation is essential for stability of the ankle joint because it keeps the lateral malleolus firmly against the lateral surface of the talus. The rough, triangular articular area on the medial surface of the inferior end of the fibula articulates with a facet on the inferior end of the tibia (Fig. 6.36). The strong **interosseous ligament** is continuous superiorly with the **interosseous membrane** and forms the principal connection between the distal ends of the tibia and fibula. The joint is also strengthened anteriorly and posteriorly by strong **anterior** and **posterior tibiofibular ligaments.** The distal, deep continuation of the posterior tibiofibular ligament—**inferior transverse ligament**—forms a strong connection between the distal ends of the tibia (medial malleolus) and fibula (lateral malleolus). Slight movement of the distal tibiofibular joint occurs to accommodate the talus during dorsiflexion of the foot. The **arteries of distal tibiofibular joint** are from the perforating branch of the fibular artery (Table 6.7) and from medial malleolar branches of the anterior and posterior tibial arteries. The **nerves of distal tibiofibular joint** are from the deep fibular, tibial, and saphenous nerves.

ANKLE JOINT

The ankle joint (talocrural) articulation is a *hinge type of synovial joint.* It is located between the distal ends of the tibia and fibula and the superior part of the talus (Fig. 6.37).

Articular Surfaces

The inferior ends of the tibia and fibula (along with the inferior transverse ligament) form a *mortise* (deep socket) into which the pulley-shaped **trochlea of talus** fits. The trochlea (L. pulley) is the rounded superior articular surface of the talus. The medial surface of the lateral malleolus articulates with the lateral surface of the talus. *The tibia articulates with the talus in two places:*

- Its inferior surface forms the roof of the mortise (deep socket)
- Its medial malleolus articulates with the medial surface of the talus.

The malleoli grip the talus tightly as it rocks anteriorly and posteriorly in the mortise during movements of the ankle joint. The grip of the malleoli is strongest during dorsiflexion of the foot because this movement forces the wider, anterior part of the trochlea posteriorly, spreading the tibia and fibula slightly apart. This spreading is limited by the strong **interosseous ligament** and the **tibiofibular ligaments** that unite the tibia and fibula (Fig. 6.38). *The ankle joint is relatively unstable during plantarflexion because the trochlea is narrower posteriorly and therefore lies loosely within the mortise.*

Articular Capsule

The *fibrous capsule of the ankle joint* is thin anteriorly and posteriorly but is supported on each side by strong ligaments. It is attached proximally to the borders of the tibial and malleolar articular surfaces and distally to the talus. The *synovial membrane* lining the fibrous capsule ascends as a short vertical recess between the tibia and fibula.

Ligaments

The fibrous capsule is reinforced laterally by the **lateral ligament,** which consists of three parts (Fig. 6.38*A*):

- **Anterior talofibular ligament**—a flat, weak band that extends anteromedially from the lateral malleolus to the neck of the talus
- **Posterior talofibular ligament**—a thick, fairly strong band that runs horizontally medially and slightly posteriorly from the malleolar fossa of the fibula to the lateral tubercle of the talus
- **Calcaneofibular ligament**—a round cord that passes posteroinferiorly from the tip of the lateral malleolus to the lateral surface of the calcaneus.

The fibrous capsule is reinforced medially by the large, strong **medial ligament** (deltoid ligament) that attaches proximally to the me-

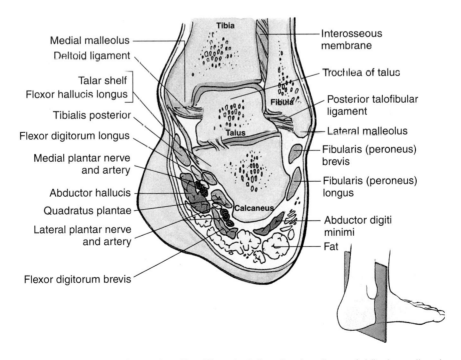

FIGURE 6.37 **Ankle joint.** Coronal section. The orientation drawing (lower right) shows the plane of the coronal section.

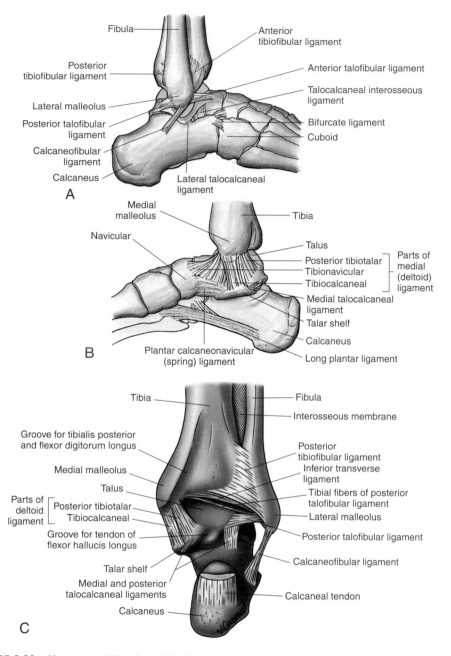

FIGURE 6.38 **Ligaments of the distal tibiofibular, ankle, and talocalcaneal joints. A.** Lateral view. **B.** Medial view. **C.** Posterior view.

dial malleolus and fans out from it to attach distally to the talus, calcaneus, and navicular (Fig. 6.38*B*) forming the:

- Tibionavicular ligament
- Anterior and posterior tibiofibular ligaments
- Tibiocalcaneal ligament.

The medial ligament stabilizes the ankle joint during eversion of the foot and prevents subluxation (partial dislocation) of the ankle joint.

Movements

The main movements of the ankle joint are dorsiflexion and plantarflexion. When the foot is plantarflexed, some rotation, abduction, and adduction of the ankle joint are possible. Structures limiting movements of the ankle joint are outlined in Table 6.17.

- **Dorsiflexion of ankle is produced by muscles in the anterior compartment of the leg** (Table 6.9). Dorsiflexion is usually limited by passive resistance of the triceps surae to stretching and by tension in the medial and lateral ligaments.
- **Plantarflexion of ankle is produced by muscles in the posterior compartment of the leg** (Table 6.10). In toe dancing by ballet dancers, for example, the dorsum of the foot is in line with the anterior surface of the leg.

Arteries and Nerves

The *arteries supplying the ankle joint* derive from malleolar branches of the **fibular and anterior and posterior tibial arteries** (Table 6.7). The *nerves supplying the ankle joint* are derived from the **tibial nerve and deep fibular nerve**.

ANKLE INJURIES
The ankle is the most frequently injured major joint in the body. Ankle sprains (tearing fibers of ligaments) are most common. A *sprained ankle* is nearly always an *inversion injury* (i.e., the foot is forcefully inverted during transfer of weight onto the plantarflexed foot). In severe ankle sprains, many fibers of the lateral ligament are torn, either partially or completely, resulting in *instability of the ankle joint.* The two most frequently torn parts of the lateral ligament are the calcaneofibular and anterior talofibular ligaments. In severe sprains, the lateral

malleolus is usually fractured. A *Pott fracture-dislocation of the ankle* occurs when the foot is forcibly everted. This pulls on the extremely strong medial ligament, often fracturing the medial malleolus. The talus then moves laterally, shearing off the lateral malleolus or, more commonly, breaking the fibula superior to the distal tibiofibular joint. If the tibia is carried anteriorly, the posterior margin of the distal end of the tibia is also sheared off by the talus.

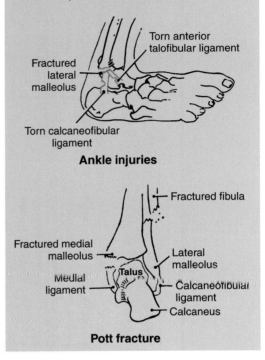

Ankle injuries

Pott fracture

JOINTS OF FOOT

The joints of the foot involve the tarsals, metatarsals, and phalanges (Fig. 6.39, Tables 6.18 and 6.19). The important intertarsal

---

TABLE 6.17. STRUCTURES LIMITING MOVEMENTS OF ANKLE JOINT

Movement	Limiting Structures
Plantarflexion	*Ligaments:* anterior talofibular, anterior part of medial, anterior articular capsule Contact of talus with tibia Tension of dorsiflexors of ankle
Dorsiflexion	*Ligaments:* medial, calcaneofibular, posterior talofibular, posterior articular capsule Contact of talus with tibia Tension of plantarflexors of ankle

Modified from Clarkson HM: *Musculoskeletal Assessment. Joint Range of Motion and Manual of Muscle Strength,* 2nd ed. Baltimore: Lippincott Williams & Wilkins 2000.

TABLE 6.18. JOINTS OF FOOT

Joint	Type	Articular Surface	Articular Capsule	Ligaments	Movements	Blood Supply	Nerve Supply
Subtalar	Plane type of synovial joint	Inferior surface of body of talus articulates with superior surface of calcaneus	Fibrous capsule is attached to margins of articular surfaces	Medial, lateral, and posterior talocalcaneal ligaments support capsule; interosseous talocalcaneal ligament binds bones together	Inversion and eversion of foot	Posterior tibial and fibular arteries	Plantar aspect, medial or lateral plantar nerves; dorsal aspect, deep fibular nerve
Talocalcaneonavicular	Synovial joint; talonavicular part is ball and socket type	Head of talus articulates with calcaneus and navicular bones	Fibrous capsule incompletely encloses joint	Plantar calcaneonavicular ("spring") ligament supports head of talus	Gliding and rotatory movements are possible	Anterior tibial artery via lateral tarsal artery	
Calcaneocuboid	Plane type of synovial joint	Anterior end of calcaneus articulates with posterior surface of cuboid	Fibrous capsule encloses joint	Dorsal calcaneocuboid ligament, plantar calcaneocuboid ligament, and long plantar ligament support fibrous capsule	Inversion and eversion of foot	Anterior tibial artery via lateral tarsal artery	

Joint	Type of joint	Articulation	Fibrous capsule	Ligaments	Movements	Artery	Nerves
Tarsometatarsal	Plane type of synovial joint	Anterior tarsal bones articulate with bases of metatarsal bones	Fibrous capsule encloses joint	Dorsal, plantar, and interosseous ligaments	Gliding or sliding	Lateral tarsal artery, a branch of dorsal artery of foot	Deep fibular, medial and lateral plantar, and sural nerves
Intermetatarsal	Plane type of synovial joint	Bases of metatarsal bones articulate with each other	Fibrous capsule encloses each joint	Dorsal, plantar, and interosseous ligaments bind bones together	Little individual movement of bones possible	Lateral metatarsal artery, a branch of dorsalis pedis artery	Digital nerves
Metatarsophalangeal	Condyloid type of synovial joint	Heads of metatarsal bones articulate with bases of proximal phalanges	Fibrous capsule encloses each joint	Collateral ligaments support capsule on each side; plantar ligament supports plantar part of capsule	Flexion, extension, and some abduction, adduction, and circumduction	Lateral tarsal artery, a branch of dorsal artery of foot	Digital nerves
Interphalangeal	Hinge type of synovial joint	Head of one phalanx articulates with base of one distal to it	Fibrous capsule encloses each joint	Collateral and plantar ligaments support joints	Flexion and extension	Digital branches of plantar arch	Digital nerves

joints are the *transverse tarsal joint* and the *subtalar joint*. Inversion and eversion of the foot are the main movements involving these joints. The other joints of the foot are relatively small and are so tightly joined by ligaments that only slight movement occurs between them. All foot bones are united by dorsal and plantar ligaments. The **transverse tarsal joint** is formed by the combined talonavicular part of the talocalcaneonavicular and calcaneocuboid joints—two separate joints aligned transversely. The **subtalar joint** (talocalcaneal joint) occurs where the talus rests on and articulates with the calcaneus (Fig. 6.39). The subtalar joint is a synovial joint that is surrounded by an articular capsule that is attached near the margins of the articular facets. The *fibrous capsule of the subtalar joint* is weak but is supported by medial, lateral, posterior, and interosseous talocalcaneal ligaments (Fig. 6.38). The **medial talocalcaneal ligament** connects the medial tubercle of the posterior process of the talus with the posterior portion of the talar shelf (sustentaculum tali); the **lateral talocalcaneal ligament** is parallel to and deeper than the calcaneofibular ligament. The **posterior talocalcaneal ligament** is a short band, the fibers of which radiate from a narrow attachment on

the lateral tubercle of the talus to the upper and medial part of the calcaneus. The **talocalcaneal interosseous ligament** is blended with the anterior part of the fibrous capsule of the subtalar joint and with the posterior part of the capsule of the talocalcaneonavicular joint. It is a strong band that connects the adjacent surfaces of the talus and calcaneus along the oblique tarsal grooves. The *synovial membrane of the subtalar joint* is separate from the other tarsal joints.

The **major plantar tarsal ligaments** (Figs. 6.38*B* and 6.40) are:

- **Long plantar ligament** that passes from the plantar surface of the calcaneus to the

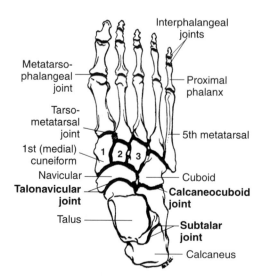

FIGURE 6.39 Joints of the foot. The important intertarsal joints are the transverse tarsal (calcaneocuboid and talonavicular joints) and subtalar joints.

Interphalangeal joints
Metatarso-phalangeal joint
Proximal phalanx
Tarso-metatarsal joint
5th metatarsal
1st (medial) cuneiform
Navicular
Cuboid
Talonavicular joint
Calcaneocuboid joint
Talus
Subtalar joint
Calcaneus

HALLUX VALGUS
Hallux valgus is a foot deformity characterized by lateral deviation of the great toe (L. hallux). In some people the deviation is so great that the 1st toe overlaps the 2nd toe. These persons are unable to move their 1st digit away from their 2nd digit because the sesamoid bones (Fig. 6.27*D*) under the head of the 1st metatarsal are displaced and lie in the space between the heads of the 1st and 2nd metatarsals.

Hammer Toe
Hammer toe is a deformity in which the proximal phalanx is permanently dorsiflexed at the metatarsophalangeal joint and the middle phalanx is plantarflexed at the interphalangeal joint. The distal phalanx is also flexed or extended, giving the digit (usually the 2nd) a hammerlike appearance. This deformity may result from weakness of the lumbricals and interossei, which flex the metatarsophalangeal joints and extend the interphalangeal joints (Table 6.11).

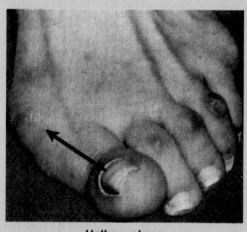

Hallux valgus
(arrow indicates change of alignment of great toe)

TABLE 6.19.   STRUCTURES LIMITING MOVEMENTS OF FOOT AND TOES

Movement	Joint	Limiting Structures
Inversion	Subtalar, transverse tarsal	*Ligaments:* lateral collateral ligament of ankle, talocalcaneal, lateral articular capsule Tension of evertor muscles of ankle
Eversion	Subtalar, transverse tarsal	*Ligaments:* medial collateral ligaments, medial talocalcaneal, medial articular capsule Tension of tibialis posterior, flexor hallucis longus, flexor digitorum longus Contact of talus with calcaneus
Flexion	MTP PIP DIP	MTP: Tension of posterior articular capsule, extensor muscles, collateral ligaments PIP: Soft tissue apposition, tension of collateral ligaments and posterior articular capsule DIP: Tension in collateral and oblique retinacular ligaments, and dorsal articular capsule
Extension	MTP PIP DIP	MTP: Tension of plantar articular capsule, plantar ligaments, and flexor muscles PIP: Tension in plantar articular capsule DIP: Ligaments and plantar articular capsule
Abduction	MTP	*Ligaments:* collateral ligaments, medial articular capsule Tension of adductor muscles Skin between web spaces
Adduction	MTP	Apposition of toes

MTP: metatarsophalangeal joints; PIP: proximal interphalangeal joints; DIP: distal interphalangeal joints (toes 2–5).
Modified from Clarkson HM: *Musculoskeletal Assessment. Joint Range of Motion and Manual of Muscle Strength,* 2nd ed. Baltimore: Lippincott Williams & Wilkins 2000.

groove for fibularis longus on the cuboid (p. 323). Some fibers extend to the bases of the metatarsals, forming a tunnel for the fibularis longus tendon. The long plantar ligament is important in maintaining the arches of the foot.

- **Plantar calcaneocuboid ligament** (short plantar ligament) that is deep to the long plantar ligament. It extends from the anterior aspect of the inferior surface of the calcaneus to the inferior surface of the cuboid.
- **Plantar calcaneonavicular ligament** (spring ligament) that extends from the talar shelf to the posteroinferior surface of the navicular. This ligament plays an important role in maintaining the longitudinal arch of the foot and in bearing weight transferred from the talar head.

The structures limiting movement of the joints are summarized in Table 6.19.

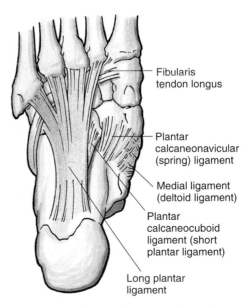

FIGURE 6.40   Plantar ligaments. Deep dissection of the right foot.

Labels:
Fibularis tendon longus
Plantar calcaneonavicular (spring) ligament
Medial ligament (deltoid ligament)
Plantar calcaneocuboid ligament (short plantar ligament)
Long plantar ligament

ARCHES OF FOOT

The tarsal and metatarsal bones are arranged in longitudinal and transverse arches that add to the weight-bearing capability and resiliency of the foot. *The arches act as shock absorbers for supporting the body weight and for propelling the body during movement.* The resilient arches make it adaptable to surface and weight changes. The weight of the body is transmitted to the talus from the tibia. Then it is transmitted posteroinferiorly to the calcaneus and anteroinferiorly to the heads of the 2nd to 5th metatarsals and the sesamoid bones associated with the head of the 1st metatarsal (Fig. 6.41*A*).

Between these weight-bearing points are the relatively elastic arches of the foot that become slightly flattened by the body weight during standing, but they normally resume their curvature (recoil) when body weight is removed (e.g., during sitting). The **longitudinal arch** is composed of medial and lateral parts (Fig. 6.41*B*). Functionally, both parts act as a unit with the transverse arch, spreading the weight in all directions. The **medial longitudinal arch** is higher and more important. This arch is composed of the calcaneus, talus, navicular, three cuneiforms, and three metatarsals. *The talar head is the keystone of the medial longitudinal arch.* The **tibialis anterior,** attaching to the 1st metatarsal and medial

cuneiform (Fig. 6.21*B*), helps strengthen the medial longitudinal arch. The **fibularis longus tendon**, passing from lateral to medial, also helps support this arch (Fig. 6.40). The **lateral longitudinal arch** is much flatter than the medial part of the arch and rests on the ground during standing. It is composed of the calcaneus, cuboid, and lateral two metatarsals. The **transverse arch** runs from side to side. It is formed by the cuboid, cuneiforms, and bases of the metatarsals. The medial and lateral parts of the longitudinal arch serve as pillars for the transverse arch. The tendon of the fibularis longus, crossing the sole of the foot obliquely, helps to maintain the curvature of the transverse arch.

The integrity of the bony arches of the foot is maintained by the:

- Shape of interlocking bones
- Strength of the plantar ligaments, especially the plantar calcaneonavicular (spring) ligament, and the long and short plantar ligaments
- Plantar aponeurosis
- Action of muscles through their tonus and the bracing action of their tendons.

Of these factors, the plantar ligaments and plantar aponeurosis bear the greatest stress and are most important in maintaining the arches.

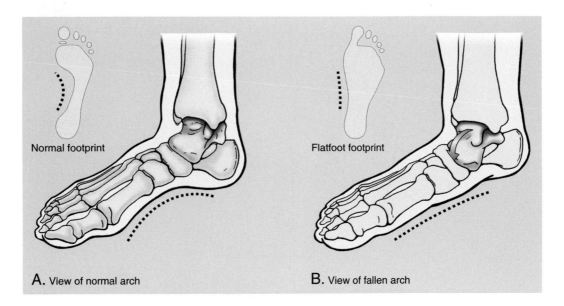

Normal footprint

A. View of normal arch

Flatfoot footprint

B. View of fallen arch

FLATFEET

Flatfeet in adolescents and adults result from "fallen arches," usually the medial parts of the longitudinal arches. When a person is standing, the plantar ligaments and plantar aponeurosis stretch somewhat under the body weight. If these ligaments become abnormally stretched during long periods of standing, the plantar calcaneonavicular ligament can no longer support the head of the talus. Consequently, the talar head displaces inferomedially and becomes prominent. As a result, some flattening of the medial part of the longitudinal arch occurs, along with lateral deviation of the forefoot. In the common type of flatfoot, the foot resumes its arched form when weight is removed from it.

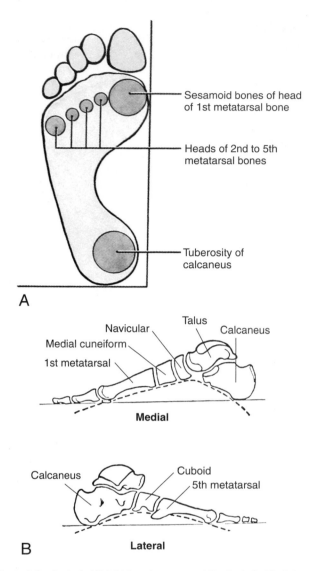

FIGURE 6.41   **Arches of the foot. A.** Weight-bearing areas of the foot. **B.** Medial and lateral longitudinal arches of the foot.

MEDICAL IMAGING OF LOWER LIMB

Radiographs of the pelvis and hip may show bone and joint abnormalities. In an *AP projection of the hip joint* (Fig. 6.42), the person is in the supine position on the radiographic table. The central x-ray beam is centered over the hip joint (see orientation). Superimposed on the femoral head is the *posterior rim of the acetabulum* (PR). At the junction of the femoral neck and shaft, the greater *trochanter* may be seen. Between the trochanters is an oblique line cast by the superimposed intertrochanteric line and crest (IC).

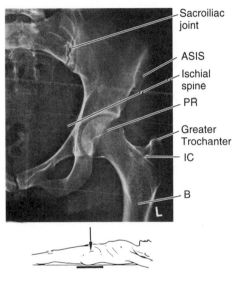

FIGURE 6.42 **Radiograph of a normal hip joint.** AP projection. *IC,* intertrochanteric crest; *B,* shaft of the femur; *PR,* posterior rim of the acetabulum; *ASIS,* anterior superior iliac spine.

Several radiographic projections (e.g., AP and lateral) are necessary to evaluate the knee joint properly (Fig. 6.43). In an AP projection, the person is in the supine position with the knee extended. The central x-ray beam is directed through the joint cavity. Identify the **femoral and tibial condyles** and observe the joint cavity that appears large because the menisci are not visible. They can be visualized if

air or an opaque fluid is injected into the joint cavity. The *intercondylar fossa* is opposite the medial and lateral tubercles of the **intercondylar eminence** of the proximal tibia. Note that the articular surfaces of the **tibial condyles** are

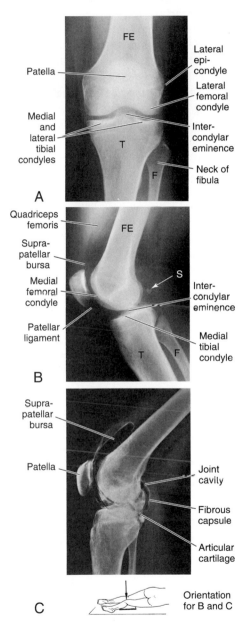

FIGURE 6.43 **Images of the knee joint. A.** AP radiograph. **B.** Lateral radiograph of the flexed knee. *FE,* femur; *T,* tibia; *F,* fibula; *S,* fabella. **C.** Arthrogram of the knee joint. Lateral projection with the joint slightly flexed.

concave. When a contrast medium is injected into the knee joint cavity, the extent of the synovial membrane is visible (Fig. 6.43*C*). Observe that the large **suprapatellar bursa** is continuous with the joint cavity. Note that the dense compact bone of the femur and leg bones appears transparent.

The common radiographs of the ankle and foot are lateral and AP. A lateral radiograph is taken with the lateral malleolus placed against the x-ray film cassette (Fig. 6.44). Observe the convex surface of the trochlea of **talus** (T) articulating with the malleoli of the tibia and fibula (shadows of malleoli are visible). Also observe the **neck** (N) and **head** (H) of talus, the disc-shaped **navicular** (Na), and the talonavicular joint. The **calcaneus** (Ca) and **cuboid** (C) articulate at the calcaneocuboid joint. The **tarsal sinus** (TS)—the space between the calcaneus and talus—contains the talocalcaneal interosseous ligament (Fig. 6.38*A*).

Magnetic resonance imaging (MRI) produces images of exquisite resolution of the limbs without the use of radiation. MRI scanning requires the patient to keep the limbs motionless for 5 to 10 min. MRIs show much

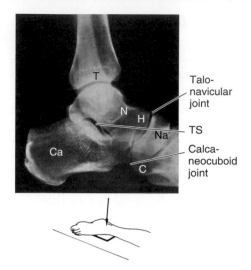

FIGURE 6.44 **Radiograph of the left ankle.** Lateral projection.

more detail in the soft tissues than do radiographs or CTs. MRIs are helpful in evaluating the menisci, collateral ligaments, and cruciate ligaments of the knee joint (Fig. 6.35*B*). It is the procedure of choice for assessing internal derangements of the knee.

7 Upper Limb

*T*he upper limb (extremity) is characterized by its mobility and ability to grasp
and manipulate. These characteristics are most
notable in the hand (L. manus). *The upper
limb consists of four segments* (Fig. 7.1):

- **Pectoral girdle** (shoulder girdle)—the
  bony ring, incomplete posteriorly, formed
  by the **scapulae** and **clavicles** and
  completed anteriorly by the **manubrium** of
  the sternum
- **Arm**—the part between the shoulder and
  elbow containing the **humerus**

- **Forearm**—the part between the elbow and
  wrist containing the **ulna** and **radius**
- **Hand**—the manual part distal to the
  forearm containing the **carpus, metacarpus,**
  and **phalanges;** the hand consists of the
  wrist, palm, dorsum, and fingers (digits).

BONES OF UPPER LIMB

The pectoral girdle and the free parts of the
limb form the superior part of the *appendicular
skeleton*—bones of the limbs (Figs. 7.2 and 7.3).

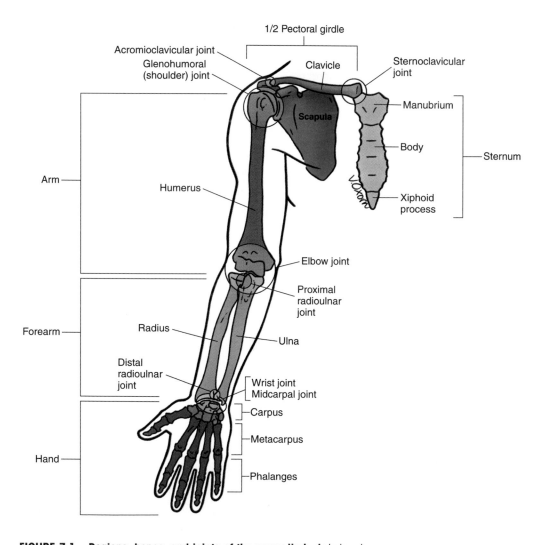

FIGURE 7.1 **Regions, bones, and joints of the upper limb.** Anterior view.

The **pectoral girdle** connects free parts of the limb to the *axial skeleton*—bones of head and trunk. Although very mobile, the pectoral girdle is supported, stabilized, and propelled by muscles that attach to the ribs, sternum, and vertebrae.

PECTORAL GIRDLE

The **clavicle** (collar bone) connects the upper limb to the trunk. Its **sternal end** articulates with the **manubrium** of the sternum at the **sternoclavicular (SC) joint** (Fig. 7.1). Its **acromial end** articulates with the **acromion** of the scapula at the **acromioclavicular (AC) joint.** The medial two thirds of the **shaft** (body) of the clavicle are convex anteriorly (Figs. 7.2*A* and 7.3), whereas the lateral third is flattened and concave anteriorly. These curvatures increase the resilience of the clavicle and give it the appearance of an elongated capital "S." *The doubly curved clavicle:*

- Serves as a strut (rigid support) keeping the limb away from the thorax so that the arm has maximum freedom of motion
- Forms one of the boundaries of the *cervicoaxillary canal* (passageway between neck and arm), affording protection to the *neurovascular bundle* (nerves and vessels) supplying the upper limb

- Transmits shocks (traumatic impacts) from the upper limb to the axial skeleton.

Although a long bone, the *clavicle has no medullary (marrow) cavity.* It consists of spongy bone with a shell of compact bone.

The **scapula** (shoulder blade) is a triangular flat bone that lies on the posterolateral aspect of the thorax, overlying the 2nd to 7th ribs. The triangular **body of scapula** is thin and translucent superior and inferior to the **spine of scapula** (Fig. 7.3, *A* and *B*). The concave **costal surface** (related to the ribs) of the scapula has a large **subscapular fossa;** the convex **posterior surface** is unevenly divided by the **spine of scapula** into a small **supraspinous fossa** and a much larger **infraspinous fossa.** The spine, a thick projecting ridge, continues laterally as the flat expanded **acromion of scapula,** which forms the subcutaneous "point of the shoulder" and articulates with the acromial end of the clavicle. Superolaterally, the lateral surface forms the **glenoid cavity of scapula** (Fig. 7.4), which articulates with the **head of humerus** at the **glenohumeral joint** (shoulder joint). The beaklike **coracoid process** is superior to the glenoid cavity and projects anterolaterally. The scapula has medial, lateral, and superior **borders** and superior, lateral, and in-

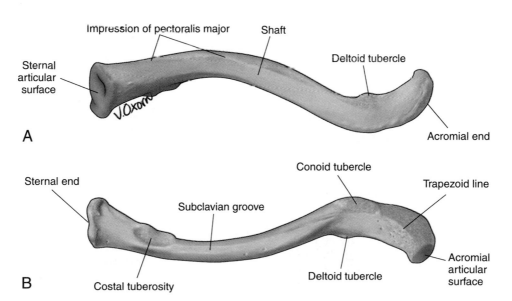

FIGURE 7.2 **Right clavicle. A.** Superior surface. **B.** Inferior surface.

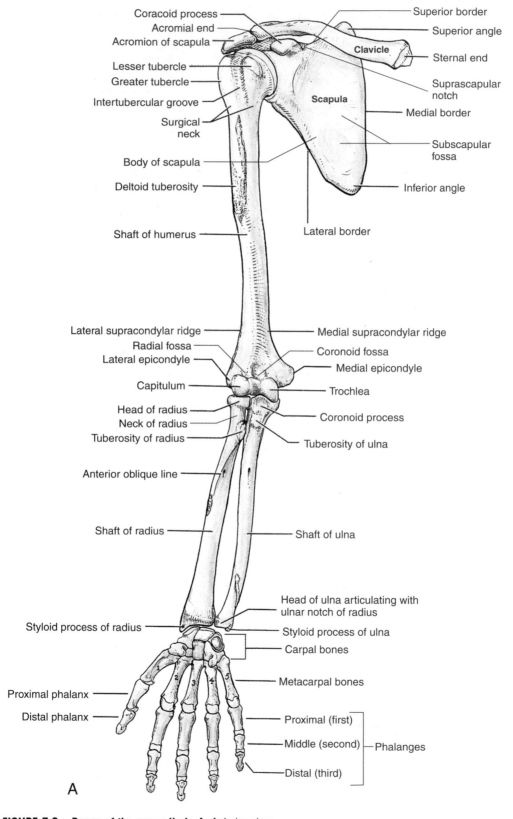

Coracoid process

Acromial end

Acromion of scapula

Lesser tubercle

Greater tubercle

Intertubercular groove

Surgical neck

Body of scapula

Deltoid tuberosity

Shaft of humerus

Lateral supracondylar ridge

Radial fossa

Lateral epicondyle

Capitulum

Head of radius

Neck of radius

Tuberosity of radius

Anterior oblique line

Shaft of radius

Styloid process of radius

Proximal phalanx

Distal phalanx

Superior border

Superior angle

Clavicle

Sternal end

Suprascapular notch

Scapula

Medial border

Subscapular fossa

Inferior angle

Lateral border

Medial supracondylar ridge

Coronoid fossa

Medial epicondyle

Trochlea

Coronoid process

Tuberosity of ulna

Shaft of ulna

Head of ulna articulating with ulnar notch of radius

Styloid process of ulna

Carpal bones

Metacarpal bones

Proximal (first)

Middle (second)

Phalanges

Distal (third)

A

FIGURE 7.3 **Bones of the upper limb. A.** Anterior view.

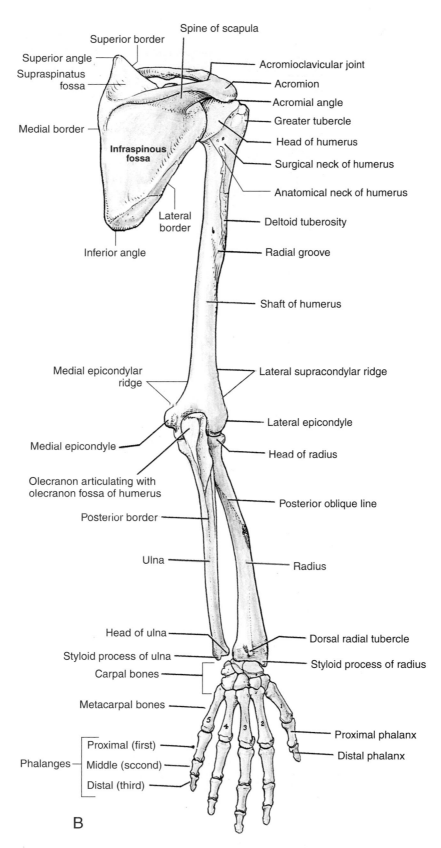

Superior border
Spine of scapula
Superior angle
Supraspinatus fossa
Acromioclavicular joint
Acromion
Acromial angle
Greater tubercle
Head of humerus
Surgical neck of humerus
Anatomical neck of humerus
Deltoid tuberosity
Radial groove
Shaft of humerus
Medial border
Infraspinous fossa
Lateral border
Inferior angle
Medial epicondylar ridge
Lateral supracondylar ridge
Lateral epicondyle
Head of radius
Medial epicondyle
Olecranon articulating with olecranon fossa of humerus
Posterior oblique line
Posterior border
Ulna
Radius
Head of ulna
Dorsal radial tubercle
Styloid process of ulna
Styloid process of radius
Carpal bones
Metacarpal bones
5   4   3   2
Proximal phalanx
Distal phalanx
Proximal (first)
Phalanges — Middle (sccond)
Distal (third)

B

FIGURE 7.3   *Continued.* **B.** Posterior view.

ferior **angles.** The superior border is marked by the **suprascapular notch** (Fig. 7.3*A*). The *lateral angle of scapula* is the thick truncated part of the scapula where the glenoid cavity is located.

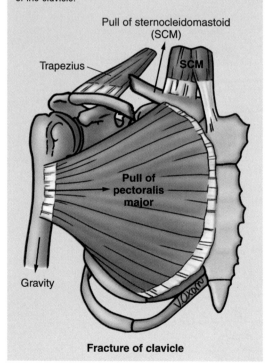
HUMERUS

The humerus (arm bone) articulates with the scapula at the glenohumeral joint and the radius and ulna at the elbow joint (Fig. 7.1). The ball-shaped **head of humerus** articulates with the **glenoid cavity** of the scapula. The **intertubercular groove** (bicipital groove) of the proximal end of the humerus separates the **lesser tubercle** from the **greater tubercle**. Just distal to the humeral head, the **anatomical neck of humerus** separates the head from the tubercles. Distal to the tubercles is the narrow **surgical neck of humerus,** which is where the humerus narrows to become the shaft (body). The **shaft of humerus** has two prominent features, the **deltoid tuberosity** laterally and the **radial groove** for the radial nerve and deep artery of arm posteriorly. The sharp medial and lateral **supracondylar ridges** end distally in prominent medial and lateral **epicondyles** (Fig. 7.3*B*). The distal end of the humerus has two articular surfaces, a lateral **capitulum** (L. little head) for articulation with the head of the radius and a medial **trochlea** (L. pulley) for articulation with the **trochlear notch of ulna** (Fig. 7.5).

Superior to the trochlea anteriorly is the **coronoid fossa** to accommodate the **coronoid process** of the ulna during full flexion of the elbow, and posteriorly the **olecranon fossa** to accommodate the **olecranon** of the ulna during extension of the elbow. Superior to the capitulum anteriorly is the shallow **radial fossa** for the edge of the head of the radius when the elbow is flexed.

ULNA AND RADIUS

The **ulna**—*the stabilizing bone of the forearm*—is the medial and longer of the two forearm bones (Fig. 7.3). Its proximal end has two prominent projections, the **olecranon** posteriorly and the **coronoid process** anteriorly. The anterior surface of the olecranon forms the posterior wall of the **trochlear notch,** which articulates with the trochlea of humerus. On the lateral side of the coronoid process is a smooth, rounded concavity, the **radial notch,** which articulates with the head of radius (Fig. 7.5). Inferior to the coronoid process is the **tuberosity of ulna.** Proximally, the **shaft (body) of ulna** is thick but it tapers, diminishing in diameter distally. At its narrow distal end is the

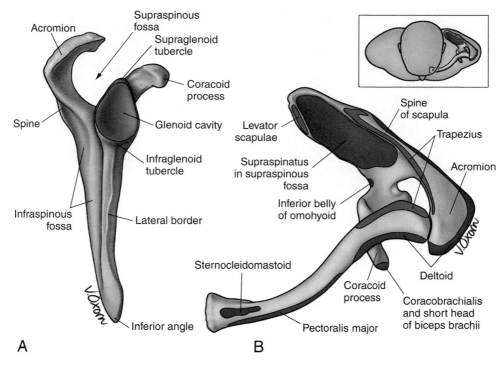

FIGURE 7.4   **Right scapula. A.** Lateral view. **B.** Superior view (including the clavicle).

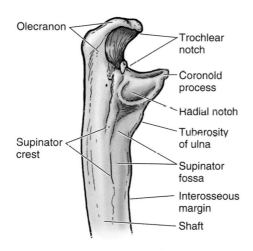

FIGURE 7.5   **Proximal part of the ulna.** Lateral view.

disclike, rounded **head of ulna** and a small, conical **ulnar styloid process** (Fig. 7.3).

The **radius** is the lateral and shorter of the two forearm bones. Its proximal end consists of a cylindrical **head,** a short **neck,** and an

oval projection from the medial surface—the **radial tuberosity** (Fig. 7.3A). Proximally, the smooth superior aspect of the **head of radius** is concave for articulation with the capitulum of humerus. The head also articulates medially with the **radial notch of ulna** (Fig. 7.5). The **neck of radius** is the narrow part between the head and radial tuberosity. The **radial tuberosity** separates the proximal end (head and neck) from the shaft (body). The **shaft of radius** has a lateral convexity and gradually and progressively enlarges in girth as it passes distally. The medial aspect of the distal end of the radius forms a concavity, the **ulnar notch of radius,** which accommodates the head of ulna. The **styloid process of radius** projects from the lateral aspect of its distal end. This process is much larger than the **ulnar styloid process** and extends approximately a finger's breadth further distally. The **dorsal radial tubercle** lies between two of the shallow grooves for passage of the tendons of forearm muscles.

FRACTURE OF HUMERUS, ULNA, AND RADIUS

Fractures of the surgical neck of the humerus are common in elderly persons and usually result from falls on the elbow when the arm is abducted. *Transverse fractures of the shaft of humerus* (**A**) frequently result from a direct blow to the arm. Fracture of the distal part of the humerus, near the supracondylar ridges, is a *supracondylar fracture* (**B**). Because nerves are in contact with the humerus (**C**), they may be injured when the associated part of the humerus is fractured.

- Surgical neck—axillary nerve
- Radial groove—radial nerve
- Distal humerus—median nerve
- Medial epicondyle—ulnar nerve.

Fractures of the shafts of the ulna and radius may occur simultaneously. Usually there is considerable displacement of the fractured bones. In fractures of the ulna, the shaft angulates posteriorly, whereas in fracture of the radius the distal fragment is pronated and pulled medially by the attached muscles. *Fracture of the distal end of the radius is the most common fracture in persons older than 50 years.* When a person falls on an outstretched hand with the forearm pronated, the main force moves through the carpus to the distal end of the radius and then proximally to the humerus, scapula, and clavicle. During such falls, fractures may occur in any of these bones, but the radius tends to break proximal to the wrist joint, producing a **Colles fracture.** The distal fragment of the radius is displaced dorsally and often comminuted (broken into pieces). The fragments are displaced posteriorly and superiorly, overlapping and producing shortening of the radius. The clinical manifestation is often referred to as the "dinner fork deformity." Normally, the radial styloid process projects further distally than the ulnar styloid process; consequently, when a Colles fracture occurs, this relationship is reversed because of shortening of the radius.

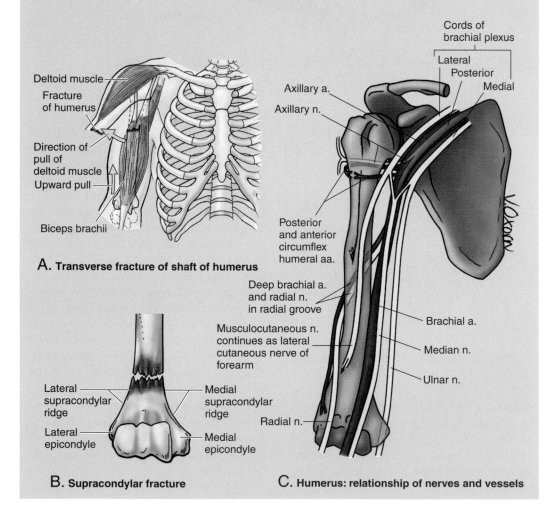

A. Transverse fracture of shaft of humerus

B. Supracondylar fracture

C. Humerus: relationship of nerves and vessels

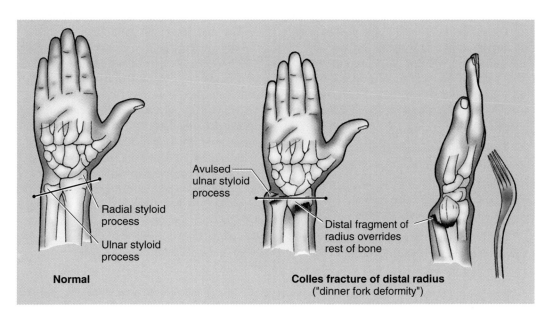

Radial styloid process

Ulnar styloid process

Normal

Avulsed ulnar styloid process

Distal fragment of radius overrides rest of bone

Colles fracture of distal radius
("dinner fork deformity")

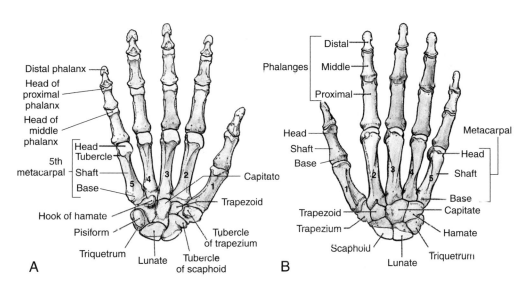

Distal phalanx

Head of proximal phalanx

Head of middle phalanx

5th metacarpal

Head
Tubercle
Shaft
Base

Hook of hamate

Pisiform

Triquetrum   Lunate   Tubercle of scaphoid

Capitato

Trapezoid

Tubercle of trapezium

A

Phalanges   Distal
              Middle
              Proximal

Head
Shaft
Base

Trapezoid
Trapezium

Scaphoid

Metacarpal

Head
Shaft

Base
Capitate

Hamate

Triquetrum

Lunate

B

FIGURE 7.6   Bones of the hand. A. Anterior view. **B.** Posterior view.

BONES OF HAND

The **carpus**—the skeleton of the wrist—is composed of eight **carpal bones** (carpals) arranged in two rows of four each (Fig. 7.6). These small bones give flexibility to the wrist. The carpus is markedly convex from side to side posteriorly and concave anteriorly. Augmenting movement at the wrist, the two rows of carpals glide on each other; each carpal also glides on those adjacent to it. From lateral to medial, the four bones in the proximal row of carpals are the:

- **Scaphoid**—a boat-shaped bone
- **Lunate**—a moon-shaped bone
- **Triquetrum**—a three-cornered (L. triquetrus) bone
- **Pisiform**—a pea-shaped bone that lies on the palmar surface of the triquetrum.

The proximal surfaces of the proximal row of carpals articulate with the inferior end of the radius and articular disc of the wrist joint. The distal surfaces of these bones articulate with the distal row of carpals. From lateral to medial, the four bones in the distal row of carpals are the:

- **Trapezium**—a four-sided bone
- **Trapezoid**—a wedge-shaped bone
- **Capitate**—a bone with a rounded head
- **Hamate**—a wedge-shaped bone, which has a hooked process, the **hook of hamate.**

The proximal surfaces of the distal row of carpals articulate with the proximal row of carpals, and their distal surfaces articulate with the metacarpals. The skeleton of the hand between the carpus and phalanges—the **metacarpus**—is composed of five **metacarpals.** Each metacarpal consists of a **shaft** (body) and two ends. The distal end or **head of the metacarpal** articulates with the proximal phalanx and forms a "knuckle of the fist." The proximal end or **base of the metacarpal** articulates with a carpal. Each finger (digit) has three **phalanges** (proximal, middle, and distal) except for the first (thumb), which has only two (proximal and distal). Each phalanx has a **base** proximally, a **head** distally, and a **shaft** (body) between the base and head.

FRACTURES OF HAND

Fractures of the hand are common and disability can result if normal relationships of the bones are not restored. *Fracture of the scaphoid is the most common injury of the wrist,* especially as a result of a fall on the palm with the hand abducted. Pain occurs primarily on the lateral side of the wrist, especially during dorsiflexion and abduction of the hand. Because of poor blood supply to the proximal part of the scaphoid, union of the fractured parts may take several months. *Avascular necrosis of the proximal fragment of the scaphoid* (pathological death of bone resulting from poor blood supply) may occur and produce *degenerative joint disease* of the wrist. *Fracture of the necks of the 1st and 2nd metacarpals* often is referred to as a "boxer's fracture." In unskilled fighters, the neck of the more mobile 5th metacarpal commonly is fractured when they strike a blow with the fist clenched.

Crushing injuries may produce multiple metacarpal fractures, resulting in instability of the hand. Similar injuries of the distal phalanges are common (e.g., when a finger is caught in a car door). A *fracture of a distal phalanx* is usually comminuted and a painful hematoma (collection of blood) develops. Fractures of the proximal and middle phalanges usually are the result of crushing or hyperextension injuries.

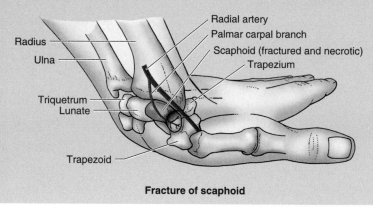

Fracture of scaphoid

Surface Anatomy of Upper Limb Bones

The **clavicle** is subcutaneous and can be palpated throughout its length (**A**). Its sternal end projects superior to the manubrium. Between the elevated sternal ends of the clavicle is the **jugular notch.** The acromial end of the clavicle often rises higher than the acromion, forming a palpable elevation at the **AC joint.** The acromial end can be palpated 2 to 3 cm medial to the lateral border of the acromion, particularly when the upper limb is swung back and forth. The **coracoid process of scapula** can be felt deeply at the lateral end of the clavicle. The **acromion** of the scapula is felt easily and may be visible. The lateral and posterior borders of the acromion meet to form the **acromial angle**—the point from which the length of the upper limb is measured (**B**). Inferior to the acromion, the **deltoid muscle** forms the rounded curve of the shoulder. The **crest of the spine of scapula** is subcutaneous and can be palpated. *When the upper limb is in the anatomical position:*

- The superior angle of the scapula lies at the level of T2 vertebra.
- The medial end of the root of the scapular spine is opposite the spinous process of T3 vertebra.
- The inferior angle of the scapula lies at the level of T7 vertebra, near the inferior border of the 7th rib and 7th intercostal space.

The **medial border of scapula** is palpable inferior to the root of the spine of the scapula as it crosses the 2nd to 7th ribs. The **lateral border of scapula** is not easily palpated because it is covered by the proximal attachment of the teres muscles. The **inferior angle of scapula** is easily felt and is often visible. The **greater tubercle of humerus** may be felt with the person's arm by the side on deep palpation through the deltoid, inferior to the lateral border of the acromion. In this position, the tubercle is the most lateral bony point of the shoulder. When the arm is abducted, the greater tubercle disappears beneath the acromion and is no longer palpable. The location of the **intertubercular groove,** between the greater and lesser tubercles, is identifiable during flexion and extension of the elbow joint by palpation of the tendon of the long head of

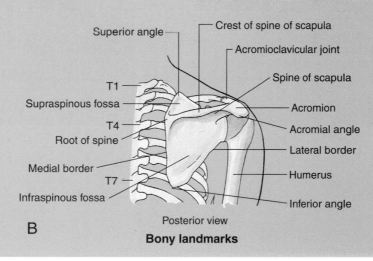

Coracoid process of scapula
Clavicle
Jugular notch
AC joint
Acromion
Manubrium
Humerus
Body of sternum
Xiphoid process

A   **Anterior view**

Superior angle
Crest of spine of scapula
Acromioclavicular joint
T1
Spine of scapula
Supraspinous fossa
Acromion
T4
Acromial angle
Root of spine
Lateral border
Medial border
Humerus
T7
Infraspinous fossa
Inferior angle

B

Posterior view
Bony landmarks

Continued

the biceps brachii as it moves through the sulcus. The **shaft of humerus** may be felt with varying distinctness through the muscles surrounding it. No part of the proximal part or the humeral body is subcutaneous. The **medial and lateral epicondyles** of the humerus are palpated easily at the medial and lateral aspects of the elbow. The *ulnar nerve* feels like a thick cord and produces an uncomfortable sensation when it is compressed as it passes posterior to the medial epicondyle.

The **olecranon** and posterior border of the ulna can be palpated easily (**C**), whereas when the elbow is flexed, the olecranon forms the apex of an approximately equilateral triangle, of which the epicondyles form the angles at its base. The **head of radius** can be palpated and felt to rotate in the depression on the posterolateral aspect of the extended elbow, just distal to the lateral epicondyle of the humerus. The **radial styloid process** can be palpated easily on the lateral side of the wrist (**D**); it is larger and approximately 1 cm more distal than the ulnar styloid process. The **head of ulna** forms a rounded subcutaneous prominence that can be easily seen and felt on the medial part of the dorsal aspect of the wrist.

The **scaphoid** and **trapezium** (**E**) can be palpated at the proximal end of the **thenar eminence** (ball of thumb) when the hand is extended. The **metacarpals,** although covered by the long extensor tendons of the digits, can be palpated on the dorsum of the hand. The **heads of metacarpals** form the knuckles of the fist; the 3rd metacarpal head is the most prominent. The dorsal aspects of the phalanges can be palpated easily. The **pisiform** can be felt on the anterior aspect of

the medial border of the wrist (**F**) and can be moved from side to side when the hand is relaxed. The **hook of hamate** can be palpated on deep pressure over the medial side of the palm, about 2 cm distal and slightly lateral to the pisiform.

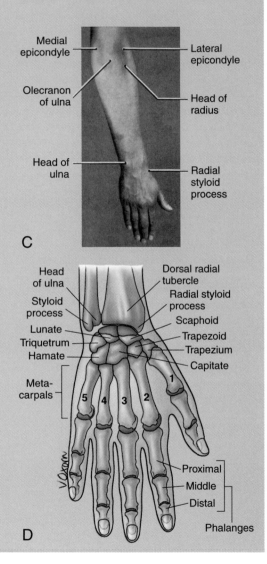

C

D

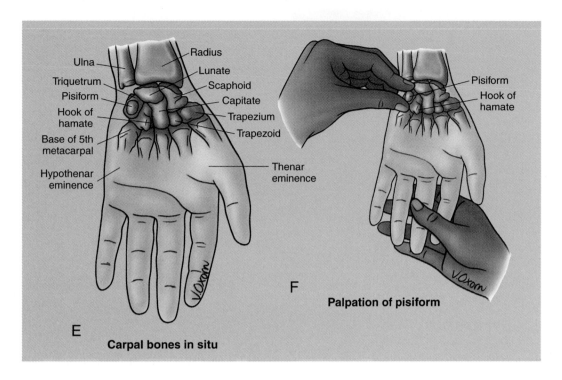

Ulna — Radius — Lunate — Triquetrum — Scaphoid — Pisiform — Capitate — Hook of hamate — Trapezium — Base of 5th metacarpal — Trapezoid — Hypothenar eminence — Thenar eminence

Pisiform — Hook of hamate

F

Palpation of pisiform

E

Carpal bones in situ

SUPERFICIAL STRUCTURES OF UPPER LIMB

Deep to the skin is subcutaneous tissue (superficial fascia), an irregular layer of loose connective tissue usually consisting primarily of a fatty layer. Deep fascia is a thin fibrous membrane, devoid of fat, that invests the muscles. If nothing (no muscle or tendon, for example) intervenes between the skin and bone, the deep fascia usually attaches to bone.

FASCIA OF UPPER LIMB

The **pectoral fascia** attaches to the clavicle and sternum, invests the pectoralis major, and is continuous inferiorly with the fascia of the abdominal wall. The pectoral fascia leaves the lateral border of the pectoralis major and becomes the **axillary fascia** (Fig. 7.7A), which forms the floor of the axilla (armpit). A fascial layer—the **clavipectoral fascia**—ascends from the axillary fascia, encloses the pectoralis minor and subclavius muscles, and then attaches to the clavicle. The part of the clavipectoral fascia

superior to the pectoralis minor—the **costocoracoid membrane**—is pierced by the lateral pectoral nerve that primarily supplies the pectoralis major (p. 437). The part of the clavipectoral fascia inferior to the pectoralis minor—the **suspensory ligament of axilla**—supports the axillary fascia and pulls it and the skin inferior to it upward during abduction of the arm.

The **brachial fascia**—a sheath of deep fascia—encloses the arm (L. brachium) like a sleeve (Fig. 7.7B); it is continuous superiorly with the pectoral and axillary layers of fascia. The brachial fascia is attached inferiorly to the epicondyles of the humerus and the olecranon of the ulna and is continuous with the **antebrachial fascia**, the deep fascia of the forearm (Fig. 7.7C). Two intermuscular septa—the **medial and lateral intermuscular septa**—extend from the deep surface of the brachial fascia and attach to the shaft and medial and lateral supracondylar ridges of the humerus, dividing the arm into **anterior** (flexor) and **posterior** (extensor) **fascial compartments,** each of which contains muscles serving similar functions, nerves, and the blood vessels that supply them.

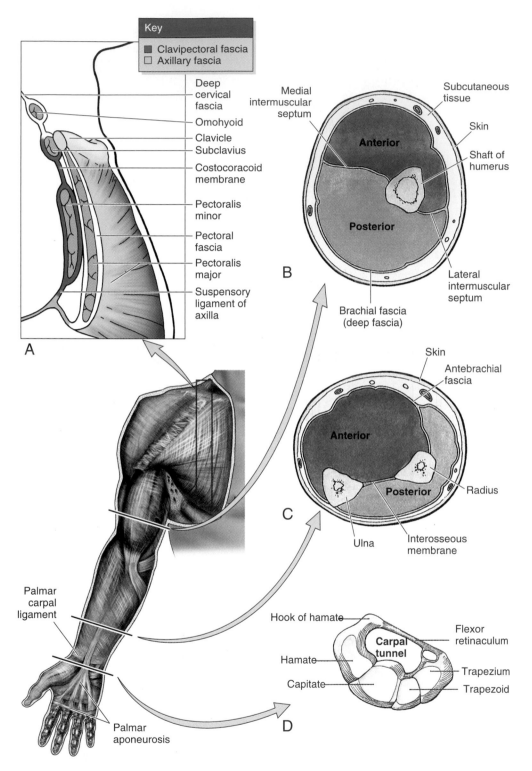

FIGURE 7.7 Fascia of the upper limb. A. Sagittal section showing axillary fascia and fascia of the pectoral region. **B.** Transverse section of the arm showing its fascial compartments. **C.** Transverse section of the forearm showing its fascial compartments. **D.** Transverse section through the distal row of the carpal bones and flexor retinaculum to show the carpal tunnel.

The **antebrachial fascia** invests the forearm muscles. It is continuous with the brachial fascia and with the deep fascia of the hand. The antebrachial fascia is attached posteriorly to the olecranon and the subcutaneous border of the ulna. The forearm is organized into anterior and posterior compartments separated by the **interosseous membrane** connecting the radius and ulna (Fig. 7.7C). The antebrachial fascia thickens posteriorly over the distal ends of the radius and ulna to form a transverse band, the **extensor retinaculum** (p. 457), which retains the extensor tendons in position. The antebrachial fascia also forms an anterior thickening—the **palmar carpal ligament.** Immediately distal but at a deeper level, the antebrachial fascia is continued as the **flexor retinaculum** (transverse carpal ligament). This fibrous band extends between the anterior prominences of the outer carpal bones and converts the anterior concavity of the carpus into a **carpal tunnel** through which the flexor tendons and median nerve pass (Fig. 7.7D). The **deep fascia of hand** is continuous through the extensor and flexor retinacula with the antebrachial fascia. The central part of the palmar fascia—the **palmar aponeurosis**—is thick, tendinous, and triangular.

CUTANEOUS NERVES OF UPPER LIMB

Cutaneous nerves in the subcutaneous tissue supply the skin of the upper limb. The **dermatomes** of the limb follow a general pattern that is easy to understand if one notes that developmentally the limbs grow as lateral protrusions of the trunk, with the 1st digit (thumb or great toe) located on the cranial side. Observe the progression of the segmental innervation (dermatomes) of the various cutaneous areas around the limb (Fig. 7.8, A and B):

- C3 and C4 nerves supply the region at the base of the neck extending laterally over the shoulder
- C5 nerve supplies the arm laterally (i.e., superior aspect of the outstretched limb)
- C6 nerve supplies the forearm laterally and the thumb
- C7 nerve supplies the middle and ring fingers and the middle of the posterior surface of the limb

- C8 nerve supplies the little finger, the medial side of the hand, and the forearm (i.e., the inferior aspect of the outstretched limb)
- T1 nerve supplies the middle of the forearm to the axilla
- T2 nerve supplies a small part of the arm and the skin of the axilla.

The cutaneous nerves to the shoulder are derived from the *cervical plexus*—a nerve network in the neck consisting of a series of nerve loops formed between adjacent anterior primary rami of the first four cervical nerves (see Chapter 9). Most cutaneous nerves of the upper limb are derived from the **brachial plexus**—a major nerve network formed by the anterior rami of the 5th cervical to the 1st thoracic spinal nerves (see Table 7.4). *The cutaneous nerves of the arm and forearm are as follows* (Fig. 7.8):

- The **supraclavicular nerves** (C3, C4) pass superficial to the clavicle, immediately deep to the platysma, and supply the skin over the clavicle and the superolateral aspect of the pectoralis major.
- The **posterior cutaneous nerve of arm,** a branch of the radial nerve, supplies the skin on the posterior surface of the arm.
- The **posterior cutaneous nerve of forearm,** also a branch of the radial nerve, supplies the skin on the posterior surface of the forearm.
- The **superior lateral cutaneous nerve of arm,** the terminal branch of the axillary nerve, emerges from beneath the posterior margin of the deltoid to supply skin over the lower part of this muscle and on the lateral side of the midarm.
- The **inferior lateral cutaneous nerve of arm,** a branch of the radial nerve, supplies the skin over the inferolateral aspect of the arm; it is frequently a branch of the posterior cutaneous nerve of the forearm.
- The **lateral cutaneous nerve of forearm,** the terminal branch of the musculocutaneous nerve, supplies the skin on the lateral side of the forearm.
- The **medial cutaneous nerve of arm** arises from the *medial cord of the brachial plexus,* often uniting in the axilla with the lateral cutaneous branch of the 2nd intercostal nerve. It supplies the skin on the medial side of the arm.

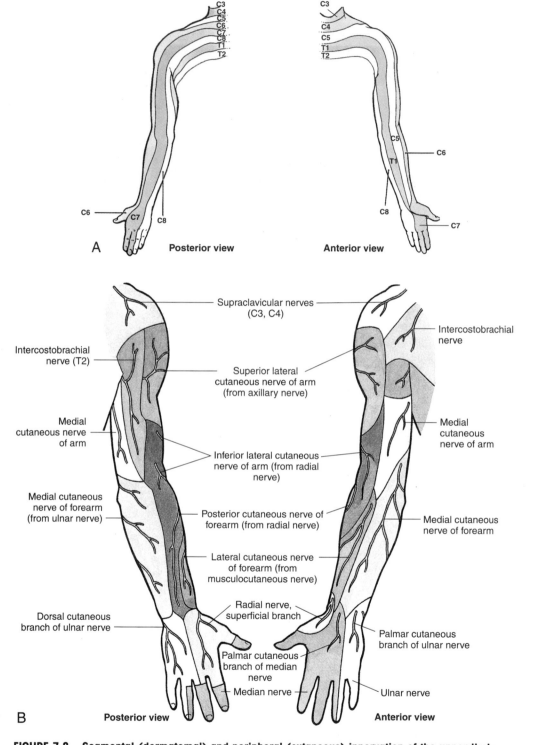

FIGURE 7.8 **Segmental (dermatomal) and peripheral (cutaneous) innervation of the upper limb.** **A.** Posterior and anterior views showing dermatome distribution. **B.** Similar views of the upper limb showing distribution of the cutaneous nerves, which usually contain fibers from more than one spinal nerve.

- The **intercostobrachial nerve,** a lateral cutaneous branch of the 2nd intercostal nerve from T2, also contributes to the innervation of the skin on the medial surface of the arm.
- The **medial cutaneous nerve of forearm** arises from the medial cord of the brachial plexus and supplies the skin on the anterior and medial surfaces of the forearm.

SUPERFICIAL VESSELS OF UPPER LIMB

The main superficial veins of the upper limb—the **cephalic** and **basilic veins**—originate in the subcutaneous tissue on the dorsum of the hand from the **dorsal venous network** (Fig. 7.9B). **Perforating veins** form communications between the superficial and deep veins. The **cephalic vein** ascends from the lateral aspect of the dorsal venous network, proceeding

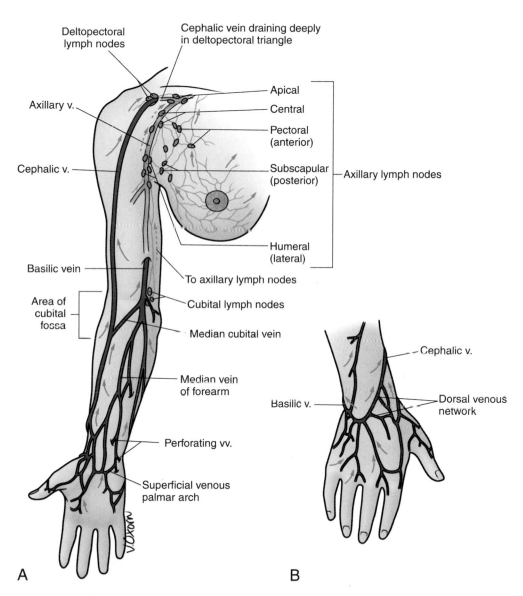

FIGURE 7.9 **Superficial venous and lymphatic drainage of the upper limb. A.** Anterior view of the upper limb showing the cephalic and basilic veins and their tributaries. *Green arrows,* superficial lymphatic drainage to the lymph nodes. **B.** Dorsal view of the hand showing the dorsal venous network.

along the lateral border of the wrist and the anterolateral surface of the forearm and arm. Anterior to the elbow the cephalic vein communicates with the **median cubital vein,** which passes obliquely across the anterior aspect of the elbow and joins the **basilic vein.** Superiorly the cephalic vein passes between the deltoid and pectoralis major muscles and enters the **deltopectoral triangle,** where it pierces the clavipectoral fascia and drains into the axillary vein. The **basilic vein** ascends from the medial end of the dorsal venous network along the medial side of the forearm and inferior arm. It then passes deeply, piercing the brachial fascia to merge with the accompanying veins (L. venae comitantes) of the brachial artery to form the **axillary vein** (Fig. 7.9A). The **median vein of forearm** ascends in the forearm between the cephalic and basilic veins; it may join the basilic vein in the cubital fossa.

VENIPUNCTURE

Because of the prominence and accessibility of the superficial veins, they are commonly used for *venipuncture* (puncture of the vein to draw blood or inject a solution). By applying a tourniquet to the arm, the venous return is occluded and the veins distend and usually are visible and/or palpable. Once a vein is punctured, the tourniquet is removed so that when the needle is removed the vein will not bleed extensively. The **median cubital vein** commonly is used for venipuncture. The veins forming the *dorsal venous network* and the cephalic and basilic veins arising from it commonly are used for long-term introduction of fluids (*intravenous feeding*). The cubital veins are also a site for the introduction of cardiac catheters to secure blood samples from the great vessels and chambers of the heart.

Superficial lymphatic vessels arise from *lymphatic plexuses* in the fingers, palm, and dorsum of the hand and ascend with superficial veins (Fig. 7.9). Some lymphatic vessels accompanying the basilic vein enter the **cubital lymph nodes** in the cubital fossa. Efferent vessels from these nodes ascend in the arm and terminate in the **humeral group of axillary nodes.** Most lymphatic vessels accompanying the cephalic vein cross the proximal part of the arm and anterior aspect of the shoulder to enter the **apical group of axillary nodes.** Some

vessels enter the **deltopectoral lymph nodes. Deep lymphatic vessels,** less numerous than superficial vessels, accompany major deep veins and terminate in the humeral group of axillary nodes.

ANTERIOR THORACOAPPENDICULAR MUSCLES

Four anterior thoracoappendicular muscles move the pectoral girdle: *pectoralis major, pectoralis minor, subclavius,* and *serratus anterior* (Fig. 7.10). The attachments, nerve supply, and main actions of these muscles are given in Table 7.1. The fan-shaped **pectoralis major** covers the superior part of the thorax. It has **clavicular** and **sternocostal heads.** The latter head is much larger, and its lateral border is responsible for the muscular mass that forms most of the *anterior wall of the axilla,* with its inferior border forming the **anterior axillary fold** (p. 430). The pectoralis major and deltoid diverge slightly from each other superiorly and, along with the clavicle, form the **deltopectoral triangle** (Fig. 7.10A). The triangular-shaped **pectoralis minor** lies in the anterior wall of the axilla (Fig. 7.10B), where it is largely covered by the pectoralis major. *The pectoralis minor stabilizes the scapula* and is used, for example, when stretching the limb forward to touch an object that is just out of reach. With the coracoid process, the pectoralis minor forms a "bridge" under which vessels and nerves pass to the arm (see Fig. 7.14). *Thus, the pectoralis minor is a useful anatomical and surgical landmark for structures in the axilla* (e.g., the axillary artery).

The **subclavius** lies almost horizontally when the arm is in the anatomical position. This small, round muscle is located inferior to the clavicle and affords some protection to the subclavian artery (e.g., if the clavicle fractures). The **serratus anterior** overlies the lateral part of the thorax and forms the medial wall of the axilla (Fig. 7.10C). This muscle was given its name because of the saw-toothed appearance of its fleshy digitations.

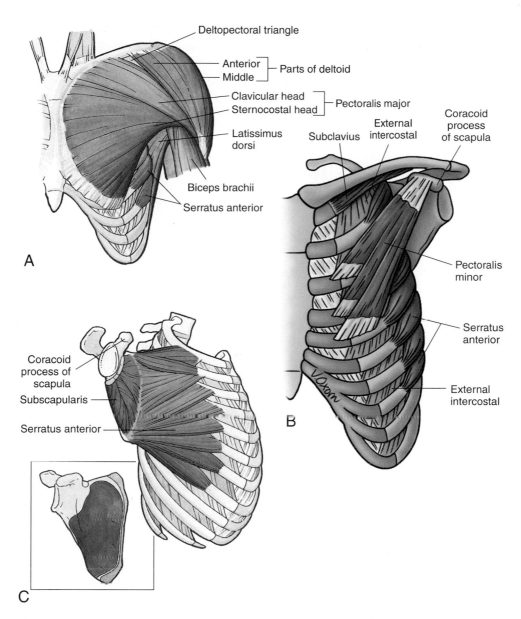

FIGURE 7.10 **Pectoral region and axilla. A.** Thoracoappendicular muscles. Anterior view. **B.** Pectoralis minor and subclavius. Anterior view. **C.** Serratus anterior and subscapularis. Lateral view. *Inset,* scapular attachments of the subscapularis (*red*) and serratus anterior (*blue*).

TABLE 7.1. ANTERIOR THORACOAPPENDICULAR MUSCLES

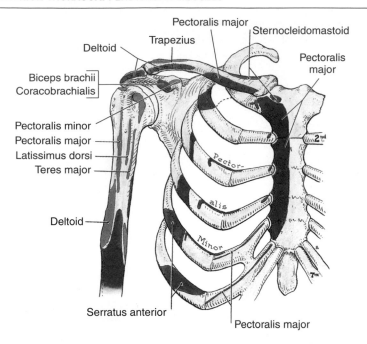

Muscle	Proximal Attachment	Distal Attachment	Innervation[a]	Main Action(s)
Pectoralis major	*Clavicular head:* anterior surface of medial half of clavicle *Sternocostal head:* anterior surface of sternum, superior six costal cartilages, and aponeurosis of external oblique muscle	Lateral lip of intertubercular groove of humerus	Lateral and medial pectoral nerves: clavicular head (C5 and **C6**), sternocostal head (**C7, C8,** and T1)	Adducts and medially rotates humerus Draws scapula anteriorly and inferiorly *Acting alone:* clavicular head flexes humerus and sternocostal head extends it from flexed position
Pectoralis minor	3rd to 5th ribs near their costal cartilages	Medial border and superior surface of coracoid process of scapula	Medial pectoral nerve (C8 and T1)	Stabilizes scapula by drawing it inferiorly and anteriorly against thoracic wall
Subclavius	Junction of 1st rib and its costal cartilage	Inferior surface of middle third of clavicle	Nerve to subclavius (**C5** and C6)	Anchors and depresses clavicle
Serratus anterior	External surfaces of lateral parts of 1st to 8th ribs	Anterior surface of medial border of scapula	Long thoracic nerve (C5, **C6,** and **C7**)	Protracts scapula and holds it against thoracic wall; rotates scapula

[a]Numbers indicate spinal cord segmental innervation (e.g., C5 and C6 indicate that nerves supplying clavicular head of pectoralis major muscle are derived from 5th and 6th cervical segments of spinal cord). Boldface indicates main segmental innervation. Damage to these segments, or to motor nerve roots arising from them, results in paralysis of muscles concerned.

By keeping the scapula closely applied to the thoracic wall, the serratus anterior (L. serratus, a saw) anchors this bone, enabling other muscles to use it as a fixed bone for movements of the humerus.

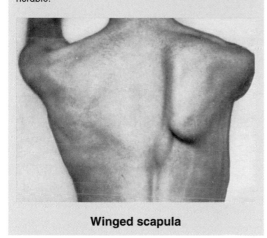

Winged scapula

POSTERIOR THORACOAPPENDICULAR AND SCAPULOHUMERAL MUSCLES

The posterior (cervico-) thoracoappendicular muscles (superficial and intermediate groups of *extrinsic back muscles*) attach the superior appendicular skeleton (of the upper limb) to the axial skeleton (of the trunk). The *intrinsic back muscles,* which maintain posture and control movements of the vertebral column, are described in Chapter 5. *The shoulder mus-cles are divided into three groups* (Figs. 7.11 and 7.12, Table 7.2):

- *Superficial (cervico-) posterior thoracoappendicular (extrinsic shoulder) muscles:* trapezius and latissimus dorsi
- *Deep posterior (cervico-) thoracoappendicular (extrinsic shoulder) muscles:* levator scapulae and rhomboids
- *Scapulohumeral (intrinsic shoulder) muscles:* deltoid, teres major, and the four rotator cuff muscles (supraspinatus, infraspinatus, teres minor, and subscapularis).

The attachments, nerve supply, and main actions of these muscles are given in Table 7.2. The **trapezius** provides a direct attachment of the pectoral girdle to the trunk. This large, triangular muscle covers the posterior aspect of the neck and the superior half of the trunk (Fig. 7.11). The trapezius attaches the pectoral girdle to the skull and cervicothoracic vertebral column and assists in suspending the upper limb. *The fibers of the trapezius are divided into three parts that have different actions:*

- Superior (cervico-occipital) fibers— elevate the scapula (e.g., when squaring shoulders)
- Middle (upper thoracic) fibers—retract the scapula (i.e., pull it posteriorly)
- Inferior (middle thoracic) fibers—depress the scapula and lower shoulder.

The **latissimus dorsi** is a large, fan-shaped muscle that passes from the trunk to the humerus and acts directly on the glenohumeral (shoulder) joint and indirectly on the pectoral girdle (scapulothoracic "joint"). In conjunction with the pectoralis major, the latissimus dorsi raises the trunk to the arm, which occurs when the limb is fixed and the body moves, as when performing chin-ups (hoisting oneself on an overhead bar, for example). These movements are also used when the trunk is fixed and the limb moves, as when chopping wood, paddling a canoe, and swimming. The superior third of the **levator scapulae** lies deep to the sternocleidomastoid; the inferior third is deep to the trapezius. True

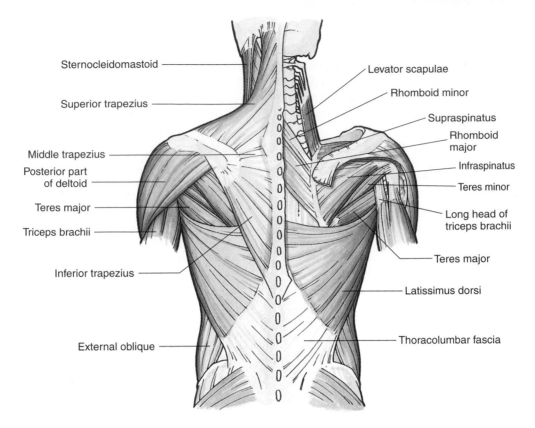

FIGURE 7.11 **Posterior thoracoappendicular and scapulohumeral muscles.** Posterior view. *Left side,* superficial extrinsic shoulder muscles; *right side,* deeper dissection.

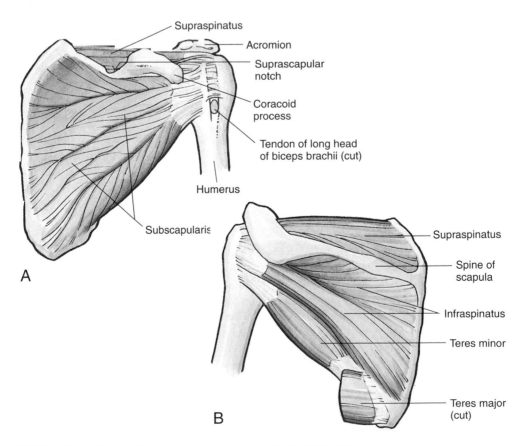

FIGURE 7.12 **Rotator cuff muscles. A.** Anterior view. **B.** Posterior view.

to its name, *the levator scapulae elevates the scapula, or its medial border, which rotates the scapula so that the glenoid cavity is depressed (tilted inferiorly)*. It also assists in retracting the scapula and fixing it against the trunk and in flexing the neck laterally.

The two **rhomboids** (major and minor) lie deep to the trapezius (Fig. 7.11) and form broad bands of parallel muscle bundles that pass inferolaterally from the vertebrae to the medial border of the scapula. The **rhomboid major** is approximately three to four times wider than the thicker **rhomboid minor** lying superior to it. The rhomboids assist the serratus anterior in holding the scapula against the thoracic wall and fixing the scapula during movements of the upper limb.

The six **scapulohumeral muscles** (Fig. 7.11, Table 7.2)—deltoid, teres major, supraspinatus, infraspinatus, subscapularis, and teres minor—are relatively short muscles that pass from the scapula to the humerus in two layers and act on the glenohumeral joint. Four of the scapulohumeral muscles—supraspinatus, infraspinatus, teres minor, and subscapularis—are called **rotator cuff muscles** because *they form a musculotendinous cuff around the glenohumeral joint* (Fig. 7.12). All except the supraspinatus are rotators of the humerus. The supraspinatus, besides being part of the rotator cuff, initiates and assists the deltoid in abduction of the arm. When the arm is fully adducted, the line of pull of the deltoid coincides with the axis of the humerus; thus, it pulls directly upward on the bone and cannot initiate abduction. The deltoid is, however, able to act as a shunt muscle, resisting inferior displacement of the head of the humerus from the glenoid cavity. From the fully adducted position, abduction must be initiated by the supraspinatus or by leaning on the side, allowing gravity to do so. The deltoid becomes fully effective as an abductor following the initial 15° of abduction. The tendons of the rotator cuff muscles blend with the articular capsule of the glenohumeral joint, reinforcing it as the *musculotendinous rotator cuff*, which protects the joint and gives it stability by holding the head of the humerus firmly against the glenoid cavity. *Bursae around the glenohumeral joint*—between the tendons of the rotator cuff muscles and the fibrous capsule of the joint—reduce friction on the tendons passing over the bones or other areas of resistance.

ATROPHY OF DELTOID

Atrophy of the deltoid occurs when the axillary nerve is severely injured (e.g., as might occur when the surgical neck of the humerus is fractured). As the deltoid atrophies, the rounded contour of the shoulder disappears. This gives the shoulder a flattened appearance and produces a slight hollow inferior to the acromion. To test the strength of the deltoid clinically, the person abducts the arm against resistance, starting from approximately 15°. Inability to abduct the arm indicates an axillary nerve injury.

Subacromial Bursitis and Rupture of Supraspinatus Tendon

The tendon of the supraspinatus is separated from the coracoacromial ligament, acromion, and deltoid by the subacromial bursa. When this bursa is inflamed—subacromial bursitis—abduction of the arm is painful. *Rupture of the supraspinatus tendon* is the most common injury of the rotator cuff. For a description of rotator cuff injuries, see page 485.

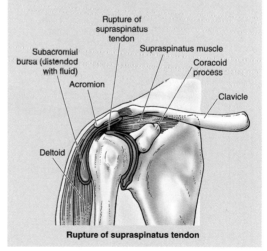

Rupture of supraspinatus tendon

TABLE 7.2. POSTERIOR THORACOAPPENDICULAR AND SCAPULOHUMERAL MUSCLES

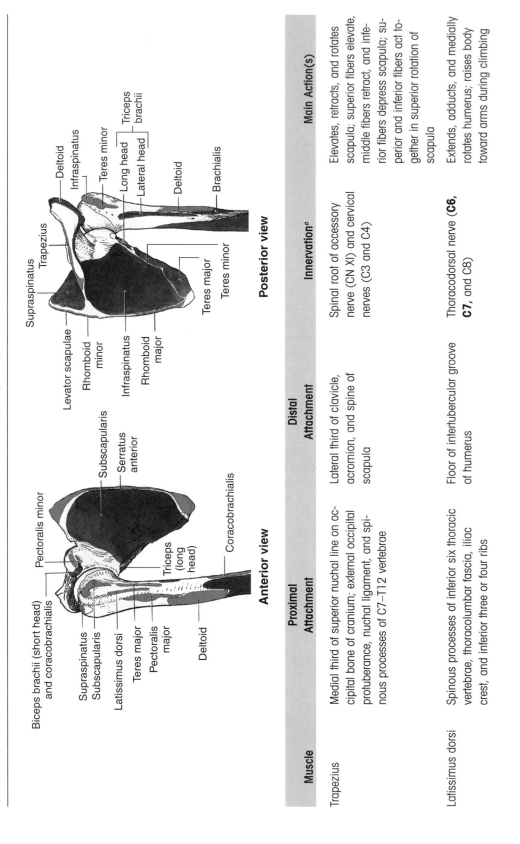

Anterior view

Posterior view

Muscle	Proximal Attachment	Distal Attachment	Innervation[a]	Main Action(s)
Trapezius	Medial third of superior nuchal line on occipital bone of cranium; external occipital protuberance, nuchal ligament, and spinous processes of C7–T12 vertebrae	Lateral third of clavicle, acromion, and spine of scapula	Spinal root of accessory nerve (CN XI) and cervical nerves (C3 and C4)	Elevates, retracts, and rotates scapula; superior fibers elevate, middle fibers retract, and inferior fibers depress scapula; superior and inferior fibers act together in superior rotation of scapula
Latissimus dorsi	Spinous processes of inferior six thoracic vertebrae, thoracolumbar fascia, iliac crest, and inferior three or four ribs	Floor of intertubercular groove of humerus	Thoracodorsal nerve (**C6, C7,** and **C8**)	Extends, adducts, and medially rotates humerus; raises body toward arms during climbing

Muscle	Proximal Attachment	Distal Attachment	Innervation	Main Action
Levator scapulae	Posterior tubercles of transverse processes of C1–C4 vertebrae	Superior part of medial border of scapula	Dorsal scapular (C5) and cervical (C3 and C4) nerves	Elevates scapula and tilts its glenoid cavity inferiorly by rotating scapula
Rhomboid minor and major	*Minor*: nuchal ligament and spinous processes of C7 and T1 vertebrae *Major*: spinous processes of T2–T5 vertebrae	Medial border of scapula from level of spine to inferior angle	Dorsal scapular nerve (C4 and **C5**)	Retract scapula and rotate it to depress glenoid cavity; fix scapula to thoracic wall
Deltoid	Lateral third of clavicle, acromion, and spine of scapula	Deltoid tuberosity of humerus	Axillary nerve (**C5** and C6)	*Anterior part*: flexes and medially rotates arm *Middle part*: abducts arm *Posterior part*: extends and laterally rotates arm
Supraspinatus[b]	Supraspinous fossa of scapula	Superior facet on greater tubercle of humerus	Suprascapular nerve (C4, **C5**, and C6)	Initiates and helps deltoid to abduct arm and acts with rotator cuff muscles[b]
Infraspinatus[b]	Infraspinous fossa of scapula	Middle facet on greater tubercle of humerus	Suprascapular nerve (**C5** and C6)	Laterally rotate arm; help to hold humeral head in glenoid cavity of scapula
Teres minor[b]	Superior part of lateral border of scapula	Inferior facet on greater tubercle of humerus	Axillary nerve (**C5** and C6)	
Teres major	Dorsal surface of inferior angle of scapula	Medial lip of intertubercular groove of humerus	Lower subscapular nerve (**C6** and C7)	Adducts and medially rotates arm
Subscapularis[b]	Subscapular fossa	Lesser tubercle of humerus	Upper and lower subscapular nerves (C5, **C6**, and C7)	Medially rotates arm and adducts it; helps to hold humeral head in glenoid cavity

[a]See Table 7.1 for explanation of nomenclature.

[b]Collectively, the supraspinatus, infraspinatus, teres minor, and subscapularis muscles are referred to as the rotator cuff muscles. Their prime function during all movements of the glenohumeral (shoulder) joint is to hold the head of humerus in the glenoid cavity of the scapula.

Surface Anatomy of Posterior Thoracoappendicular and Scapulohumeral Muscles

The large vessels and nerves to the upper limb pass posterior to the convexity in the clavicle (*CL*). The **deltopectoral triangle** (*D*) is the slightly depressed area just inferior to the lateral part of the clavicle. The deltopectoral triangle is bounded by the clavicle superiorly, the deltoid laterally, and the **clavicular head of pectoralis major** (*C*) medially. When the arm is abducted and then adducted against resistance, the two heads of the **pectoralis major** (*C* and *ST*) are obvious in a lean individual. As this muscle extends from the thoracic wall to the arm, it forms the **anterior axillary fold** (*AX*). Digitations of a well-developed **serratus anterior** (*SA*) appear inferolateral to the pectoralis major. The **coracoid process** of scapula is covered by the **anterior part of deltoid** (*AD*); however, the tip of the process can be felt on deep palpation in the deltopectoral triangle. *The coracoid process is used as a bony landmark when performing a brachial plexus block* (injection of local anesthetic solution), and the

position of the process is important in diagnosing shoulder dislocations.

The **deltoid** forms the contour of the shoulder and, as its name indicates, is shaped like an inverted Greek letter delta (V) when viewed laterally. The superior border of the **latissimus dorsi** and a part of the **rhomboid major** are overlapped by the **trapezius.** The triangle formed by the borders of these three muscles is the **triangle of auscultation.** When the scapulae are drawn anteriorly by folding the arms across the thorax and the trunk is flexed, the auscultatory triangles enlarge as the bordering muscles rotate and the 6th intercostal spaces become subcutaneous; consequently, respiratory sounds in the triangle are clearly audible with a stethoscope.

The **teres major** forms a raised oval area on the inferolateral third of the dorsum of the scapula when the arm is adducted against resistance. The **posterior axillary fold** (*PX*) is formed by the teres major and the tendon of the latissimus dorsi.

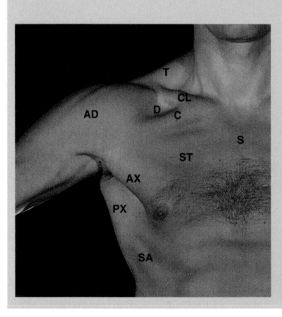

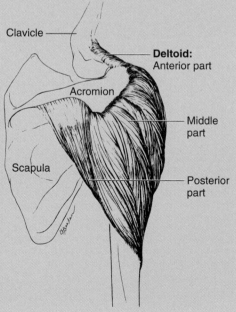

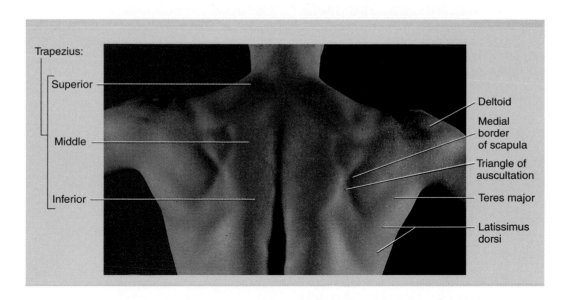

AXILLA

The axilla (armpit) is the pyramidal space inferior to the glenohumeral joint and superior to the skin and axillary fascia at the junction of the arm and thorax (Fig. 7.13). The shape and size of the axilla varies depending on the position of the arm; it almost disappears when the arm is fully abducted. *The axilla provides a passageway for vessels and nerves going to and from the upper limb.* The axilla has an apex, base, and four walls (Figs. 7.10, 7.13, and 7.14), three of which are muscular:

- *Apex of the axilla*—the entrance from neck to axilla—lies between the 1st rib, clavicle, and superior edge of the subscapularis

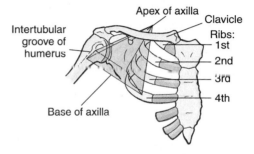

FIGURE 7.13   Location of axilla. Anterior view.

- *Base of the axilla* is formed by the concave skin, subcutaneous tissue, and axillary fascia extending from the arm to the thoracic wall

- *Anterior wall of the axilla* is formed by the pectoralis major and minor and the pectoral and clavipectoral fascia associated with them
- *Posterior wall of the axilla* is formed chiefly by the scapula and subscapularis on its anterior surface and inferiorly by the teres major and latissimus dorsi
- *Medial wall of the axilla* is formed by the thoracic wall (1st to 4th ribs and intercostal muscles) and the overlying serratus anterior
- *Lateral wall of the axilla* is the narrow bony wall formed by the *intertubercular groove* of the humerus.

AXILLARY VESSELS

The **axillary artery** begins at the lateral border of the 1st rib as the continuation of the **subclavian artery** and ends at the inferior border of the teres major (Fig. 7.14, Table 7.3). The axillary artery passes posterior to the pectoralis minor into the arm and becomes the **brachial artery** when it passes distal to the inferior border of the teres major. *For descriptive purposes, the axillary artery is divided into three parts relative to the pectoralis minor* (the part number also indicates its number of branches):

- **First part of axillary artery**—located between the lateral border of the 1st rib and the medial border of the pectoralis minor—is enclosed in the **axillary sheath** (see Fig. 7.16D) along with the axillary vein and cords of the brachial plexus. It has one branch, the *superior thoracic artery.*
- **Second part of axillary artery**—lies posterior to the pectoralis minor and has two branches, the *thoracoacromial* and *lateral thoracic arteries,* which pass medial and lateral to the muscle, respectively.
- **Third part of axillary artery**—extends from the lateral border of the pectoralis minor to the inferior border of the teres major. It has three branches, the *subscapular*—the largest branch of the axillary artery—opposite which the *anterior circumflex humeral* and *posterior circumflex humeral arteries* arise.

The **axillary vein** lies on the medial side of the axillary artery (see Fig. 7.16). *This large vein is formed by the union of the brachial veins*—the companion veins of the brachial artery—and the basilic vein at the inferior border of the teres major. The axillary vein ends at the lateral border of the 1st rib, where it becomes the **subclavian vein.** The axillary vein receives tributaries that correspond to the branches of the axillary artery with a few minor exceptions.

COMPRESSION OF AXILLARY ARTERY

Compression of the third part of this artery against the humerus may be necessary when profuse bleeding occurs (e.g., resulting from a stab wound in the axilla). If arterial compression is required at a more proximal site, the axillary artery can be compressed at the lateral border of the 1st rib by exerting downward pressure in the angle between the clavicle and the attachment of the SCM.

Arterial Anastomoses Around Scapula

Many *arterial anastomoses*—communications between arteries—occur around the scapula (Table 7.3). Several arteries join to form networks on the anterior and posterior surfaces of the scapula—the dorsal scapular, suprascapular, and subscapular (via its circumflex scapular branch). The importance of the collateral circulation that is possible through these anastomoses becomes apparent when ligation of a lacerated subclavian or axillary artery is necessary. For example, the axillary artery may have to be ligated between the 1st rib and subscapular artery. In this case, the direction of blood flow in the subscapular artery is reversed, enabling blood to reach the third part of the axillary artery. *Note that the subscapular artery receives blood through several anastomoses with the suprascapular artery, transverse cervical artery, and intercostal arteries.* Slow occlusion of an artery (e.g., resulting from disease) often enables sufficient collateral circulation to develop, preventing *ischemia* (deficiency of blood). Sudden occlusion usually does not allow sufficient time for adequate collateral circulation to develop; as a result, ischemia of the upper limb occurs. *Ligation of the axillary artery distal to the subscapular artery and proximal to the deep artery of the arm (L. profunda brachii) cuts off the blood supply to the arm because the collateral circulation is inadequate.*

INJURY TO AXILLARY VEIN

Wounds in the axilla often involve the axillary vein because of its large size and exposed position. When the arm is fully abducted, the axillary vein overlaps the axillary artery anteriorly. A wound in the proximal part of the vein (which does not collapse because of its attachment to adjacent bony structures) is particularly dangerous not only because of profuse bleeding but also due to the risk of air entering the vein and producing *air emboli* (bubbles) in the blood.

TABLE 7.3. BRANCHES OF SUBCLAVIAN, AXILLARY, AND BRACHIAL ARTERIES

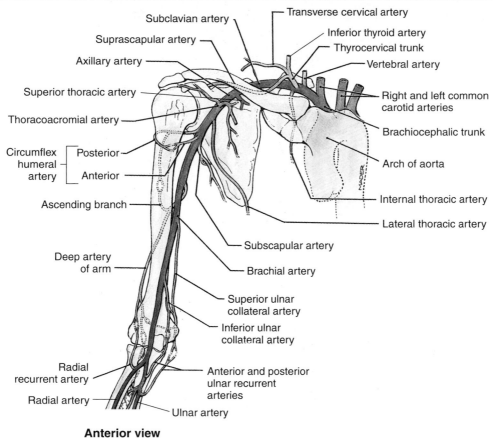

Subclavian artery
Suprascapular artery
Axillary artery
Superior thoracic artery
Thoracoacromial artery
Circumflex humeral artery — Posterior, Anterior
Ascending branch
Deep artery of arm
Radial recurrent artery
Radial artery
Ulnar artery

Transverse cervical artery
Inferior thyroid artery
Thyrocervical trunk
Vertebral artery
Right and left common carotid arteries
Brachiocephalic trunk
Arch of aorta
Internal thoracic artery
Lateral thoracic artery
Subscapular artery
Brachial artery
Superior ulnar collateral artery
Inferior ulnar collateral artery
Anterior and posterior ulnar recurrent arteries

Anterior view

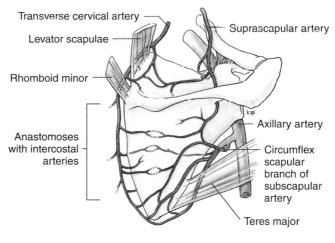

Transverse cervical artery
Levator scapulae
Rhomboid minor
Anastomoses with intercostal arteries
Suprascapular artery
Axillary artery
Circumflex scapular branch of subscapular artery
Teres major

Posterior view

continued

TABLE 7.3. *CONTINUED*

Artery	Origin	Course
Vertebral	Superior aspect of first part of subclavian artery	Ascends through transverse foramina of cervical vertebrae, except for C7, and enters the cranium through the foramen magnum
Internal thoracic	Inferior surface of subclavian artery	Descends, inclining anteromedially, posterior to sternal end of clavicle and first costal cartilage, and enters thorax
Thyrocervical trunk	Anterior aspect of first part of subclavian artery	Ascends as a short, wide trunk and gives rise to inferior thyroid, suprascapular, ascending cervical, and transverse cervical arteries
Suprascapular	Thyrocervical trunk	Passes inferolaterally over anterior scalene muscle and phrenic nerve, crosses subclavian artery and brachial plexus, and runs laterally posterior and parallel to clavicle; it then passes to posterior aspect of scapula and supplies supraspinatus and infraspinatus
Superior thoracic	Only branch of first part of axillary artery	Runs anteromedially along superior border of pectoralis minor and passes between it and pectoralis major to thoracic wall; helps supply 1st and 2nd intercostal spaces
Thoracoacromial	Second part of axillary artery, deep to pectoralis minor	Runs around superomedial border of pectoralis minor, pierces clavipectoral fascia, and divides into four branches
Lateral thoracic	Second part of axillary artery	Descends along axillary border of pectoralis minor and follows it onto thoracic wall
Subscapular	Third part of axillary artery	Descends along lateral border of subscapularis and axillary border of scapula to its inferior angle, where it passes onto thoracic wall
Circumflex scapular artery	Subscapular artery	Curves around axillary border of scapula and enters infraspinous fossa
Thoracodorsal	Subscapular artery	Continues course of subscapular artery and accompanies thoracodorsal nerve
Anterior and posterior circumflex humeral	Third part of axillary artery	These arteries anastomose to form a circle around surgical neck of humerus; larger posterior circumflex humeral artery passes through quadrangular space with axillary nerve
Deep artery of arm	Brachial artery near its origin	Accompanies radial nerve in radial groove of humerus and takes part in anastomosis around elbow
Ulnar collateral (superior and inferior)	Superior ulnar collateral artery arises from brachial artery near middle of arm; inferior ulnar collateral artery arises from brachial artery just superior to elbow	Superior ulnar collateral artery accompanies ulnar nerve to posterior aspect of elbow; inferior ulnar collateral artery divides into anterior and posterior branches; both ulnar collateral arteries take part in anastomosis around elbow

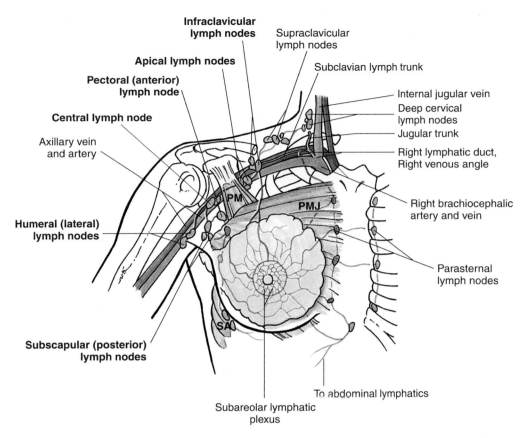

FIGURE 7.14 **Axillary lymph nodes.** Anterior view. *PM,* pectoralis minor; *PMJ,* pectoralis major; *SA,* serratus anterior.

AXILLARY LYMPH NODES

Many lymph nodes are found in the fibrofatty connective tissue of the axilla. **There are five principal groups of axillary lymph nodes:** apical, pectoral, subscapular, humeral, and central (Fig. 7.14).

The **apical group of axillary nodes** consists of nodes at the apex of the axilla, located along the medial side of the axillary vein and the first part of the axillary artery. *The apical group receives lymph from all other groups of axillary nodes* as well as from lymphatics accompanying the proximal cephalic vein. Efferent vessels from the apical group of nodes unite to form the **subclavian lymphatic trunk,** which may join the jugular and bronchomediastinal trunks on the right side to form the **right lymphatic duct,** or it may enter the **right venous angle** independently. On the left side,

the subclavian trunk most commonly joins the *thoracic duct* (p. 115).

The **pectoral (anterior) group of axillary nodes** consists of nodes that lie along the medial wall of the axilla, around the lateral thoracic vein and inferolateral border of the pectoralis minor. The pectoral group receives lymph mainly from the anterior thoracic wall, including the breast. Efferent lymphatic vessels from these nodes pass to the central and apical groups of nodes.

The **subscapular (posterior) group of axillary nodes** consists of nodes that lie along the *posterior axillary fold* (p. 430) and subscapular blood vessels. This group of nodes receives lymph from the ipsilateral upper quadrant of the back. Efferent lymphatic vessels pass from these nodes to the central and apical groups of nodes.

The **humeral (lateral) group of axillary nodes** consists of nodes that lie along the lateral wall of the axilla, around the distal part of the axillary vein. *This group of nodes receives nearly all the lymph from the upper limb,* except that carried by lymphatic vessels accompanying the cephalic vein, which drains to the central and apical groups of nodes.

The **central group of axillary nodes** consists of large nodes situated deep to the pectoralis minor in the central part of the axilla, in association with the second part of the axillary artery. *The central group of nodes receives lymph from the pectoral, subscapular, and humeral groups of axillary nodes.* Efferent vessels from the central group pass to the apical group of nodes.

BRACHIAL PLEXUS

The brachial plexus (L. a braid) is a major network of nerves supplying the upper limb. *The brachial plexus is formed by the union of the anterior primary rami of C5 through C8 nerves and the greater part of the anterior ramus of the T1 nerve* (Figs. 7.15 and 7.16, Table 7.4). The merging of the rami constitute the **roots of brachial plexus,** which are located in the posterior triangle of the neck. As they emerge from the **scalene hiatus** (triangular gap bounded by anterior and middle scalene muscles and the 1st rib to which the muscles attach), *the roots of the brachial plexus unite in the neck to form three trunks:*

- C5 and C6 roots combine to form the superior trunk

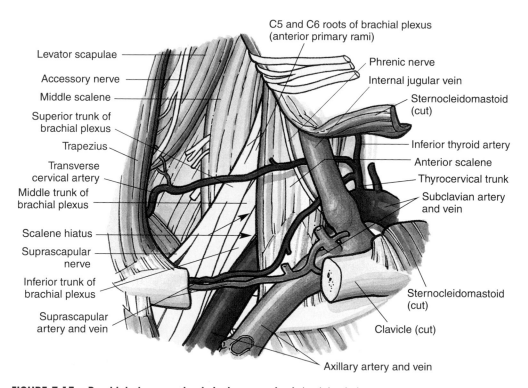

FIGURE 7.15 Brachial plexus and subclavian vessels. Anterolateral view.

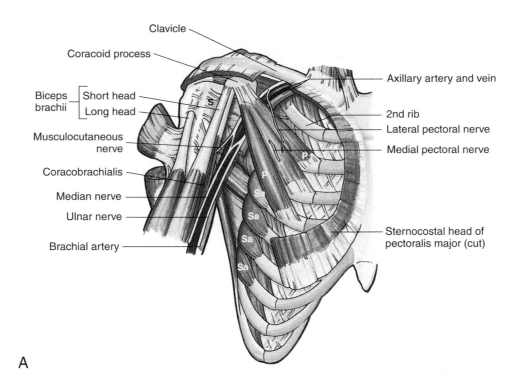

Clavicle

Coracoid process

Biceps brachii — Short head
— Long head

Musculocutaneous nerve

Coracobrachialis

Median nerve

Ulnar nerve

Brachial artery

Axillary artery and vein

2nd rib

Lateral pectoral nerve

Medial pectoral nerve

Sternocostal head of pectoralis major (cut)

A

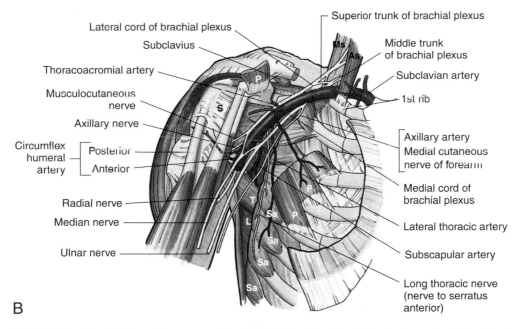

Lateral cord of brachial plexus

Subclavius

Thoracoacromial artery

Musculocutaneous nerve

Axillary nerve

Circumflex humeral artery — Posterior
— Anterior

Radial nerve

Median nerve

Ulnar nerve

Superior trunk of brachial plexus

Middle trunk of brachial plexus

Subclavian artery

1st rib

Axillary artery
Medial cutaneous nerve of forearm

Medial cord of brachial plexus

Lateral thoracic artery

Subscapular artery

Long thoracic nerve (nerve to serratus anterior)

B

FIGURE 7.16 **Boundaries and contents of the axilla. A.** Anterior view. **B.** Posterior and medial walls of the axilla showing the axillary artery and brachial plexus. Anterior view. *S,* subscapularis; *Sa,* serratus anterior; *As,* anterior scalene; *Ms,* middle scalene; *T,* teres major; *L,* latissimus dorsi; *P,* pectoralis minor.

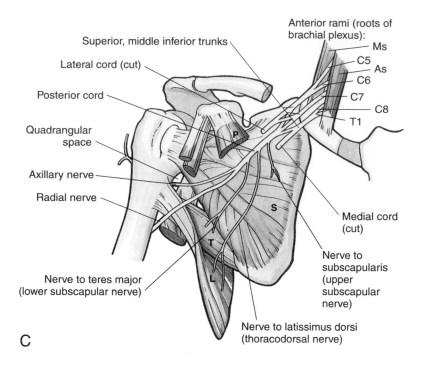

C

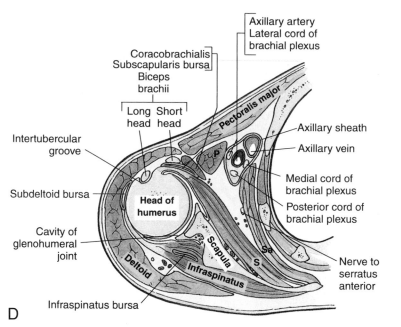

D

FIGURE 7.16 *Continued.* **C.** Posterior wall of the axilla demonstrating the posterior cord of the brachial plexus and its branches. Anterior view. **D.** Transverse section of the shoulder and axilla. *S,* subscapularis; *Sa,* serratus anterior; *As,* anterior scalene; *Ms,* middle scalene; *T,* teres major; *L,* latissimus dorsi; *P,* pectoralis minor.

- **C7** root remains alone as the **middle trunk**
- **C8 and T1 roots** combine to form the **inferior trunk.**

The trunks of the brachial plexus run posterior to the clavicle, passing from the neck into the axilla through the *cervicoaxillary canal.* As they cross the 1st rib, **all three trunks divide into anterior and posterior divisions of the plexus.** Nerve fibers in the anterior divisions are destined for the anterior aspect of the limb, and those in posterior divisions are destined for the posterior aspect of the limb. *Within the axilla, the divisions of the brachial plexus form three cords:*

- Anterior divisions of the superior and middle trunks merge to form the **lateral cord** of the plexus.
- Anterior division of the inferior trunk becomes the **medial cord** of the plexus.
- Posterior divisions of all three trunks become the **posterior cord** of the plexus.

The cords of the brachial plexus are named for their position in relation to the axillary artery (e.g., the lateral cord is lateral to the axillary artery). **The brachial plexus is divided into supraclavicular and infraclavicular branches by the clavicle** (Table 7.4).

- *Supraclavicular branches of the brachial plexus arise from the anterior rami* (roots) *and superior trunk of the plexus* (dorsal scapular nerve, long thoracic nerve, nerve to subclavius, and suprascapular nerve) and are approachable through the neck.
- *Infraclavicular branches of the brachial plexus arise from the cords of the brachial plexus* and are approachable through the axilla.

The **cords of brachial plexus** give rise to most of the named peripheral nerves that result from the plexus formation. The **lateral cord of brachial plexus,** lying lateral to the axillary artery and carrying nerve fibers primarily from C5 through C7 anterior rami (roots), **has three branches:**

- One side branch—*lateral pectoral nerve*
- Two terminal branches—*musculocutaneous nerve* and *lateral root of the median nerve.*

The **lateral pectoral nerve** (C5, **C6,** and C7) pierces the clavipectoral fascia to supply the *pectoralis major* (Fig. 7.16A, Table 7.4). The **musculocutaneous nerve** (C5 through C7) exits the axilla by piercing the coracobrachialis—supplying this muscle as it traverses it. The musculocutaneous nerve passes between the biceps brachii and brachialis, supplying both. Thus, *the musculocutaneous nerve supplies all muscles in the anterior compartment of the arm.* It then continues as the lateral cutaneous nerve of the forearm (Fig. 7.8B). The **median nerve** is formed by the union of the lateral and medial roots from the lateral and medial cords of the brachial plexus, respectively. *The median nerve supplies primarily flexor muscles in the anterior compartment of the forearm,* the skin of part of the hand, and five hand muscles.

The **medial cord of brachial plexus,** lying medial to the axillary artery and carrying nerve fibers from C8 and T1 roots, **has five branches:**

- Three side branches—medial pectoral nerve, medial cutaneous nerve of the arm, and medial cutaneous nerve of the forearm
- Two terminal branches—*ulnar nerve* and *medial root of the median nerve.*

The **medial pectoral nerve** (**C8,** T1) is a slender nerve that usually passes through the *pectoralis minor,* supplying it and then continuing to supply mainly the sternocostal part of the *pectoralis major* (Fig. 7.16A, Table 7.4). Although called the medial pectoral nerve because it arises from the medial cord, *the nerve is located lateral to the lateral pectoral nerve.* The **medial cutaneous nerve of arm** (C8, T1) supplies the skin on the medial side of the arm and the superior part of the forearm (Fig. 7.8B). The **medial cutaneous nerve of forearm** (C8, T1) runs between the axillary artery and vein and supplies the skin on the medial side of the forearm. The **ulnar nerve** (C8, T1, and sometimes C7) traverses the arm to reach the forearm without branching and supplies one and a half muscles in the anterior compartment (flexor carpi ulnaris and ulnar part of flexor digitorum profundus).

TABLE 7.4. BRACHIAL PLEXUS AND NERVES OF UPPER LIMB

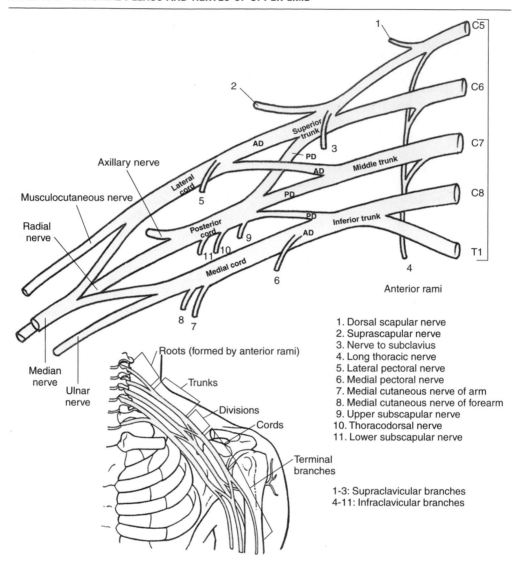

Observe that three nerves (musculocutaneous, median, and ulnar) are arranged like limbs of a capital M. Also observe anterior divisions (*AD*) and posterior divisions (*PD*).

1. Dorsal scapular nerve
2. Suprascapular nerve
3. Nerve to subclavius
4. Long thoracic nerve
5. Lateral pectoral nerve
6. Medial pectoral nerve
7. Medial cutaneous nerve of arm
8. Medial cutaneous nerve of forearm
9. Upper subscapular nerve
10. Thoracodorsal nerve
11. Lower subscapular nerve

1-3: Supraclavicular branches
4-11: Infraclavicular branches

Nerve	Origin	Course	Distribution
Supraclavicular branches			
Dorsal scapular	Anterior ramus of C5 with a frequent contribution from C4	Pierces scalenus medius, descends deep to levator scapulae, and enters deep surface of rhomboids	Innervates rhomboids and occasionally supplies levator scapulae
Long thoracic	Anterior rami of C5–C7	Descends posterior to C8 and T1 rami and passes distally on external surface of serratus anterior	Innervates serratus anterior
Nerve to subclavius	Superior trunk receiving fibers from C5 and C6 and often C4	Descends posterior to clavicle and anterior to brachial plexus and subclavian artery	Innervates subclavius and sternoclavicular joint
Suprascapular	Superior trunk receiving fibers from C5 and C6 and often C4	Passes laterally across posterior triangle of neck, through scapular notch under superior transverse scapular ligament	Innervates supraspinatus, infraspinatus, and glenohumeral (shoulder) joint

TABLE 7.4. *CONTINUED*

Nerve	Origin	Course	Distribution
Infraclavicular branches			
Lateral pectoral	Lateral cord receiving fibers from C5–C7	Pierces clavipectoral fascia to reach deep surface of pectoral muscles	Primarily supplies pectoralis major but sends a loop to medial pectoral nerve that innervates pectoralis minor
Musculocutaneous	Lateral cord receiving fibers from C5–C7	Enters deep surface of coraco-brachialis and descends between biceps brachii and brachialis	Innervates coracobrachialis, biceps brachii, and brachialis; continues as lateral cutaneous nerve of forearm
Median	Lateral root is a continuation of lateral cord, receiving fibers from C6 and C7; medial root is a continuation of medial cord receiving fibers from C8 and T1	Lateral root joins medial root to form median nerve lateral to axillary artery	Innervates flexor muscles in forearm (except flexor carpi ulnaris, ulnar half of flexor digitorum profundus, and five hand muscles)
Medial pectoral	Medial cord receiving fibers from C8 and T1	Passes between axillary artery and vein and enters deep surface of pectoralis minor	Innervates the pectoralis minor and part of pectoralis major
Medial cutaneous nerve of arm	Medial cord receiving fibers from C8 and T1	Runs along the medial side of axillary vein and communicates with intercostobrachial nerve	Supplies skin on medial side of arm
Medial cutaneous nerve of forearm	Medial cord receiving fibers from C8 and T1	Runs between axillary artery and vein	Supplies skin over medial side of forearm
Ulnar	A terminal branch of medial cord receiving fibers from C8 and T1 and often C7	Passes down medial aspect of arm and runs posterior to medial epicondyle to enter forearm	Innervates one and one half flexor muscles in forearm, most small muscles in hand, and skin of hand medial to a line bisecting 4th digit (ring finger)
Upper subscapular	Branch of posterior cord receiving fibers from C5 and C6	Passes posteriorly and enters subscapularis	Innervates superior portion of subscapularis
Thoracodorsal	Branch of posterior cord receiving fibers from **C6, C7,** and C8	Arises between upper and lower subscapular nerves and runs inferolaterally to latissimus dorsi	Innervates latissimus dorsi
Lower subscapular	Branch of posterior cord receiving fibers from C5 and C6	Passes inferolaterally, deep to subscapular artery and vein to subscapularis and teres major	Innervates inferior portion of subscapularis and teres major
Axillary	Terminal branch of posterior cord receiving fibers from C5 and C6	Passes to posterior aspect of arm through quadrangular space[a] in company with posterior circumflex humeral artery and then winds around surgical neck of humerus; gives rise to lateral cutaneous nerve of arm	Innervates teres minor and deltoid, glenohumeral joint, and skin over inferior part of deltoid
Radial	Terminal branch of posterior cord receiving fibers from C5–C8 and T1	Descends posterior to axillary artery; enters radial groove with deep brachial artery to pass between long and medial heads of triceps	Innervates triceps brachii, anconeus, brachioradialis, and extensor muscles of forearm; supplies skin on posterior aspect of arm and forearm via posterior cutaneous nerves of arm and forearm

[a]*Quadrangular space* is bounded superiorly by subscapularis and teres minor, inferiorly by teres major, and medially by long head of triceps and laterally by humerus (Fig. 7.16C).

The ulnar nerve continues into the hand, where it supplies most of the intrinsic muscles and skin on the medial side of the hand. The medial root of the medial cord unites with the lateral root of the lateral cord to form the **median nerve,** the distribution of which has been described already.

The **posterior cord of brachial plexus** (Fig. 7.16*C,* Table 7.4), carrying fibers from C5 to T1 roots, **has five branches:**

- Three side branches—upper subscapular, thoracodorsal, and lower subscapular nerves
- Two terminal branches—*axillary* and *radial nerves.*

The **upper subscapular nerve** (C5, C6) supplies the subscapularis; the **thoracodorsal nerve (C6, C7,** C8) supplies the latissimus dorsi; and the **lower subscapular nerve** (C5, C6,) supplies the teres major as well as the inferior part of the subscapularis. The **axillary nerve** (C5, C6) supplies the teres minor as it exits the axilla through the **quadrangular space** (see Fig. 7.18*A*)—bounded superiorly by the subscapularis and teres minor, inferiorly by the teres major, medially by the long head of triceps, and laterally by the humerus. The axillary nerve then supplies the deltoid from its deep posterior aspect and continues as the **superior lateral cutaneous nerve of arm,** supplying skin over the inferior half of the deltoid (Fig. 7.8*B*). The **radial nerve** (C5 through C8, T1)—*the largest branch of the brachial plexus—supplies all the extensor muscles of the posterior compartments of the upper limb* and skin on the posterior aspect of the arm and forearm.

ARM

The arm lies between the shoulder and elbow. Two types of movement occur between the arm and forearm: flexion-extension at the humeroulnar joint and pronation-supination at the proximal radioulnar joint. The muscles performing these movements are clearly divided into anterior (*flexor*) and posterior (*extensor*) groups. The chief action of both groups is at the elbow joint, but some muscles also act at the glenohumeral joint.

MUSCLES OF ARM

Of the four arm (L. brachium) muscles, **three flexors** (biceps brachii, brachialis, and coracobrachialis) are in the *anterior compartment of the arm* (Figs. 7.7*C* and 7.17) and are supplied by the **musculocutaneous nerve** (Fig. 7.14*A*), and **one extensor** (triceps brachii) is in the *posterior compartment of the arm* and supplied by the **radial nerve** (Fig. 7.18*B*). A small muscle on the posterior aspect of the elbow, the **anconeus,** is partly blended with the triceps. See Table 7.5 for attachments, nerve supply, and main actions of the arm muscles.

The **biceps brachii** has *two heads* (as its name "biceps" indicates—bi, two + L. caput, head): a *long head* and a *short head.* When the elbow is extended, the biceps is a *simple flexor of the forearm;* however, when the elbow is flexed, the biceps is the *primary (most powerful) supinator of the forearm.* Radiating fibers from the distal attachment of the biceps tendon form the **bicipital aponeurosis** (Fig. 7.17, *A* and *B*), a triangu-

VARIATIONS OF BRACHIAL PLEXUS

Variations in the brachial plexus formation are common. In addition to the five anterior rami (C5 through C8 and T1) that form the roots of the plexus, small contributions may be made by the anterior rami of C4 or T2. When the superiormost root of the plexus is C4 and the inferiormost root is C8, it is a *prefixed brachial plexus*. Alternatively, when the superior root is C6 and the inferior root is T2, it is a *postfixed brachial plexus*. In the latter type, the inferior trunk of the plexus may be compressed by the 1st rib, producing neurovascular symptoms in the upper limb.

Variations also may occur in the formation of trunks, divisions, and cords; origin and/or combination of branches; and relations to the axillary artery and scalene muscles.

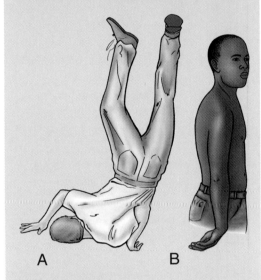

A   B

Brachial Plexus Injuries

Injuries to the brachial plexus affect movements and cutaneous sensations in the upper limb. Disease, stretching, and wounds in the posterior triangle of the neck or in the axilla may produce *brachial plexus injuries*. Signs and symptoms depend on which part of the plexus is involved. Injuries to the brachial plexus result in loss of muscular movement (*paralysis*) and loss of cutaneous sensation (*anesthesia*).

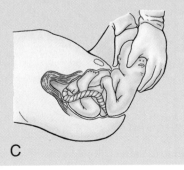

C

Injuries to superior parts of the brachial plexus (C5 and C6) usually result from an excessive increase in the angle between the neck and shoulder. These injuries can occur in a person who is thrown from a motorcycle (**A**) or a horse and lands on the shoulder in a way that widely separates the neck and shoulder. When thrown, the person's shoulder often hits something (e.g., a tree or the ground) and stops, but the head and trunk continue to move. This stretches or tears superior parts of the plexus. Injury to the superior trunk is apparent by the characteristic position of the limb (**B**)—"waiter's tip position"—Erb palsy (paralysis), in which the limb hangs by the side in medial rotation so that the palm faces posteriorly instead of medially. *Upper brachial plexus injuries* can also occur in a newborn when excessive stretching of the neck occurs during delivery (**C**).

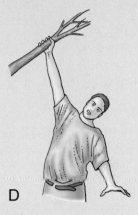

D

Injuries to inferior parts of the brachial plexus are much less common. These injuries may occur when the upper limb is suddenly pulled superiorly—for example, when a person grasps something to break a fall (**D**) or when a baby's limb is pulled excessively (**E**) during delivery. These events injure the inferior trunk of the plexus (C8 and T1) and may avulse (pull) the roots of the spinal nerves from the spinal cord. The short muscles of the hand are affected and a *clawhand* (**F**) results (atrophy of interosseous muscles of the hand with hyperextension of the metacarpophalangeal joints and flexion of the interphalangeal joints).

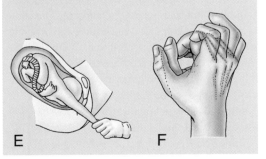

E   F

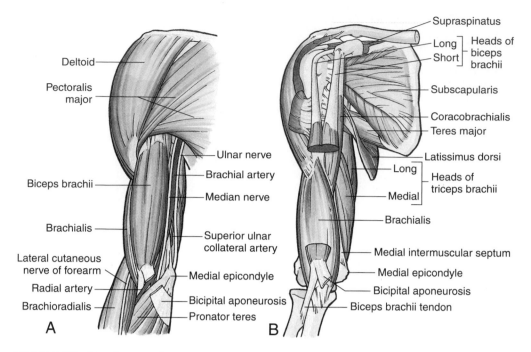

FIGURE 7.17   Muscles, arteries, and nerves of the arm. Anterior views. **A.** Muscles of the shoulder and the arm showing the brachial artery and associated nerves. **B.** Deep dissection of muscles.

lar band that passes obliquely across the cubital fossa and merges with the antebrachial fascia covering the flexor muscles in the medial side of the forearm. The **brachialis** lies posterior (deep) to the biceps. *The brachialis is the main flexor of the forearm; it flexes the forearm in all positions and during slow and quick movements.* When the forearm is extended slowly, the brachialis steadies the movement by slowly relaxing. The **coracobrachialis** in the superomedial part of the arm is a useful landmark (Fig. 7.17*B*). The musculocutaneous nerve pierces it, and the distal part of its attachment indicates the location of the nutrient foramen of the humerus. The coracobrachialis helps flex and adduct the arm and stabilize the glenohumeral joint. With the deltoid and the long head of the triceps, it serves as a shunt muscle, resisting downward dislocation of the head of the humerus. As indicated by its name, the **triceps brachii** arises by three heads— long, lateral, and medial (Figs. 7.18 and 7.19, Table 7.5). *The triceps is the main extensor of the elbow.* Because its long head crosses the glenohumeral joint, *the triceps helps stabilize the adducted glenohumeral joint by serving as a shunt*

muscle, resisting inferior displacement of the head of the humerus.

BICEPS TENDINITIS
The tendon of the long head of the biceps, enclosed by a synovial sheath, moves back and forth in the intertubercular groove of the humerus. Wear and tear of this mechanism is a common cause of shoulder pain. Inflammation of the tendon (*biceps tendinitis*) usually is the result of repetitive microtrauma. Sometimes the tendon is partially or completely dislocated from the groove. This injury occurs in athletes with a history of biceps tendinitis.

Rupture of Tendon of Long Head of Biceps
Rupture of the tendon usually results from wear and tear of an inflamed tendon (*biceps tendinitis*). Usually the tendon is torn from its attachment to the supraglenoid tubercle of the scapula. This injury commonly occurs in older athletes (e.g., baseball pitchers). The detached muscle belly forms a ball near the center of the distal part of the anterior aspect of the arm ("popeye deformity").

ARTERIES AND VEINS OF ARM

The **brachial artery** provides the main arterial supply to the arm (Figs. 7.17*A* and 7.19*A*, Table 7.3). The brachial artery, *the continuation of the axillary artery,* begins at the inferior border of

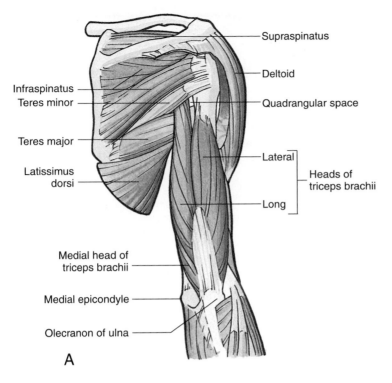

Supraspinatus

Deltoid

Infraspinatus
Teres minor

Quadrangular space

Teres major

Lateral

Heads of
triceps brachii

Latissimus
dorsi

Long

Medial head of
triceps brachii

Medial epicondyle

Olecranon of ulna

A

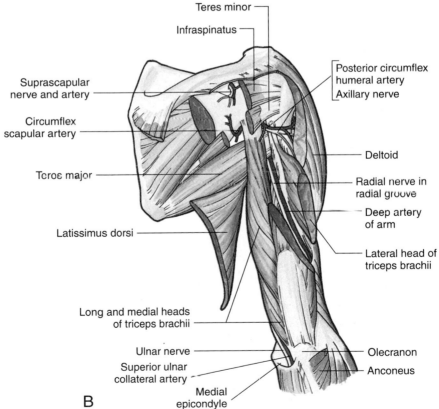

Teres minor

Infraspinatus

Posterior circumflex
humeral artery
Axillary nerve

Suprascapular
nerve and artery

Circumflex
scapular artery

Teres major

Deltoid

Radial nerve in
radial groove

Deep artery
of arm

Lateral head of
triceps brachii

Latissimus dorsi

Long and medial heads
of triceps brachii

Ulnar nerve

Superior ulnar
collateral artery

Medial
epicondyle

Olecranon

Anconeus

B

FIGURE 7.18 **Muscles, arteries, and nerves of the arm.** Posterior views. **A.** Muscles of the shoulder and arm. **B.** Deeper dissection showing arteries and nerves.

TABLE 7.5. MUSCLES OF ARM

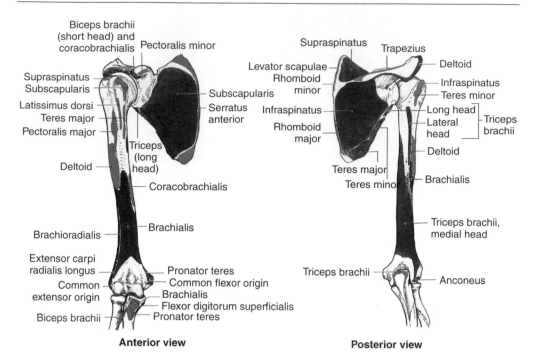

Anterior view   Posterior view

Muscle	Proximal Attachment	Distal Attachment	Innervation	Main Action(s)
Biceps brachii	*Short head:* tip of cora-coid process of scapula *Long head:* supraglenoid tubercle of scapula	Tuberosity of radius and fascia of fore-arm via bicipital aponeurosis	Musculocutaneous nerve (C5 and **C6**)	Supinates forearm and when it is supine, flexes forearm
Brachialis	Distal half of anterior surface of humerus	Coronoid process and tuberosity of ulna		Flexes forearm in all positions
Coracobrachialis	Tip of coracoid process of scapula	Middle third of me-dial surface of humerus	Musculocutaneous nerve (C5, **C6**, and C7)	Helps to flex and adduct arm
Triceps brachii	*Long head:* infraglenoid tubercle of scapula *Lateral head:* posterior surface of humerus, su-perior to radial groove *Medial head:* posterior surface of humerus, infe-rior to radial groove	Proximal end of ole-cranon of ulna and fascia of forearm	Radial nerve (C6, **C7**, and **C8**)	Extends forearm; it is chief extensor of fore-arm; long head steadies head of ab-ducted humerus
Anconeus	Lateral epicondyle of humerus	Lateral surface of olecranon and su-perior part of poste-rior surface of ulna	Radial nerve (C7, C8, and T1)	Assists triceps in ex-tending forearm; sta-bilizes elbow joint; abducts ulna during pronation

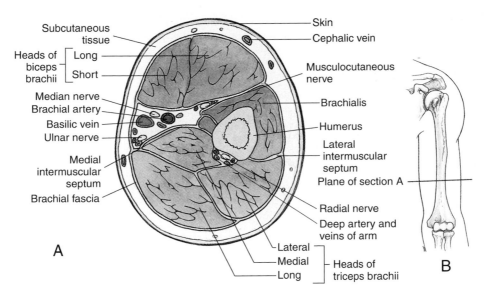

FIGURE 7.19   **Muscles and neurovascular structures of the arm. A.** Transverse section. **B.** Diagram showing the level of section **A.**

the teres major and ends in the cubital fossa opposite the neck of the radius. Under cover of the bicipital aponeurosis, *the brachial artery divides into the radial and ulnar arteries.* The brachial artery, superficial and palpable throughout its course, lies anterior to the triceps and brachialis. At first it lies medial to the humerus and then anterior to it. As it passes inferolaterally, *the brachial artery accompanies the median nerve,* which crosses anterior to the artery. During its course, the brachial artery gives rise to muscular branches and a *nutrient humeral artery* that arise from its lateral aspect. The main named branches of the brachial artery that arise from its medial aspect are the **deep artery of arm** and the superior and inferior **ulnar collateral arteries.** The latter vessels help to form the *arterial anastomoses around the elbow* (Table 7.3).

The **veins of the arm** anastomose freely with each other. Unpaired **superficial veins** course in the subcutaneous tissue (Fig. 7.19*A*). The main superficial veins—**cephalic** and **basilic veins**—are described on page 421. Paired **deep veins** accompany the arteries and share their names (e.g., brachial veins accompany the brachial artery). Both superficial and deep veins have valves, but they are more numerous in deep veins. **Perforating veins** carry blood from deep veins to superficial veins.

MEASURING BLOOD PRESSURE

A *sphygmomanometer* is used to measure arterial blood pressure. A cuff is placed around the arm and inflated with air until it compresses the brachial artery against the humerus and occludes it. A *stethoscope* is placed over the artery in the *cubital fossa,* the pressure in the cuff is gradually released, and the examiner detects the sound of blood beginning to spurt through the artery. The first audible spurt indicates *systolic blood pressure.* As the pressure is completely released, the point at which the pulse can no longer be heard indicates *diastolic blood pressure.*

Compression of Brachial Artery

The best place to compress the brachial artery to control hemorrhage is near the middle of the arm. The biceps has to be pushed laterally to detect pulsations of the artery. Because the arterial anastomoses around the elbow provide a functionally and surgically important collateral circulation, the brachial artery may be clamped distal to the inferior ulnar collateral artery without producing tissue damage (Table 7.3). The anatomical basis for this is that

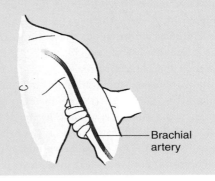

Continued

the ulnar and radial arteries still receive sufficient blood through the anastomoses. *Ischemia of the elbow and forearm* results from clamping the brachial artery proximal to the deep artery of the arm for an extended period.

Occlusion or Laceration of Brachial Artery

Although collateral pathways confer some protection against gradual temporary and partial occlusion, sudden complete occlusion or laceration of the brachial artery creates a surgical emergency because paralysis of muscles results from ischemia within a few hours. After this, fibrous scar tissue develops and causes the involved muscles to shorten permanently, producing a flexion deformity—*ischemic compartment syndrome* (Volkmann ischemic contracture). Contraction of the fingers and sometimes the wrist results in loss of hand power.

NERVES OF ARM

Four main nerves pass through the arm: median, ulnar, musculocutaneous, and radial (Figs. 7.16–7.19, Table 7.4). *The median and ulnar nerves supply no branches to the arm;* however, they supply articular branches to the elbow joint. The **median nerve** is formed in the axilla by the union of medial and lateral roots from the medial and lateral cords of the brachial plexus, respectively (Fig. 7.16, *A* and *B*). The nerve runs distally in the arm, initially on the lateral side of the brachial artery until it reaches the middle of the arm, where it crosses to the medial side and contacts the brachialis. The median nerve then descends to the *cubital fossa, where it lies deep to the bicipital aponeurosis* and median cubital vein. The **ulnar nerve** arises from the medial cord of the brachial plexus, conveying fibers mainly from C8 and T1 nerves (Fig. 7.16). It passes distally, anterior to the triceps, on the medial side of the brachial artery. *The ulnar nerve passes posterior to the medial humeral epicondyle of the humerus* (Figs. 7.17, *A* and 7.18*B*).

The **musculocutaneous nerve** arises from the lateral cord of the brachial plexus, passes through the coracobrachialis, and then runs distally between the brachialis and biceps (Fig. 7.16, *A* and *B*). *It supplies these three muscles and continues distally as* the *lateral cutaneous nerve of the forearm* (Fig. 7.8*A*; see also Fig. 7.22). The **radial nerve** arises from the posterior cord of the brachial plexus, con-

veying fibers from all roots of the plexus (Figs. 7.16, *B* and *C* and 7.18*B*). The radial nerve curves around the posterior surface in the *radial groove of the humerus* and passes to the cubital fossa. *Here the radial nerve divides into deep and superficial branches* (see Fig. 7.22). The radial nerve supplies the muscles in the posterior compartments of the arm and forearm and the overlying skin.

INJURY TO MUSCULOCUTANEOUS NERVE

Injury to the musculocutaneous nerve in the axilla is usually inflicted by a knife or bullet. The wound results in paralysis of the coracobrachialis, biceps, and brachialis; consequently, flexion of the elbow and supination of the forearm are weakened. Loss of sensation may occur on the lateral surface of the forearm supplied by the lateral cutaneous nerve of the forearm.

Injury to Radial Nerve

Injury to the radial nerve superior to the origin of its branches to the triceps brachii results in *paralysis of the triceps, brachioradialis, supinator, and extensor muscles of the wrist and fingers.* Loss of sensation occurs in areas of skin supplied by this nerve (e.g., lateral aspect of the elbow region). When the radial nerve is injured in the radial groove, the triceps usually is not completely paralyzed but it is weakened because only the medial head of the triceps is affected; however, the muscles in the posterior compartment of the forearm that are supplied by more distal branches of the radial nerve are paralyzed. *The characteristic clinical sign of radial nerve injury is wrist-drop* (inability to extend the wrist and fingers at the metacarpophalangeal joints); instead, the wrist is flexed because of unopposed tonus of the flexor muscles and gravity.

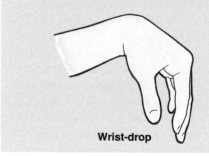

Wrist-drop

CUBITAL FOSSA

The cubital fossa is the shallow triangular depression on the anterior surface of the elbow (see Figs. 7.21 and 7.22). **The boundaries of the cubital fossa are:**

- Superiorly—imaginary line connecting the medial and lateral epicondyles

- Medially—pronator teres
- Laterally—brachioradialis.

The *floor of the cubital fossa* is formed by the brachialis and supinator muscles. The *roof of the fossa* is formed by deep fascia—reinforced by the *bicipital aponeurosis*—subcutaneous tissue and skin. **The contents of the cubital fossa are the:**

- *Terminal part of the brachial artery* and the commencement of its terminal branches, the *radial* and *ulnar arteries;* the brachial artery lies between the biceps tendon and the median nerve

- *(Deep) companion veins* of these arteries
- *Biceps tendon*
- *Median nerve.*

In the subcutaneous tissue overlying the cubital fossa are the (Figs. 7.8 and 7.9A):

- *Median cubital vein,* lying anterior to the bicipital aponeurosis, which in turn lies anterior to the brachial artery and median nerve

- *Medial and lateral cutaneous nerves* of the forearm, related to the basilic and cephalic veins.

Surface Anatomy of Arm and Cubital Fossa

The borders of the deltoid are visible when the arm is abducted against resistance. The *distal attachment of the deltoid* can be palpated on the lateral surface of the humerus. The **three heads of the triceps** form a bulge on the posterior aspect of the arm and are identifiable when the forearm is extended from the flexed position against resistance. The **triceps tendon** may be felt as it descends along the posterior aspect of the arm to the olecranon. The **biceps brachii** forms a bulge on the anterior aspect of the arm; its belly becomes more prominent when the elbow is flexed and supinated against resistance. Medial and lateral **bicipital grooves** separate the bulges formed by the biceps and triceps. The cephalic vein runs superiorly in the lateral bicipital groove and the basilic vein ascends in the medial bicipital groove. The **biceps tendon** can be palpated in the cubital fossa, immediately lateral to the midline. The proximal part of the **bicipital aponeurosis** can be palpated where it passes obliquely over the brachial artery and median nerve. The **brachial artery** may be felt pulsating deep to the medial border of the biceps.

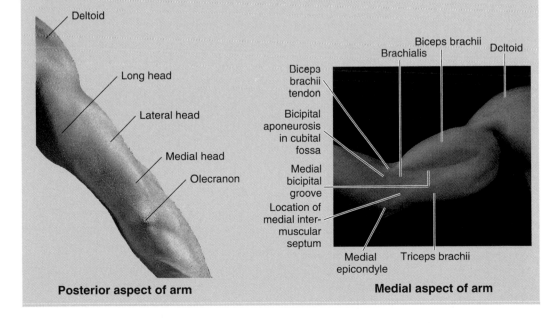

Posterior aspect of arm

- Deltoid
- Long head
- Lateral head
- Medial head
- Olecranon

Medial aspect of arm

- Biceps brachii
- Brachialis
- Deltoid
- Biceps brachii tendon
- Bicipital aponeurosis in cubital fossa
- Medial bicipital groove
- Location of medial inter-muscular septum
- Medial epicondyle
- Triceps brachii

FOREARM

The forearm lies between the elbow and wrist. It contains two bones, the **radius** and **ulna,** and many muscles, the tendons of which pass mostly to the hand (Fig. 7.20).

MUSCLES OF FOREARM

The tendons of the forearm muscles pass through the distal part of the forearm and into the hand. The radius, ulna, and the **interosseous membrane** connecting them divide the forearm into *anterior (flexor-pronator)* and *posterior (extensor-supinator) compartments* (Fig. 7.20).

- The **flexor-pronator muscles** arise by a common flexor tendon from the **medial epicondyle** (Table 7.6), which constitutes the *common flexor attachment.*
- The **extensor-supinator muscles** arise by a common extensor tendon from the **lateral epicondyle,** which constitutes the *common extensor attachment.*

Flexor-Pronator Muscles of Forearm
The flexor-pronator muscles are in the anterior compartment of the forearm (Figs. 7.20 and 7.21). The tendons of most flexor muscles pass across the anterior surface of the wrist and are held in place by the **palmar carpal ligament** and the **flexor retinaculum,** thickenings of the antebrachial fascia. The muscles are arranged in four layers and divided into two groups, superficial and deep (Table 7.6):

- **A superficial group of five muscles—** pronator teres, flexor carpi radialis, palmaris longus, flexor carpi ulnaris, and flexor digitorum superficialis (**FDS**)—the latter muscle is considered by some authors to constitute an intermediate layer. These muscles are attached, at least in part, by a *common flexor tendon* from the medial epicondyle of the humerus— the *common flexor attachment*
- **A deep group of three muscles—**flexor digitorum profundus (**FDP**), flexor pollicis longus, and pronator quadratus.

The five superficial muscles cross the elbow joint; the three deep muscles do not. See Table 7.6 for attachments, nerve supply, and main actions of the flexor-pronator muscles. *All muscles in the anterior compartment are supplied by the median and/or ulnar nerves* (most by the median nerve—only one and a half exceptions are supplied by the ulnar nerve). *Functionally, the brachioradialis is a flexor of the forearm,* but it is located in the posterior (posterolateral) or extensor compartment and thus *the brachioradialis is supplied by the radial nerve* (Table 7.7). Therefore, this muscle is a major exception to the generalization that the radial nerve supplies only extensor muscles and that all flexors lie in the anterior compartment. The **long flexors of the digits** (FDS and FDP) also flex the metacarpophalangeal and wrist joints. The FDP flexes the fingers (digits) in slow action; this action is reinforced by the FDS when speed and flexion against resistance are required. When the wrist is flexed at the same time that the metacarpophalangeal and interphalangeal joints are flexed, the long flexor muscles of the fingers are operating over a shortened distance between attachments, and the action resulting from their contraction is consequently weaker. Extending the wrist increases their operating distance, and thus their contraction is more efficient in producing a strong grip. Tendons of the long flexors pass through the distal part of the forearm, wrist, and palm and continue to the medial four fingers. The *FDS flexes the middle phalanges; the FDP flexes the distal phalanges.*

The **pronator quadratus** pronates the forearm at the radioulnar joints and also at the "intermediate" (radioulnar) syndesmosis; *it is the prime mover in pronation.* The pronator quadratus initiates pronation; it is assisted by the pronator teres when more speed and power are needed. The pronator quadratus also acts as a shunt muscle by helping the interosseous membrane hold the radius and ulna together, particularly when upward thrusts are transmitted through the wrist (e.g., during a fall on the hand).

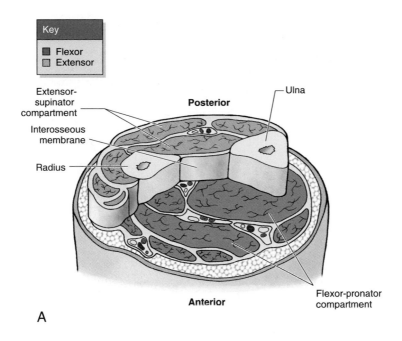

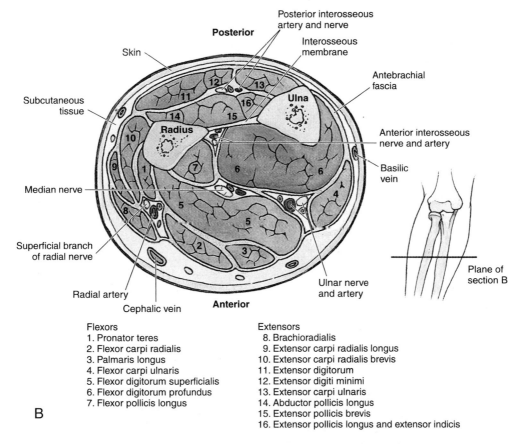

Flexors
1. Pronator teres
2. Flexor carpi radialis
3. Palmaris longus
4. Flexor carpi ulnaris
5. Flexor digitorum superficialis
6. Flexor digitorum profundus
7. Flexor pollicis longus

Extensors
8. Brachioradialis
9. Extensor carpi radialis longus
10. Extensor carpi radialis brevis
11. Extensor digitorum
12. Extensor digiti minimi
13. Extensor carpi ulnaris
14. Abductor pollicis longus
15. Extensor pollicis brevis
16. Extensor pollicis longus and extensor indicis

FIGURE 7.20   Bones, muscles, and compartments of the forearm. A. Anterosuperior view of a stepped transverse section. **B.** Transverse section.

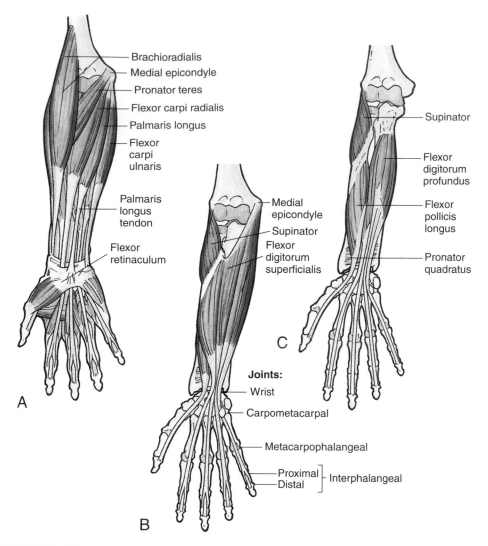

FIGURE 7.21 **Flexor muscles of the forearm.** Anterior views. **A.** First layer. **B.** Second layer. **C.** Third and fourth layers.

MUSCLE TESTING OF FDS AND FDP
To test the FDS, one finger is flexed at the proximal interphalangeal joint against resistance and the other three fingers are held in an extended position to inactivate the FDP. *To test the FDP,* the proximal interphalangeal joint is held in the extended position while the person attempts to flex the distal interphalangeal joint.

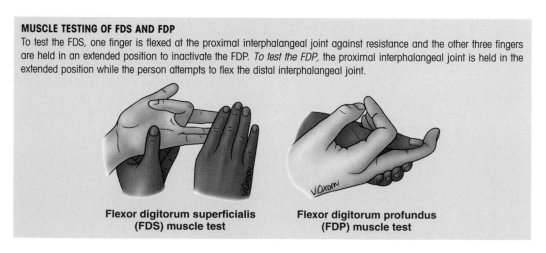

Flexor digitorum superficialis (FDS) muscle test   **Flexor digitorum profundus (FDP) muscle test**

TABLE 7.6. MUSCLES OF ANTERIOR COMPARTMENT OF FOREARM

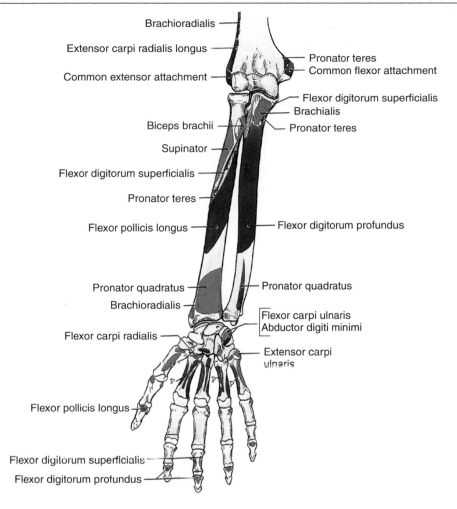

Muscle	Proximal Attachment	Distal Attachment	Innervation[a]	Main Action(s)
Superficial muscles				
Pronator teres	Medial epicondyle of humerus and coronoid process of ulna	Middle of lateral surface of radius	Median nerve (C6 and **C7**)	Pronates forearm and flexes it (at elbow)
Flexor carpi radialis	Medial epicondyle of humerus	Base of second metacarpal bone		Flexes hand and abducts it (at wrist)
Palmaris longus		Distal half of flexor retinaculum and palmar aponeurosis	Median nerve (C7 and C8)	Flexes hand (at wrist) and tightens palmar aponeurosis

continued

TABLE 7.6. *CONTINUED*

Muscle	Proximal Attachment	Distal Attachment	Innervation[a]	Main Action(s)
Flexor carpi ulnaris	*Humeral head:* medial epicondyle of humerus *Ulnar head:* olecranon and posterior border of ulna	Pisiform bone, hook of hamate, and 5th metacarpal	Ulnar nerve (C7 and **C8**)	Flexes and adducts hand (at wrist)
Flexor digitorum superficialis	*Humeroulnar head:* medial epicondyle of humerus, ulnar collateral ligament, and coronoid process of ulna *Radial head:* superior half of anterior border of radius	Bodies of middle phalanges of medial four digits	Median nerve (C7, **C8**, and T1)	Flexes middle phalanges at proximal interphalangeal joints of medial four digits; acting more strongly, it also flexes proximal phalanges at metacarpophalangeal joints and hand
Deep muscles				
Flexor digitorum profundus	Proximal three fourths of medial and anterior surfaces of ulna and interosseous membrane	Bases of distal phalanges of medial four digits	*Medial part:* ulnar nerve (**C8** and T1) *Lateral part:* median nerve (**C8** and T1)	Flexes distal phalanges at distal interphalangeal joints of medial four digits; assists with flexion of hand
Flexor pollicis longus	Anterior surface of radius and adjacent interosseous membrane	Base of distal phalanx of thumb	Anterior interosseous nerve from median nerve (**C8** and T1)	Flexes phalanges of first digit (thumb)
Pronator quadratus	Distal fourth of anterior surface of ulna	Distal fourth of anterior surface of radius		Pronates forearm; deep fibers bind radius and ulna together

[a]Numbers indicate spinal cord segmental innervation (e.g., C5 and **C7** indicate that nerves supplying the pronator teres muscle are derived from the 5th and 7th cervical segments of spinal cord). Boldface numbers indicate main segmental innervation. Damage to these segments, or to motor nerve roots arising from them, results in paralysis of muscles concerned.

Extensor Muscles of Forearm

The extensor muscles are in the posterior (extensor-supinator) compartment of the forearm, and all are innervated by the radial nerve (Figs. 7.20 and 7.22, Table 7.7). **The extensor muscles may be organized into three functional groups:**

- *Muscles that extend and abduct or adduct the hand at the wrist joint* (extensor carpi radialis longus, extensor carpi radialis brevis, and extensor carpi ulnaris)

- *Muscles that extend the medial four digits* (extensor digitorum, extensor indicis, and extensor digiti minimi)

- *Muscles that extend or abduct the 1st digit, or thumb* (abductor pollicis longus [APL], extensor pollicis brevis [EPB], and extensor pollicis longus [EPL]).

The extensor tendons are held in place in the wrist region by the **extensor retinaculum,** which prevents bowstringing of the tendons

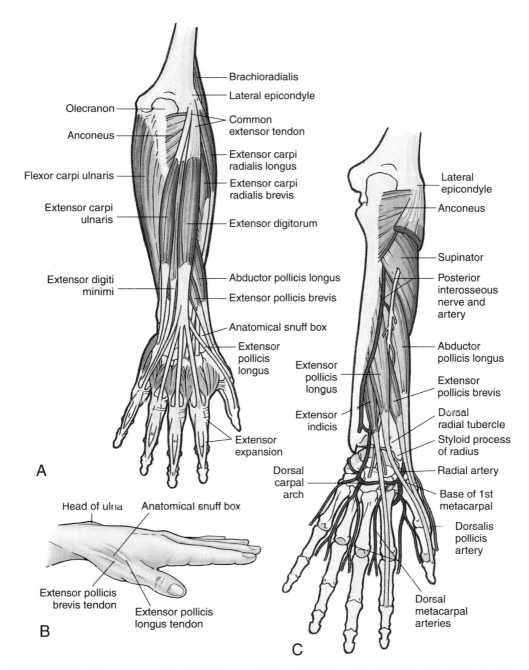

FIGURE 7.22 **Extensor muscles of the forearm. A.** Superficial dissection. Posterior view. **B.** Anatomical snuff box. **C.** Deeper dissection of the supinator and outcropping muscles showing arteries and the posterior interosseous nerve, the terminal part of the deep branch of the radial nerve.

when the hand is hyperextended at the wrist. As the tendons pass over the dorsum of the wrist, they are provided with **synovial sheaths** that reduce friction between the extensor tendons and the bones (Fig. 7.23).

The extensor muscles also may be divided into superficial and deep groups. Four *superficial extensors* (extensor carpi radialis brevis, extensor digitorum, extensor digiti minimi, and extensor carpi ulnaris) are attached by a **common extensor tendon** to the lateral epicondyle (Fig. 7.22A, Table 7.7). The proximal attachment of the other two superficial extensors (brachioradialis and extensor carpi radialis longus) is to the lateral supracondylar ridge of the humerus and adjacent lateral intermuscular septum. The four tendons of the **extensor digitorum** pass deep to the extensor retinaculum to the medial four fingers (Fig. 7.23, A and B). The flattened tendons of the index and little fingers are joined on their medial sides near the knuckles by the respective tendons of the extensor indicis and extensor digiti minimi (extensors of index and little fingers, respectively), which enable relatively independent extension of these fingers. The extensor indicis tendon enters the hand in the same tunnel as the tendons of the extensor digitorum. The tendon of the extensor digiti minimi has its own tunnel. Usually three oblique bands—**intertendinous connections** (Fig. 7.23A)—unite the four tendons of the extensor digitorum proximal to the knuckles, restricting independent actions of the middle and ring fingers. Consequently, normally no one digit can remain fully flexed as the other ones are fully extended.

The extensor tendons flatten to form **extensor expansions** ("dorsal hoods") on the dorsal aspect of digits 2 to 5 (Fig. 7.23). Each extensor expansion is a triangular tendinous aponeurosis that wraps around the dorsum and the sides of a head of the metacarpal and base of the proximal phalanx, and extending across the middle phalanx and the two interphalangeal joints to the distal phalanx. The visorlike "hood" of the expansion over the head of the metacarpal is anchored on each side to the **palmar ligament,** holding the ex-

tensor tendon in the middle of the digit. The tendinous part of the extensor expansion divides into a *median band* that passes to the base of the middle phalanx and two *lateral bands* that pass to the base of the distal phalanx. The **interosseous** and **lumbrical muscles** of the hand attach to the lateral bands of the extensor expansion (Fig. 7.23, A and C). On flexing the distal interphalangeal joint the extensor expansion becomes taut, pulling the proximal interphalangeal joint into flexion. Similarly, when the metacarpophalangeal joint is flexed by the interosseous and lumbrical muscles, the proximal and distal joints are pulled by the extensor expansions (lateral bands) into nearly complete extension (the so-called "Z-movement").

The **deep extensors of forearm** (abductor pollicis longus [**APL**], extensor pollicis brevis [**EPB**], and extensor pollicis longus [**EPL**]) act on the thumb, and the extensor indicis helps extend the index finger (Figs. 7.20B and 7.22, Table 7.7). The three muscles acting on the thumb (APL, EPB, and EPL) are deep to the superficial extensors and emerge (or "crop out") along a furrow on the lateral part of the forearm that divides the extensors. Because of this characteristic, the *APL, EPB, and EPL* are referred to as "outcropping muscles." The tendons of the APL and EPB bound the triangular **anatomical snuff box** anteriorly, and the tendon of the EPL bounds it posteriorly (Fig. 7.22, A and B). The "snuff box" is visible as a hollow on the lateral aspect of the wrist when the thumb is extended fully; this draws the APL, EPB, and EPL tendons up and produces a concavity between them. *In the anatomical snuffbox, observe that the:*

- *Radial artery* lies on the floor of the snuff box
- *Radial styloid process* can be palpated proximally in the snuff box and the base of the 1st metacarpal can be palpated distally in it
- *Scaphoid and trapezium* can be felt in the floor of the snuff box between the radial styloid process and the 1st metacarpal.

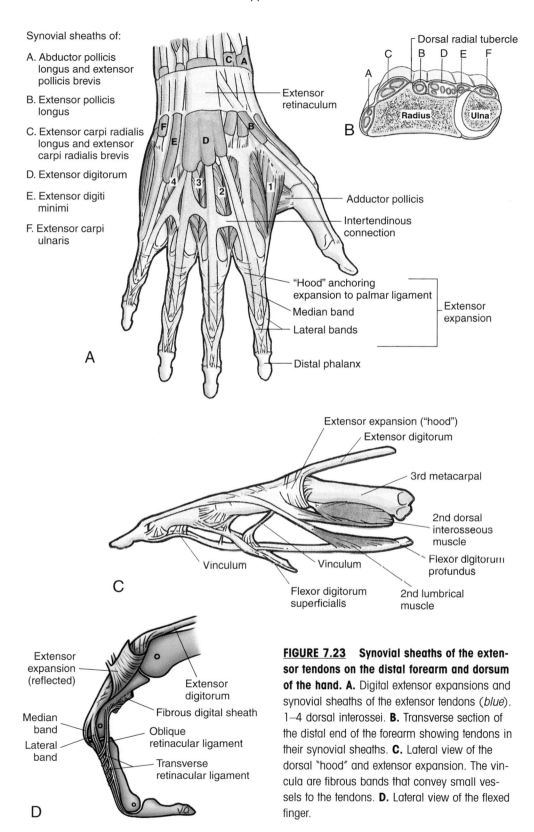

Synovial sheaths of:

A. Abductor pollicis longus and extensor pollicis brevis

B. Extensor pollicis longus

C. Extensor carpi radialis longus and extensor carpi radialis brevis

D. Extensor digitorum

E. Extensor digiti minimi

F. Extensor carpi ulnaris

Extensor retinaculum

Adductor pollicis

Intertendinous connection

"Hood" anchoring expansion to palmar ligament

Median band

Lateral bands

Extensor expansion

Distal phalanx

A

Dorsal radial tubercle

Radius   Ulna

B

Extensor expansion ("hood")

Extensor digitorum

3rd metacarpal

2nd dorsal interosseous muscle

Flexor digitorum profundus

2nd lumbrical muscle

Vinculum

Vinculum

Flexor digitorum superficialis

C

Extensor expansion (reflected)

Median band

Lateral band

Extensor digitorum

Fibrous digital sheath

Oblique retinacular ligament

Transverse retinacular ligament

D

FIGURE 7.23 Synovial sheaths of the extensor tendons on the distal forearm and dorsum of the hand. A. Digital extensor expansions and synovial sheaths of the extensor tendons (*blue*). 1–4 dorsal interossei. **B.** Transverse section of the distal end of the forearm showing tendons in their synovial sheaths. **C.** Lateral view of the dorsal "hood" and extensor expansion. The vincula are fibrous bands that convey small vessels to the tendons. **D.** Lateral view of the flexed finger.

TABLE 7.7. MUSCLES OF POSTERIOR COMPARTMENT OF FOREARM

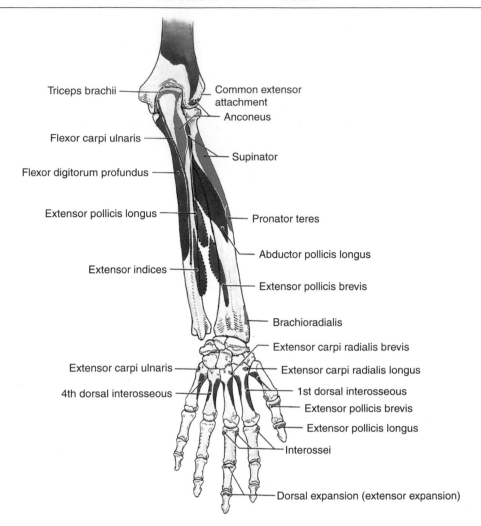

Muscle	Proximal Attachment	Distal Attachment	Innervation[a]	Main Action(s)
Brachioradialis	Proximal two thirds of lateral supracondylar ridge of humerus—the common extensor attachment	Lateral surface of distal end of radius	Radial nerve (C5, **C6**, and C7)	Flexes forearm
Extensor carpi radialis longus	Lateral supracondylar ridge	Base of 2nd metacarpal	Radial nerve (C6 and C7)	Extend and abduct hand at wrist joint
Extensor carpi radialis brevis	Lateral epicondyle of humerus—the common extensor attachment	Base of 3rd metacarpal	Deep branch of radial nerve (**C7** and C8)	Extend and abduct hand at wrist joint

TABLE 7.7. *CONTINUED*

Muscle	Proximal Attachment	Distal Attachment	Innervation[a]	Main Action(s)
Extensor digitorum	Lateral epicondyle of humerus	Extensor expansions of medial four digits	Posterior interosseous nerve (**C7** and C8), a branch of the radial nerve	Extends medial four digits at metacarpophalangeal joints; extends hand at wrist joint
Extensor digiti minimi		Extensor expansion of 5th digit		Extends 5th digit at metacarpophalangeal and interphalangeal joints
Extensor carpi ulnaris	Lateral epicondyle of humerus and posterior border of ulna	Base of 5th metacarpal		Extends and adducts hand at wrist joint
Anconeus	Lateral epicondyle humerus	Lateral surface of olecranon and superior part of posterior surface of ulna	Radial nerve (C7, C8, and T1)	Assists triceps in extending elbow joint, stabilizes elbow joint; abducts ulna during pronation
Supinator	Lateral epicondyle of humerus, radial collateral and anular ligaments, supinator fossa, and crest of ulna	Lateral, posterior, and anterior surfaces of proximal third of radius	Deep branch of radial nerve (C5 and **C6**)	Supinates forearm, i.e., rotates radius to turn palm anteriorly
Abductor pollicis longus	Posterior surfaces of ulna, radius, and interosseous membrane	Base of 1st metacarpal	Posterior interosseous nerve (C7 and **C8**)	Abducts thumb and extends it at carpometacarpal joint
Extensor pollicis brevis	Posterior surface of radius and interosseous membrane	Base of proximal phalanx of thumb		Extends proximal phalanx of thumb at carpometacarpal joint
Extensor pollicis longus	Posterior surface of middle third of ulna and interosseous membrane	Base of distal phalanx of thumb		Extends distal phalanx of thumb at metacarpophalangeal and interphalangeal joints
Extensor indicis	Posterior surface of ulna and interosseous membrane	Extensor expansion of 2nd digit		Extends 2nd digit and helps to extend hand

[a]Numbers indicate spinal cord segmental innervation (e.g., C5, **C6**, and C7 indicate that nerves supplying the brachioradialis muscle are derived from 5th to 7th cervical segments of spinal cord). Boldface numbers indicate main segmental innervation. Damage to these segments, or to motor nerve roots arising from them, results in paralysis of muscles concerned.

NERVES OF FOREARM

The major nerves of the forearm are the median, ulnar, and radial. Aside from the branches of the cutaneous nerves, two nerves supply the anterior aspect of the forearm: the median and ulnar nerves. Their origins are described in Table 7.4 and their courses and distributions are described in Table 7.8.

The **median nerve**—the principal nerve of the anterior (flexor-pronator) compartment of the forearm—enters the forearm with the brachial artery and lies medial to it. The median nerve leaves the cubital fossa by passing between the heads of the pronator teres (Fig. 7.24*B*), giving branches to them. The median nerve then passes deep to the FDS and continues distally through the middle of the forearm, between the FDS and FDP. Near the wrist, the median nerve becomes superficial by passing between the tendons of the FDS and flexor carpi radialis, deep to the palmaris longus tendon (see Fig. 7.28*A*).

The **ulnar nerve** *passes posterior to the medial epicondyle of the humerus* and enters the forearm by passing between the heads of the flexor carpi ulnaris (Fig. 7.24*A*), giving branches to them. It then passes inferiorly between the

flexor carpi ulnaris and the FDP, supplying the ulnar (medial) part of the muscle that sends tendons to digits 4 and 5. The ulnar nerve becomes superficial at the wrist, running on the medial side of the ulnar artery and the lateral side of the flexor carpi ulnaris tendon. The ulnar nerve emerges from beneath the flexor carpi ulnaris tendon just proximal to the wrist and passes superficial to the flexor retinaculum to enter the hand, where it supplies the skin on the medial side of the hand. The branches of the ulnar nerve in the forearm are described in Table 7.8.

The **radial nerve** leaves the posterior compartment of the arm to cross the anterior aspect of the lateral epicondyle of the humerus. In the cubital region, the radial nerve divides into deep and superficial branches (Fig. 7.24). The **deep branch of radial nerve** arises anterior to the lateral epicondyle and pierces the supinator. *The deep branch winds around the lateral aspect of the neck of the radius* and enters the posterior (extensor-pronator) compartment of the forearm where it continues as the **posterior interosseous nerve** (Fig. 7.22*C*, Table 7.8). The superficial branch of the radial nerve is a cutaneous and articular nerve that descends in the forearm under cover of the brachioradialis (Fig. 7.24*A*). The **superficial branch of the radial nerve** emerges in the distal part of the forearm and crosses the roof of the anatomical snuff box. It is distributed to skin on the dorsum of the hand and to a number of joints in the hand.

ARTERIES AND VEINS OF FOREARM

The brachial artery ends in the distal part of the cubital fossa by dividing into *the ulnar and radial arteries—the main arteries of the forearm* (Figs. 7.23 and 7.24). The branches of the ulnar and radial arteries are described in Table 7.9. The **ulnar artery,** the larger of the two terminal branches, *usually begins in the cubital fossa near the neck of the radius,* just medial to the biceps tendon. The artery descends through the anterior (flexor-pronator) compartment of the forearm, deep to the pronator teres. The artery then passes distally over the anterior aspect of the wrist to the palm. The **radial artery,** smaller than the ulnar artery, also *begins in the cubital fossa near the neck of the radius.*

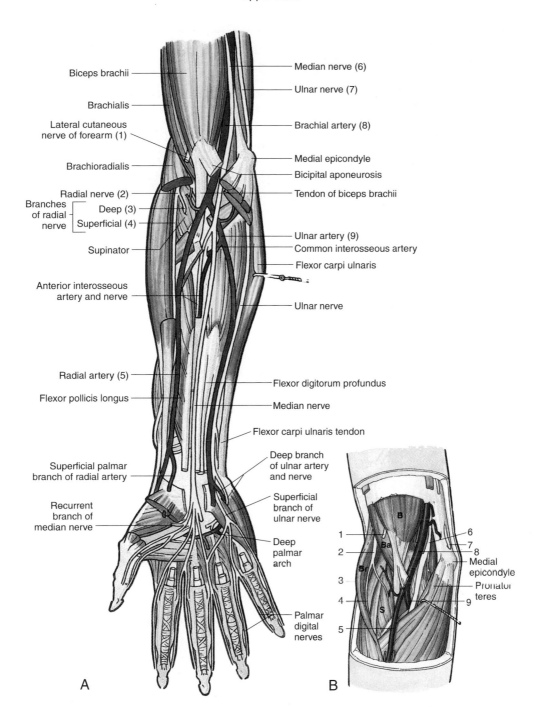

FIGURE 7.24 **Dissection of the anterior aspect of the upper limb and cubital fossa. A.** Muscles, vessels, and nerves. **B.** Contents of the cubital fossa. The *numbers* refer to structures labelled in **A.** *B,* biceps brachii; *Ba,* brachialis; *Br,* brachioradialis; *S,* supinator.

TABLE 7.8.   NERVES OF FOREARM AND HAND

Nerve	Origin	Course	Distribution
Median	By two roots from lateral (C6 and C7) and medial (C8 and T1) cords of brachial plexus	Enters cubital fossa medial to brachial artery, passes between heads of pronator teres, descends between flexor digitorum superficialis and flexor digitorum profundus, and passes close to flexor retinaculum as it passes through carpal tunnel to reach hand	
Recurrent branch of median	Arises from median as soon as it passes distal to flexor retinaculum	Loops around distal border of flexor retinaculum to reach thenar muscles	
Lateral branch of median (1)	Lateral division of median nerve as it enters palm of hand	Runs laterally supplying first lumbrical and cutaneous branches to anterior surface of thumb and lateral side of index finger	
Medial branch of median (1)	Medial division of median nerve as it enters palm of the hand	Runs medially to 2nd lumbrical muscle and sends cutaneous branches to adjacent sides of index and middle fingers and adjacent sides of middle and ring fingers	
Palmar cutaneous branch of median (2)	Median nerve just proximal to flexor retinaculum	Passes between tendons of palmaris longus and flexor carpi radialis and runs superficial to flexor retinaculum	
Anterior interosseous	Median nerve in distal part of cubital fossa	Passes inferiorly on interosseous membrane to supply flexor digitorum profundus, flexor pollicis longus, and pronator quadratus	
Ulnar (3)	Medial cord of brachial plexus (C8 and T1), but it often receives fibers from anterior ramus of C7	Passes posterior to medial epicondyle of humerus and enters forearm between heads of flexor carpi ulnaris; descends through forearm between flexor carpi ulnaris and flexor digitorum profundus; becomes superficial in distal part of forearm and passes superficial to flexor retinaculum	

Anterior view

Cutaneous nerves

Posterior view

Pronator teres
Flexor carpi radialis
Palmaris longus
Flexor digitorum superficialis
Flexor digitorum profundus (lateral half to digits 2 and 3)
Lumbricals to digits 2 and 3

Pronator teres
Flexor pollicis longus
Pronator quadratus
Thenar muscles

Anterior view
Median nerve

TABLE 7.8. *CONTINUED*

Nerve	Origin	Course	Distribution
Superficial branch of ulnar nerve	Arises from ulnar nerve at wrist as it passes between pisiform and hamate bones	Passes to palmaris brevis and to skin of medial one and one half digits	
Deep branch of ulnar nerve	Arises from ulnar nerve as described above	Supplies muscles of hypothenar eminence and then curves around inferior edge of hamate to pass deeply in palm to supply muscles shown in diagram	
Palmar cutaneous branch of ulnar nerve (4)	Ulnar nerve near middle of forearm	Descends on ulnar artery and perforates deep fascia in the distal third of forearm	
Radial	Posterior cord of brachial plexus (C5–C8 and T1)	Passes into cubital fossa and descends between brachialis and brachioradialis; at level of lateral epicondyle of humerus, it divides into superficial and deep branches	
Superficial branch of radial nerve (5)	Continuation of radial nerve after deep branch is given off	Passes distally, anterior to pronator teres and deep to brachioradialis; pierces deep fascia at wrist and passes onto dorsum of hand	
Deep branch of radial nerve	Arises from radial nerve just distal to elbow	Winds around neck of radius in supinator, enters posterior compartment as the posterior interosseous nerve	
Posterior interosseous	Terminal branch of deep branch of radial nerve	Passes deep to extensor pollicis longus and ends on interosseous membrane; supplies muscles shown in diagram	
Posterior cutaneous nerve of forearm (6)	Arises in arm from radial nerve	Perforates lateral head of triceps and descends along lateral side of arm and posterior aspect of forearm to wrist	
Lateral cutaneous nerve of forearm (7)	Continuation of musculocutaneous nerve	Descends along lateral border of forearm to wrist	
Medial cutaneous nerve of forearm (8)	Medial cord of brachial plexus, receiving fibers from C8 and T1	Runs down arm on medial side of brachial artery; pierces deep fascia in cubital fossa and runs along medial aspect of forearm	

Anterior view
Ulnar nerve

Posterior view
Radial nerve

Numbers in parentheses refer to cutaneous nerves in the top diagram on page 462.

TABLE 7.9. ARTERIES OF FOREARM

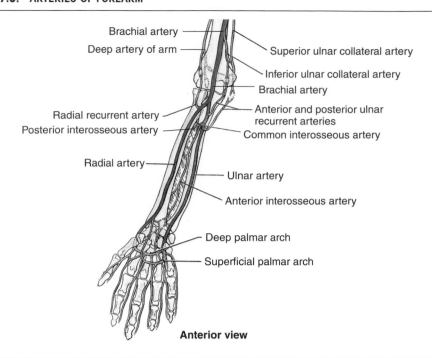

Brachial artery
Deep artery of arm
Superior ulnar collateral artery
Inferior ulnar collateral artery
Brachial artery
Radial recurrent artery
Posterior interosseous artery
Anterior and posterior ulnar recurrent arteries
Common interosseous artery
Radial artery
Ulnar artery
Anterior interosseous artery
Deep palmar arch
Superficial palmar arch

Anterior view

Artery	Course	Distribution
Ulnar	Larger terminal branch of brachial artery in cubital fossa	Passes inferomedially and then directly inferiorly, deep to pronator teres, palmaris longus, and flexor digitorum superficialis to reach medial side of forearm; passes superficial to flexor retinaculum at wrist and gives a deep palmar branch to deep arch and continues as superficial palmar arch
Anterior and posterior ulnar recurrent	Ulnar artery, just distal to elbow joint	Anterior ulnar recurrent artery passes superiorly and posterior ulnar recurrent artery passes posteriorly to anastomose with ulnar collateral and interosseous recurrent arteries
Common interosseous	Ulnar artery, just distal to bifurcation of brachial artery	After a short course, it terminates by dividing into anterior and posterior interosseous arteries
Anterior and posterior interosseous	Common interosseous artery	Pass to anterior and posterior sides of interosseous membrane: anterior interosseous artery supplies both anterior and posterior compartments in distal forearm; the posterior interosseous artery gives rise to the recurrent interosseous artery, which participates in the arterial anastomoses around the elbow
Dorsal and palmar carpal branches	Ulnar artery at level of wrist	Anastomose with corresponding branches of radial artery to form dorsal and palmar carpal arches, providing collateral circulation at wrist
Radial	Smaller terminal division of brachial artery in cubital fossa	Runs inferolaterally under cover of brachioradialis and distally lies lateral to flexor carpi radialis tendon; winds around lateral aspect of radius and crosses floor of anatomical snuff box to pierce fascia; ends by forming deep palmar arch with deep branch of ulnar artery
Radial recurrent	Lateral side of radial artery, just distal to its origin	Ascends on supinator and then passes between brachioradialis and brachialis
Dorsal and palmar carpal branches	Radial artery at level of wrist	Anastomose with corresponding branches of ulnar artery to form dorsal and palmar carpal arches, providing collateral circulation at wrist

The radial artery passes inferolaterally to the brachioradialis and lies on the anterior surface of the radius in the distal part of the forearm. It is covered only by skin and fascia and leaves the forearm by winding around the lateral aspect of the wrist and crossing the floor of the anatomical snuff box to reach the hand. There are superficial and deep veins in the forearm: *superficial veins* ascend in the subcutaneous tissue (p. 421); *deep veins* accompany the deep arteries (e.g., radial and ulnar).

HAND

The wrist—the proximal part of the hand—is at the junction of the forearm and hand (pp. 406 and 413). The *skeleton of the hand* consists of *carpals* in the wrist, *metacarpals* in the hand proper, and *phalanges* in the fingers, which are numbered from one to five beginning with the thumb and ending with the little finger.

FASCIA OF PALM

The palmar fascia is continuous with the antebrachial fascia and the fascia of the dorsum of the hand. The **palmar fascia** is thin over the thenar and hypothenar eminences, but it is thick centrally where it forms the palmar aponeurosis and in the digits where it forms the fibrous digital sheaths (Fig. 7.25*C*). The **palmar aponeurosis,** a strong, well-defined part of the palmar fascia, overlies the soft tissues of the central part of the palm and the long flexor tendons. The apex of the triangular palmar aponeurosis is continuous with the **flexor retinaculum** and **palmaris longus tendon** (Fig. 7.21*A*). Four *longitudinal digital bands* arise at the apex and radiate distally to the bases of the proximal phalanges where they become continuous with the fibrous digital sheaths (Fig. 7.25*C*). The **fibrous digital sheaths** are ligamentous tubes that enclose the superficial and deep flexor tendons and the synovial sheaths that surround them.

A **medial fibrous septum** extends deeply from the medial border of the palmar aponeurosis to the 5th metacarpal. Medial to this septum is the medial or **hypothenar compartment** containing the hypothenar muscles (Fig. 7.25*B*).

Similarly, a **lateral fibrous septum** extends deeply from the lateral border of the palmar aponeurosis to the 3rd metacarpal. Lateral to the septum is the lateral or **thenar compartment** containing the thenar muscles. Between the hypothenar and thenar compartments is the **central compartment** containing the flexor tendons and their sheaths, the lumbrical muscles, the superficial palmar arch, and the digital vessels and nerves (see Fig. 7.28*A*). A muscular plane deep to the central and hypothenar compartment is the **adductor compartment** containing the adductor pollicis muscle. Between the flexor tendons and the fascia covering the deep palmar muscles are two potential spaces, the **thenar space** and the **midpalmar space** (Fig. 7.25*A*). These spaces are bounded by fibrous septa passing from the edges of the palmar aponeurosis to the metacarpals. Between the two spaces is the especially strong lateral fibrous septum that is attached to the 3rd metacarpal (Fig. 7.25*B*).

DUPUYTREN CONTRACTURE OF PALMAR FASCIA
Dupuytren contracture is a progressive shortening, thickening, and fibrosis (increase in fibrous tissue) of the palmar fascia—especially the *palmar aponeurosis.* The fibrous degeneration of the longitudinal digital bands of the palmar aponeurosis on the medial side of the hand pulls the ring and little fingers into partial flexion at the metacarpophalangeal and proximal interphalangeal joints. The contracture is frequently bilateral and is most common in men older than 50 years.

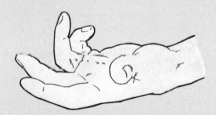

Dupuytren contracture

Hand Infections
Because the palmar fascia is thick and strong, swellings resulting from hand infections usually appear on the dorsum of the hand where the fascia is thinner. The fascial spaces determine the extent and direction of the spread of pus formed in the infected areas. Depending on the site of infection, pus will accumulate in the thenar, hypothenar, or adductor compartments. Owing to the widespread use of antibiotics, infections are rarely encountered that spread from one of these fascial compartments, but an untreated infection can spread proximally through the carpal tunnel into the forearm anterior to the pronator quadratus and its fascia.

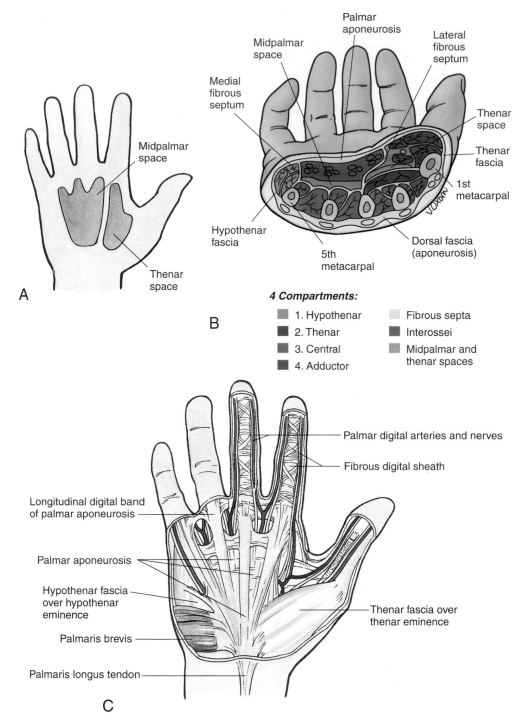

FIGURE 7.25 **Compartments, spaces, and fascia of the palm. A.** Thenar and midpalmar spaces. Anterior view. **B.** Transverse section of the palm. **C.** Palmar aponeurosis, fibrous digital sheaths, and digital nerves and vessels. Anterior view.

MUSCLES OF HAND

The intrinsic muscles of the hand are in four compartments (Figs. 7.25 and 7.27, Table 7.10):

- *Thenar muscles* in the **thenar compartment:** abductor pollicis brevis, flexor pollicis brevis, and opponens pollicis
- *Hypothenar muscles* in the **hypothenar compartment:** abductor digiti minimi, flexor digiti minimi, and opponens digiti minimi
- *Lumbricals associated with long flexor tendons* in the **central compartment**
- *Adductor pollicis* in the **adductor compartment.**

Thenar Muscles

The thenar muscles—*chiefly responsible for opposition of the thumb*—form the **thenar eminence** on the lateral surface of the palm (Figs. 7.25–7.27). The complex movement of opposition begins with the thumb in the extended position and initially involves a medial rotation of the 1st metacarpal (cupping the palm) produced by the action of the opponens pollicis at the carpometacarpal joint and then abduction, flexion, and usually adduction. The reinforcing action of the adductor pollicis and flexor pollicis longus increases the pressure that the opposed thumb can exert on the fingertips. *Normal movement of the thumb is important for the precise activities of the hand.* Because the 1st metacarpal in the thumb is more mobile than those of the other fingers, several muscles are required to control its freedom of movement. *The following movements occur at the carpometacarpal and metacarpophalangeal joints of the thumb* (Fig. 7.26):

- *Abduction:* Abductor pollicis longus (APL) and abductor pollicis brevis (APB)
- *Adduction:* adductor pollicis
- *Extension:* extensor pollicis longus (EPL), extensor pollicis brevis (EPB), and APL
- *Flexion:* flexor pollicis longus and flexor pollicis brevis
- *Opposition:* opponens pollicis, flexor pollicis brevis, adductor pollicis, and flexor pollicis longus increase pressure between the pulps of the fingers.

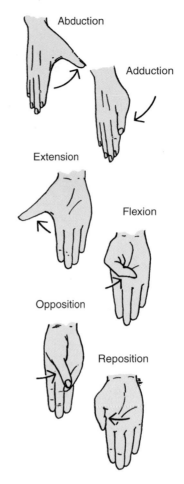

FIGURE 7.26   Thumb movements. The most complex movement, opposition, brings the tip of the thumb in contact with the pulps (pads) of the fingers (little finger here).

Hypothenar Muscles

These muscles (abductor digiti minimi, flexor digiti minimi brevis, and opponens digiti minimi) are in the hypothenar compartment and produce the **hypothenar eminence** on the medial side of the palm (Fig. 7.27, *A* and *B*). Their activities move the little finger. There is a small muscle in the subcutaneous tissue of the eminence, the **palmaris brevis** (Fig. 7.25*C*).

The palmaris brevis is not in the hypothenar compartment and it does not move the little finger. It wrinkles the skin of the hypothenar eminence, deepening the hollow of the palm, thereby aiding the palmar grip. *The palmaris brevis covers and protects the ulnar nerve and artery.* It is attached proximally to the medial border of the palmar aponeurosis and to the skin on the medial border of the hand.

Short Muscles of Hand

The short hand muscles are the lumbricals and interossei (Figs. 7.27 and 7.28, Table 7.10). The **four lumbricals** were named because of their wormlike appearance (L. *lumbricus*, earthworm). *The slender lumbricals flex the digits at the metacarpophalangeal joints and, in combination with the interossei, extend the interphalangeal joints.* The **four dorsal interossei** are located between the metacarpals; the **three palmar interossei**[1] are on the palmar surfaces of the 2nd, 4th, and 5th metacarpals. The 1st dorsal interosseous muscle is easy to palpate; oppose the thumb firmly against the index finger and it can be felt easily in the web between them. *The four dorsal interossei abduct the digits and the three palmar interossei adduct them.* A mnemonic device is to make acronyms of **D**orsal **Ab**duct (**DAB**) and **P**almar **Ad**duct (**PAD**). Acting together, the dorsal and palmar interossei and lumbricals produce flexion at the metacarpophalangeal joints and extension of the interphalangeal joints.

FLEXOR TENDONS OF EXTRINSIC MUSCLES

The tendons of the flexor digitorum superficialis (FDS) and flexor digitorum profundus (FDP) enter the **common synovial sheath** of digital flexors (Fig. 7.27). The tendons enter the central compartment of the hand and fan out to enter the respective **synovial sheaths of the digits.** The common and digital synovial sheaths enable the tendons to slide freely over the joints of the hand and relative to each other during movements of the digits. Near the base of the proximal phalanx, the tendon of the FDS splits and surrounds the tendon of the FDP (Fig. 7.28*A*). The halves of the FDS tendon are attached to the margins of the an-

---

[1]Some authors describe four palmar interossei; in so doing, they are including the deep head of the flexor pollicis brevis because of its similar innervation and placement on the thumb.

terior aspect of the base of the middle phalanx. The tendon of the FDP, after passing through the split in the FDS tendon, passes distally to attach to the anterior aspect of the base of the distal phalanx.

The **fibrous sheaths** of the digits (fibrous digital sheaths) are strong ligamentous tunnels containing the flexor tendons and their **synovial sheaths** (Figs. 7.27 and 7.28). The fibrous sheaths extend from the heads of the metacarpals to the bases of the distal phalanges. These sheaths prevent the tendons from pulling away from the concavities of the anterior aspect of the digits and the digits themselves as they flex. The fibrous sheaths combine with the phalanges to form **osseofibrous tunnels** through which the tendons pass within the digits. The fibrous sheaths have thick and thin parts; the thick parts form five **anular ligaments** and four **cruciate ligaments** (pulleys). The long flexor tendons are supplied by small blood vessels that pass to them within synovial folds (*vincula*—plural of vinculum) from the periosteum of the phalanges (Fig. 7.24*C*). The *tendon of the flexor pollicis longus passes deep to the flexor retinaculum to the thumb within its own synovial sheath.* At the head of the metacarpal, the tendon runs between two *sesamoid bones,* one in the combined tendon of the flexor pollicis brevis and abductor pollicis brevis and the other in the tendon of the adductor pollicis.

ARTERIES AND VEINS OF HAND

The ulnar and radial arteries and their branches provide all the blood to the hand (Fig. 7.28, Table 7.11). The **ulnar artery** enters the hand anterior to the flexor retinaculum between the pisiform and the hook of hamate. The ulnar artery lies lateral to the ulnar nerve. It divides into two terminal branches, the superficial palmar arch and the deep palmar branch. The **superficial palmar arch,** the main termination of the ulnar artery, gives rise to three **common palmar digital arteries** that anastomose with **palmar metacarpal arteries** from the deep palmar arch. Each common palmar digital artery di-

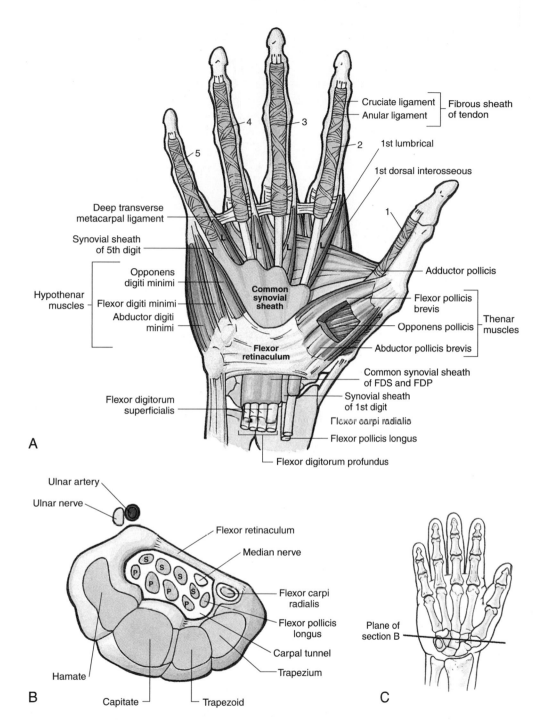

FIGURE 7.27 **Flexor tendons, common synovial sheath, fibrous sheaths, and synovial sheaths of the digits. A.** Dissection of the hand showing muscles, common synovial sheath, and synovial sheaths of digits 1 through 5 (*blue*) of the long flexor tendons. Anterior view. *L,* lumbricals. **B.** Transverse section of the wrist showing the carpal tunnel and its contents. *P,* flexor digitorum profundus (FDP); *S,* flexor digitorum superficialis (FDS). **C.** Orientation drawing.

TABLE 7.10. MUSCLES OF HAND

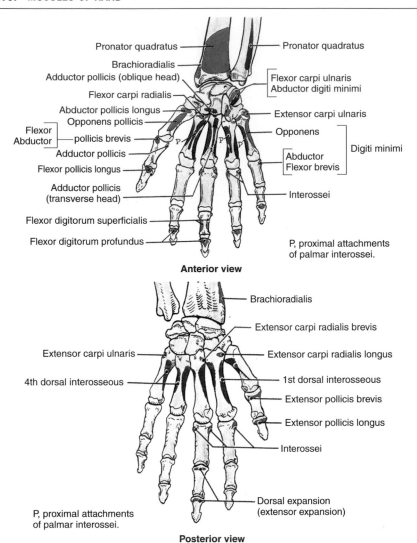

Pronator quadratus

Brachioradialis

Adductor pollicis (oblique head)

Flexor carpi radialis

Abductor pollicis longus

Opponens pollicis

Flexor
Abductor — pollicis brevis

Adductor pollicis

Flexor pollicis longus

Adductor pollicis
(transverse head)

Flexor digitorum superficialis

Flexor digitorum profundus

Pronator quadratus

Flexor carpi ulnaris
Abductor digiti minimi

Extensor carpi ulnaris

Opponens

Abductor
Flexor brevis

Digiti minimi

Interossei

P, proximal attachments
of palmar interossei.

Anterior view

Brachioradialis

Extensor carpi radialis brevis

Extensor carpi radialis longus

Extensor carpi ulnaris

4th dorsal interosseous

1st dorsal interosseous

Extensor pollicis brevis

Extensor pollicis longus

Interossei

Dorsal expansion
(extensor expansion)

P, proximal attachments
of palmar interossei.

Posterior view

Muscle	Proximal Attachment	Distal Attachment	Innervation[a]	Main Action(s)
Thenar muscles				
Abductor pollicis brevis	Flexor retinaculum and tubercles of scaphoid and trapezium	Lateral side of base of proximal phalanx of thumb	Recurrent branch of median nerve (**C8** and T1)	Abducts thumb and helps oppose it
Flexor pollicis brevis				Flexes thumb
Opponens pollicis		Lateral side of 1st metacarpal		Draws 1st metacarpal bone laterally to oppose thumb toward center of palm and rotates it medially

[a]Numbers indicate spinal cord segmental innervation (e.g., C8 and T1 indicate that nerves supplying the thenar muscles are derived from C8 and T1 segments of spinal cord). Boldface numbers indicate main segmental innervation. Damage to these segments, or to motor nerve roots rising from them, results in paralysis of muscles concerned.

TABLE 7.10. *CONTINUED*

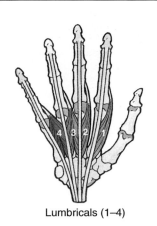

Lumbricals (1–4)

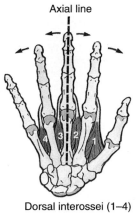

Dorsal interossei (1–4)

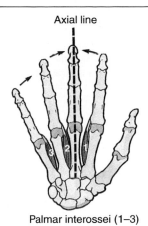

Palmar interossei (1–3)

Lumbricals and interossei

Muscle	Proximal Attachment	Distal Attachment	Innervation[a]	Main Action(s)
Adductor pollicis	*Oblique head:* bases of 2nd and 3rd metacarpals, capitate, and adjacent carpals *Transverse head:* anterior surface of body of 3rd metacarpal	Medial side of base of proximal phalanx of thumb	Deep branch of ulnar nerve (C8 and **T1**)	Adducts thumb toward middle digit
Hypothenar muscles				
Abductor digiti minimi	Pisiform	Medial side of base of proximal phalanx of digits		Abducts digit 5
Flexor digiti minimi brevis	Hook of hamate and flexor retinaculum			Flexes proximal phalanx of digit 5
Opponens digiti minimi		Medial border of 5th metacarpal		Draws 5th metacarpal anteriorly and rotates it, bringing digit 5 into opposition with thumb
Short muscles				
Lumbricals 1 and 2	Lateral two tendons of flexor digitorum profundus	Lateral sides of extensor expansions of digits 2–5	Median nerve (C8 and **T1**)	Flex digits at metacarpophalangeal joints and extend interphalangeal joints
Lumbricals 3 and 4	Medial three tendons of flexor digitorum profundus		Deep branch of ulnar nerve (C8 and **T1**)	
Dorsal interossei 1–4	Adjacent sides of two metacarpals (bipennate muscles)	Extensor expansions and bases of proximal phalanges of digits 2–4	Deep branch of ulnar nerve (C8 and **T1**)	Abduct digits from axial line and act with lumbricals to flex metacarpophalangeal joints and extend interphalangeal joints
Palmar interossei 1–3	Palmar surfaces of 2nd, 4th, and 5th metacarpals (unipennate muscles)	Extensor expansions of digits and bases of proximal phalanges of digits 2, 4, and 5		Adduct digits 2, 4, and 5 toward axial line and assist lumbricals in flexing metacarpophalangeal joints and extending interphalangeal joints

TENOSYNOVITIS

Injuries such as puncture of the palm by a rusty nail can cause *infection of the synovial sheaths of the digits*. When inflammation of the tendon and synovial sheath (*tenosynovitis*) occurs, the finger swells and movement becomes painful. Because the tendons of the 2nd, 3rd, and 4th digits nearly always have separate synovial sheaths, the infection usually is confined to the infected digit. In neglected infections, however, the proximal ends of these sheaths may rupture, allowing the infection to spread to the *midpalmar space* (Fig. 7.25A). Because the synovial sheath of the little finger is usually continuous with the *common synovial sheath*, tenosynovitis in this digit may spread to the common sheath and thus through the palm and carpal tunnel to the anterior forearm. Likewise, tenosynovitis in the thumb may spread through the continuous synovial sheath of the flexor pollicis longus (radial bursa). Just how far an infection spreads from the digits depends on variations in their connections with the common flexor sheath.

Thickening of a fibrous sheath on the palmar aspect of the digit often results in *stenosis (narrowing) of the osseofibrous tunnel of a finger*. If the tendons of the FDS and FDP enlarge (forming a nodule) proximal to the tunnel, the person is unable to extend the finger. When the finger is extended passively, a snap is audible. Flexion produces another snap as the thickened tendon moves. This condition is called *digital tenovaginitis stenosans* ("trigger finger" or "snapping finger").

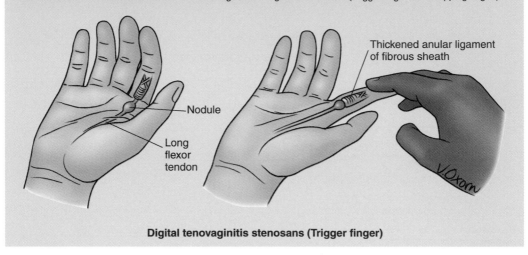

Digital tenovaginitis stenosans (Trigger finger)

vides into a pair of **proper palmar digital arteries** that run along the adjacent sides of the 2nd through 4th fingers. The **radial artery** curves dorsally around the scaphoid and trapezium in the floor of the anatomical snuff box and enters the palm by passing between the heads of the 1st dorsal interosseous muscle. It then turns medially and passes between the heads of the adductor pollicis (Fig. 7.28A). The radial artery anastomoses with the deep branch of the ulnar artery to form the **deep palmar arch.** This arch, formed mainly by the radial artery, lies across the metacarpals just distal to their bases. The deep palmar arch gives rise to three **palmar metacarpal arteries** and the **princeps pollicis** arteries, which supply the palmar surface and sides of the thumb.

The superficial and deep **palmar arches** are accompanied by superficial and deep **palmar venous arches,** respectively. The dorsal digital veins drain into three *dorsal metacarpal veins,* which unite to form a **dorsal venous network** (p. 421). Superficial to the metacarpus, this network is prolonged proximally on the lateral side as the **cephalic vein.** The **basilic vein** arises from the medial (ulnar) side of the dorsal venous network.

LACERATION OF PALMAR ARCHES

Bleeding is usually profuse when the arterial arches are lacerated. It may not be sufficient to ligate (tie off) only one forearm artery when the arches are lacerated because these vessels usually have numerous communications in the forearm and hand and thus bleed from both ends.

TABLE 7.11. ARTERIES OF HAND

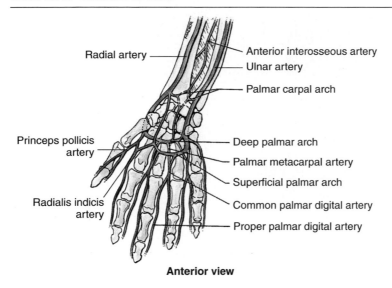

Anterior view

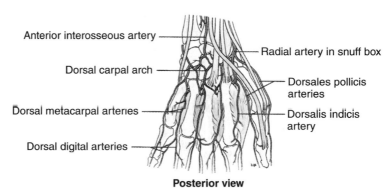

Posterior view

Artery	Origin	Course
Superficial palmar arch	Direct continuation of ulnar artery; arch is completed on lateral side by superficial branch of radial artery or another of its branches	Curves laterally deep to palmar aponeurosis and superficial to long flexor tendons; curve of arch lies across palm at level of distal border of extended thumb
Deep palmar arch	Direct continuation of radial artery; arch is completed on medial side by deep branch of ulnar artery	Curves medially deep to long flexor tendons and is in contact with bases of metacarpals
Common palmar digitals	Superficial palmar arch	Pass distally on lumbricals to webbings of digits
Proper palmar digitals	Common palmar digital arteries	Run along sides of digits 2–5
Princeps pollicis	Radial artery as it turns into palm	Descends on palmar aspect of 1st metacarpal and divides at the base of proximal phalanx into two branches that run along sides of thumb
Radialis indicis	Radial artery but may arise from princips pollicis artery	Passes along lateral side of index finger to its distal end
Dorsal carpal arch	Radial and ulnar arteries	Arches within fascia on dorsum of hand

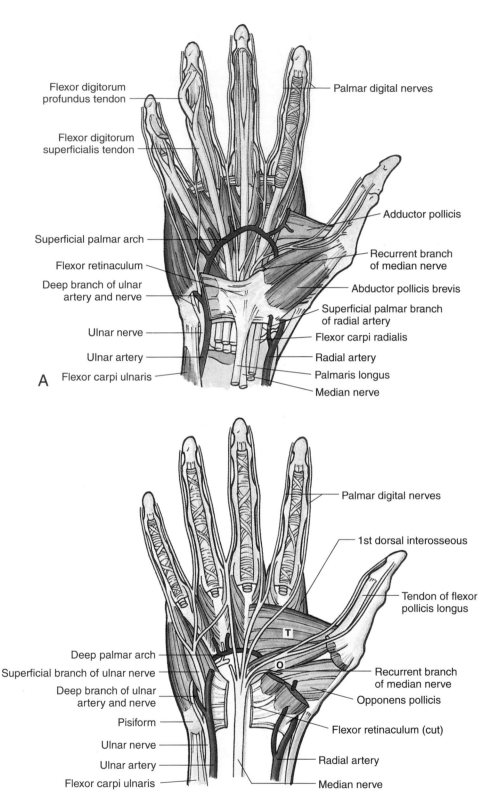

FIGURE 7.28 Palmar arches and nerves. A. Superficial dissection of the palm of the hand, showing the superficial palmar arch and the distribution of the median and ulnar nerves. Anterior view. **B.** Deeper dissection showing the deep palmar arch and the deep branch of the ulnar nerve. Anterior view. *T,* transverse head of adductor pollicis; *O,* oblique head of adductor pollicis.

NERVES OF HAND

The median, ulnar, and radial nerves supply the hand (Figs. 7.22*B* and 7.24, Table 7.8). The **median nerve** enters the hand through the carpal tunnel, deep to the flexor retinaculum (Figs. 7.27 and 7.28), along with the tendons of the flexors digitorum superficialis and profundus and the flexor pollicis longus. The **carpal tunnel** is the passageway deep to the flexor retinaculum between the tubercles of the scaphoid and the trapezoid bones on the lateral side and the pisiform and the hook of hamate on the medial side. *Distal to the carpal tunnel, the median nerve supplies the three thenar muscles and the 1st and 2nd lumbricals.* It also sends sensory fibers to the skin on the entire palmar surface, the sides of the first three digits, the lateral half of the 4th digit, and the dorsum of the distal halves of these digits. Note, however, that the palmar branch, which supplies the central palm, arises proximal to the carpal tunnel and does not traverse the tunnel (i.e., it runs superficial to the flexor retinaculum). Thus, although this skin lies distal to the tunnel, it does not lose sensation when *carpal tunnel syndrome* develops.

The **ulnar nerve** leaves the forearm by emerging from deep to the tendon of the flexor carpi ulnaris (Figs. 7.27 and 7.28, Table 7.8). It passes distally to the wrist, where it is bound by fascia to the anterior surface of the flexor retinaculum. It then passes alongside the lateral border of the pisiform; the ulnar artery is on its lateral side. Just proximal to the wrist, the ulnar nerve gives off a *palmar cutaneous branch* that passes superficial to the flexor retinaculum and palmar aponeurosis; it supplies skin on the medial side of the palm. The ulnar nerve also gives off a *dorsal cutaneous branch* that supplies the medial half of the dorsum of the hand, the 5th digit, and the medial half of the 4th digit. The ulnar nerve ends at the distal border of the flexor retinaculum by dividing into superficial and deep branches (Fig. 7.28*B*). The **superficial branch of ulnar nerve** supplies cutaneous branches to the anterior surfaces of the medial one and a half digits. The **deep branch of ulnar nerve** supplies the hypothenar muscles, the medial two lumbricals, the adductor pollicis, and all the interossei. The deep branch also supplies several joints (wrist, intercarpal, carpometacarpal, and intermetacarpal). *The ulnar nerve is referred to as the nerve of fine movements because it innervates muscles that are concerned with intricate hand movements.*

The **radial nerve** supplies no hand muscles. Its terminal branches, superficial and deep, arise in the cubital fossa (Fig. 7.24, Table 7.8). The *superficial branch of the radial nerve* is the direct continuation of the radial nerve along the anterolateral aspect of the forearm and is entirely sensory. It travels under cover of the brachioradialis and then pierces the deep fascia near the dorsum of the wrist to supply the skin and fascia over the lateral two thirds of the dorsum of the hand, the dorsum of the thumb, and the proximal parts of the index and middle fingers.

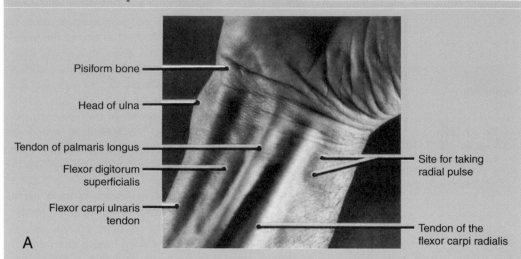

Pisiform bone

Head of ulna

Tendon of palmaris longus

Flexor digitorum
superficialis

Flexor carpi ulnaris
tendon

Site for taking
radial pulse

Tendon of the
flexor carpi radialis

A

A common place for measuring the pulse rate—**radial pulse**—is where the radial artery lies on the anterior surface of the distal end of the radius, lateral to the tendon of the flexor carpi radialis (**A**). Here the artery can be compressed against the radius, where it lies between the tendons of the flexor carpi radialis and abductor pollicis longus. The tendons of the flexor carpi radialis and palmaris longus can be palpated and usually observed by flexing the closed fist against resistance. *The tendon of the palmaris longus serves as a guide to the median nerve, which lies deep to it.* The **tendon of flexor carpi radialis** may be seen and palpated anterior to the wrist, a little lateral to its middle. The **tendon of flexor carpi ulnaris** can be palpated as it crosses the anterior aspect of the wrist near the medial side and inserts into the pisiform. *The flexor carpi ulnaris tendon serves as a guide to the ulnar nerve and artery.* The tendons of the FDS can be palpated as the digits are alternately flexed and extended.

The tendons of the APL and EPB muscles indicate the anterior boundary of the **anatomical snuff box** and the tendon of the EPL indicates the posterior boundary of the box (**B**). The radial artery passes through the snuff box, where its pulsations may be felt.

If the dorsum of the hand is examined with the wrist extended against resistance and the digits abducted, the *tendons of the extensor digitorum* to the fingers stand out (**B**). These tendons are not visible far beyond the knuckles because they flatten here to form the extensor expansions. Under the loose subcutaneous tissue and extensor tendons, the metacarpals can be palpated. The palmar skin presents several more or less constant *flexion creases* where the skin is firmly bound to the deep fascia (**C**). The **distal wrist crease** indicates the proximal border of the flexor retinaculum. The transverse palmar creases indicate where the skin folds during flexion of the hand. The **proximal palmar crease** commences on the lateral border of the palm, superficial to the bodies of the 3rd through 5th metacarpals. The **distal palmar crease** begins at or near the cleft between the index and middle fingers and crosses the palm with a slight convexity, superficial to the heads of the 2nd through 4th metacarpals. Each of the medial four digits usually has three transverse flexion creases. The **proximal digital crease** is located at the root of the digit, approximately 2 cm distal to the metacarpophalangeal joint. The proximal digital crease of the thumb crosses obliquely, proximal to the 1st metacarpophalangeal joint. The **middle digital crease** lies over the proximal interphalangeal joint, and the **distal digital crease** lies proximal to the distal interphalangeal joint. The thumb, having two phalanges, has only two flexion creases.

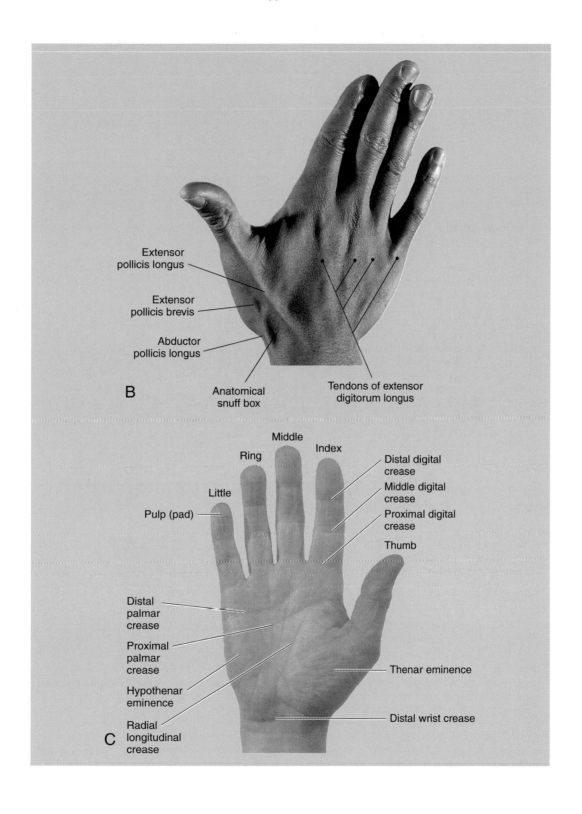

Extensor pollicis longus

Extensor pollicis brevis

Abductor pollicis longus

Anatomical snuff box

Tendons of extensor digitorum longus

B

Middle

Ring

Index

Little

Pulp (pad)

Distal digital crease

Middle digital crease

Proximal digital crease

Thumb

Distal palmar crease

Proximal palmar crease

Hypothenar eminence

Radial longitudinal crease

Thenar eminence

Distal wrist crease

C

LACERATION OF WRIST

Accidental laceration of the wrist often causes median nerve injury because this nerve is relatively close to the surface. In *attempted suicides by wrist slashing,* the median nerve is commonly injured just proximal to the flexor retinaculum. This results in paralysis of the thenar muscles and the first two lumbricals. Hence, opposition of the thumb is not possible and fine control movements of the 2nd and 3rd digits are impaired. *Ape hand* refers to a deformity that is marked by thumb movements being limited to flexion and extension of the thumb in the plane of the palm because of the inability to oppose and the limited abduction of the thumb. Sensation is also lost over the thumb and adjacent two and a half digits.

Trauma to Median Nerve

Median nerve injury resulting from a perforating wound in the elbow region results in loss of flexion of the proximal and distal interphalangeal joints of the 2nd and 3rd digits ("hand of benediction"). The ability to flex the metacarpophalangeal joints of these digits is also affected because digital branches of the median nerve supply the 1st and 2nd lumbricals. The *recurrent branch of the median nerve* supplying the thenar muscles lies superficially (Fig. 7.28B) and may be severed by relatively minor lacerations involving the thenar eminence. Severance of the recurrent branch of the median nerve paralyzes the thenar muscles, and the thumb loses much of its usefulness.

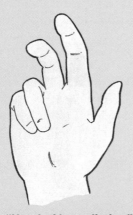

"Hand of benediction"

Ulnar Nerve Injury

Ulnar nerve injury commonly occurs where the nerve passes posterior to the medial epicondyle of the humerus. The injury results when the lateral part of the elbow hits a hard surface, fracturing the medial epicondyle. Ulnar nerve injury occurring at the elbow, wrist, or in the hand may result in extensive motor and sensory loss to the hand with accompanying impaired power of adduction. On flexing the wrist joint, the hand is drawn to the lateral (radial) side by the flexor carpi radialis in the absence of the "balance" provided by the flexor carpi ulnaris. *After ulnar nerve injury, persons are likely to have difficulty making a fist because*

of paralysis of most intrinsic hand muscles. In addition, their metacarpophalangeal joints become hyperextended and they cannot flex their 4th and 5th digits at the distal interphalangeal joints when they try to make a fist; nor can they extend their interphalangeal joints when they try to straighten their fingers. This results in a characteristic *clawhand appearance.* Compression of the ulnar nerve also may occur at the wrist where it passes between the pisiform and the hook of hamate. The depression between these bones is converted by the *pisohamate ligament* into an osseofibrous tunnel (Guyon canal). *Compression of the ulnar nerve* in this canal results in hypesthesia—diminished sensitivity to stimulation—in the medial one and one half digits and weakness of the intrinsic hand muscles.

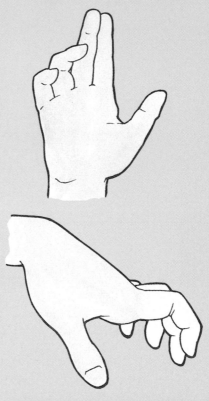

Ulnar nerve injury (clawhand)

Radial Nerve Injury

Although the radial nerve supplies no muscles in the hand, radial nerve injury in the arm can produce serious disability of the hand. The characteristic handicap is *paralysis of the extensor muscles of the forearm* (Table 7.7). The hand is flexed at the wrist and lies flaccid, a condition known as **wrist-drop** (p. 448). The digits also remain in the flexed position at the metacarpophalangeal joints. The radial nerve has only a small area of exclusive cutaneous supply to the hand. The extent of anesthesia is minimal, even in serious radial nerve injuries, and usually is confined to a small area on the lateral part of the dorsum of the hand.

JOINTS OF UPPER LIMB

The *pectoral girdle* involves the sternoclavicular, acromioclavicular, and glenohumeral (shoulder) joints. Generally, these joints move at the same time. Functional defects in any of these joints impair movements of the pectoral girdle. Mobility of the scapula is essential for the freedom of movement of the upper limb. When testing the range of motion of the pectoral girdle, both scapulothoracic (movement of the scapula on the thoracic wall) and glenohumeral movements must be considered (Fig. 7.29). When elevating the arm, the movement occurs in a 2:1 ratio; for every 3° of elevation, approximately 2° occurs at the glenohumeral joint and 1° at the scapulothoracic movement ("scapulo-humeral rhythm").

STERNOCLAVICULAR JOINT

This synovial articulation is between the sternal end of the clavicle and the manubrium of the sternum and the cartilage of the 1st rib. The SC joint is a saddle type of joint but functions as a ball-and-socket joint (Fig. 7.30). The SC joint is divided into two compartments by an **articular disc.** The disc is firmly attached to the anterior and posterior **SC ligaments**—thickenings of the fibrous capsule of the joint—as well as to the **interclavicular ligament**—a thickened part of the superior aspect of the fibrous capsule prolonged across the manubrium to become continuous with that of the contralateral joint. The great strength of the SC joint is a consequence of these attachments. Thus, although the articular disc serves as a shock absorber of forces transmitted along the clavicle from the upper limb, dislocation of the clavicle is unusual whereas fracture is common. The SC joint—the only articulation between the upper limb and the axial skeleton—can be readily palpated because the sternal end of the clavicle lies superior to the manubrium. The **fibrous capsule**—the fibrous part of the articular capsule—surrounds the SC joint, including the epiphysis at the sternal end of the clavicle. The fibrous capsule is attached to the margins of the articular surfaces, including the periphery of the articular disc. A *synovial membrane* lines the fibrous part of the articular capsule and both surfaces of the articular disc. Anterior and posterior **SC ligaments** reinforce the articular capsule anteriorly and posteriorly. The **costoclavicular ligament**—an extra-articular ligament of the SC joint—anchors the inferior surface of the sternal end of the clavicle to the 1st rib and its costal cartilage, limiting elevation of the pectoral girdle. Although the SC joint is extremely strong, it is significantly mobile to allow movements of the pectoral girdle and upper limb. During full elevation of the limb, the clavicle is raised to approximately a 60° angle. *The SC joint moves in several directions: anteriorly, posteriorly, and inferiorly*, up to 24 to 30° along its long axis. The SC joint is supplied by internal thoracic and suprascapular arteries (Table 7.3). Branches of the medial supraclavicular nerve and the nerve to the subclavius supply the SC joint (Table 7.4).

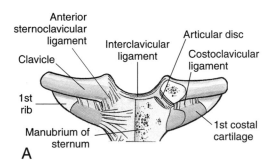
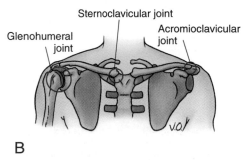

FIGURE 7.29   Sternoclavicular (SC) joints. Anterior view. **A.** Section of the left joint showing the articular disc dividing the joint into two compartments. **B.** Pectoral girdle. Orientation drawing for **A.**

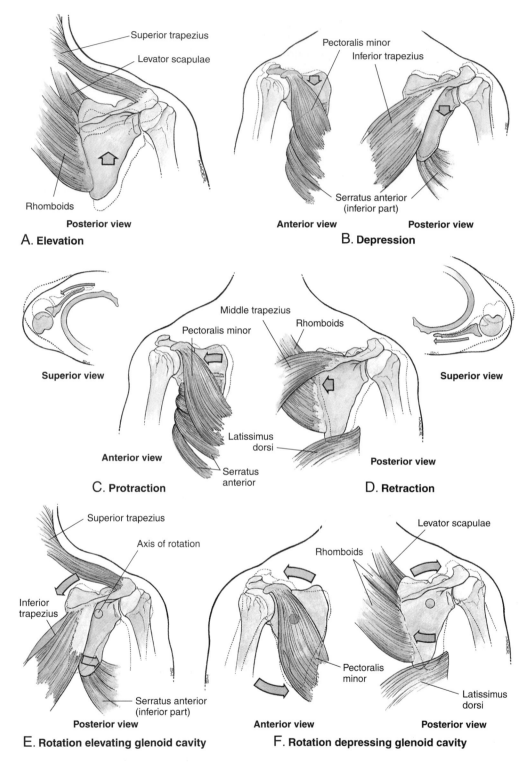

FIGURE 7.30   **Scapular movements.** The scapula moves on the thoracic wall at the conceptual "scapu-lothoracic joint." **A.** Elevation. **B.** Depression. **C.** Protraction. **D.** Retraction. **E.** Rotation elevating the glenoid cavity. **F.** Rotation depressing the glenoid cavity. *Dotted lines* represent the starting position of each movement.

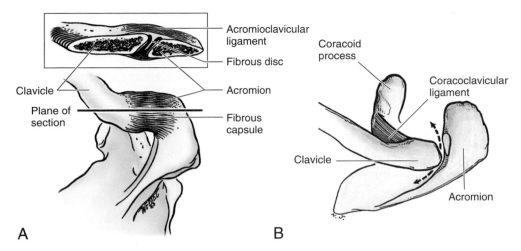

FIGURE 7.31   **Acromioclavicular (AC) joints. A.** Superior view of the right joint. *Inset,* coronal section of the acromioclavicular joint showing its fibrous capsule and disc. **B.** Diagram demonstrating the function of the coracoclavicular ligament. Superior view.

ACROMIOCLAVICULAR JOINT

The acromial end of the clavicle articulates with the acromion. The articular surfaces, covered with fibrocartilage, are separated by an incomplete wedge-shaped **articular disc.** The AC joint is a plane synovial joint (Fig. 7.31). It is located 2 to 3 cm from the point of the shoulder formed by the lateral part of the acromion of the scapula. The sleevelike, relatively loose *fibrous part of the articular capsule*—**fibrous capsule**—is attached to the margins of the articular surfaces. A *synovial membrane* lines the fibrous capsule. Although relatively weak, the articular capsule is strengthened superiorly by fibers of the trapezius (Fig. 7.29*A*). Most of its "strength" comes from coracoclavicular ligaments. They maintain its integrity and prevent the acromion from being driven under the clavicle even when the AC joint is separated.

The **AC ligament,** a fibrous band extending from the acromion to the clavicle, strengthens the AC joint superiorly (Fig. 7.32, *C* and *D*). The strong extra-articular **coracoclavicular ligament** (subdivided into conoid and trapezoid ligaments), located several cm from the AC joint, anchors the clavicle to the coracoid process of the scapula. The apex of the vertical **conoid ligament** is attached to the root of the coracoid process in front of the scapular notch. Its wide attachment (base) is to the

conoid tubercle on the inferior surface of the clavicle. The nearly horizontal **trapezoid ligament** is attached to the superior surface of the coracoid process and extends laterally and posteriorly to the trapezoid line (p. 407) on the inferior surface of the clavicle. *The conoid and trapezoid ligaments suspend the free upper limb from the strut formed by the clavicle,* passively bearing its weight.

The acromion of the scapula rotates on the acromial end of the clavicle. These movements are associated with motion at the conceptual scapulothoracic joint where the scapula moves on the thoracic wall. *No muscles cross the AC joint connecting the articulating bones to move the AC joint.* The thoracoappendicular muscles that attach to and move the scapula cause the acromion to move on the clavicle (Table 7.12). Factors limiting scapular movements are listed in Table 7.12. The AC joint is supplied by the suprascapular and thoracoacromial arteries (Table 7.3). Supraclavicular, lateral pectoral, and axillary nerves supply the AC joint (Table 7.4).

GLENOHUMERAL JOINT

The glenohumeral (shoulder) joint is a ball-and-socket synovial joint between the **humeral head** and the **glenoid cavity** of the

TABLE 7.12. STRUCTURES LIMITING MOVEMENTS OF SCAPULA

Movement	Limiting Structures (Tension)
Elevation	*Ligaments:* costoclavicular, inferior sternoclavicular, articular capsule *Muscles:* inferior trapezius, pectoralis minor, subclavius
Depression	*Ligaments:* sternoclavicular, interclavicular, articular disc *Muscles:* superior trapezius, levator scapulae *Bony opposition* between clavicle and 1st rib
Protraction	*Ligaments:* trapezoid, posterior sternoclavicular, posterior part of costoclavicular
Retraction	*Ligaments:* conoid ligament, anterior part of costoclavicular, anterior sternoclavicular *Muscles:* serratus anterior, pectoralis minor
Rotation depressing glenoid cavity	*Ligament:* conoid *Muscles:* serratus anterior
Rotation elevating glenoid cavity	*Ligaments:* trapezoid *Muscles:* levator scapulae, rhomboids

Modified from Clarkson HM: *Musculoskeletal Assessment: Joint Range of Motion and Manual of Muscle Strength,* 2nd ed. Baltimore: Lippincott Williams & Wilkins, 2000.

DISLOCATION OF AC JOINT

Although its extrinsic (coracoclavicular) ligament is strong, the AC joint itself is weak and easily injured by a direct blow. In contact sports such as football, soccer, and hockey, it is not uncommon for *dislocation of the AC joint* to result from a hard fall on the shoulder with the impact taken by the acromion, or from a fall on the outstretched upper limb. Dislocation of the AC joint also can occur when a hockey player is driven violently into the boards. The AC injury, often called a "shoulder separation," is severe when both the AC and coracoclavicular ligaments are torn. When the coracoclavicular ligament tears, the shoulder separates (falls away) from the clavicle because of the weight of the upper limb. Dislocation of the AC joint makes the acromion more prominent and the clavicle may move superior to this process.

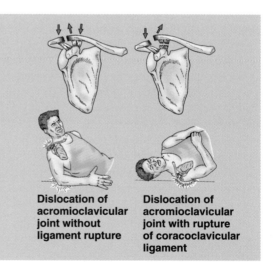

Dislocation of acromioclavicular joint without ligament rupture

Dislocation of acromioclavicular joint with rupture of coracoclavicular ligament

---

scapula. The relatively shallow glenoid cavity (Fig. 7.32) is deepened by the fibrocartilaginous **glenoid labrum** (L. lip). Both articular surfaces are covered with hyaline **articular cartilage.** The loose *fibrous part of the articular capsule*—**fibrous capsule**—surrounds the glenohumeral joint and is attached medially to the margin of the glenoid cavity and later-

ally to the anatomical neck of the humerus. The **synovial membrane** lines the fibrous capsule and forms a sheath for the tendon of the long head of the biceps brachii.

Ligaments of Glenohumeral Joint

The **glenohumeral ligaments** strengthen the anterior aspect of the articular capsule and the

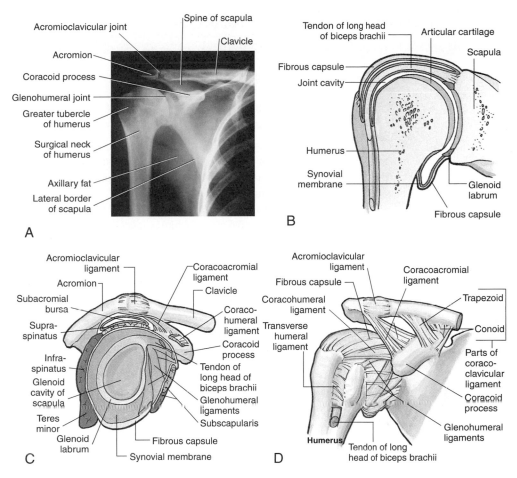

FIGURE 7.32   Glenohumeral and acromioclavicular joints. A. Radiograph of the glenohumeral and acromioclavicular joints. **B.** Coronal section illustrating the articulating bones and articular capsule of the glenohumeral joint. **C.** Lateral view of the scapula showing the glenoid cavity and the glenohumeral ligaments. **D.** Ligaments of the glenohumeral and SC joints. Anterior view.

coracohumeral ligament strengthens the capsule superiorly (Fig. 7.32, *C* and *D*). These ligaments are intrinsic ligaments—part of the fibrous capsule. The capsule is also thickened by the **transverse humeral ligament;** it strengthens the capsule and bridges the gap between the greater and lesser tubercles of the humerus. The **coracoacromial arch** is an extrinsic, protective structure formed by the smooth inferior aspect of the **acromion** and **coracoid process** of the scapula, with the **coracoacromial ligament** spanning between them (Fig. 7.32C). *The coracoacromial arch overlies the head of the humerus, preventing its superior displacement from the glenoid cavity.* The coracoacromial arch is so strong that a forceful superior thrust of the humerus will not fracture it; the shaft of the humerus or clavicle fractures first.

Movements of Glenohumeral Joint

The glenohumeral joint has more freedom of movement than any other joint in the body. This freedom results from the laxity of its articular capsule and the large size of the humeral head compared with the small size of the glenoid cavity. The glenohumeral joint allows movements around the three axes and permits flexion-extension, abduction-adduction, medial and lateral rotation, and circumduction. See

TABLE 7.13.   STRUCTURES LIMITING MOVEMENTS OF PECTORAL GIRDLE

Movement	Joint(s)	Limiting Structures (Tension)
Flexion (0–180°)	Sternoclavicular Acromioclavicular Glenohumeral Scapulothoracic	*Ligaments:* posterior part of coracohumeral, trapezoid, and posterior part of articular capsule of glenohumeral joint *Muscles:* rhomboids, levator scapulae, extensor and external rotator muscles, rotator muscles of glenohumeral joint
Abduction (0–180°)	Sternoclavicular Acromioclavicular Glenohumeral Scapulothoracic	*Ligaments:* middle and inferior glenohumeral, trapezoid, and inferior part of articular capsule of glenohumeral joint *Muscles:* rhomboids, levator scapulae, adductor muscles of glenohumeral joint *Bony apposition* between greater tubercle of humerus and superior part of glenoid cavity/labrum or lateral aspect of acromion
Extension	Glenohumeral	*Ligaments:* anterior part of coracohumeral and anterior part of articular capsule of glenohumeral joint *Muscles:* clavicular head of pectoralis major
Medial (internal) rotation	Glenohumeral	*Ligaments:* posterior glenohumeral articular capsule *Muscles:* infraspinatus and teres minor
Lateral (external) rotation	Glenohumeral	*Ligaments:* glenohumeral, coracohumeral, anterior glenohumeral articular capsule *Muscles:* latissimus dorsi, teres major, pectoralis major, subscapularis

Modified from Clarkson HM: *Musculoskeletal Assessment: Joint Range of Motion and Manual of Muscle Strength,* 2nd ed. Baltimore: Lippincott Williams & Wilkins, 2000.

Table 7.13 for structures limiting movements of the glenohumeral joint. The muscles producing movements of the joint are the *thoracoappendicular muscles,* which may act indirectly on the joint (i.e., they act on the pectoral girdle), and the *scapulohumeral muscles,* which act directly on the joint (p. 425).

- *Chief flexors of the glenohumeral joint*—pectoralis major (clavicular part) and deltoid (anterior part), assisted by the coracobrachialis and biceps brachii
- *Chief extensor of the glenohumeral joint*—latissimus dorsi
- *Chief abductor of the glenohumeral joint*—deltoid, especially its central fibers (following initiation of movement by the supraspinatus)
- *Chief adductors of the glenohumeral joint*—pectoralis major and latissimus dorsi
- *Chief medial rotator of the glenohumeral joint*—subscapularis
- *Chief lateral rotator of the glenohumeral joint*—infraspinatus.

Other muscles serve the glenohumeral joint as *shunt muscles,* acting to resist dislocation without producing movement at the joint. The tonus of the *rotator cuff muscles* holds the large head of the humerus in the relatively shallow glenoid cavity. The glenohumeral joint is supplied by the anterior and posterior **circumflex humeral arteries** and branches of the **suprascapular artery** (Table 7.3). The *suprascapular, axillary,* and *lateral pectoral nerves* supply the glenohumeral joint.

There are several bursae around the glenohumeral joint. The bursae are located where tendons rub against bone, ligaments, or other tendons and where skin moves over a bony prominence. Some of them communicate with the joint cavity; hence, opening a bursa may mean entering the cavity of the joint. The **subacromial bursa** (Fig. 7.32C) is between the acromion and the fibrous capsule of the joint. This bursa facilitates movement of the supraspinatus tendon under the coracoacromial arch and of the deltoid over the fibrous capsule and the greater tubercle of the humerus. The *subdeltoid bursa* is between the deltoid and the fibrous capsule. It may be combined with the subacromial bursa. The *subscapular bursa* is located between the tendon of the subscapularis and the neck of the scapula. This bursa protects the tendon where it passes inferior to the root of the coracoid process and over the neck of the scapula. It usually communicates with the cavity of the joint through an opening in the fibrous capsule.

DISLOCATION OF GLENOHUMERAL JOINT

Because of its freedom of movement and instability, the glenohumeral joint is commonly dislocated by direct or indirect injury. *Anterior dislocation of the glenohumeral joint* occurs most often in young adults, particularly athletes. It is usually caused by excessive extension and lateral rotation of the humerus. The head of the humerus is driven inferoanteriorly, and the fibrous capsule and glenoid labrum may be stripped from the anterior aspect of the glenoid cavity. A hard blow to the humerus when the glenohumeral joint is fully abducted tilts the head of the humerus inferiorly onto the inferior weak part of the articular capsule. This may tear the articular capsule and dislocate the joint so that the humeral head comes to lie inferior to the glenoid cavity and anterior to the infraglenoid tubercle. Subsequently, the strong flexor and abductor muscles of the glenohumeral joint usually pull the humeral head anterosuperiorly into a subcoracoid position. Unable to use the arm, the person commonly supports it with the other hand. The axillary nerve may be injured when the glenohumeral joint dislocates because of its close relation to the inferior part of the articular capsule of this joint.

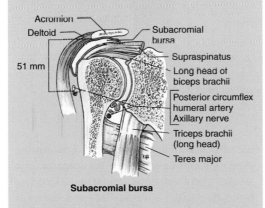

Acromion
Deltoid
Subacromial bursa
51 mm
Supraspinatus
Long head of biceps brachii
Posterior circumflex humeral artery
Axillary nerve
Triceps brachii (long head)
Teres major

Subacromial bursa

Supraspinatus Tendinitis

Inflammation and calcification of the subacromial bursa result in pain, tenderness, and limitation of movement of the glenohumeral joint. This condition is also known as *calcific scapulohumeral bursitis.* Calcium deposits in the supraspinatus tendon may irritate the subacromial bursa, producing an inflammatory reaction—*subacromial bursitis* (p. 427). As long as the glenohumeral joint is adducted, no pain usually results because in this position the painful lesion is away from the inferior surface of the acromion. The pain—felt during abduction of the arm—usually develops in persons 50 years and older after unusual or excessive use of the glenohumeral joint (e.g., during a tennis game).

Rotator Cuff Injuries

The musculotendinous rotator cuff is commonly injured during repetitive use of the upper limb above the horizontal (e.g., while throwing a baseball and/or in racquet sports, swimming, and weight lifting). *Recurrent inflammation of the rotator cuff,* especially the relatively avascular area of the supraspinatus tendon, is a common cause of shoulder pain and tears of the rotator cuff. Repetitive use of the rotator cuff muscles may allow the humeral head and rotator cuff to impinge on the coracoacromial arch, producing irritation of the arch and inflammation of the rotator cuff. Tendon degeneration and rupture of the rotator cuff may occur.

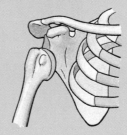

Anterior dislocation of right shoulder

ELBOW JOINT

The elbow joint is a compound hinge synovial joint—located 2 to 3 cm inferior to the humeral epicondyles—between the humerus and the forearm bones. The spool-shaped **trochlea** and spheroidal **capitulum** of the humerus articulate with the **trochlear notch** of the ulna and concave superior aspect of the **head of radius,** respectively; therefore there are *humeroulnar* and *humeroradial articulations* (Fig. 7.33, *A* and *C*). The fibrous part of the articular capsule—**fibrous capsule**—surrounding the joint is attached to the humerus at the margins of the lateral and medial ends of the articular surfaces of the capitulum and trochlea. Anteriorly and posteriorly the capsule is carried superiorly, proximal to the coronoid and olecranon fossae. The **synovial membrane** lines the fibrous capsule and intracapsular parts of the humerus. It is continuous inferiorly with the synovial membrane of the proximal radioulnar joint. The articular capsule is weak anteriorly and posteriorly but is strengthened on each side by ligaments.

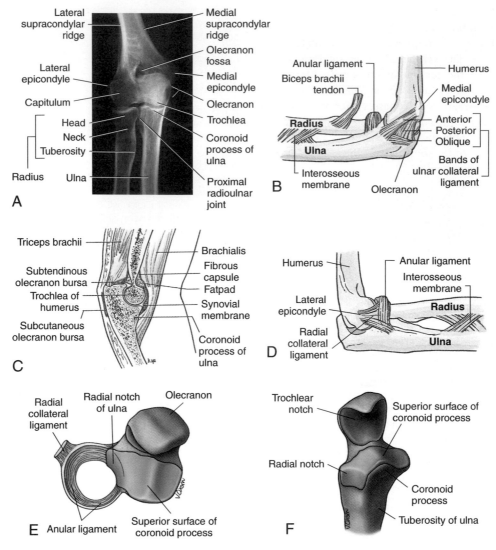

FIGURE 7.33 **Elbow and proximal radioulnar joints. A.** Anteroposterior radiograph. **B.** Ligaments. Medial view. **C.** Sagittal section of the elbow joint. **D.** Ligaments. Lateral view. **E.** Anular ligament attached to the radial notch of the ulna. Superior view. **F.** Articular surfaces of ulna. Anterolateral view.

Ligaments of Elbow Joint

The **collateral ligaments** of the elbow joint are strong triangular bands that are medial and lateral *thickenings of the fibrous capsule* (Fig. 7.33, *B, D,* and *E*). The lateral **radial collateral ligament** extends from the lateral epicondyle of the humerus and blends distally with the **anular ligament of radius.** This ligament encircles and holds the head of the radius in the radial notch of the ulna, forming the proximal radioulnar joint and permitting pronation and supination of the forearm. The medial **ulnar collateral ligament**—extending from the medial epicondyle of the humerus to the coronoid process and olecranon of the ulna—consists of three bands. The *anterior cordlike band* is the strongest; the *posterior fanlike band* is the weakest; and the slender *oblique band* deepens the socket for the trochlea of the humerus.

Movements of Elbow Joint

The movements of the elbow joint are flexion and extension. The long axis of the fully extended ulna makes an angle of approximately 170° with the long axis of the humerus—the **carrying angle** (Fig. 7.34). The obliquity of the angle is more pronounced in women than in men. See Table 7.14 for structures limiting movements of the elbow joint. The muscles moving the elbow joint cross the elbow and extend to the forearm and hand:

- *Chief flexors of the elbow joint*—brachialis, biceps brachii, and brachioradialis, in order of decreasing strength, assisted by the pronator teres when flexion is resisted
- *Chief extensors of the elbow joint*—triceps brachii, especially its medial head, assisted by the anconeus.

The **arteries supplying the elbow** are derived from the anastomosis of arteries around the elbow joint (Table 7.8). The **nerves supplying the elbow joint** are the musculocutaneous, radial, and ulnar nerves. **The two important bursae around the elbow** (Figs. 7.33C and 7.35) **are the:**

- *Subtendinous olecranon bursa (triceps bursa),* located between the olecranon and triceps tendon
- *Subcutaneous olecranon bursa,* located in the subcutaneous connective tissue over the olecranon.

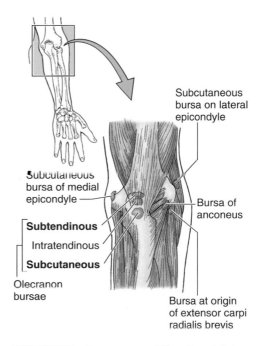

FIGURE 7.35   Bursae around the elbow joint.
Posterior view. The main bursae are in boldface.

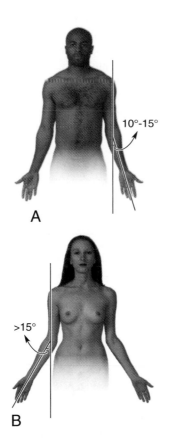

FIGURE 7.34   Carrying angle of the elbow joint.
Anterior view. **A.** Male. **B.** Female. Note the angle is greater in the woman.

BURSITIS OF ELBOW
Subtendinous olecranon bursitis results from excessive friction between the triceps tendon and olecranon, for example, resulting from repeated flexion-extension of the forearm as occurs during certain assembly line jobs. The pain is severe during flexion of the forearm because of pressure exerted on the inflamed subtendinous olecranon bursa by the triceps tendon. The subcutaneous olecranon bursa is exposed to injury during falls on the elbow and to infection from abrasions of the skin covering the olecranon. Repeated excessive pressure and friction produces a friction *subcutaneous olecranon bursitis* (e.g., "student's elbow").

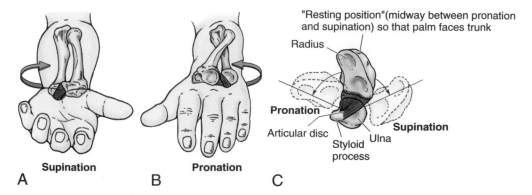

FIGURE 7.36   Supination and pronation of the forearm and hand. A. Supination. **B.** Pronation. **C.** Inferior surface of the radius, ulna, and articular disc. The articular disc (triangular ligament) of the distal radioulnar joint has a broad attachment to the radius but a narrow attachment to the styloid process of ulna, which serves as the pivot point for the rotary movement.

Avulsion of Medial Epicondyle

Avulsion of the medial epicondyle in children can result from a fall that causes severe abduction of the extended elbow. The resulting traction on the ulnar collateral ligament pulls the medial epicondyle distally. The anatomical basis of avulsion of the medial epicondyle is that the epiphysis for the medial epicondyle may not fuse with the distal end of the humerus until up to age 20. *Traction injury of the ulnar nerve* is a complication of the abduction type of avulsion of the medial epicondyle.

Dislocation of Elbow Joint

Posterior dislocation of the elbow joint may occur when children fall on their hands with their elbows flexed. Dislocations of the elbow may result from hyperextension or a blow that drives the ulna posteriorly or posterolaterally. The distal end of the humerus is driven through the weak anterior part of the fibrous capsule as the radius and ulna dislocate posteriorly.

RADIOULNAR JOINTS

The **proximal radioulnar joint** is between the head of the radius and the ring formed by the radial notch of the ulna and the anular ligament (Fig. 7.33, *B* and *E*). The *fibrous part of the articular capsule*—**fibrous capsule**—encloses the proximal radioulnar joint and is continuous with that of the elbow joint. The **synovial membrane** lines the fibrous capsule and nonarticulating aspects of the bones and is an inferior prolongation of the synovial membrane of the elbow joint (Fig. 7.33*C*). The **anular ligament** attaches to the ulna, anterior and posterior to the radial notch, forming a collar that, with the radial notch, forms a ring that completely *encircles the*

head of the radius. The deep surface of the anular ligament is lined with synovial membrane, which continues distally as a *sacciform recess* on the neck of the radius. During pronation and supination (Fig. 7.36), the head of the radius rotates within the anular ligament. **Supination** turns the palm anteriorly (or superiorly when the forearm is flexed). **Pronation** turns the palm posteriorly (or inferiorly when the forearm is flexed). During pronation and supination it is the radius that rotates. See Table 7.14 for structures limiting movements of the proximal radioulnar joint.

Supination is produced by the supinator (when resistance is absent) and by the biceps brachii (when resistance is present)—with some assistance from the extensor pollicis longus and extensor carpi radialis. *Pronation is produced by the pronator quadratus (primarily) and pronator teres (secondarily)*—with some assistance from the flexor carpi radialis, palmaris longus, and brachioradialis (when the forearm is in the midprone position).

The **distal radioulnar joint** is a pivot synovial joint between the head of ulna and the ulnar notch on the radius (Fig. 7.36, Table 7.15). The distal end of the radius rotates around the relatively fixed distal end of the ulna. A fibrocartilaginous **articular disc** binds the ends of the ulna and radius together. The base of the disc attaches to the medial edge of the ulnar notch of radius, and its apex is attached to the lateral side of the base of the styloid process of ulna. The

TABLE 7.14.   STRUCTURES LIMITING MOVEMENTS OF THE ELBOW AND RADIOULNAR JOINTS

Movement	Joint(s)	Limiting Structures (Tension)
Humeroulnar Humeroradial	Extension	*Muscles:* flexor muscles of elbow *Articular capsule:* anteriorly *Bony apposition* between olecranon of ulna and olecranon fossa of humerus
Humeroulnar Humeroradial	Flexion	*Muscle:* triceps brachii *Articular capsule:* posteriorly *Soft tissue apposition* between anterior forearm and arm *Bony apposition* between head of radius and radial fossa of humerus
Humeroradial Proximal radioulnar Distal radioulnar Interosseous membrane	Pronation	*Muscles:* supinator, biceps brachii *Ligaments:* quadrate, dorsal inferior radioulnar, interosseous membrane *Bony apposition* of the radius on ulna
Humeroradial Proximal radioulnar Distal radioulnar	Supination	*Muscles:* pronator teres, pronator quadratus *Ligaments:* quadrate, anterior inferior radioulnar, interosseous membrane

Modified from Clarkson HM: *Musculoskeletal Assessment: Joint Range of Motion and Manual of Muscle Strength*, 2nd ed. Baltimore: Lippincott Williams & Wilkins, 2000.

proximal surface of the triangular disc articulates with the distal aspect of the head of the ulna. Hence, the joint cavity is L-shaped in a coronal section, with the vertical bar of the "L" between the radius and ulna and the horizontal bar between the ulna and articular disc. The articular disc separates the cavity of the distal radioulnar joint from the cavity of the wrist joint. The *fibrous part of the articular capsule*—**fibrous capsule**—encloses the joint but is deficient superiorly. The **synovial membrane** extends superiorly between the radius and ulna to form another **sacciform recess** (Table 7.15). Like the proximal one, this redundancy of the synovial membrane accommodates the twisting of the capsule that occurs when the distal end of the radius travels around the relatively fixed distal end of the ulna during pronation and supination of the forearm. See Table 7.14 for structures limiting movements of the distal radioulnar joint. **Anterior** and **posterior ligaments** strengthen the fibrous capsule. These relatively weak transverse bands extend from the radius to the ulna across the anterior and posterior surfaces of the joint. The muscles producing movements of the distal radioulnar joint are discussed with the proximal radioulnar joint.

Arteries and Nerves

The proximal radioulnar joint is supplied by the anterior and posterior **interosseous arteries** (Table 7.9). The *ulnar* and *anterior interosseous arteries* supply the distal radioulnar joint. The proximal radioulnar joint is supplied by the **musculocutaneous, median,** and **radial nerves.** Pronation is essentially a function of the median nerve, whereas supination is a function of the musculocutaneous and radial nerves. The anterior and posterior **interosseous nerves** supply the distal radioulnar joint.

SUBLUXATION AND DISLOCATION OF RADIAL HEAD

Preschool children, particularly girls, are vulnerable to transient subluxation (incomplete dislocation) of the head of the radius ("pulled elbow"). The history of these cases is typical. The child is suddenly lifted (jerked) by the upper limb when the forearm is pronated (e.g., when lifting a child into a bus). The child may cry out and refuse to use the limb, which is protected by holding it with the elbow flexed and the forearm pronated. The sudden pulling of the upper limb tears the distal attachment of the anular ligament, where it is loosely attached to the neck of the radius (Fig. 7.33*E*). The radial head then moves distally, partially out of the torn anular ligament. The proximal part of the torn ligament may become trapped between the head of the radius and the capitulum of the humerus. The source of pain is the pinched anular ligament.

TABLE 7.15. JOINTS OF HAND

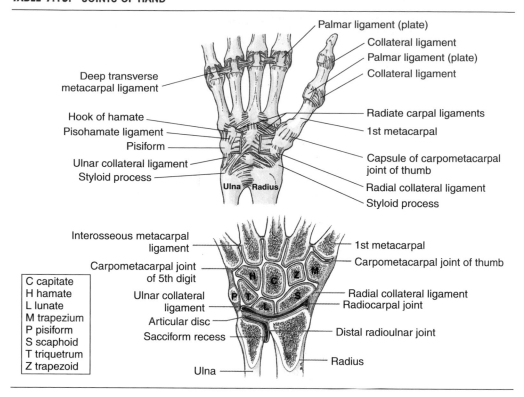

	Metacarpophalangeal Joints	Interphalangeal Joints
Type	Condyloid synovial joints	Hinge synovial joints
Articulation	Heads of metacarpals articulate with base of proximal phalanges (Fig. 7.37)	Heads of phalanges articulate with bases of more distally located phalanges (Fig. 7.37)
Articular capsule	Fibrous capsule encloses each joint and a synovial membrane attaches to margins of each joint	Fibrous capsule encloses each joint and a synovial membrane attaches to margins of each joint
Ligaments	Strong palmar ligaments are attached to phalanges and metacarpals; deep transverse metacarpal ligaments unite 2nd to 5th joints that hold heads of metacarpals together; collateral ligaments pass from heads of metacarpals to bases of phalanges	Ligaments are similar to those of metacarpophalangeal joints, except that they unite phalanges
Movements	Flexion-extension, abduction-adduction, and circumduction of 2nd to 5th digits; flexion-extension of thumb occurs but abduction-adduction is limited	Flexion-extension
Blood supply	Deep digital arteries that arise from superficial palmar arches	Digital arteries
Neve supply	Digital nerves that arise from ulnar and medial nerves	Digital nerves arising from ulnar and medial nerves

TABLE 7.15. *CONTINUED*

	Wrist (Radiocarpal) Joint	Carpal (Intercarpal) Joints	Carpometacarpal and Intermetacarpal Joints
Type	Condyloid synovial joint	Plane synovial joint	Plane synovial joints, except for carpometacarpal joint of thumb, which is a saddle-shaped synovial joint
Articulation	Distal end of radius and its articular disc articulate with the proximal row of carpal bones with the exception of pisiform	Between carpal bones of proximal row Joints between carpal bones of distal row The *midcarpal joint* is the synovial joint between the proximal joint and distal rows of carpal bones The *pisiform joint* is the synovial joint between the pisiform and triquetrum	Carpals and metacarpals articulate with each other as do metacarpals; carpometacarpal joint of thumb is between trapezium and base of 1st metacarpal
Articular capsule	Fibrous capsule surrounds joint and attaches to distal ends of radius and ulna and proximal row of carpal bones	Fibrous capsule surrounds joints; the pisiform joint is separate from other carpal joints	Fibrous capsule surrounds joints
Ligaments	Anterior and posterior ligaments strengthen fibrous capsule; ulnar collateral ligament attaches to styloid process of ulna and triquetrum; radial collateral ligament attaches to styloid process of radius and scaphoid	Carpal bones are united by anterior, posterior, and interosseous ligaments	Bones are united by anterior, posterior, and interosseous ligaments
Movements	Flexion-extension, abduction-adduction, and circumduction	A small amount of gliding movement is possible; flexion and abduction of hand occur at midcarpal joint	Flexion-extension and abduction-adduction of carpometacarpal joint of 1st digit; almost no movement occurs at 2nd and 3rd digits; 4th digit is slightly mobile; and 5th digit is very mobile
Blood supply	Dorsal and palmar carpal arches	Dorsal and palmar carpal arches	Dorsal and palmar metacarpal arteries and deep carpal and deep palmar arches
Nerve supply	All these joints are supplied by the anterior interosseous branch of median nerve, posterior interosseous branch of radial nerve, and dorsal and deep branches of ulnar nerve		

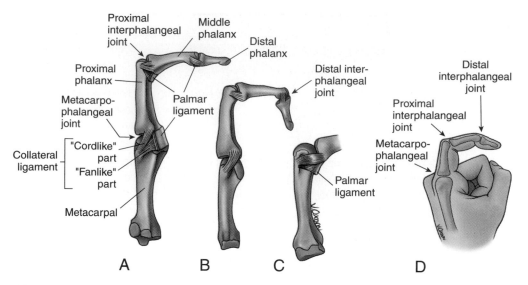

FIGURE 7.37 **Collateral ligaments of the metacarpophalangeal (MCP) and interphalangeal (IP) joints.** Lateral views. **A.** Extended MCP and distal IP joints. **B.** Flexed distal IP joint. **C.** Flexed MCP joint location. **D.** Drawing of a flexed left index finger showing its phalanges and the location of the MCP and IP joints. Lateral view.

JOINTS OF HAND

The joints of the hand (Figs. 7.37 and 7.38, Tables 7.15–7.17) include the:

- *Wrist (radiocarpal) joint*
- *Carpal (intercarpal) joints*
- Carpometacarpal joints
- Intermetacarpal joints
- Metacarpophalangeal joints
- Interphalangeal joints.

HAND JOINT INJURIES

Most wrist injuries occur as a result of falling on an outstretched hand. *Colles fracture* of the distal radius with displacement and/or angulation of the distal fragment dorsally is discussed on page 412. *Skier's thumb* refers to rupture or chronic laxity of the collateral ligament of the 1st metacarpophalangeal joint. The injury results from hyperabduction of the metacarpophalangeal joint of the thumb, which occurs when the thumb is held by the ski pole while the rest of the hand hits the ground. *Dislocation of the proximal interphalangeal joint* is the most common hand joint dislocation. This injury may be serious because digital nerves and vessels run along the sides of the fingers.

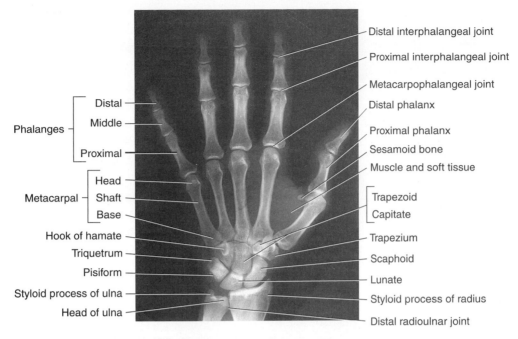

FIGURE 7.38 **Anteroposterior radiograph of the wrist and hand.** Notice the wide "joint space" at the distal end of the ulna because of the radiolucent articular disc. (Courtesy of Dr. E.L. Lansdown, Professor of Medical Imaging, University of Toronto, Toronto, Ontario, Canada.)

TABLE 7.16. STRUCTURES LIMITING MOVEMENTS OF WRIST AND CARPAL JOINTS

Movement	Limiting Structures (Tension)
Flexion	*Ligaments:* posterior radiocarpal and posterior part of articular capsule of joint
Extension	*Ligaments:* anterior radiocarpal and anterior part of articular capsule of joint *Bony apposition* between radius and carpal bones
Abduction	*Ligaments:* ulnar collateral ligament and medial part of articular capsule of joint *Bony apposition* between styloid process of radius and scaphoid
Adduction	*Ligaments:* radial collateral and lateral part of articular capsule of joint

Modified from Clarkson HM: *Musculoskeletal Assessment: Joint Range of Motion and Manual of Muscle Strength,* 2nd ed. Baltimore: Lippincott Williams & Wilkins, 2000.

TABLE 7.17. STRUCTURES LIMITING MOVEMENTS OF DIGITS

Movement	Joint(s)	Limiting Structures (Tension)
Flexion	CMC (thumb)	*Ligaments:* posterior part of articular capsule of joint *Muscles:* extensor and abductor pollicis brevis *Apposition* between thenar eminence and palm
	MCP (digits 1–5)	*Ligaments:* collateral, posterior part of articular capsule of joint *Apposition* between proximal phalanx and metacarpal
	PIP (digits 2–5)	*Ligaments:* collateral, posterior part of articular capsule of joint *Apposition* between middle and proximal phalanges
	DIP (digits 2–5)	*Ligaments:* collateral, oblique retinacular, and posterior part of articular capsule of joint
	IP (thumb)	*Ligaments:* collateral and posterior part of articular capsule of joint *Apposition* between distal and proximal phalanges
Extension	CMC (thumb)	*Ligaments:* anterior part of articular capsule of joint *Muscles:* 1st dorsal interosseous, flexor pollicis brevis
	MCP (digits 1–5) PIP and DIP (digits 2–5) IP (thumb)	*Ligaments:* anterior part of articular capsule of joint, palmar ligament
Abduction	CMC and MCP	*Muscles:* 1st dorsal interosseous adductor pollicis *Fascia and skin* of 1st web space
	MCP (digits 2–5)	*Ligaments:* collateral *Fascia and skin* of web spaces
Adduction	CMC and MCP (thumb)	Apposition between thumb and index finger
	MCP (digits 2–5)	Apposition between adjacent digits

CMC, carpometacarpal joint; *MCP,* metacarpophalangeal joint; *PIP,* proximal interphalangeal joint; *DIP,* distal interphalangeal joint; *IP,* interphalangeal joint.
Modified from Clarkson HM: *Musculoskeletal Assessment: Joint Range of Motion and Manual of Muscle Strength,* 2nd ed. Baltimore: Lippincott Williams & Wilkins, 2000.

MEDICAL IMAGING OF UPPER LIMB

Radiological examinations of the upper limb focus mainly on bony structures because muscles, tendons, and nerves are not well visualized. In addition to the usual anteroposterior (AP) view of the glenohumeral joint, an axial projection of the shoulder is often examined to obtain another view of the glenohumeral joint. To obtain an axial projection, the patient is asked to abduct the arm and extend the shoulder over the x-ray film cassette. In Figure 7.39, observe the acromion, glenoid cavity, humeral head, coracoid process, and suprascapular notch. Radiographs of the upper limb are also shown in Figures 7.32*A*, 7.33*A*, and 7.38.

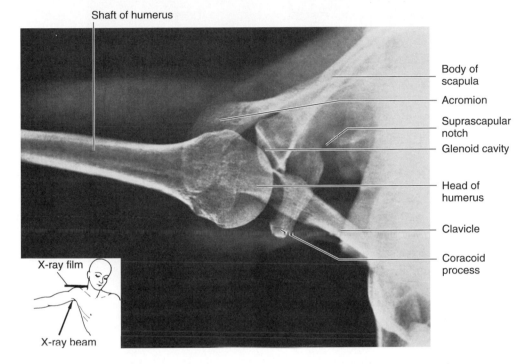

Shaft of humerus

Body of scapula

Acromion

Suprascapular notch

Glenoid cavity

Head of humerus

Clavicle

Coracoid process

X-ray film

X-ray beam

FIGURE 7.39   Axial projection of the glenohumeral joint. The orientation drawing shows how the radiograph was taken.

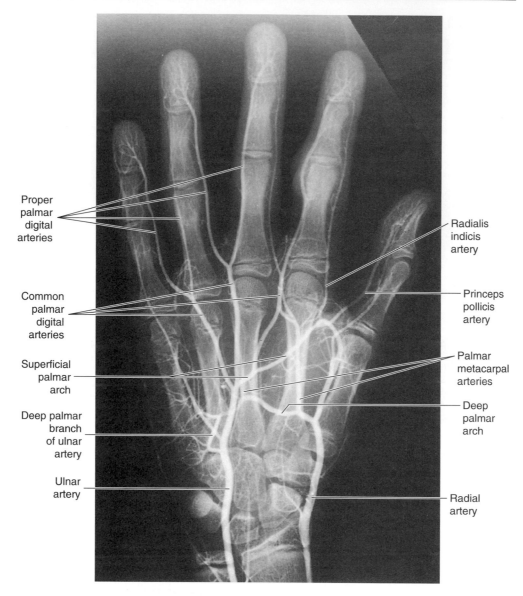

Proper palmar digital arteries

Radialis indicis artery

Common palmar digital arteries

Princeps pollicis artery

Superficial palmar arch

Palmar metacarpal arteries

Deep palmar branch of ulnar artery

Deep palmar arch

Ulnar artery

Radial artery

FIGURE 7.40 Angiogram of the wrist and hand. Observe the superficial and deep palmar arterial arches. (Courtesy of Dr. D. Armstrong, Associate Professor of Medical Imaging, University of Toronto, Toronto, Ontario, Canada.)

Arteriography (visualization of the arteries) is used to detect vascular injuries, ischemia, and variations of arteries. Arteriograms are produced by injecting a dye into an artery as a radiograph is taken (Fig. 7.40). When interest is in a specific artery, the dye is injected directly into it, usually through a catheter. Arteriography may be used to determine the patency of arteries before and after surgical procedures in the upper limb to repair injuries resulting from trauma.

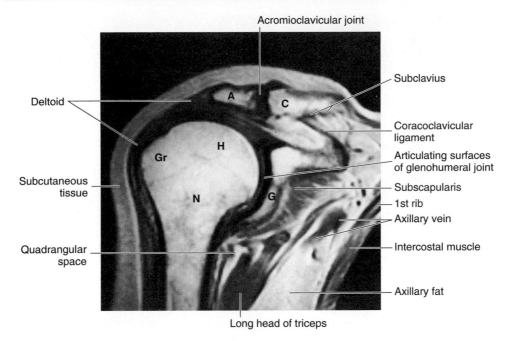

FIGURE 7.41 **Coronal MRI of the glenohumeral and acromioclavicular (AC) joints.** The "white" (signal intense) parts of the identified bones are the fatty matrix of cancellous bone; the thin black outlines (absence of signal) of the bones are the compact bone that forms their outer surface. *A*, acromion; *C*, clavicle; *Gr*, greater tubercle of humerus; *N*, surgical neck of humerus; *G*, glenoid cavity; *H*, head of humerus.

Magnetic resonance imaging (MRI) produces images with good resolution of soft tissues of the limbs (Fig. 7.41). The limb must be kept motionless for the 5 to 10 minutes required for scanning. This technique produces cross-sectional, coronal, and sagittal images. MRI has the advantage that it does not involve the use of x-rays.

8 Head

*T*he head consists of the cranium (skull), face, scalp, teeth, brain, cranial nerves, meninges (membranous coverings of the brain), cerebrospinal fluid (CSF), special sense organs, and other structures such as blood vessels and lymphatics. The head is also where food is ingested and air is inspired and expired. Learning the features of the cranium initially serves as an important framework that facilitates the understanding of the complicated head region.

CRANIUM

The cranium, consisting of a series of bones (Fig. 8.1), forms the skeleton of the head. The two parts of the cranium are the **neurocranium** (brain box) and **viscerocranium** (facial skeleton). *The neurocranium encloses the brain and its meninges,* proximal parts of the cranial nerves, and blood vessels. *The neurocranium is formed by eight bones: a frontal bone,* paired *parietal bones,* paired *temporal bones,* an *occipital bone, a sphenoid bone,* and an *ethmoid bone.* The neurocranium has a domelike roof—the **calvaria** (skullcap)—and a **cranial base** (see Fig. 8.3). The *viscerocranium* contains the orbits (eye sockets) and nasal cavities and includes the maxilla and mandible (upper and lower jaws). *The viscerocranium consists of 14 bones: lacrimal bones (2), nasal bones (2), maxillae (2), zygomatic bones (2), palatine bones (2), inferior nasal conchae (2), mandible (1), and vomer (1).*

ANTERIOR ASPECT

Features of the anterior aspect of the cranium are the frontal and zygomatic bones, orbits, nasal region, maxillae, and mandible (Fig. 8.1*A*). The **frontal bone** forms the skeleton of the forehead, articulating inferiorly with nasal and zygomatic bones. The intersection of the frontal and nasal bones at the bridge of the nose is the **nasion** (L. nasus, nose). The **supraorbital margin** of the frontal bone has a **supraorbital foramen,** or **notch** in some cases. Just superior to the supraorbital margin is a ridge—the **superciliary arch.** Within the orbits are the superior and inferior **orbital fissures** and **optic canals.** The prominences of the cheek are formed by the **zygomatic bones.** Inferior to the nasal bones are the pear-shaped **piriform apertures** (anterior nasal apertures). Through these openings the bony **nasal septum** can be observed, dividing the nasal cavity into right and left parts. On the lateral wall of each nasal cavity are curved bony plates, the **nasal conchae** (the middle and inferior conchae are shown).

The two **maxillae** form the whole upper jaw; they are united at the **intermaxillary suture.** Their **alveolar processes** contain the *dental alveoli* (tooth sockets) and constitute the supporting bone for the **maxillary teeth.** The maxillae surround most of the piriform apertures and form the infraorbital margins medially. They have a broad connection with the zygomatic bones laterally and have an **infraorbital foramen** inferior to each orbit. The **mandible** is the U-shaped bone forming the lower jaw; it has alveolar processes for the **mandibular teeth.** Inferior to the second premolar teeth are **mental foramina.** Forming the prominence of the chin is the **mental protuberance,** a triangular elevation of bone inferior to the **mandibular symphysis** (L. symphysis menti), the region where the halves of the fetal bone fused.

LATERAL ASPECT

The lateral aspect of the cranium is formed by both neurocranial and viscerocranial bones (Fig. 8.1*B*). The main features of the neurocranial part include the **temporal fossa,** which is bounded superiorly and posteriorly by inferior and superior **temporal lines,** anteriorly by the **frontal** and **zygomatic bones,** and inferiorly by the **zygomatic arch.** The zygomatic arch is formed by the union of the *temporal process of the zygomatic bone* and the *zygomatic process of the temporal bone.* In the anterior part of the temporal fossa, superior to

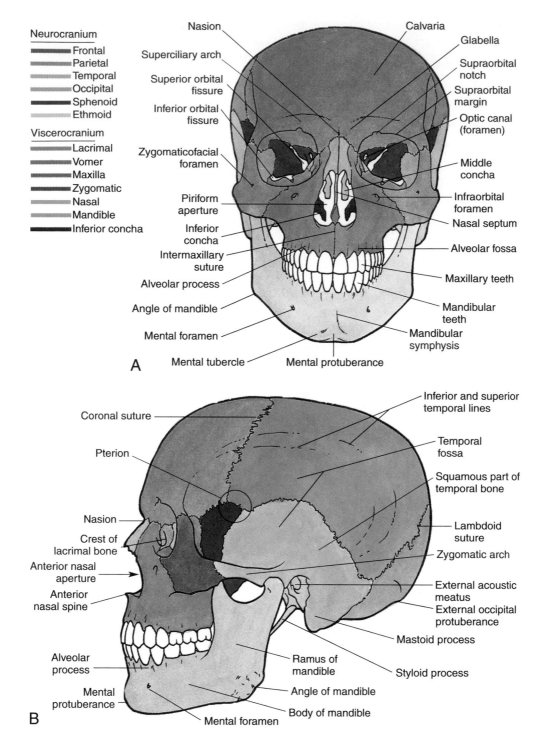

FIGURE 8.1 **Adult cranium (skull). A.** Anterior aspect. **B.** Lateral aspect. Within the temporal fossa, observe the **pterion**—the area of junction of four bones.

the midpoint of the zygomatic arch, is the **pterion**—*the point at which the frontal, parietal, sphenoid (greater wing), and temporal bones are united by an H-shaped formation of sutures.* The **external acoustic opening** is the entrance to the **external acoustic meatus** (canal), which leads to the tympanic membrane (eardrum). The **mastoid process** of the temporal bone lies posteroinferior to the external acoustic meatus. Anteromedial to the mastoid process is the slender **styloid process** of the temporal bone. The **mandible** has a horizontal curved part, the **body,** and a vertical part, the **ramus.** The junction of the body and ramus is the **angle** of the mandible.

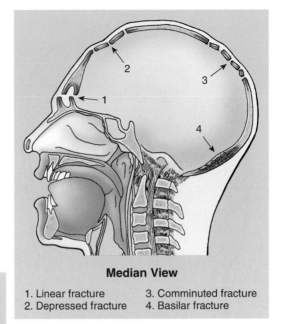

Median View

1. Linear fracture   3. Comminuted fracture
2. Depressed fracture   4. Basilar fracture

FRACTURES OF CALVARIA

The pterion is an important clinical landmark because it overlies the anterior branches of the middle meningeal vessels, which lie in the grooves on the internal aspect of the lateral wall of the calvaria. A blow to the side of the head may fracture the thin bones forming the pterion, rupturing the anterior branch of the middle meningeal artery. *The resulting extradural collection of blood (usually an* epidural hematoma*) exerts pressure on the underlying cerebral cortex. Untreated middle meningeal artery hemorrhage may cause death in a few hours. The convexity of the calvaria distributes and thereby minimizes the effects of a blow to it. However, hard blows to the head in thin areas of the cranium are likely to produce* depressed fractures, *in which a fragment of bone is depressed inward to compress or injure the brain. In* comminuted fractures, *the bone is broken into several pieces.* Linear fractures, *the most frequent type, usually occur at the point of impact, but fracture lines often radiate away from it in two or more directions. If the area of the calvaria is thick at the site of impact, the bone usually bends inward without fracturing; however, a fracture may occur some distance from the site of direct trauma where the calvaria is thinner. In a* contrecoup ('counterblow') fracture, *the fracture occurs on the opposite side of the cranium rather than at the point of impact.*

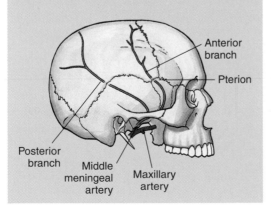

Anterior branch

Pterion

Posterior branch

Middle meningeal artery

Maxillary artery

POSTERIOR ASPECT

The rounded posterior aspect of the cranium or **occiput** (L. back of head) is formed by the occipital bone, parts of the parietal bones, and mastoid parts of the temporal bones (Fig. 8.2*A*). The **external occipital protuberance** is usually an easily palpable elevation in the median plane. The **superior nuchal line,** marking the superior limit of the neck, extends laterally from each side of this protuberance; the **inferior nuchal line** is less distinct. In the center of the occiput, the **lambda** indicates the junction of the sagittal and lambdoid sutures. The lambda can sometimes be felt as a depression.

SUPERIOR ASPECT

The superior aspect of the cranium, usually somewhat oval in form, broadens posterolaterally at the **parietal eminences** (Fig. 8.2*B*). The four bones forming the *calvaria*—the domelike roof of the neurocranium—are visible from this aspect: the frontal bone anteriorly, the right and left parietal bones laterally, and the occipital bone posteriorly. The **coronal suture** separates the frontal and parietal bones; the **sagittal suture** separates the parietal bones; and the **lambdoid suture** separates

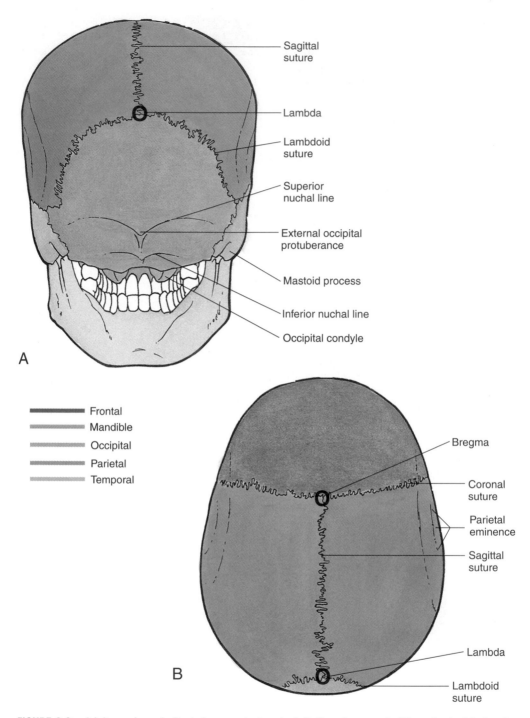

FIGURE 8.2   **Adult cranium. A.** Posterior aspect of occiput. **B.** Superior aspect of the calvaria (skullcap).

the parietal and temporal bones from the occipital bone. The **bregma** is the landmark formed by the intersection of the sagittal and coronal sutures. The *vertex*—the superior (topmost) point of the cranium—is near the midpoint of the sagittal suture.

CRANIAL BASE

The **external aspect of the cranial base** or basicranium shows the *alveolar arch of the maxillae* (U-shaped free inferior border formed by the alveolar processes that surround and support the maxillary teeth), the **palatine processes** of the maxillae, and the palatine, sphenoid, vomer, temporal, and occipital bones (Fig. 8.3). The **hard palate** is formed by the **palatine processes of the maxillae** anteriorly and the **horizontal plates of the palatine bones** posteriorly. Posterior to the central incisor teeth is the **incisive fossa.** Posterolaterally are the greater and lesser **palatine foramina.** The posterior edge of the palate forms the inferior boundary of the choanae (posterior nasal apertures). The **vomer,**

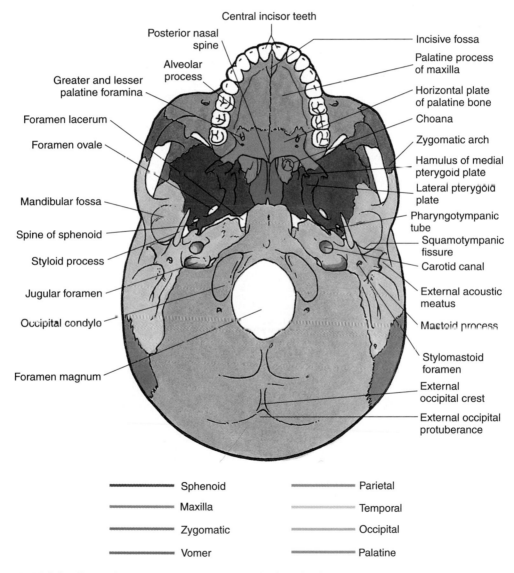

Central incisor teeth
Posterior nasal spine
Alveolar process
Greater and lesser palatine foramina
Foramen lacerum
Foramen ovale
Mandibular fossa
Spine of sphenoid
Styloid process
Jugular foramen
Occipital condyle
Foramen magnum

Incisive fossa
Palatine process of maxilla
Horizontal plate of palatine bone
Choana
Zygomatic arch
Hamulus of medial pterygoid plate
Lateral pterygoid plate
Pharyngotympanic tube
Squamotympanic fissure
Carotid canal
External acoustic meatus
Mastoid process
Stylomastoid foramen
External occipital crest
External occipital protuberance

Sphenoid
Maxilla
Zygomatic
Vomer
Parietal
Temporal
Occipital
Palatine

FIGURE 8.3   **External aspect of the cranial base (basicranium).**

a thin flat bone, makes a major contribution to the bony **nasal septum** (Fig. 8.1*A*). Located centrally, between the frontal, temporal, and occipital bones, is the **sphenoid bone,** which consists of a body from which three pairs of processes arise: the **greater and lesser wings** and the **pterygoid processes** (Fig. 8.4*B*). The pterygoid processes, consisting of medial and lateral **pterygoid plates,** extend inferiorly on each side from the junction of the body and greater wings. The groove for the cartilaginous part of the *pharyngotympanic tube* (auditory tube) lies me-

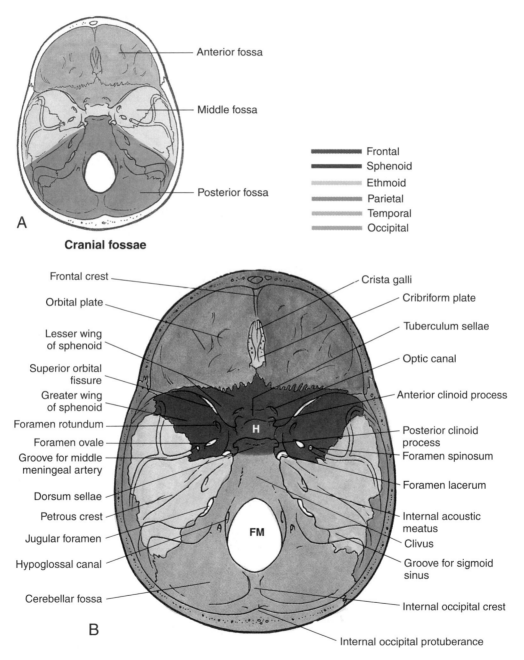

FIGURE 8.4 Internal aspect of the cranial base. Superior view. **A.** Cranial fossae: anterior, middle, posterior. **B.** Bones and foramina of fossae. *H,* hypophysial fossa; *FM,* foramen magnum.

dial to the **spine of the sphenoid.** Depressions in the temporal bone—the **mandibular fossae** (Fig. 8.3)—accommodate the condyles of the mandible when the mouth is closed. The cranial base is formed posteriorly by the **occipital bone,** which articulates with the sphenoid centrally and anteriorly. The parts of the occipital bone encircle the large **foramen magnum.** On the lateral parts of the occipital bone are two large protuberances, the **occipital condyles.** The large opening between the occipital bone and the petrous part of the temporal bone is the **jugular foramen** (difficult to observe unless examined from an oblique angle). The entrance to the **carotid canal** is located just anterior to the jugular foramen. The **mastoid process** of the temporal bone is ridged because of the muscles that attach to it. The **stylomastoid foramen** lies posterior to the base of the styloid process.

The **internal aspect of the cranial base** has three steplike levels formed by three **cranial fossae** (anterior, middle, and posterior) that form the bowl-shaped floor of the cranial cavity (Fig. 8.4*A*). The anterior cranial fossa is at the highest level, and the posterior cranial fossa is at the lowest level. The **anterior cranial fossa** is formed by the frontal bone anteriorly and laterally, the ethmoid bone centrally, and the body and lesser wings of the sphenoid posteriorly (Fig. 8.4*B*). The greater part of the anterior cranial fossa is formed by ridged **orbital plates of the frontal bone,** which support the frontal lobes of the brain and form the roofs of the orbits. The **frontal crest** is a median bony extension of the frontal bone, and the **crista galli** (cock's comb) is a median ridge of bone that projects superiorly from the ethmoid. On each side of the crista galli is the sievelike **cribriform plate** of the ethmoid.

The butterfly-shaped **middle cranial fossa** is composed of deep depressions on each side of the sella turcica (Turkish saddle), which is located on the upper surface of the body of the sphenoid. The **sella turcica** is surrounded by the anterior and posterior **clinoid processes** ("clinoid" means "bedpost"). *The saddlelike sella turcica is composed of three parts:*

- **Tuberculum sellae** ("saddle horn"), the slight elevation anteriorly on the body of the sphenoid

- **Hypophysial fossa,** a saddlelike depression for the pituitary gland (L. hypophysis cerebri) in the middle
- **Dorsum sellae** ("back of saddle") posteriorly, a square plate of bone on the body of the sphenoid forming the posterior part of the sella turcica.

The bones forming the larger, lateral parts of the middle cranial fossa are the **greater wings of the sphenoid,** squamous parts of the **temporal bones** laterally, and **petrous parts of the temporal bones** posteriorly. The lateral parts of the middle cranial fossa are posteroinferior to the anterior cranial fossa and support the temporal lobes of the brain. The boundary between the middle and posterior cranial fossae is formed by the **petrous crests of the temporal bones** laterally and the **dorsum sellae** of the sphenoid medially. The sharp posterior margins of the **lesser wings of the sphenoid** overhang the anteriormost part of the middle cranial fossa. The wings end medially in two posteriorly directed projections, the **anterior clinoid processes.** The **foramen lacerum** lies posterolateral to the **hypophysial fossa.** The **optic canal** lies between the root of the lesser wing, and the **superior orbital fissure** is an opening between the greater and lesser wings. In Figure 8.4, observe the location of the **foramen rotundum** (round foramen), **foramen ovale** (oval foramen), and **foramen spinosum** (spinous foramen).

The **posterior cranial fossa,** the largest and deepest of the cranial fossae, contains the cerebellum, pons, and medulla oblongata (p. 525). This fossa is formed largely by the occipital bone but parts of the sphenoid and temporal bones make smaller contributions to it. The broad grooves in this fossa are formed by the transverse and **sigmoid sinuses.** At the center of the posterior cranial fossa is the **foramen magnum.** Posterior to this large foramen, the **internal occipital crest** is a landmark that divides the posterior part of the fossae into two **cerebellar fossae;** the crest ends superiorly in the **internal occipital protuberance.** At the bases of the petrous crests (ridges) of the temporal bones are the **jugular foramina.** The **hypoglossal canals** for the hypoglossal nerves (CN XII) lie between the anterolateral margin of the foramen magnum and jugular foramina.

FACE

The face is the anterior aspect of the head from the forehead to the chin (including the eyes, nose, mouth, and cheeks; excludes the ears). The basic shape of the face is determined by the underlying bones, the facial muscles, and the subcutaneous tissue. The skin of the face is thin, pliable, and firmly attached to the underlying cartilages of the external ear and nose.

MUSCLES OF FACE

The muscles of the face are in the subcutaneous tissue; they move the skin and change facial expressions to convey mood (Table 8.1). Most muscles attach to bone or fascia and produce their effects by pulling the skin. The *muscles of facial expression* also surround the orifices of the mouth, eyes, and nose and act as sphincters and dilators that close and open the orifices. The **orbicularis oris** is the sphincter of the mouth and is the first of a series of sphincters associated with the alimentary (digestive) tract. The **buccinator** (L. trumpeter), active in smiling, also keeps the cheek taut, thereby preventing it from folding and being injured during chewing; it also works with the tongue to hold food between the teeth for chewing. The buccinator is also active during sucking, whistling, and blowing (e.g., when playing a wind instrument).

NERVES OF FACE

The cutaneous nerves of the neck extend upward onto some regions of the face. Cutaneous branches of the cervical nerves from the *cervical plexus* (see Fig. 9.3A) extend over the ear, the posterior aspect of the neck, and much of the parotid region (area overlying the angle of the mandible). The **trigeminal nerve** (CN V) is the *sensory nerve for the face* and the *motor nerve for the muscles of mastication* and several other small muscles (Table 8.2). Three large groups of peripheral processes from nerve cell bodies comprising the **trigeminal ganglion**—the large sensory ganglion of CN V—form the **ophthalmic nerve** (CN V_1), the **maxillary nerve** (CN V_2), and the sensory component of the **mandibular nerve** (CN V_3). These nerves are named according to their main regions of termination—the eye, maxilla, and mandible, respectively. The first two divisions (CN V_1 and CN V_2) are wholly sensory; CN V_3 is largely sensory but also conveys fibers of the motor root of CN V. *The major cutaneous branches of the ophthalmic nerve (CN V_1) (Table 8.2) are the:*

- Lacrimal nerve
- Supraorbital nerve
- Supratrochlear nerve
- Infratrochlear nerve
- External nasal nerves.

The major cutaneous branches of the maxillary nerve (CN V_2) are the:

- Infraorbital nerve
- Zygomaticotemporal nerve
- Zygomaticofacial nerve.

The major cutaneous branches of the mandibular nerve (CN V_3) are the:

- Auriculotemporal nerve
- Buccal nerve
- Mental nerve.

The **motor nerves of the face** are the *facial nerve (CN VII)* to the muscles of facial expression and the *mandibular nerve (CN V_3)* to the muscles of mastication (p. 547)—masseter, temporal, medial, and lateral pterygoids—and to the mylohyoid (p. 567), anterior belly of digastric (see Table 9.3), tensor veli palatini (p. 558), and tensor tympani (p. 583). The **facial nerve (CN VII)** exits the cranium via the **stylomastoid**

TABLE 8.1. MUSCLES OF FACE

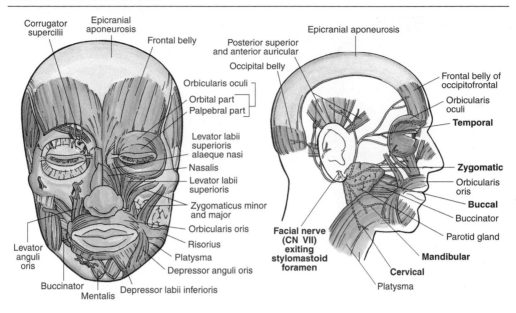

(All these muscles are supplied by the facial nerve (CN VII).

Muscle[a]	Origin	Insertion	Action(s)
Orbicularis oculi	Medial orbital margin, medial palpebral ligament, and lacrimal bone	Skin around margin of orbit; tarsal plate (see Fig. 8.16)	Closes eyelids and assists flow of lacrimal fluid by closing palpebral fissure (aperture between eyelids) in a medial to lateral direction (palpebral part gently closes eyelids, orbital part tightly closes eyelids)
Orbicularis oris	Some fibers arise near median plane of maxilla superiorly and mandible inferiorly; other fibers arise from deep surface of skin	Mucous membrane of lips	As sphincter of oral opening, it compresses and protrudes lips (e.g., purses them during whistling and sucking)
Buccinator	Mandible, pterygomandibular raphe, and alveolar processes of maxilla and mandible	Angle of mouth	Presses cheek against molar teeth, thereby aiding chewing; expels air from oral cavity as occurs when playing a wind instrument
Platysma	Superficial fascia of deltoid and pectoral regions	Mandible, skin of cheek, angle of mouth, and orbicularis oris	Depresses mandible and tenses skin of lower face and neck

[a]The frontal belly of the occipitofrontal muscle of the scalp elevates the eyebrows and the skin of the forehead.
Boldface type indicates facial nerve and its branches.

TABLE 8.2. SENSORY NERVES OF FACE AND SCALP

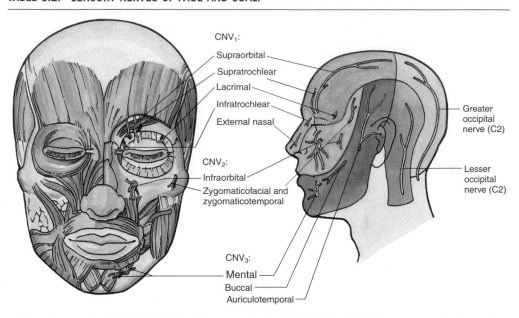

Nerve	Origin	Course	Distribution
Frontal	Ophthalmic nerve (CN V_1)	Crosses orbit on superior aspect of levator palpebrae superioris; divides into supraorbital and supratrochlear branches	Skin of forehead, scalp, upper eyelid, and nose; conjunctiva of upper lid and mucosa of frontal sinus
Supraorbital	Continuation of frontal nerve (CN V_1)	Emerges through supraorbital notch, or foramen, and breaks up into small branches	Mucous membrane of frontal sinus and conjunctiva (lining) of upper eyelid, skin of forehead as far as vertex
Supratrochlear	Frontal nerve (CN V_1)	Passes superiorly on medial side of supraorbital nerve and divides into two or more branches	Skin in middle of forehead to hairline
Infratrochlear	Nasociliary nerve (CN V_1)	Follows medial wall of orbit to upper eyelid	Skin and conjunctiva (lining) of upper eyelid
Lacrimal	Ophthalmic nerve (CN V_1)	Passes through palpebral fascia of upper eyelid near lateral angle (canthus) of eye	Lacrimal gland and small area of skin and conjunctiva of lateral part of upper eye
External nasal	Anterior ethmoidal nerve (CN V_1)	Runs in nasal cavity and emerges on face between nasal bone and lateral nasal cartilage	Skin on dorsum of nose, including tip of nose

Continued

TABLE 8.2. *CONTINUED*

Nerve	Origin	Course	Distribution
Zygomatic	Maxillary nerve (CN V$_2$)	Arises in floor of orbit, divides into zygomaticofacial and zygomaticotemporal nerves, which traverse foramina of same name	Skin over zygomatic arch and anterior temporal region; carries postsynaptic parasympathetic fibers from pterygopalatine ganglion to lacrimal nerve
Infraorbital	Terminal branch of maxillary nerve (CN V$_2$)	Runs in floor of orbit and emerges at infraorbital foramen	Skin of cheek, lower lid, lateral side of nose and inferior septum and upper lip; upper premolar incisors and canine teeth; mucosa of maxillary sinus and upper lip
Auriculotemporal	Mandibular nerve (CN V$_3$)	From posterior division of CN V$_3$, it passes between neck of mandible and external acoustic meatus to accompany superficial temporal artery	Skin anterior to ear and posterior temporal region, tragus and part of helix of auricle, and roof of exterior acoustic meatus and upper tympanic membrane
Buccal	Mandibular nerve (CN V$_3$)	From the anterior division of CN V$_3$ in infratemporal fossa, it passes anteriorly to reach cheek	Skin and mucosa of cheek, buccal gingiva adjacent to 2nd and 3rd molar teeth
Mental	Terminal branch of inferior alveolar nerve (CN V$_3$)	Emerges from mandibular canal at mental foramen	Skin of chin and lower lip and mucosa of lower lip

foramen (Fig. 8.3, Table 8.1). Its extracranial branches (temporal, zygomatic, buccal, mandibular, cervical, and posterior auricular nerves) supply the superficial muscle of the neck and chin (platysma), muscles of facial expression, muscle of the cheek (buccinator), muscles of the ear (auricular), and muscles of the scalp (occipital and frontal bellies of occipitofrontal muscle).

TRIGEMINAL NEURALGIA

Trigeminal neuralgia (tic douloureux) is a sensory disorder of the sensory root of CN V that is characterized by sudden attacks of excruciating, lightening-like jabs of facial pain. A *paroxysm* (sudden sharp pain) can last for 15 minutes or more. The maxillary nerve is most frequently involved, then the mandibular nerve, and, least frequently, the ophthalmic nerve. The pain often is initiated by touching a sensitive *trigger zone of the skin*. The cause of trigeminal neuralgia is unknown; however, some

investigators believe that most affected persons have an anomalous blood vessel that compresses the sensory root of CN V. When the aberrant artery is moved away from the root, the symptoms usually disappear. In some cases it is necessary to section the sensory root for relief of trigeminal neuralgia.

Lesions of Trigeminal Nerve

Lesions of the entire trigeminal nerve cause widespread anesthesia involving the:

- Corresponding anterior half of the scalp
- Face, except for an area around the angle of the mandible
- Cornea and conjunctiva
- Mucous membranes of the nose and paranasal sinuses, mouth, and anterior part of the tongue
  Paralysis of the muscles of mastication also occurs.

Bell Palsy

The most common nontraumatic cause of facial palsy or paralysis is inflammation of the facial nerve near the

Continued

stylomastoid foramen. This produces edema (swelling) and compression of the nerve in the facial canal (Bell palsy [Bell's palsy]). The loss of tonus of the orbicularis oculi causes the lower lid to evert (turn away from the surface of the eye) so that the cornea on the affected side is not adequately hydrated—lubricated with lacrimal fluid (tears)—making it vulnerable to ulceration. *Persons with Bell palsy cannot whistle, blow a wind instrument, or chew effectively.* The palsy weakens or paralyzes the buccinator and orbicularis oris, the cheek and lip muscles that aid chewing by holding food between occlusal surfaces of the teeth and out of the oral vestibule (gutter between the teeth and cheek). Food accumulates there during chewing and often must be continually removed with a finger. Displacement of the mouth is produced by contraction of unopposed contralateral facial muscles and by drooping of the corner of the mouth by the unopposed pull of gravity, resulting in food and saliva dribbling out of the side of the mouth. People frequently dab their eyes and mouth with a handkerchief to wipe the fluid (tears and saliva), which runs from the drooping lid and mouth.

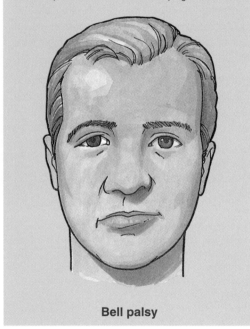

Bell palsy

VASCULATURE OF FACE

Most arteries supplying the face are branches of the *external carotid artery*. The **facial artery** provides the major arterial supply to the face (Fig. 8.5*A*, Table 8.3). It arises from the external carotid artery and winds its way to the inferior border of the mandible, just anterior to the masseter. It then courses over the face to the medial angle (canthus) of the eye. Enroute,

the facial artery sends branches to the upper and lower lips (superior and inferior **labial arteries**), to the side of the nose (**lateral nasal artery**), and then terminates as the **angular artery,** which supplies the medial angle of the eye. The **superficial temporal artery** is the smaller terminal branch of the external carotid artery; the other branch is the maxillary artery. The superficial temporal artery emerges on the face between the temporomandibular joint (TMJ) and the ear and ends in the scalp by dividing into **frontal** and **parietal branches** (Fig. 8.5*A*). The **transverse facial artery** arises from the superficial temporal artery (see Fig. 8.26) within the parotid gland and crosses the face superficial to the masseter. It divides into numerous branches that supply the parotid gland and duct, the masseter, and the skin of the face.

The **facial vein** (Fig. 8.5, *B* and *C*) provides the major venous drainage of the face. It begins at the medial angle of the eye as the **angular vein** formed by the union of the **supraorbital** and **supratrochlear veins.** The facial vein then runs inferoposteriorly through the face, posterior to the facial artery. As it runs, it receives the *deep facial vein* that drains the **pterygoid venous plexus** of the infratemporal fossa. Inferior to the margin of the mandible, the facial vein is usually joined by the anterior branch of the retromandibular vein. The facial vein drains into the **internal jugular vein** (IJV) directly or indirectly. The **superficial temporal vein** drains the forehead and scalp and receives tributaries from the veins of the temple and face. Near the auricle, the superficial temporal vein enters the parotid gland (Fig. 8.5*A*). The **retromandibular vein** (Fig. 8.5, *B* and *C*), formed by the union of the superficial temporal vein and the **maxillary vein,** descends within the parotid gland, superficial to the external carotid artery and deep to the facial nerve. The retromandibular vein divides into an anterior branch that unites with the facial vein and a posterior branch that joins the **posterior auricular vein** to form the **external jugular vein.** The external jugular vein crosses the superficial surface of the sternocleidomastoid muscle to enter the subclavian vein in the root of the neck.

Lymphatic vessels of the face accompany other facial vessels (Fig. 8.6). Those from the lateral part of the face, including the eyelids,

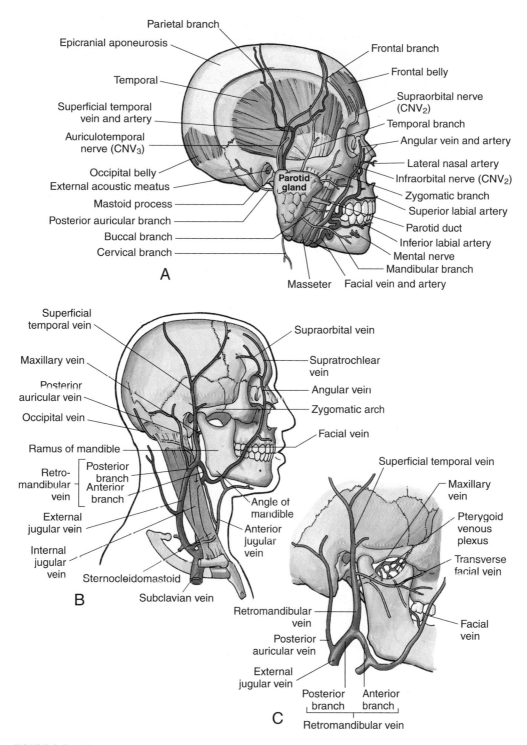

FIGURE 8.5 **Vasculature and nerves of face.** Lateral views. **A.** Vessels and nerves. **B.** Venous drainage of the head and neck. **C.** Veins and pterygoid venous plexus.

TABLE 8.3. ARTERIES OF FACE AND SCALP

Artery	Origin	Course	Distribution
Facial	External carotid artery	Ascends deep to submandibular gland, winds around inferior border of mandible and enters face	Muscles of facial expression and face
Superior labial	Facial artery near angle of mouth	Runs medially in upper lip	Upper lip and ala (side) and septum of nose
Inferior labial	Facial artery near angle of mouth	Runs medially in lower lip	Lower lip and chin
Lateral nasal	Facial artery as it ascends alongside nose	Passes to ala of nose	Skin on ala and dorsum of nose
Angular	Terminal branch of facial artery	Passes to medial angle (canthus) of eye	Superior part of cheek and lower eyelid
Superficial temporal	Smaller terminal branch of external carotid artery	Ascends anterior to ear to temporal region and ends in scalp	Facial muscles and skin of frontal and temporal regions
Transverse facial	Superficial temporal artery within parotid gland	Crosses face superficial to masseter and inferior to zygomatic arch	Parotid gland and duct, muscles and skin of face
Mental	Terminal branch of inferior alveolar artery	Emerges from mental foramen and passes to chin	Facial muscles and skin of chin
Supraorbital	Terminal branch of ophthalmic artery, a branch of internal carotid artery	Passes superiorly from supraorbital foramen	Muscles and skin of forehead and scalp
Supratrochlear	Terminal branch of ophthalmic artery, a branch of internal carotid artery	Passes superiorly from supratrochlear notch	Muscles and skin of scalp

drain inferiorly to the **parotid lymph nodes.** Lymph from the deep parotid nodes drains into the **deep cervical lymph nodes.** Lymphatic vessels in the upper lip and lateral parts of the lower lip drain into the **submandibular lymph nodes,** whereas lymphatic vessels in the chin and the central part of the lower lip drain into the **submental lymph nodes.**

PULSES OF FACIAL ARTERIES
The *pulse of the facial artery* can be palpated where the artery winds around the inferior border of the mandible. Because of the numerous anastomoses between the branches of the facial artery and other arteries of the face,

compression of the facial artery on one side does not stop all bleeding from a lacerated facial artery or one of its branches. In lacerations of the lip, pressure must be applied on both sides of the cut to stop the bleeding. In general, facial wounds bleed freely but heal quickly. The *pulse of the superficial temporal artery* can be palpated as the artery passes anterior to the ear and crosses the zygomatic arch to supply the scalp.

Carcinoma of Lip
Carcinoma of the lip usually involves the lower lip. Overexposure to sunshine over many years, as occurs with outdoor workers, and smoking are common features of the histories in these cases. Cancer cells from the central part of the lip spread initially to the submental lymph nodes, whereas cancer cells from lateral parts of the lip drain initially to the submandibular lymph nodes.

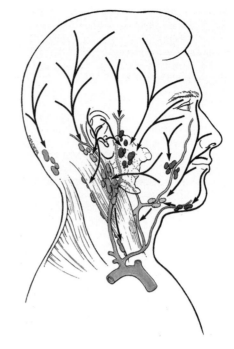

Lymph nodes:

▬▬▬ Occipital
▬▬▬ Mastoid (retroauricular)
▬▬▬ Parotid
▬▬▬ Buccal
▬▬▬ Submental
▬▬▬ Submandibular
▬▬▬ Jugulo-omohyoid
▬▬▬ Superficial cervical
▬▬▬ Deep cervical

FIGURE 8.6   Lymphatic drainage of the head and neck. Lateral view. *Arrows,* direction of lymph flow.

PAROTID GLAND

The parotid gland—the largest of the salivary glands (p. 568)—is enclosed within a tough fascial capsule, the *parotid sheath,* a continuation of the investing layer of deep cervical fascia. The parotid gland has an irregular shape because the area it occupies, the *parotid bed,* is anteroinferior to the external acoustic meatus (Fig. 8.5A), where it is wedged between the *ramus of the mandible* (which it engulfs) and the *mastoid process.* The inferiorly directed apex of the gland is posterior to the *angle of the mandible* and its base is related to the *zygomatic arch.* The **parotid duct** passes anteriorly and horizontally from the anterior edge of the gland. At the anterior border of the masseter (Fig. 8.5A), the duct turns medially, pierces the buccinator, and enters the oral cavity opposite the second maxillary molar tooth. *Structures within the parotid gland,* from superficial to deep, are the **facial nerve** and its branches, the **retromandibular vein** (Fig. 8.5B), and the *external carotid artery.* On the parotid sheath and within the gland are **parotid lymph nodes** (Fig.

8.6), which receive lymph from the forehead, lateral parts of the eyelids, temporal region, lateral surface of the auricle, anterior wall of the external acoustic meatus, and the middle ear. Lymph from the parotid nodes drains into the upper **deep cervical lymph nodes.**

The *great auricular nerve* (C2 and C3), a branch of the cervical plexus (see Fig. 9.3A), innervates the *parotid sheath* and the overlying skin. The **auriculotemporal nerve,** a branch of CN V₃, is closely related to the parotid gland and passes superior to it with the superficial temporal vessels (Fig. 8.5A, Table 8.1). The parasympathetic component of the *glossopharyngeal nerve* (CN IX) supplies secretory fibers to the parotid gland; the fibers are conveyed from the *otic ganglion* by the auriculotemporal nerve. Stimulation of these fibers produces saliva. Sympathetic fibers are derived from the cervical ganglia through the *external carotid nerve plexus* on the external carotid artery. *Sensory nerve fibers* pass to the gland through the great auricular and auriculotemporal nerves.

SCALP

The scalp consists of skin and subcutaneous tissue that covers the neurocranium from the superior nuchal lines on the occipital bone to the supraorbital margins of the frontal bone. Laterally, the scalp extends over the temporal fascia to the zygomatic arches. *The scalp consists of five layers,* the first three of which constitute the *scalp proper* and are connected intimately, thus moving as a unit (e.g., when wrinkling the forehead). Each letter in the term **scalp** serves as a memory key for one of its five layers that cover the neurocranium (Fig. 8.7*A*):

- **S**kin, thin except in the occipital region, contains many sweat and sebaceous glands and hair follicles; it has an abundant arterial supply and good venous and lymphatic drainage.
- **C**onnective tissue, forming the thick, *dense, richly vascularized, subcutaneous layer* that is well supplied with cutaneous nerves.

- **A**poneurosis—the *epicranial aponeurosis* (L. galea aponeurotica)—*a strong tendinous sheet that covers the calvaria* like a helmet (L. galea) between the frontal and occipital bellies of the occipitofrontal muscle (Fig. 8.5*A*) and the superior auricular muscle; collectively the aponeurosis and muscles inserting into it form the *epicranius muscle.*
- **L**oose connective tissue, somewhat like a sponge because it has many potential spaces that may distend with fluid resulting from injury or infection; this layer allows free movement of the scalp proper over the underlying calvaria.
- **P**ericranium, a dense layer of connective tissue that forms the external periosteum of the calvaria; it is firmly attached but can be stripped fairly easily from the calvaria of living persons, except where the pericranium is continuous with the fibrous tissue in the cranial sutures.

Innervation of the scalp (Fig. 8.7*B*, Table 8.2) anterior to the auricles is by branches of all three divisions of the **trigeminal nerve** (CN V_1, CN V_2, CN V_3). Posterior to the auricles, innervation of the scalp is by *spinal cutaneous nerves* (C2 and C3).

The **arteries of the scalp** run in layer two—the dense, richly vascularized subcutaneous layer of the scalp between the skin and the epicranial aponeurosis. They are held by the dense connective tissue in such a way that they tend to remain open when cut, and, because of abundant anastomoses, severed arteries bleed from both ends. The arteries derive from the *external carotid arteries* through the **occipital, posterior auricular,** and **superficial temporal arteries** and from the *internal carotid arteries* by way of the **supratrochlear** and **supraorbital arteries** (Fig. 8.7*B*, Table 8.3). Arteries of the scalp supply very little blood to the bones of the calvaria; these bones are supplied by the middle meningeal artery (p. 501). Hence, loss of the scalp does not produce necrosis (death) of the bones forming the calvaria.

Venous drainage of superficial parts of the scalp is through the accompanying veins of the scalp—the **supraorbital** and **supratrochlear veins,** which begin in the forehead and descend

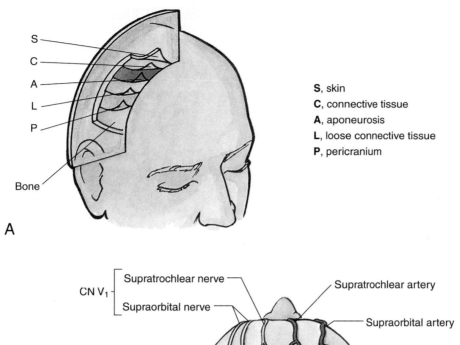

S, skin
C, connective tissue
A, aponeurosis
L, loose connective tissue
P, pericranium

FIGURE 8.7 **Scalp. A.** Layers. **B.** Arteries and nerves. Superior view.

to unite at the medial angle of the eye to form the **angular vein** that becomes the **facial vein** at the inferior margin of the orbit (Fig. 8.5, *B* and *C*). The **superficial temporal veins** and **posterior auricular veins** drain the scalp anterior and posterior to the auricles, respectively. The occipital veins drain the occipital region of the scalp. **Venous drainage of deep parts of the scalp** occurs via **emissary veins** that communicate with the dural sinuses (p. 519) and in the temporal region through *deep temporal veins* that are tributaries of the *pterygoid venous plexus.*

Lymphatic drainage of the face and scalp is into the *superficial ring (pericervical collar) of lymph nodes*—the submental, submandibular, parotid, mastoid (or retroauricular), and occipital—that is, nodes located at the junction of the head and neck (Fig. 8.6). *There are no lymph nodes in the scalp.* Lymph from the superficial ring of nodes drains into the **deep cervical lymph nodes** along the IJV.

SCALP INJURIES AND INFECTIONS

Because the scalp arteries arising at the sides of the head are well protected by dense connective tissue and anastomose freely, *a partially detached scalp* may be replaced with a reasonable chance of healing as long as one of the vessels supplying the scalp remains intact. During an *attached craniotomy*—removal of a segment of the calvaria with a soft tissue *scalp flap* to expose the cranial cavity—the incisions usually are made convex upward, and the superficial temporal artery is included in the flap. Consequently, surgical scalp flaps are made so that they remain attached inferiorly to preserve the nerves and vessels and to promote good healing.

The first three layers of the scalp, the *scalp proper,* are often regarded clinically as a single layer because they remain together when a scalp flap is made during a *craniotomy* (surgical opening of the cranium), as well as when part of the scalp is torn off during accidents. Nerves and vessels of the scalp enter inferiorly and ascend through the second (connective tissue) layer of the scalp to the skin.

The loose connective tissue layer (fourth layer) is considered the dangerous area of the scalp because pus or blood spreads easily through its potential spaces. Infection in this layer can also pass into the cranial cavity through **emissary veins** (Fig. 8.8*A*) that pass through the parietal foramina in the calvaria and infect intracranial structures (e.g., brain). Such an infection cannot pass posteriorly into the neck because the occipital belly of the occipitofrontalis muscle attaches to the occipital bone and mastoid parts of the temporal bones. A scalp infection cannot spread laterally beyond the zygomatic arches because the epicranial aponeurosis is continuous with the temporal fascia covering the temporal muscle that attaches to these arches (Fig. 8.5*A*). An infection or fluid (e.g., pus or blood) can enter the eyelids and the root of the nose because the frontal belly of the occipitofrontalis muscle inserts into the skin and dense subcutaneous tissue and does not attach to the bone. Consequently, a black eye can result from an injury to the scalp or forehead. Most blood enters the upper eyelid, but some may enter the lower one.

Scalp lacerations are the most common type of head injury requiring surgical care. These wounds bleed profusely because the arteries anastomose across the midline and bleed from both ends. The arteries do not retract when lacerated; instead, they are held open by the dense fibrous tissue in the second layer of the scalp. Hence, unconscious patients may bleed to death from scalp lacerations if bleeding is not controlled (e.g., by sutures).

CRANIAL MENINGES

The cranial meninges—internal to the neurocranium—protect the brain and form the supporting framework for arteries, veins, and venous sinuses. *The cranial meninges consist of three layers (Fig. 8.8):*

- **Dura mater** (dura)—an external thick, *dense fibrous membrane*
- **Arachnoid mater** (arachnoid)—an intermediate, *delicate membrane*
- **Pia mater** (pia)—an internal *delicate, vascular membrane.*

The meninges enclose the **cerebrospinal fluid** (CSF), a liquid similar to blood plasma in constitution; CSF provides nutrients but has less protein and a different ion concentration. *CSF is formed predominantly by the choroid plexuses* within the four ventricles of the brain (see Fig. 8.13). CSF leaves the ventricular system of the brain and enters the **subarachnoid space** between the arachnoid and pia mater, where it cushions and nourishes the brain.

DURA MATER

The **dura mater** (dura) is adherent to the internal surface of the cranium and is described as a two-layered membrane (Fig. 8.8):

- An *external periosteal layer,* formed by the periosteum covering the internal surface of the calvaria
- An *internal meningeal layer,* a strong fibrous membrane that is continuous at the foramen magnum with the dura covering the spinal cord.

The internal meningeal layer of the dura draws away from the external periosteal layer of the dura to form **dural infoldings** (reflections), which separate the regions of the brain from each other. These infoldings divide the cranial cavity into compartments and support parts of the brain (Fig. 8.9). The dural infoldings include the **cerebral falx, cerebellar tentorium, cerebellar falx,** and **sellar diaphragm.**

The **cerebral falx** (L. falx cerebri), the largest dural infolding, is a sickle-shaped partition that

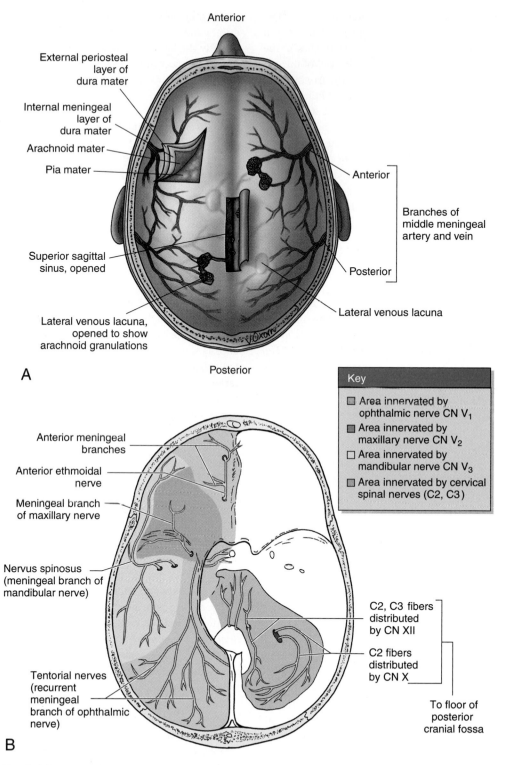

Anterior

External periosteal
layer of
dura mater

Internal meningeal
layer of
dura mater

Arachnoid mater

Pia mater

Anterior

Branches of
middle meningeal
artery and vein

Posterior

Superior sagittal
sinus, opened

Lateral venous lacuna

Lateral venous lacuna,
opened to show
arachnoid granulations

A   Posterior

Key
☐ Area innervated by
   ophthalmic nerve CN V_1
☐ Area innervated by
   maxillary nerve CN V_2
☐ Area innervated by
   mandibular nerve CN V_3
☐ Area innervated by cervical
   spinal nerves (C2, C3)

Anterior meningeal
branches

Anterior ethmoidal
nerve

Meningeal branch
of maxillary nerve

Nervus spinosus
(meningeal branch of
mandibular nerve)

C2, C3 fibers
distributed
by CN XII

C2 fibers
distributed
by CN X

To floor of
posterior
cranial fossa

Tentorial nerves
(recurrent
meningeal
branch of ophthalmic
nerve)

B

FIGURE 8.8   Dura mater and arachnoid granulations. A. Meningeal vessels. Superior view. **B.** Innervation of the dura in the cranial base.

lies in the *longitudinal cerebral fissure* (Fig. 8.9*A*) and separates the right and left cerebral hemispheres. The cerebral falx attaches in the median plane to the internal surface of the calvaria, from the *frontal crest* of the frontal bone and the crista galli of the ethmoid bone anteriorly to the internal occipital protuberance posteriorly. The cerebral falx ends posteriorly by becoming continuous with the cerebellar tentorium. The **cerebellar tentorium** (L. tentorium cerebelli), the second largest dural infolding (Fig. 8.9), is a wide crescentic septum that separates the occipital lobes of the cerebral hemispheres from the cerebellum. The cerebellar tentorium attaches rostrally to the clinoid processes of the sphenoid bone, rostrolaterally to the crest of the petrous part of the temporal bone, and posterolaterally to the internal surface of the occipital bone and part of the parietal bone where they are grooved by the transverse sinuses. *The cerebral falx attaches to the cerebellar tentorium in the midline and holds it up, giving it a tentlike appearance* (L. tentorium, tent). The concave anteromedial border of the tentorium is free, producing a gap—the **tentorial notch** (incisure)—through which the brainstem extends from the posterior into the middle cranial fossa (Fig. 8.9*A*).

The **cerebellar falx** is a vertical dural infolding that lies inferior to the cerebellar tentorium in the posterior part of the posterior cranial fossa; it partially separates the cerebellar hemispheres. The **sellar diaphragm** (L. diaphragma sellae), the smallest dural infolding, is a circular sheet of dura that is suspended between the clinoid processes; it *forms a roof over the hypophysial fossa* (Fig. 8.9*B*). The sellar diaphragm covers the *pituitary gland* and has an aperture for passage of the *infundibulum* (pituitary stalk) and hypophysial veins.

Dural venous sinuses (e.g., superior and inferior sagittal sinuses) are endothelial-lined spaces between the periosteal and meningeal layers of the dura mater (Figs. 8.8–8.11). They form mainly where dural infoldings (septa) attach. Large veins from the surface of the brain empty into these sinuses, and all blood from the brain ultimately drains through them into the IJVs. **Arachnoid granulations** (collections of arachnoid villi) are tufted prolongations of the arachnoid that protrude through the meningeal layer of the dura mater into the dural venous sinuses (Figs. 8.8*A* and 8.11), especially the lateral lacunae, and effect transfer of CSF to the venous system.

The **superior sagittal sinus** lies in the convex attached (superior) border of the cerebral falx. It begins at the crista galli and ends near the internal occipital protuberance at the **confluence of sinuses** (Fig. 8.9*A*). The superior sagittal sinus receives the superior cerebral veins and communicates on each side through slitlike openings with the **lateral lacunae**—lateral expansions of the superior sagittal sinus (Figs. 8.8*A* and 8.11). The **inferior sagittal sinus,** much smaller than the superior sagittal sinus, runs in the inferior, free concave border of the cerebral falx and ends by merging with the **great cerebral vein** to form the straight sinus.

The **straight sinus** runs inferoposteriorly along the line of attachment of the cerebral falx to the cerebellar tentorium to join the confluence of sinuses. The **transverse sinuses** pass laterally from the **confluence of sinuses** in the posterior attached margin of the cerebellar tentorium, grooving the occipital bones and the posteroinferior angles of the parietal bones. The transverse sinuses leave the cerebellar tentorium at the posterior aspect of the petrous temporal bone and become the sigmoid sinuses.

The **sigmoid sinuses** follow S-shaped courses in the posterior cranial fossa, forming deep grooves in the temporal and occipital bones (Fig. 8.9*B*). Each sigmoid sinus turns anteriorly and then continues as the IJV after transversing the jugular foramen. The **occipital sinus** lies in the attached border of the cerebellar falx and ends superiorly in the confluence of sinuses. The occipital sinus communicates inferiorly with the *internal vertebral (epidural) venous plexus* (p. 292).

The **cavernous sinus** (Figs. 8.9 and 8.10*B*) is situated bilaterally on each side of the sella turcica on the upper body of the sphenoid bone. Each sinus extends from the superior orbital fissure anteriorly to the apex of the petrous part of the temporal bone posteriorly. The cavernous sinus receives blood from the superior and inferior ophthalmic veins, the superficial middle cerebral vein, and the sphenoparietal sinus. The venous channels in the cavernous sinuses communicate with each other through

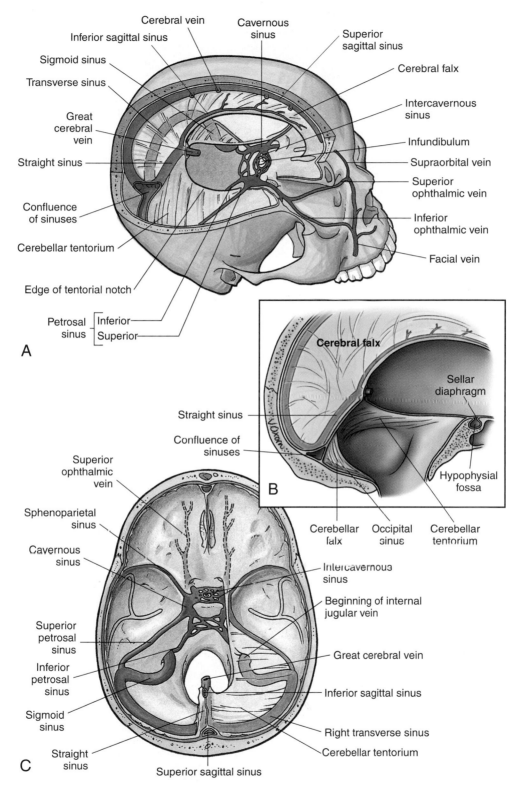

FIGURE 8.9 **Dural infoldings (reflections) and dural venous sinuses. A.** Right superolateral view. **B.** Lateral view. **C.** Superior view.

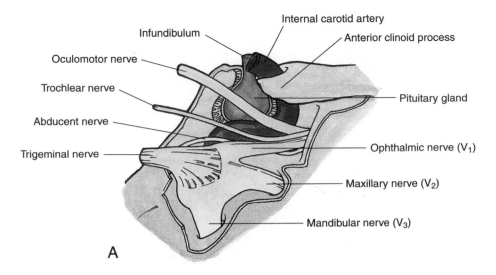

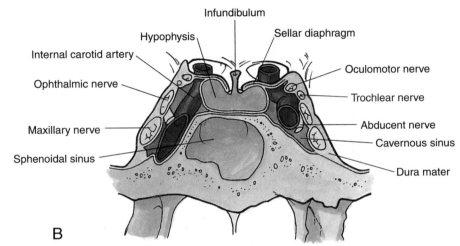

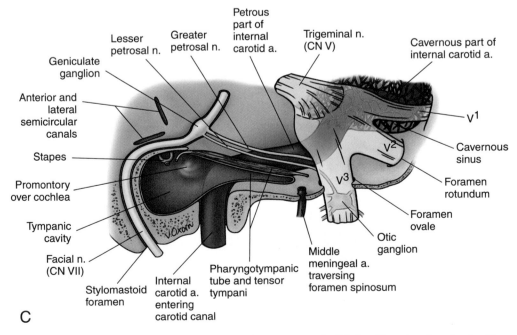

FIGURE 8.10 **Internal carotid artery and associated structures. A.** Relationships of oculomotor, trochlear, trigeminal, and abducent nerves. Lateral view. **B.** Coronal section of the cavernous sinuses. **C.** Petrous and cavernous parts of the internal carotid artery. Lateral view.

intercavernous sinuses. The cavernous sinuses drain posteroinferiorly through the superior and inferior **petrosal sinuses** and via emissary veins to the **pterygoid plexuses** (Fig. 8.5*C*). The **internal carotid artery** (Fig. 8.10), accompanied by its sympathetic plexus, courses through the cavernous sinus and is crossed by the abducent nerve (CN VI). From superior to inferior, the lateral wall of each cavernous sinus (Fig. 8.10B) contains the oculomotor nerve (CN III), trochlear nerve (CN IV), and CN V$_1$ and CN V$_2$ divisions of the trigeminal nerve.

The **superior petrosal sinuses** (Fig. 8.9) run from the posterior ends of the cavernous sinuses to join the transverse sinuses where these sinuses curve inferiorly to form the sigmoid sinuses. Each superior petrosal sinus lies in the anterolateral attached margin of the cerebellar tentorium, which attaches to the superior border of the petrous part of the temporal bone (petrous crest). The **inferior petrosal sinuses** also commence at the posterior end of the cavernous sinus inferiorly. The inferior petrosal sinuses drain the cavernous sinuses directly into the origin of the IJVs. The *basilar plexus* (sinus) connects the inferior petrosal sinuses and communicates inferiorly with the internal vertebral (epidural) venous plexus (Chapter 5). **Emissary veins** connect the dural venous sinuses with veins outside the cranium (Fig. 8.11*A*). The size and number of emissary veins vary.

THROMBOPHLEBITIS
The *facial veins make clinically important connections with the cavernous sinus through the superior ophthalmic veins* (Fig. 8.9*A*). Blood from the medial angle of the eye, nose, and lips usually drains inferiorly into the facial vein. However, because the facial vein has no valves, blood may pass superiorly to the superior ophthalmic vein and enter the cavernous sinus. In people with *thrombophlebitis of the facial vein* (inflammation of the vein with secondary thrombus formation), pieces of a thrombus may produce *thrombophlebitis of the cavernous sinuses*. Infection of the facial veins spreading to the dural venous sinuses may be initiated by squeezing pustules ("pimples") on the side of the nose and upper lip.

Metastasis of Tumor Cells
The basilar and occipital sinuses communicate through the foramen magnum with the *internal vertebral venous plexuses* (p. 292). Because these venous channels are valveless, compression of the thorax, abdomen, or pelvis—as occurs during heavy coughing and straining—may force venous blood from these regions into the vertebral venous

system and subsequently into the dural venous sinuses. As a result, pus in abscesses and tumor cells from the trunk may spread to the vertebrae and brain via these venous interconnections.

Fractures of Cranial Base
Fractures of the cranial base may tear the internal carotid artery within the cavernous sinus, producing an *arteriovenous fistula*. Arterial blood rushes into the cavernous sinus, enlarging it and forcing blood into the connecting veins, especially the superior ophthalmic veins. As a result, the eye protrudes (*exophthalmos*) and the conjunctiva becomes engorged (*chemosis*). The protruding eye pulsates in synchrony with the radial pulse, a phenomenon known as *pulsating exophthalmos*. Because CNs III, IV, V$_1$, V$_2$, and VI lie in or close to the lateral wall of the cavernous sinus (Fig. 8.10), they may also be affected when the sinus is injured. The attachment of the periosteal layer of the dura mater to the floor of the cranium is firmer than it is to the calvaria. Consequently, a blow to the head can detach the dura from the calvaria without fracturing the bones. A basal fracture usually tears the dura and arachnoid, resulting in leakage of CSF (e.g., into neck).

The **arteries of the dura** supply more blood to the calvaria than they do to the dura. The largest of the meningeal arteries, the **middle meningeal artery** (Fig. 8.8*A*), is a branch of the maxillary artery. The middle meningeal artery enters the cranial cavity through the *foramen spinosum*, runs laterally on the floor of the middle cranial fossa, and turns superoanteriorly on the greater wing of the sphenoid, where it divides into anterior and posterior branches. The anterior branch runs superiorly to the pterion and then curves posteriorly to ascend toward the vertex of the cranium. The posterior branch runs posterosuperiorly and ramifies over the posterior aspect of the cranium. The **veins of the dura** (Fig. 8.8*A*) accompany the meningeal arteries.

Innervation of the dura is largely by the three divisions of CN V (Fig. 8.8*B*). Sensory branches are also conveyed from the vagus (CN X) and hypoglossal (CN XII) nerves, but the fibers probably are peripheral branches from sensory ganglia of the superior three cervical nerves. The sensory endings are more numerous in the dura along each side of the superior sagittal sinus and in the tentorium cerebelli than they are in the floor of the cranium. Pain fibers are also numerous where arteries and veins pierce the dura.

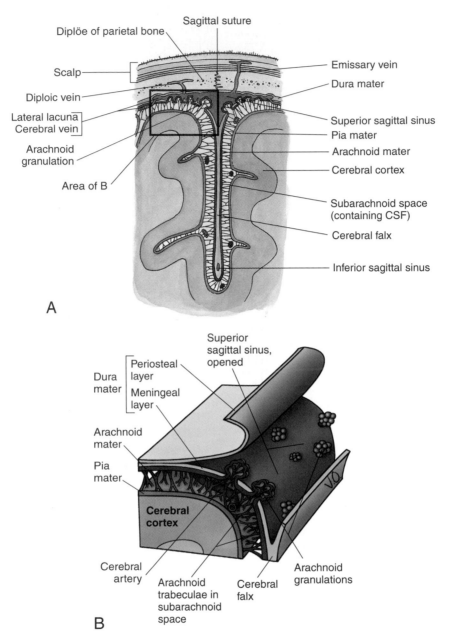

FIGURE 8.11   Cranial meninges. A. Coronal section of the cranium and brain showing the superior sagittal sinus and meninges. **B.** Meninges and subarachnoid (leptomeningeal) space.

DURAL ORIGIN OF HEADACHES

The dura is sensitive to pain, especially where it is related to the dural venous sinuses and meningeal arteries. Consequently, pulling on arteries at the base of the cranium or on veins near the vertex where they pierce the dura causes pain. Although the causes of headache are numerous, distention of the scalp or meningeal vessels (or both) is believed to be one cause. Many headaches appear to be dural in original, such as the headache occurring after a *lumbar spinal puncture for removal of CSF* (see Chapter 5) that is thought to result from stimulation of sensory nerve endings in the dura. When CSF is removed, the brain sags slightly, pulling on the dura; this may cause pain and headache. For this reason, patients are advised to lie inclined, with their heads lower than their trunk (Trendelenburg position), after a lumbar puncture to minimize or prevent headaches.

PIA AND ARACHNOID MATER

The pia-arachnoid (leptomeninx—combined pia mater and arachnoid mater) develops from a single layer of mesenchyme surrounding the embryonic brain. Fluid-filled spaces form within this embryonic connective tissue and coalesce to form the **subarachnoid space** (Fig. 8.11). Web-like **arachnoid trabeculae** (supporting bundles of fibers) pass between the arachnoid and pia. The *avascular arachnoid mater,* closely applied to the meningeal layer of the dura, is held against the inner surface of the dura by the pressure of the CSF. The **pia mater** adheres to the surface of the brain and follows its contours. When the cerebral arteries penetrate the cerebral cortex, the pia follows them for a short distance, forming a pial coat and a periarterial space. Although it is commonly stated that the brain "floats" in CSF, the brain (within its pial lining) is suspended in the CSF-filled subarachnoid space by the **arachnoid trabeculae.**

MENINGEAL SPACES

Three meningeal spaces relate to the cranial meninges:

- *The dura-cranium interface (extradural or epidural "space")* is normally not an actual space but only a potential one between the cranial bones and the periosteal layer of the dura because the dura is attached to the bones. It becomes a real space only pathologically—for example, when blood from torn meningeal vessels pushes the periosteum from the cranium and accumulates.
- *The dura-arachnoid junction or interface* ("subdural space") is likewise normally only a potential space that may develop in the dural border cell layer of the dura after a blow to the head (Haines, 2002).
- The *subarachnoid space,* between the arachnoid and pia, is an actual space that contains CSF, trabecular cells, arteries, and veins.

HEAD INJURIES

Extradural or epidural hemorrhage between the endosteal layer of the dura and the calvaria may follow a blow to the head. Typically, a brief concussion results, followed by a lucid interval of some hours. This is succeeded by drowsiness and coma. Most bleeding from the torn meningeal arteries results in an *extradural* or *epidural hematoma*—a slow, localized accumulation of blood. As the blood mass increases, compression of the brain occurs, necessitating evacuation of the blood and occlusion of the bleeding vessels.

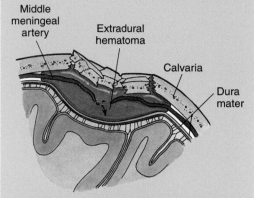

Extradural or epidural hematoma

A dural border hematoma classically is called a *subdural hematoma;* however, this is a misnomer because there is no naturally occurring space at the dura-arachnoid junction. Although the dura and arachnoid are normally adjacent and are usually encountered as two surfaces of a single membrane, blood may collect in the abnormal space that forms when trauma separates them. *Dural border hemorrhage* usually follows a blow to the head that jerks the brain inside the cranium and injures it. The precipitating trauma may be trivial or forgotten. Displacement of the brain is greatest in elderly people in whom some shrinkage of the brain has occurred. *Dural border hemorrhage is typically venous in origin* and commonly results from the tearing of a cerebral vein as it enters the superior sagittal sinus.

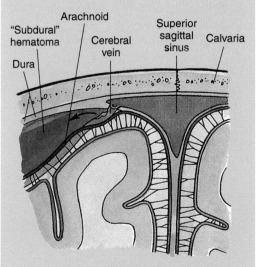

Dural border (subdural) hematoma

Continued

Subarachnoid hemorrhage is an extravasation (escape) of blood into the subarachnoid space. Most of these hemorrhages result from rupture of a *saccular aneurysm* (dilation of an intracranial blood vessel). Subarachnoid hemorrhages are also associated with head trauma involving cranial fractures and cerebral lacerations. Bleeding into the subarachnoid space results in meningeal irritation, which produces a severe headache, stiff neck, and, often, loss of consciousness.

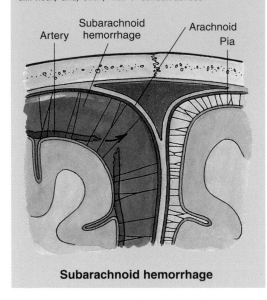

Subarachnoid hemorrhage

BRAIN

The brain, composed of the *cerebrum, cerebellum,* and *brainstem* (midbrain, pons, and medulla oblongata), is lodged in the cranial cavity. The roof of the cranial cavity is formed by the *calvaria* and its floor is formed by the *cranial base.* The following brief discussion of the gross structure of the brain shows how the brain relates to the cranium, cranial nerves, meninges, and CSF.

SUBDIVISIONS OF BRAIN

When the calvaria and dura mater are removed, **gyri** (folds), **sulci** (grooves), and **fissures** of the cerebral cortex are visible through the delicate pia-arachnoid layers. The sulci and fissures of the brain are distinctive landmarks that subdivide the cerebral hemispheres into smaller areas—lobes and gyri (Fig. 8.12). The **cerebrum**—

the principal subdivision of the brain—includes the cerebral hemispheres and diencephalon but not the cerebellum and brainstem.

- The **cerebral hemispheres** (telencephalon) form the largest part of the brain, occupying the anterior and middle cranial fossae and extending posteriorly over the cerebellar tentorium and cerebellum. The cavity in each hemisphere, a *lateral ventricle,* is part of the *ventricular system of the brain* (Fig. 8.13).

- The **diencephalon**—composed of the epithalamus, thalamus, and hypothalamus—forms the central core of the brain and surrounds the 3rd ventricle, the cavity between the right and left halves of the diencephalon.

- The **midbrain** (mesencephalon)—the rostral part of the brainstem—lies at the junction of the middle and posterior cranial fossae. The cavity of the midbrain forms a narrow canal—the **cerebral aqueduct**—that conducts CSF from the lateral and 3rd ventricles to the 4th ventricle.

- The **pons**—the part of the brainstem between the midbrain rostrally and the medulla oblongata caudally—lies in the anterior part of the posterior cranial fossa; the cavity in the pons forms the superior part of the 4th ventricle.

- The **medulla oblongata** (medulla)—the caudal part of the brainstem that is continuous with the spinal cord—lies in the posterior cranial fossa. The cavity of the medulla forms the inferior part of the 4th ventricle, which leads to and ends as the central canal of the spinal cord.

- The **cerebellum**—the large brain mass lying dorsal to the pons and medulla and ventral to the posterior part of the cerebrum—lies beneath the cerebellar tentorium in the posterior cranial fossa; it consists of two hemispheres.

Eleven of twelve cranial nerves arise from the brain (Fig. 8.14A). They have motor, parasympathetic, and/or sensory functions. Generally, these nerves are surrounded by a *dural sheath* as they leave the cranium; the dural sheath becomes continuous with the connective tissue of the epineurium. For a summary of the cranial nerves, see Chapter 10.

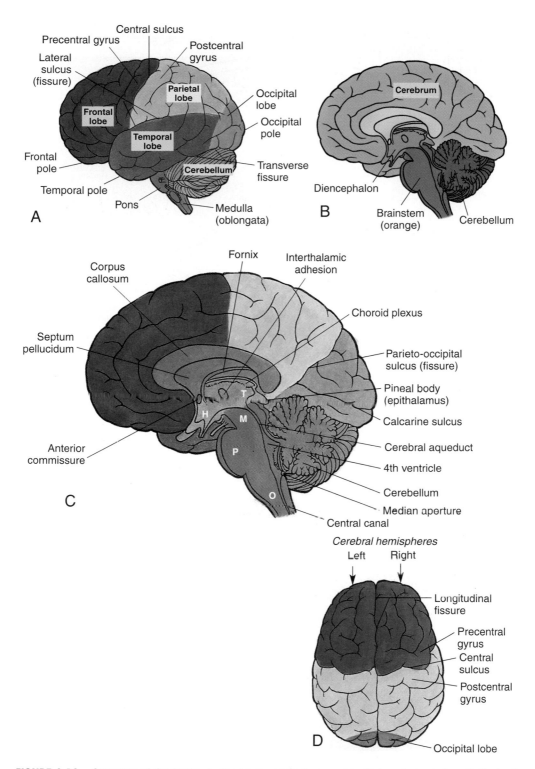

FIGURE 8.12   **Structure of the brain. A.** Cerebrum, cerebellum, and brainstem. Lateral view. **B.** Parts of the brain. Median section. **C.** Features and lobes of the brain. Median section. *Arrow*, site of interventricular foramen. *T*, thalamus; *H*, hypothalamus; *M*, midbrain; *P*, pons; *O*, medulla oblongata. **D.** Superior view of the right and left cerebral hemispheres.

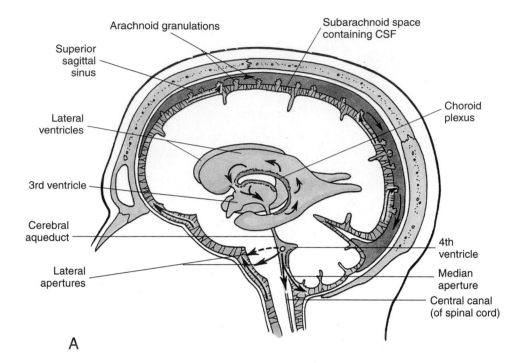

Arachnoid granulations

Subarachnoid space containing CSF

Superior sagittal sinus

Choroid plexus

Lateral ventricles

3rd ventricle

Cerebral aqueduct

4th ventricle

Lateral apertures

Median aperture

Central canal (of spinal cord)

A

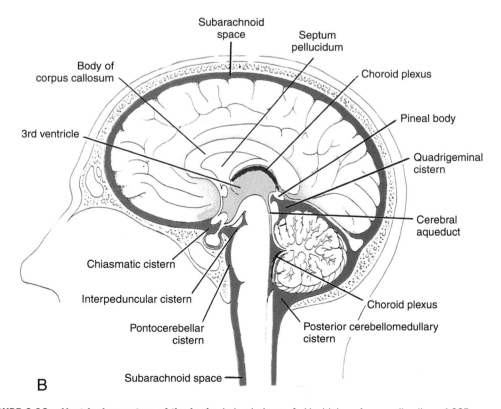

Subarachnoid space

Septum pellucidum

Body of corpus callosum

Choroid plexus

Pineal body

3rd ventricle

Quadrigeminal cistern

Cerebral aqueduct

Chiasmatic cistern

Interpeduncular cistern

Pontocerebellar cistern

Posterior cerebellomedullary cistern

Choroid plexus

Subarachnoid space

B

FIGURE 8.13   Ventricular system of the brain. Lateral views. **A.** Ventricles. *Arrows,* direction of CSF flow. **B.** Subarachnoid cisterns.

VENTRICULAR SYSTEM OF BRAIN

The ventricular system of the brain consists mainly of two lateral ventricles and the midline 3rd and 4th ventricles connected by the **cerebral aqueduct** (Fig. 8.13*A*). The **lateral ventricles** (1st and 2nd ventricles) open into the 3rd ventricle through the *interventricular foramina* (of Monro). The **3rd ventricle** is a slitlike cavity between the right and left halves of the diencephalon. The **4th ventricle** lying in the posterior parts of the pons and medulla extends inferoposteriorly. It is continuous with the central canal in the inferior part of the medulla and with the central canal in the spinal cord. *CSF drains from the 4th ventricle through a single median and paired lateral apertures into the subarachnoid space.* These apertures are the only means by which CSF enters the subarachnoid space. If they are blocked, the ventricles distend, producing compression of the cerebral hemispheres. At certain places, mainly at the base of the brain, the arachnoid and pia mater are widely separated by large pools (cisterns) of CSF (Fig. 8.13*B*). **Major subarachnoid cisterns include the:**

- **Posterior cerebellomedullary cistern** (cisterna magna)—the largest of the cisterns—is between the cerebellum and the medulla and receives CSF from the apertures of the 4th ventricle

- **Pontocerebellar cistern** (pontine cistern)—a space on the lateral aspects of the pons at its junction with the cerebellum
- **Interpeduncular cistern** (basal cistern)—between the cerebral peduncles of the midbrain and the structures of the interpeduncular fossa—*contains the cerebral arterial circle* (of Willis)
- **Chiasmatic cistern** (cistern of optic chiasm)—inferior and anterior to the *optic chiasm*
- **Quadrigeminal cistern** (cistern of the great cerebral vein, superior cistern)—between the posterior part of the corpus callosum and the superior surface of the cerebellum.

The main source of CSF secretion is the choroid plexus (Fig. 8.13, *A* and *B*). **Choroid plexuses**—vascular fringes of pia mater covered by cuboidal epithelial cells—are located in the roofs of the 3rd and 4th ventricles and on the floors of the bodies and inferior horns of the lateral ventricles. Although choroid plexuses are the main source of CSF, there are exchanges between blood plasma and CSF elsewhere (e.g., across the lining of the ventricles). From the subarachnoid cisterns, some CSF passes inferiorly into the subarachnoid space around the spinal cord and posterosuperiorly over the cerebellum. However, most CSF flows into the interpeduncular and quadrigeminal cisterns. CSF from the various cisterns spreads superiorly through the sulci and fissures on the medial and superolateral surfaces of the cerebral hemispheres. CSF also passes into the extensions of the subarachnoid space around the cranial nerves. *The main site of CSF absorption into the venous system* is through the **arachnoid granulations**—protrusions of arachnoid villi into the walls of dural venous sinuses, especially the superior sagittal sinus and its lateral lacunae (Figs. 8.8*A* and 8.13*A*).

Hydrocephalus

Overproduction of CSF, obstruction of its flow, or interference with its absorption results in an excess of CSF in the ventricles and enlargement of the head, a condition known as *hydrocephalus*. Although a condition generally related to a fetus or infant, hydrocephalus also occurs in the adult. Excess CSF dilates the ventricles, thins the brain, and separates the cranial bones.

Leakage of CSF

Fractures in the floor of the middle cranial fossa may result in leakage of CSF from the ear (*CSF otorrhea*) if the meninges superior to the middle ear are torn and the tympanic membrane (eardrum) is ruptured. Fractures in the floor of the anterior cranial fossa may involve the cribriform plate of the ethmoid, resulting in leakage of CSF through the nose (*CSF rhinorrhea*). CSF otorrhea and CSF rhinorrhea present a risk of *meningitis* because an infection may spread to the meninges from the ear or nasal cavities.

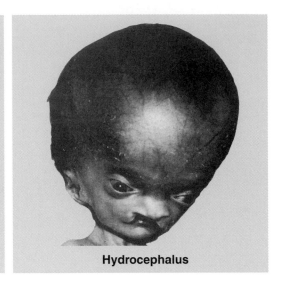

Hydrocephalus

VASCULATURE OF BRAIN

The **arterial supply to the brain** derives from the internal carotid and vertebral arteries (Fig. 8.14, Table 8.4). The **internal carotid arteries** arise in the neck from the common carotid arteries. The **anterior** and **middle cerebral arteries** are terminal branches of the internal carotid. The **vertebral arteries** begin in the root of the neck as branches of the first part of the subclavian arteries and unite at the caudal border of the pons to form the **basilar artery,** so-named because of its close relationship to the cranial base. The basilar artery runs through the pontocerebellar cistern to the superior border of the pons, where it ends by dividing into the two **posterior cerebral arteries.** In general, each cerebral artery supplies a surface and a pole of the brain as follows:

* The **anterior cerebral artery** supplies most of the medial and superior surfaces and the frontal pole

TABLE 8.4.   ARTERIAL SUPPLY TO BRAIN

Artery	Origin	Distribution
Vertebral	Subclavian artery	Cranial meninges and cerebellum
Posterior inferior cerebellar	Vertebral artery	Posteroinferior aspect of cerebellum
Basilar	Formed by junction of vertebral arteries	Brainstem, cerebellum, and cerebrum
Pontine	Basilar artery	Numerous branches to brainstem
Anterior inferior cerebellar		Inferior aspect of cerebellum
Superior cerebellar		Superior aspect of cerebellum
Internal carotid	Common carotid artery at superior border of thyroid cartilage	Gives branches in cavernous sinus and provides primary supply to brain
Anterior cerebral	Internal carotid artery	Cerebral hemispheres, except for occipital lobes
Middle cerebral	Continuation of the internal carotid artery distal to anterior cerebral artery	Most of lateral surface of cerebral hemispheres
Posterior cerebral	Terminal branch of basilar artery	Inferior aspect of cerebral hemisphere and occipital lobe
Anterior communicating	Anterior cerebral artery	Cerebral arterial circle
Posterior communicating	Posterior cerebral artery	Cerebral arterial circle

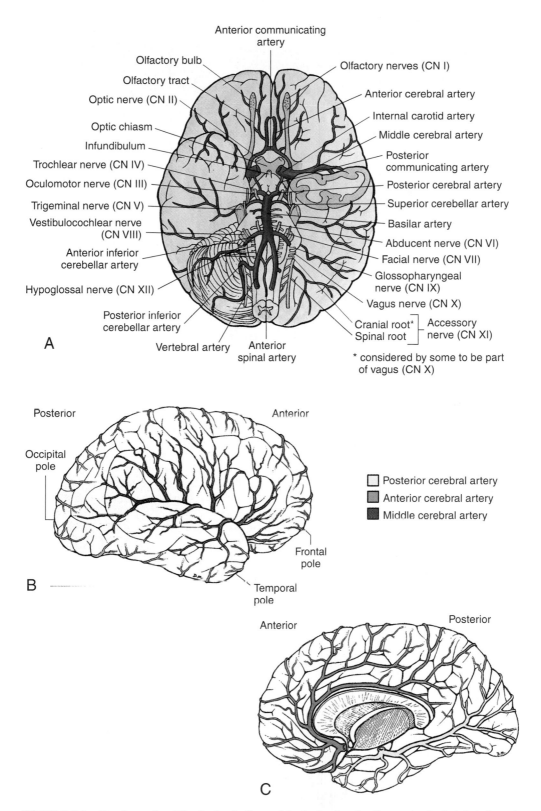

FIGURE 8.14 **Blood supply of the brain. A.** Base of the brain showing the cerebral arterial circle and cranial nerves. Inferior view. **B.** Right lateral view of the right hemisphere. **C.** Medial view of the right hemisphere.

- The **middle cerebral artery** supplies the lateral surface and temporal pole
- The **posterior cerebral artery** supplies the inferior surface and occipital pole.

The **cerebral arterial circle** (of Willis) at the base of the brain is an important anastomosis between four arteries (two vertebrals and two internal carotids) that supply the brain (Fig. 8.14*A*). **The circle is formed by the posterior cerebral, posterior communicating, internal carotid, anterior cerebral, and anterior communicating arteries.** Variations in the origin and size of the vessels forming the circle are common (e.g., about one person in three has one posterior cerebral artery as a branch of the internal carotid artery).

Venous drainage of the brain from superficial and deep veins enters the *dural venous sinuses* (Fig. 8.9), which drain into the *IJVs*. The cerebral veins on the superolateral surface of the brain drain into the superior sagittal sinus; cerebral veins on the posteroinferior aspect drain into the straight, transverse, and superior petrosal sinuses.

VASCULAR STROKES

The cerebral arterial circle is an important means of collateral circulation in the event one of the arteries forming the circle is obstructed. In elderly persons, the anastomoses are often inadequate when a large artery (e.g., internal carotid) is suddenly occluded; as a result, a vascular stroke results. The most common causes of vascular strokes are spontaneous *cerebrovascular accidents* such as cerebral thrombosis, cerebral hemorrhage, cerebral embolism, and subarachnoid hemorrhage. *Hemorrhagic stroke* follows from rupture of an artery or an aneurysm. The most common type of aneurysm is a *berry aneurysm,* occurring in the vessels of or near the cerebral arterial circle and the medium-sized arteries at the base of the brain. In time, especially in persons with high blood pressure (hypertension), the weak part of the arterial wall expands and may rupture, allowing blood to enter the subarachnoid space.

Transient Ischemic Attacks

Transient ischemic attacks (TIAs) refer to neurological symptoms resulting from ischemia (deficient blood supply) of the brain. The symptoms of a TIA may be ambiguous: staggering, dizziness, light-headedness, fainting, and par-esthesia (e.g., tingling in a limb). Most attacks last a few minutes only, but some persist for an hour or more.

The 12 *cranial nerves* associated with the brain (Fig. 8.14*A*) are described and illustrated in Chapter 10.

ORBIT

The orbit (eye socket) is a pyramidal, bony cavity in the facial skeleton with its base (the *orbital opening*) anterior and its apex posterior (Fig. 8.15). The orbits contain and protect the eyeballs and their muscles, nerves, and vessels, together with most of the lacrimal apparatus. **The orbit has four walls and an apex:**

- The *superior wall (roof) of the orbit* is approximately horizontal and is formed mainly by the **orbital part of the frontal bone,** which separates the orbital cavity from the anterior cranial fossa. Near the apex of the orbit, the superior wall is formed by the lesser wing of the sphenoid. The *lacrimal gland* occupies the **fossa for the lacrimal gland** in the orbital part of the frontal bone.
- The *medial wall of the orbit* is formed by the **ethmoid bone,** along with contributions from the **frontal, lacrimal, and sphenoid bones;** anteriorly, the *paper-thin medial wall* is indented by the **fossa for the lacrimal sac** and the proximal part of the nasolacrimal duct.

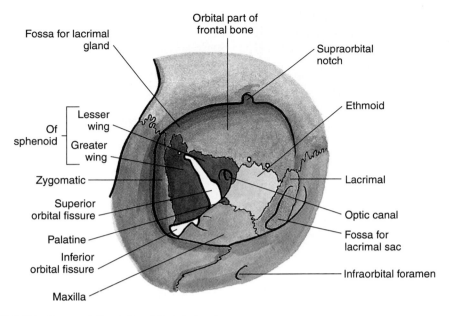

FIGURE 8.15   Bones of the right orbit. Anterior view.

- The *lateral wall of the orbit* is formed by the **frontal process of the zygomatic bone** and the **greater wing of the sphenoid.** The lateral wall is the strongest and thickest wall and it is most vulnerable to blows and direct trauma. It separates the orbit from the temporal and middle cranial fossae.

- The *inferior wall (floor) of the orbit* is formed mainly by the **maxilla** and partly by the **zygomatic** and **palatine bones;** the thin inferior wall is partly separated from the lateral wall of the orbit by the **inferior orbital fissure.** The inferior wall slants inferiorly from the apex of the orbit to the inferior orbital margin.

- The *apex of the orbit* is at the optic canal, just medial to the superior orbital fissure.

The bones forming the orbit are lined with *periorbita* (periosteum of the orbit), which forms the **fascial sheath of the eyeball** (Fig. 8.16*A*). The periorbita is continuous at the **optic canal** and **superior orbital fissure** with the periosteal layer of the dura. The periorbita is also continuous over the orbital margins and through the inferior orbital fissure with the periosteum covering the external surface of the cranium (pericranium).

FRACTURE OF ORBIT

Because of the thinness of the medial and inferior walls of the orbit, an anterior blow to the eye may fracture these walls. Indirect traumatic injury that displaces the orbital walls is a "blowout fracture." Fractures of the medial wall may involve the ethmoidal and sphenoidal sinuses, whereas fractures in the inferior wall may involve the maxillary sinus (p. 576). Although the superior wall is stronger than the medial and inferior walls, it is thin enough to be translucent and may be readily penetrated. Thus, a sharp object may pass through it into the frontal lobe of the brain.

Exophthalmos

Tumors in the orbit produce *exophthalmos*—protrusion of the eyeball. The easiest entrance to the orbital cavity for a tumor in the middle cranial fossa is through the superior orbital fissure. *Hyperthyroidism* also may produce exophthalmos, resulting from the increased volume of the orbital contents, such as the orbital musculature and fat.

EYELIDS AND LACRIMAL APPARATUS

The **eyelids** (L. palpebrae) protect the cornea and eyeball from injury (e.g., dust). When closed, the eyelids cover the eyeball anteriorly, thereby protecting it from injury and excessive light (Fig. 8.16). The eyelids also keep the cornea moist by spreading the lacrimal fluid (tears). The eyelids are movable folds that are

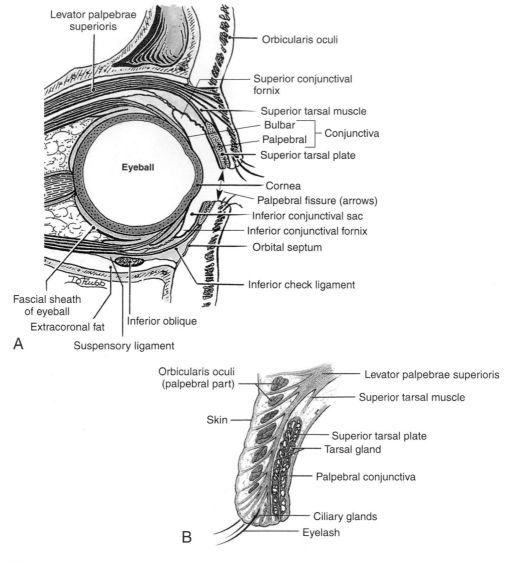

FIGURE 8.16 Orbit and eyelids. Sagittal sections. **A.** Orbital contents. **B.** Superior (upper) eyelid.

covered externally by thin skin and internally by **palpebral conjunctiva**—the mucous membrane investing the posterior surface of the eyelids. The palpebral conjunctiva is reflected onto the eyeball, where it is continuous with the **bulbar conjunctiva.** This part of the conjunctiva is thin and transparent and attaches loosely to the anterior surface of the eye. The bulbar conjunctiva is loose and wrinkled over the sclera and contains small blood vessels. The bulbar conjunctiva is adherent to the periphery of the cornea. The **conjunctival sac** is the space bound by the conjunctival membrane between the *palpebral*

and *bulbar conjunctiva.* The lines of reflection of the palpebral conjunctiva onto the eyeball form deep recesses, the **superior** and **inferior conjunctival fornices.** The eyelids are strengthened by dense bands of connective tissue, the superior and inferior **tarsal plates** (tarsi). Fibers of the **orbicularis oculi** muscle are in the subcutaneous tissue superficial to these plates and deep to the skin of the eyelid. Embedded in the tarsal plates are **tarsal glands** (see Fig. 8.18*B*), the lipid secretion of which lubricates the edges of the eyelids and prevents them from sticking together when they close. This secretion also forms a barrier that lacrimal fluid normally does not spill across. The **eyelashes** (L. cilia) are in the margins of the eyelids. The large *sebaceous glands* associated with the eyelashes are the **ciliary glands.** The upper and lower eyelids meet at the *angles of the eye* (canthi). Thus, each eye has medial and lateral angles.

In the **medial angle (corner) of the eye** is a relatively deep region, the **lacrimal lake,** within which is the **lacrimal caruncle,** a small mound of moist, pink modified skin (Fig. 8.17A). Lateral to the caruncle is a **semilunar conjunctival fold** (L. plica semilunaris) that slightly overlaps the eyeball. When the edge of the inferior eye-

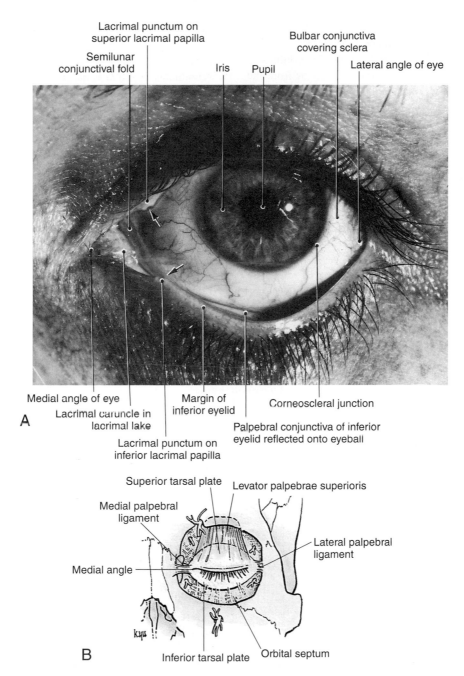

A

Lacrimal punctum on superior lacrimal papilla

Semilunar conjunctival fold

Iris

Pupil

Bulbar conjunctiva covering sclera

Lateral angle of eye

Medial angle of eye

Lacrimal caruncle in lacrimal lake

Margin of inferior eyelid

Corneoscleral junction

Palpebral conjunctiva of inferior eyelid reflected onto eyeball

Lacrimal punctum on inferior lacrimal papilla

B

Superior tarsal plate

Levator palpebrae superioris

Medial palpebral ligament

Lateral palpebral ligament

Medial angle

Inferior tarsal plate

Orbital septum

FIGURE 8.17   Eye and eyelids. A. Surface anatomy. Anterior view. **B.** Skeleton of eyelids. Anterior view.

lid is everted, a small pit called the **lacrimal punctum** (*arrows*) is visible at its medial end on the summit of a small elevation called the **lacrimal papilla.** A similar punctum and papilla are on the upper eyelid.

Between the nose and the medial angle of the eye is the **medial palpebral ligament,** which connects to the medial aspect of the tarsal plates and provides the origin and insertion for the orbicularis oculi muscle (Fig. 8.17*B*). A similar **lateral palpebral ligament** attaches the eyelids to the lateral margin of the orbit. The **orbital septum** is a weak membrane that spans from the tarsal plates to the margins of the orbit, where it

becomes continuous with the periosteum. It keeps the orbital fat contained and can limit the spread of infection to and from the orbit.

The lacrimal apparatus consists of (Figs. 8.17 and 8.18):

- *Lacrimal glands,* which secrete lacrimal fluid (tears)
- *Lacrimal ducts,* which convey lacrimal fluid from the lacrimal glands to the conjunctival sac
- *Lacrimal canaliculi* (L. small canals), each commencing at a *lacrimal punctum* (opening) on the *lacrimal papilla* near the

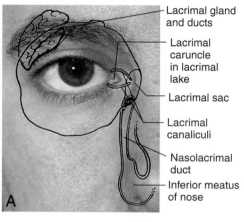

Lacrimal gland and ducts

Lacrimal caruncle in lacrimal lake

Lacrimal sac

Lacrimal canaliculi

Nasolacrimal duct

Inferior meatus of nose

A

FIGURE 8.18   Lacrimal apparatus.
Anterior views. **A.** Surface anatomy.
B. Dissection of the eye and nose.

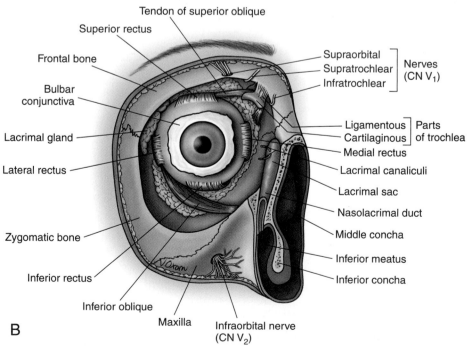

Tendon of superior oblique

Superior rectus

Frontal bone

Bulbar conjunctiva

Lacrimal gland

Lateral rectus

Zygomatic bone

Inferior rectus

Inferior oblique

Maxilla

Infraorbital nerve (CN V$_2$)

B

Supraorbital
Supratrochlear   Nerves (CN V$_1$)
Infratrochlear

Ligamentous   Parts
Cartilaginous   of trochlea
Medial rectus

Lacrimal canaliculi

Lacrimal sac

Nasolacrimal duct

Middle concha

Inferior meatus

Inferior concha

medial angle of the eye, which conveys the lacrimal fluid from the *lacrimal lake*—a triangular space at the medial angle of the eye where the tears collect—in the *lacrimal sac,* the dilated superior part of the nasolacrimal duct

- *Nasolacrimal duct,* which conveys the lacrimal fluid to the nasal cavity.

The almond-shaped **lacrimal gland** lies in the **fossa for the lacrimal gland** in the superolateral part of each orbit. **Lacrimal fluid** or **tears**—the production of which is stimulated by parasympathetic impulses from CN VII—enters the conjunctival sac through up to 12 **lacrimal ducts** that open into the **superior conjunctival fornix** (Fig. 8.16*A*)—the superior line of reflection of the palpebral conjunctiva to the eyeball. After passing over the eyeball—due in large part to the way the eye closes from lateral to medial—the lacrimal fluid enters the **lacrimal lake** at the medial angle of the eye from which it drains by capillary action through the **lacrimal puncta** and **lacrimal canaliculi** to the lacrimal sac. From this sac, the lacrimal fluid passes to the nasal cavity through the **nasolacrimal duct** (Fig. 8.18). Here it flows back to the nasopharynx and is swallowed. However, when the fluid (tears) increases as a result of emotion or other causes, it flows anteriorly over the lipid barrier on the edge of the eyelids and onto the cheeks. The eye also blinks when the cornea becomes dry, and the eyelids carry a moisturizing film of fluid over the cornea. Foreign material such as dust is also carried to the medial angle of the eye where it can be removed.

The **nerve supply of the lacrimal gland** is both sympathetic and parasympathetic. *The presynaptic, parasympathetic secretomotor fibers are conveyed from the facial nerve by the greater petrosal nerve to the nerve of the pterygoid canal that brings them to the pterygopalatine ganglion,* where they synapse with the cell body of the postsynaptic fiber (p. 569). Vasoconstrictive, postsynaptic sympathetic fibers brought from the *superior cervical ganglion* by the *internal carotid plexus* and deep petrosal nerve join the parasympathetic fibers forming the nerve of the pterygoid canal and traverse the *pterygopalatine ganglion.* Branches of the

zygomatic nerve (from the maxillary nerve) then bring both types of fibers to the lacrimal branch of the ophthalmic nerve (CN V₁), by which they enter the gland.

INJURY TO FACIAL NERVE SUPPLYING EYELIDS

Damage to the facial nerve (CN VII) involves paralysis of the orbicularis oculi muscle, preventing the eyelids from closing fully. Normal rapid protective blinking of the eye is also lost. The loss of tonus of the muscle in the lower eyelid causes the lid to fall away (become everted) from the surface of the eye. This leads to drying of the cornea and leaves it unprotected from dust and small particles. Thus, irritation of the unprotected eyeball results in excessive but inefficient *lacrimation* (tear formation).

Inflammation of Palpebral Glands

Any of the glands in the eyelid may become inflamed and swollen from infection or obstruction of their ducts. If the *ducts of the ciliary glands* become obstructed, a painful red suppurative (puss-producing) swelling—a *sty*—develops on the eyelid. Cysts of the ciliary glands—*chalazia*—also may form.

ORBITAL CONTENTS

The contents of the orbit are the eyeball, optic nerve, ocular muscles, fascia, nerves, vessels, fat, lacrimal gland, and conjunctival sac. **The eyeball has three layers** (Fig. 8.19):

- The outer *fibrous layer*—the **sclera** and **cornea**
- The middle *vascular (pigmented) layer*—the **choroid, ciliary body,** and **iris**
- The *inner layer*—the **retina**—consisting of optic and nonvisual parts.

The **sclera** is the opaque part of the fibrous coat covering the posterior five-sixths of the eyeball. The anterior part of the sclera is visible through the transparent bulbar conjunctiva as the "white of the eye." The **cornea** is the transparent part of the fibrous coat covering the anterior one-sixth of the eyeball. The **choroid**—a dark brown membrane between the sclera and retina—forms the largest part of the vascular layer of the eyeball and lines most of the sclera. It terminates anteriorly in the **ciliary body.** The choroid attaches firmly to the pigment layer of the retina, but it can be stripped easily from the sclera. The **ciliary body**—which is muscular as well as vascular—connects the choroid with the circumference

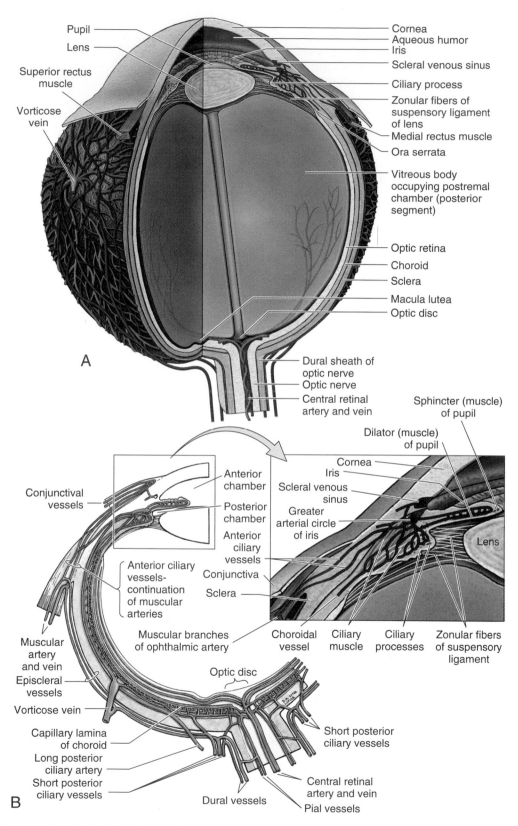

FIGURE 8.19 Eyeball. **A.** Parts of the eyeball. **B.** Partial horizontal section of the right eyeball.

of the iris. Folds on its internal surface—the **ciliary processes**—secrete *aqueous humor,* which fills the chambers of the eye. The **anterior chamber of the eye** is the space between the cornea anteriorly and the iris/pupil posteriorly. The **posterior chamber of the eye** is the space between the iris/pupil anteriorly and the lens and ciliary body posteriorly. The **iris,** which literally lies on the anterior surface of the lens, is a *thin contractile diaphragm* with a central aperture—the **pupil**—for transmitting light. When a person is awake, the size of the pupil varies continually to regulate the amount of light entering the eye. Two muscles control the size of the pupil: the **sphincter pupillae** closes the pupil and the **dilator pupillae** opens it (Fig. 8.19*B*).

Grossly, the **retina** consists of three parts: the optic part, ciliary part, and iridial part. The **optic retina,** which receives the visual light rays, has two layers: a neural layer and a pigmented layer. The *neural layer* is the light-receptive part. The *pigmented layer* reinforces the light-absorbing property of the choroid in reducing the scattering of light in the eye. The *ciliary* and *iridial parts of the retina* are anterior continuations of the pigmented layer and a layer of supporting cells over the ciliary body and the posterior surface of the iris, respectively. In the **fundus** (posterior part of the eye) is a circular depressed area—the **optic disc**—where the optic nerve enters the eyeball. Because it contains nerve fibers and no photoreceptors, *the optic disc is insensitive to light.* Just lateral to the optic disc is the **macula lutea.** The yellow color of the macula is apparent only when the retina is examined with red-free light. *The macula—a small area of the retina with special photoreceptor cones—is specialized for acuity of vision.* At the center of the macula is a depression—the *fovea centralis* (L. central pit)—*the area of most acute vision.* The functional optic retina terminates anteriorly along the **ora serrata** (L. serrated edge), an irregular border slightly posterior to the ciliary body. The ora serrata marks the anterior termination of the light-receptive part of the retina. Except for the cone and rod cells of the retina, the retina is supplied by the **central artery of the retina** (Fig. 8.19*A*), a branch of the ophthalmic artery. A corresponding system of retinal veins unites to form the **central vein of the retina.**

OPHTHALMOSCOPY

Physicians view the fundus of the eye with an *ophthalmoscope.* The retinal arteries and veins radiate over the fundus from the optic disc. Observe the pale, oval optic disc with retinal vessels radiating from its center in this view of the retina seen through an ophthalmoscope. An increase in CSF pressure slows venous return from the retina, causing *edema of the retina* (fluid accumulation in the retina). Normally, the optic disc is flat and does not form a papilla. *Papilledema* (edema of the papilla) results from increased intracranial pressure, which increases CSF pressure in the extension of the subarachnoid space around the optic nerve. Continued increased pressure may result in blindness.

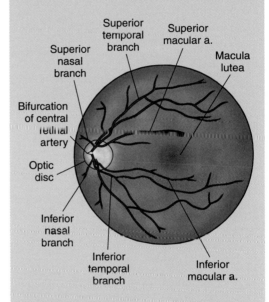

Detachment of Retina

The developing layers of the retina are separated in the embryo by an intraretinal space. During the early fetal period, the embryonic layers fuse, obliterating the intraretinal space. Although the pigmented layer becomes firmly fixed to the choroid, its attachment to the neural layer is not firm. Consequently, detachment of the retina may follow a blow to the eye, reverting to the state that existed in the embryo. A *detached retina* usually results from seepage of fluid between the neural and pigmented layers of the retina, perhaps days or even weeks after trauma to the eye. Persons with a retinal detachment may complain of the perception of flashes of light. Laser treatment of the detached area may prevent permanent loss of vision, depending on the size of the affected area and the timing of identification of the retinal detachment.

On their way to the retina, light waves pass through the **refractive media of the eye:** the cornea, aqueous humor, lens, and vitreous humor in the vitreous body (Fig. 8.19*A*). The **cornea** is the circular area of the anterior part of the outer fibrous coat of the eyeball; it is largely responsible for refraction of light that enters the eye. It is transparent, avascular, and sensitive to touch. The cornea is supplied by the *ophthalmic nerve* (CN V$_1$) and is nourished by the aqueous humor, lacrimal fluid, and oxygen absorbed from the air and capillaries at its periphery (corneoscleral junction or limbus). The **aqueous humor** in the chambers of the eyeball is produced by the **ciliary processes.** This watery solution provides nutrients for the avascular cornea and lens. After passing through the pupil from the posterior chamber into the anterior chamber (Fig. 8.19*B*), the aqueous humor drains into the **scleral venous sinus** (L. sinus venosus sclerae, canal of Schlemm).

The **lens**—posterior to the iris and anterior to the vitreous humor—is a transparent biconvex structure enclosed in a capsule. The *lens capsule* is anchored by the **suspensory ligaments of the lens** to the **ciliary bodies** and is encircled by the **ciliary processes.** The convexity of the lens, particularly its anterior surface, constantly varies to focus near or distant objects on the retina. Contraction of the **ciliary muscle** in the ciliary body changes the shape of the lens (Fig. 8.19*B*). Stretched within the circle of the relaxed ciliary body, the attachments around its periphery pull the lens relatively flat, enabling far vision. When parasympathetic stimulation causes the smooth muscle of the circular ciliary body to contract, the circle—like a sphincter—becomes smaller in size and the tension on the lens is reduced, allowing the lens to round up. The increased convexity is for near vision. In the absence of parasympathetic stimulation, the ciliary muscles relax again and the lens is pulled into its flatter, far vision shape. The **vitreous humor** is enclosed in the meshes of the **vitreous body,** a transparent jellylike substance filling the interior of the eyeball, posterior to the lens and retina. In addition to transmitting light, the vitreous humor holds the retina in place and supports the lens.

CORNEAL ABRASIONS AND LACERATIONS
Foreign objects such as dirt and sand produce *corneal abrasions* (scratches) that cause sudden, stabbing eye pain and excess lacrimal fluid. Opening and closing the eyelids is also painful. *Corneal lacerations* are caused by sharp objects such as fingernails.

Corneal Ulcers and Transplants
When the sensory innervation of the cornea is damaged, the cornea can be injured easily by foreign particles, such as sand, that may produce *corneal ulcers*. Patients with scarred or opaque corneas often receive homologous *corneal transplants*. Corneal implants of nonreactive plastic material are also used.

Presbyopia and Cataracts
As people get older, their lenses become harder and more flattened. These changes gradually reduce the focusing power of the lenses—*presbyopia*. Some elderly people also experience a loss of transparency (clouding) of the lens from areas of opaqueness (*cataracts*). Replacing a severely affected lens with a small prescription plastic lens currently is a common surgical procedure.

Glaucoma
When drainage of aqueous humor is reduced significantly, pressure builds up in the chambers of the eye—glaucoma. Compression of the neural layer of the retina occurs if aqueous humor production is not reduced to maintain normal intraocular pressure. The danger relates primarily to the slow gradual process without exhibiting symptoms. Untreated glaucoma results in irreversible blindness.

The **muscles of the orbit** are the **levator palpebrae superioris,** four **recti** (superior, inferior, medial, and lateral), and two **oblique** (superior and inferior). These muscles work together to move the superior (upper) eyelids and eyes. Their attachments, nerve supply, and actions are illustrated in Figures 8.20 and 8.21 and in Table 8.5. The **levator palpebrae superioris**—the *elevator muscle of the superior eyelid*—broadens into a wide aponeurosis as it approaches its distal attachment to the *superior tarsal plate* (Figs. 8.16 and 8.17*B*). This muscle is the antagonist of the orbicularis oculi, the sphincter of the palpebral fissure. A layer of smooth muscle, the **superior tarsal muscle** extends from the aponeurosis of the levator to the superior tarsal plate; it is innervated by sympathetic nerve fibers and helps the levator in elevating the superior eyelid and may cause the eye to be opened more widely during a sympathetic response (e.g., fright).

TABLE 8.5. MUSCLES OF ORBIT

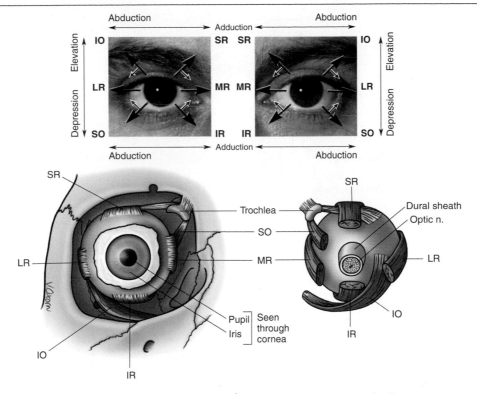

Individual anatomical actions of muscles us studied anatomically

It is essential to appreciate that all muscles are continuously involved in eye movements; thus, the individual actions are not usually tested clinically. **SR**, superior rectus (CN III); **LR**, lateral rectus (CN VI); **IR**, inferior rectus (CN III); **IO**, inferior oblique (CN III); **MR**, medial rectus (CN III); **SO**, superior oblique (CN IV). *Small arrows* lying perpendicular to *larger arrows* in (**A**) indicate rotation around the A-P axis; movement of the superior pole of the eyeball toward the midline is medial rotation (intorsion), while movement of the superior pole away from the midline is lateral rotation (extorsion).

Muscle	Origin	Insertion	Innervation	Action(s)
Levator palpebrae superioris	Lesser wing of sphenoid, superior and anterior to optic canal	Tarsal plate and skin of superior eyelid	Oculomotor nerve; deep layer (superior tarsal muscle) is supplied by sympathetic fibers	Elevates superior eyelid
Superior rectus	Common tendinous ring	Sclera just posterior to cornea	Oculomotor nerve	Elevates, adducts, and rotates eyeball medially
Inferior rectus				Depresses, adducts, and rotates eyeball medially
Lateral rectus			Abducent nerve	Abducts eyeball
Medial rectus			Oculomotor nerve	Adducts eyeball
Superior oblique	Body of sphenoid bone	Its tendon passes through a fibrous ring or trochlea and changes its direction and inserts into sclera deep to superior rectus muscle	Trochlear nerve	Abducts, depresses, and medially rotates eyeball
Inferior oblique	Anterior part of floor of orbit	Sclera deep to lateral rectus muscle	Oculomotor nerve	Abducts, elevates, and laterally rotates eyeball

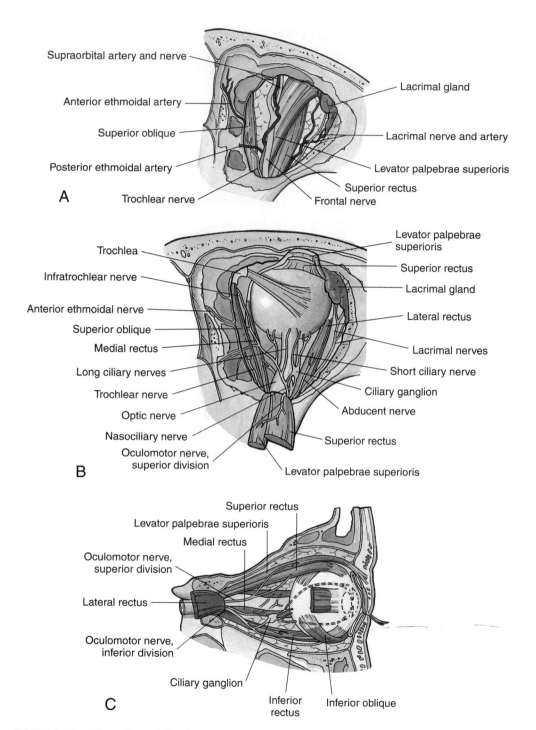

Supraorbital artery and nerve

Anterior ethmoidal artery

Superior oblique

Posterior ethmoidal artery

Lacrimal gland

Lacrimal nerve and artery

Levator palpebrae superioris

Superior rectus

A   Trochlear nerve   Frontal nerve

Trochlea

Infratrochlear nerve

Anterior ethmoidal nerve

Superior oblique

Medial rectus

Long ciliary nerves

Trochlear nerve

Optic nerve

Nasociliary nerve

Oculomotor nerve,
  superior division

Levator palpebrae
  superioris

Superior rectus

Lacrimal gland

Lateral rectus

Lacrimal nerves

Short ciliary nerve

Ciliary ganglion

Abducent nerve

Superior rectus

B   Levator palpebrae superioris

Superior rectus

Levator palpebrae superioris

Medial rectus

Oculomotor nerve,
  superior division

Lateral rectus

Oculomotor nerve,
  inferior division

Ciliary ganglion

C   Inferior   Inferior oblique
       rectus

FIGURE 8.20   Dissections of the right orbit. A. Superior view of a superficial dissection showing muscles, nerves, and vessels. **B.** Similar view of a deep dissection. **C.** Lateral view.

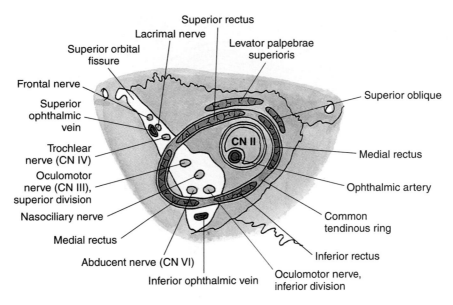

FIGURE 8.21 **Structures in the apex of the right orbit.** Observe the nerves that enter the orbit through the superior orbital fissure.

The **four recti muscles** arise from a fibrous cuff, the **common tendinous ring** (Fig. 8.21), which surrounds the optic canal and part of the superior orbital fissure. Structures that enter the orbit through this canal and the adjacent part of the fissure lie at first in the cone of recti. The lateral and medial recti lie in the same horizontal plane, and the superior and inferior recti lie in the same (oblique) vertical plane. All four recti attach to the sclera on the anterior half of the eyeball. The actions of the recti muscles are described and illustrated in Table 8.5:

• The **medial and lateral recti** move the pupil medially (adduction) and laterally (abduction), respectively
• The **superior rectus** moves the pupil superiorly (elevation)

• The **inferior rectus** moves the pupil inferiorly (depression).

However, neither the superior rectus nor the inferior rectus pulls directly parallel to the long axis of the eyeball (neutral axis of gaze). As a result, both of these recti tend to move the pupil medially (adduction). This medial pull of the superior and inferior recti normally is balanced by a similar tendency of the oblique muscles to move the pupil laterally (abduction). The **inferior oblique** directs the pupil laterally and superiorly; therefore, when it works synergistically with the superior rectus, pure elevation of the pupil occurs. Similarly, the **superior oblique** directs the pupil inferiorly and laterally; therefore, when it works synergistically with the inferior rectus, pure depression of the pupil results.

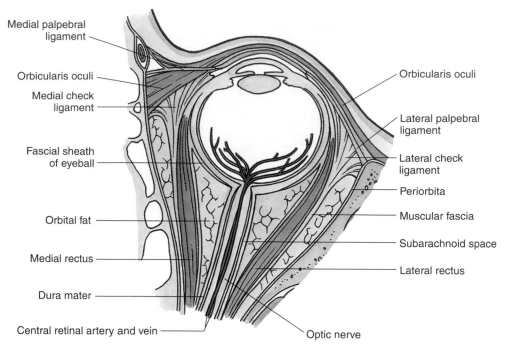

FIGURE 8.22 **Horizontal section of the right orbit.** Viewed superiorly, showing the fascial sheath of the eyeball.

The **fascial sheath of the eyeball** (bulbar sheath, Tenon capsule) envelops the eyeball from the optic nerve nearly to the *corneoscleral junction* (Figs. 8.17*A* and 8.22). The facial sheath is pierced by the tendons of the extraocular muscles and is reflected onto each as a tubular muscular sheath. Triangular expansions from the sheaths of the medial and lateral recti—medial and lateral **check ligaments**—attach to the lacrimal and zygomatic bones, respectively, limiting abduction and adduction. A blending of the check ligaments with the fascia of the inferior rectus and inferior oblique muscles forms a hammocklike sling, the **suspensory ligament,** which supports the eyeball (Fig. 8.19). A potential space between the eyeball and the fascial sheath allows the eyeball to move inside the cuplike sheath. A similar check ligament from the fascial sheath of the inferior rectus retracts the inferior eyelid when the gaze is directed downward. Because the sheaths of the superior rectus and levator palpebrae superioris are fused, the superior eyelid is elevated when the gaze is directed upward.

The **nerves of the orbit,** in addition to the *optic nerve* (CN II), include those that enter through the *superior orbital fissure* (Figs. 8.20 and 8.21) and supply the muscles of the eyeball (oculomotor, *CN III;* trochlear, *CN IV;* and abducent, *CN VI*).

- CN III (oculomotor nerve) supplies the levator palpebrae superioris, superior rectus, medial rectus, inferior rectus, and inferior oblique
- CN IV (trochlear nerve) supplies the superior oblique
- CN VI (abducent nerve) supplies the lateral rectus.

In summary, all muscles of the orbit are supplied by CN III, except the superior oblique and lateral rectus, which are supplied by CN IV and CN VI, respectively. A memory device is: **LR$_6$, SO$_4$, AO$_3$** (**L**ateral **R**ectus, **CN VI**, **S**uperior **O**blique, **CN IV**, **A**ll **O**thers, **CN III**). Several branches of the *ophthalmic nerve* (CN V$_1$) also pass through the superior orbital fissure and supply structures in the orbit.

- The **lacrimal nerve** arises in the lateral wall of the cavernous sinus and passes to the lacrimal gland, giving sensory branches to the conjunctiva and skin of the superior eyelid; its distal part also carries secretomotor fibers conveyed to it from the zygomatic nerve (CN V_2).

- The **frontal nerve** enters the orbit through the superior orbital fissure and divides into the supraorbital and supratrochlear nerves, which provide sensory innervation to the superior eyelid, scalp, and forehead.

- The **nasociliary nerve,** the sensory nerve to the eyeball, also supplies several branches to the orbit as well as to the face, paranasal sinuses, and anterior cranial fossa. The **infratrochlear nerve,** a terminal branch of the nasociliary nerve, supplies the eyelids, conjunctiva, skin of the nose, and lacrimal sac. The anterior and posterior **ethmoidal nerves,** also branches of the nasociliary nerve, supply the mucous membrane of the sphenoidal and ethmoidal sinuses and the nasal cavities (p. 576) and the dura of the anterior cranial fossa.

- The **long ciliary nerves** are branches of the nasociliary nerve (CN V_1). The **short ciliary nerves** are branches of the ciliary ganglion (Fig. 8.20, *B* and *C*). The **ciliary ganglion** is a very small group of nerve cell bodies lying between the optic nerve and the lateral rectus toward the posterior limit of the orbit. The **short ciliary nerves** consist of postsynaptic parasympathetic fibers originating in the ciliary ganglion, afferent fibers from the nasociliary nerve that pass through the ganglion, and postsynaptic sympathetic fibers that also pass through it. The **long ciliary nerves** transmit postsynaptic sympathetic fibers to the dilator pupillae and afferent fibers from the iris and cornea.

OCULOMOTOR AND ABDUCENT NERVE PALSY

Complete oculomotor nerve palsy affects most of the ocular muscles, the levator palpebrae superioris, and the sphincter pupillae. The superior eyelid droops (ptosis) and cannot be raised voluntarily because of the unopposed orbicularis oculi, supplied by the facial nerve. Paralysis of CN VII does not cause ptosis but does prevent folding of the eyelids. The pupil is also fully dilated and nonreactive because of the unopposed dilator pupillae. The pupil is fully abducted (**A**) and depressed ("down and out") because of the unopposed lateral rectus and superior oblique muscles, respectively. A le-

sion of the abducent nerve results in loss of lateral gaze to the ipsilateral side because of paralysis of the lateral rectus muscle. On forward gaze the eye is diverted medially (**B**) because of the lack of normal resting tone in the lateral rectus, resulting in diplopia (double vision).

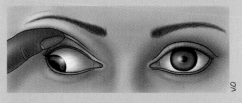

Right eye: Downward and outward gaze, dilated pupil, eyelid manually elevated due to ptosis   Left

Right oculomotor (CN III) nerve palsy

A

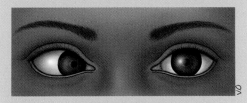

Right   Left eye: Does not abduct

Direction of gaze ———————→

Left abducent (CN VI) nerve palsy

B

Horner Syndrome

Interruption of a cervical sympathetic trunk results in paralysis of the *superior tarsal muscle* (p. 538) supplied by sympathetic fibers, causing ptosis. Other signs of Horner syndrome are a constricted pupil, sinking, redness, and dryness of the eye, and increased temperature of the face on the affected side.

Paralysis of Extraocular Muscles

One or more extraocular muscles may be paralyzed by disease in the brainstem or by head injury; this results in *diplopia* (double vision). Paralysis of a muscle is apparent by limitation of eye movement in the field of action of the muscle and by the production of two images (diplopia) when one attempts to use the muscle.

The **arteries of the orbit** are mainly from the **ophthalmic artery** (Figs. 8.20–8.23, Table 8.6); the **infraorbital artery** also contributes to the supply of this region. The **central retinal artery,** a branch of the ophthalmic artery inferior to the optic nerve, runs within the dural sheath of this nerve until it approaches the eyeball (Figs.

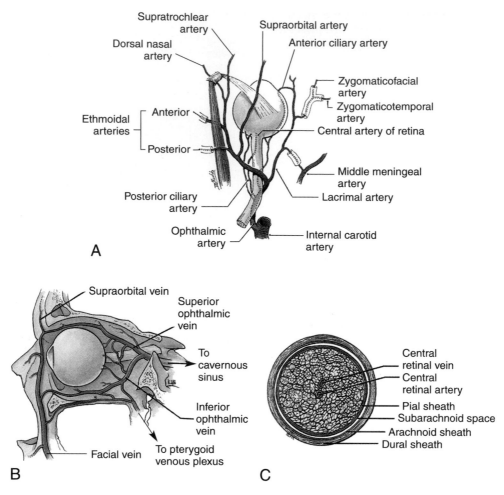

FIGURE 8.23 **Vasculature of the orbit. A.** Superior view of the arteries of the right orbit. **B.** Lateral view of the veins of the right orbit. **C.** Transverse section of the optic nerve and coverings (sheaths).

8.22 and 8.23C). The central retinal artery pierces the optic nerve and runs within it to emerge at the optic disc. Branches of this artery spread over the internal surface of the retina. *The terminal branches of the central retinal artery are end arteries that provide the only blood supply to most of the retina* (Fig. 8.19). The nonvascular layer of the retina, which includes the photoreceptor cells (cones and rods), is supplied by the **capillary lamina of the choroid.** Of the eight or so posterior ciliary arteries—also branches of the ophthalmic artery—six **short posterior ciliary arteries** directly supply the choroid. Two **long posterior ciliary arteries,** one on each side of the eyeball, pass between the sclera and choroid to anastomose with the **an-**terior ciliary arteries—continuations of the muscular branches of the ophthalmic artery—supplying the ciliary plexus.

The **veins of the orbit** are tributaries of the **superior** and **inferior ophthalmic veins** that pass through the superior orbital fissure and enter the **cavernous sinus** (Fig. 8.23B). The inferior ophthalmic vein also drains to the **pterygoid venous plexus**, especially when the head is erect (p. 511). The **central retinal vein** usually enters the cavernous sinus directly, but it may join one ophthalmic vein (Fig 8.23B). The **vorticose veins** from the middle vascular layer of the eyeball drain into the ophthalmic veins (Fig. 8.19A). The **scleral venous sinus** is a vascular structure encircling the anterior chamber

TABLE 8.6.   ARTERIES OF ORBIT

Artery	Origin	Course and Distribution
Ophthalmic	Internal carotid artery	Traverses optic foramen to reach orbital cavity
Central retinal artery		Runs in dural sheath of optic nerve and pierces nerve near eyeball; appears at center of optic disc; supplies neural retina (except cones and rods)
Supraorbital		Passes superiorly and posteriorly from supraorbital foramen to supply forehead and scalp
Supratrochlear		Passes from supraorbital margin to forehead and scalp
Lacrimal		Passes along superior border of lateral rectus muscle to supply lacrimal gland, conjunctiva, and eyelids
Dorsal nasal	Ophthalmic artery	Courses along dorsal aspect of nose and supplies its surface
Short posterior ciliaries		Pierce sclera at periphery of optic nerve to supply choroid, which in turn supplies the cones and rods of neural retina
Long posterior ciliaries		Pierce sclera to supply ciliary body and iris
Posterior ethmoidal		Passes through posterior ethmoidal foramen to posterior ethmoidal cells
Anterior ethmoidal		Passes through anterior ethmoidal foramen to anterior cranial fossa; supplies anterior and middle ethmoidal cells, frontal sinus, nasal cavity, and skin on dorsum of nose
Infraorbital	Third part of maxillary artery	Passes along infraorbital groove and foramen to face
Anterior ciliary	Ophthalmic artery	Pierces sclera at the periphery of iris and forms network in iris and ciliary body

of the eye through which the aqueous humor is returned to the blood circulation.

BLOCKAGE OF CENTRAL RETINAL ARTERY
Because terminal branches of the central retinal artery are end arteries, obstruction of them by emboli—plugs composed of detached thrombi (clots)—results in instant blindness. The extent of blindness is determined by the area normally supplied beyond the blockage.

Blockage of Central Retinal Vein
Because the central vein of the retina enters the cavernous sinus, *thrombophlebitis* of this sinus may result in passage of thrombi to the central retinal vein and produce clotting in the small retinal veins. Blockage of the central retinal vein usually results in slow loss of vision.

TEMPORAL REGION

The temporal region includes the temporal and infratemporal fossae—superior and inferior to the zygomatic arch, respectively (Fig. 8.24, *A* and *B*).

TEMPORAL FOSSA

The boundaries of the oval temporal fossa (Fig. 8.24, *A* and *C*), in which most of the temporal (L. temporalis) muscle is located, are:

- Posteriorly and superiorly—superior and inferior temporal lines
- Anteriorly—frontal and zygomatic bones
- Laterally—zygomatic arch
- Inferiorly—infratemporal crest.

The *floor of the temporal fossa* is formed by parts of the four bones (frontal, sphenoid, temporal, parietal) that form the **pterion.** The fan-shaped **temporal muscle** arises from the floor and the tough overlying **temporal fascia,** which comprises the *roof of the temporal fossa* (see Fig. 8.26, Table 8.7). The temporal fascia extends from the superior temporal line to the zygomatic arch. When the powerful masseter—attached to the inferior border of the arch—contracts, exerting a

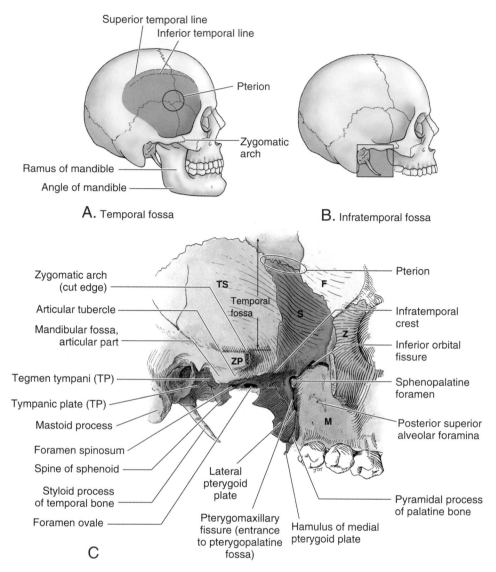

A. Temporal fossa

B. Infratemporal fossa

Zygomatic arch (cut edge)

Articular tubercle

Mandibular fossa, articular part

Tegmen tympani (TP)

Tympanic plate (TP)

Mastoid process

Foramen spinosum

Spine of sphenoid

Styloid process of temporal bone

Foramen ovale

Lateral pterygoid plate

Pterygomaxillary fissure (entrance to pterygopalatine fossa)

Hamulus of medial pterygoid plate

Pterion

Infratemporal crest

Inferior orbital fissure

Sphenopalatine foramen

Posterior superior alveolar foramina

Pyramidal process of palatine bone

Temporal fossa

C

FIGURE 8.24   Right temporal and infratemporal fossae. Lateral views. **A.** Temporal fossa. **B.** Infratemporal fossa. **C.** Bony boundaries of the fossae. The mandible and most of the zygomatic arch have been removed. *TS,* squamous part of temporal bone; *F,* frontal bone; *S,* sphenoid; *Z,* zygomatic bone; *ZP,* zygomatic process of temporal bone; *TP,* tympanic part of temporal bone; *M,* maxilla.

strong downward pull on the arch, the temporal fascia provides resistance.

INFRATEMPORAL FOSSA

The infratemporal fossa is an irregularly shaped space deep and inferior to the zygomatic arch, deep to the ramus of the mandible,

and posterior to the maxilla. *The boundaries of the fossa* (Fig. 8.24, *B* and *C*) are:

- Laterally—ramus of the mandible
- Medially—lateral pterygoid plate
- Anteriorly—posterior aspect of the maxilla
- Posteriorly—tympanic plate and mastoid and styloid processes of the temporal bone

TABLE 8.7. MUSCLES ACTING ON TEMPOROMANDIBULAR JOINT

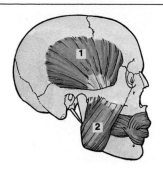
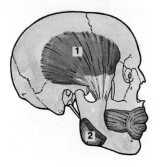
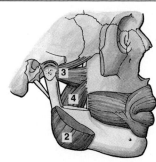

Muscle	Origin	Insertion	Innervation	Main Action(s)
Temporal (1) (L. temporalis)	Floor of temporal fossa and deep surface of temporal fascia	Tip and medial surface of coronoid process and anterior border of ramus of mandible	Deep temporal branches of mandibular nerve (CN V₃)	Elevates mandible, closing jaws; its posterior fibers retrude mandible after protrusion
Masseter (2)	Inferior border and medial surface of zygomatic arch	Lateral surface of ramus of mandible and its coronoid process	Mandibular nerve via masseteric nerve that enters its deep surface	Elevates and protrudes mandible, thus closing jaws; deep fibers retrude it
Lateral pterygoid (3)	*Superior head:* infratemporal surface and infratemporal crest of greater wing of sphenoid bone *Inferior head:* lateral surface of lateral pterygoid plate	Neck of mandible, articular disc, and capsule of temporomandibular joint	Mandibular nerve (CN V₃) via lateral pterygoid nerve from anterior trunk, which enters its deep surface	*Acting together,* they protrude mandible and depress chin; *Acting alone* and alternatively, they produce side-to-side movements of mandible
Medial pterygoid (4)	*Deep head:* medial surface of lateral pterygoid plate and pyramidal process of palatine bone *Superficial head:* tuberosity of maxilla	Medial surface of ramus of mandible, inferior to mandibular foramen	Mandibular nerve (CN V₃) via medial pterygoid nerve	*Acting together,* they help to elevate mandible, closing jaws; they help to protrude mandible; *Acting alone,* they protrude side of jaw; *Acting alternately,* they produce a grinding motion

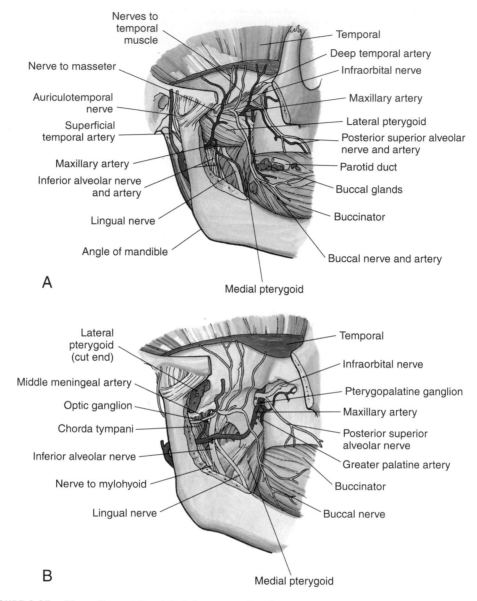

FIGURE 8.25   Dissections of the right infratemporal region. Lateral views. **A.** Superficial. **B.** Deep.

- Superiorly—inferior (infratemporal) surface of the greater wing of the sphenoid bone
- Inferiorly—attachment of the medial pterygoid muscle to the mandible (Table 8.7).

The *contents of the infratemporal fossa* (Fig. 8.25) are the inferior part of the **temporal muscle** (L. temporalis), the lateral and medial **pterygoid muscles,** the **maxillary artery,** the **pterygoid venous plexus,** the **mandibular, inferior alveolar,**

lingual, buccal, and **chorda tympani nerves,** and the **otic ganglion.**

The **temporal muscle** is attached proximally to the temporal fossa and distally to the tip and medial surface of the coronoid process and anterior border of the ramus of the mandible (Fig. 8.25, Table 8.7). It elevates the mandible (closes the lower jaw); its posterior fibers retrude (retract) the protruded mandible. The two-headed **lateral pterygoid muscle** passes posteriorly with its upper head attaching to the capsule and disc of the TMJ and the lower head attaching primarily to the pterygoid fovea at the condylar process of the mandible. The **medial pterygoid muscle** lies on the medial aspect of the ramus of the mandible. Its two heads embrace the inferior head of the lateral pterygoid and then unite (Fig. 8.25*A*). The medial pterygoid passes inferoposteriorly and attaches to the medial surface of the mandible near its angle. The attachments, nerve supply, and actions of the pterygoid muscles are described in Table 8.7.

The **maxillary artery**—*the larger of the two terminal branches of the external carotid artery*—arises posterior to the neck of the mandible, courses anteriorly deep to the neck of the mandibular condyle, and then passes superficial or deep to the lateral pterygoid (Fig. 8.25*A*). The artery passes medially from the infratemporal fossa through the **pterygomaxillary fissure** to enter the **pterygopalatine fossa** (Fig. 8.24). *The maxillary artery is thus divided into three parts by its relation to the lateral pterygoid muscle* (Figs. 8.25 and 8.26).

Branches of the first or retromandibular part of the maxillary artery are the:

- *Deep auricular artery* to the external acoustic meatus
- *Anterior tympanic artery* to the tympanic membrane
- *Middle meningeal artery* to the dura and calvaria
- *Accessory meningeal arteries* to the cranial cavity
- *Inferior alveolar artery* to the mandible, gingivae (gums), teeth, and floor of the mouth.

Branches of the second or pterygoid part of the maxillary artery are the:

- *Deep temporal arteries,* anterior and posterior, which ascend to supply the temporal muscle
- *Pterygoid arteries,* which supply the pterygoid muscles

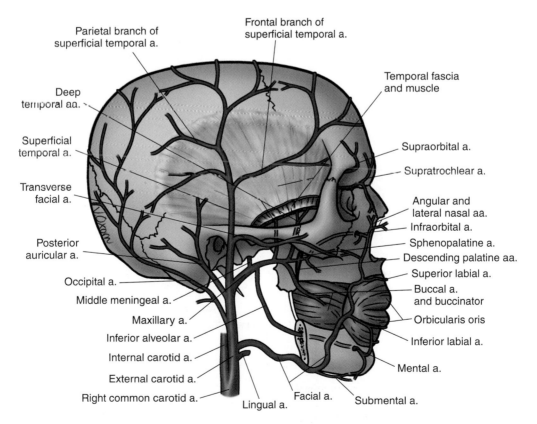

FIGURE 8.26 **External carotid artery and its branches.** Lateral view.

- *Masseteric artery,* which passes laterally through the mandibular notch to supply the masseter muscle
- *Buccal artery,* which supplies the buccinator muscle and mucosa of the cheek.

Branches of the third or pterygopalatine part of the maxillary artery are the:

- *Posterior superior alveolar artery,* which supplies the maxillary molar and premolar teeth, the buccal gingiva, and the lining of the maxillary sinus
- *Infraorbital artery,* which supplies the inferior eyelid, lacrimal sac, infraorbital region of the face, side of the nose, and the upper lip
- *Descending palatine artery,* which supplies the mucous membrane and glands of the palate (roof of the mouth) and palatine gingiva

- *Artery of pterygoid canal,* which supplies the superior part of the pharynx, the pharyngotympanic (auditory) tube, and the tympanic cavity
- *Pharyngeal artery,* which supplies the roof of the pharynx, the sphenoidal sinus, and the inferior part of the pharyngotympanic tube
- *Sphenopalatine artery,* the termination of the maxillary artery, which supplies the lateral nasal wall, the nasal septum, and the adjacent paranasal sinuses.

The **pterygoid venous plexus** (Fig. 8.27) occupies most of the infratemporal fossa. The plexus drains anteriorly to the facial vein via the deep facial vein but mainly drains posteriorly via the maxillary and then the retromandibular veins.

The **mandibular nerve** (CN V$_3$) receives the motor root of the trigeminal nerve (CN V)

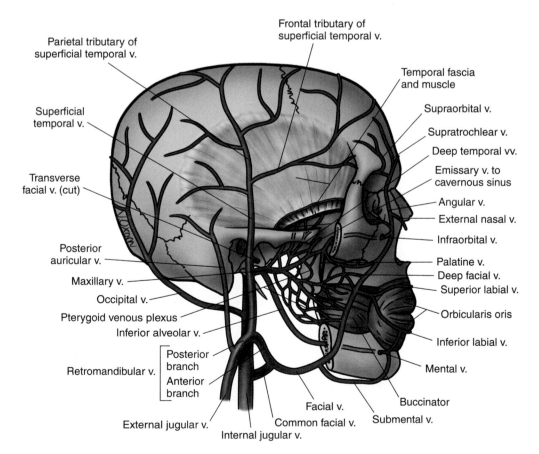

FIGURE 8.27   Venous drainage of the face and infratemporal fossa. Lateral view.

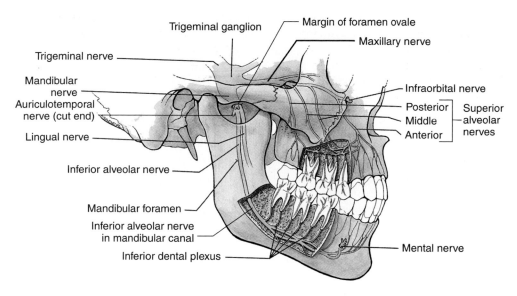

FIGURE 8.28 **Alveolar nerves and innervation of the teeth.** Right lateral view.

and descends through the foramen ovale to enter the infratemporal fossa, dividing almost immediately into anterior and posterior trunks (Fig. 8.25*B*). The branches of the large posterior trunk are the auriculotemporal, inferior alveolar, and lingual nerves (Fig. 8.28). The smaller anterior division gives rise to the **buccal nerve** and branches to the four muscles of mastication (temporal, masseter, and pterygoids) but not the buccinator, which is supplied by the facial nerve (CN VII).

The **otic ganglion** (parasympathetic) is in the infratemporal fossa (Fig. 8.25*B*), just inferior to the foramen ovale, medial to the mandibular nerve, and posterior to the medial pterygoid muscle. Presynaptic parasympathetic fibers, derived mainly from the glossopharyngeal nerve (CN IX), synapse in the otic ganglion. Postsynaptic parasympathetic fibers, which are secretory to the parotid gland, pass from the ganglion to this gland through the auriculotemporal nerve (p. 513).

The **auriculotemporal nerve** (Fig. 8.25, Table 8.2) arises via two roots that encircle the middle meningeal artery and then unite into a single trunk. The trunk divides into numerous branches, the largest of which passes posteriorly, medial to the neck of the mandible, and supplies sensory fibers to the auricle and temporal region. The auriculotemporal nerve also sends articular fibers to the TMJ and parasympathetic secretomotor fibers to the parotid gland.

The **inferior alveolar nerve** enters the mandibular foramen and passes through the **mandibular canal** forming the **inferior dental plexus** (Fig. 8.28), which sends branches to all mandibular teeth on that side. The *nerve to the mylohyoid muscle,* a small branch of the inferior alveolar nerve, is given off just before the nerve enters the mandibular foramen. A branch of the inferior dental plexus, the **mental nerve,** passes through the mental foramen and supplies the skin and mucous membrane of the lower lip, the skin of the chin, and the vestibular gingiva of the mandibular incisor teeth.

The **lingual nerve** lies anterior to the inferior alveolar nerve (Figs. 8.25 and 8.28). It is sensory to the anterior two thirds of the tongue, the floor of the mouth, and the lingual gingivae. It enters the mouth between the medial pterygoid and the ramus of the mandible and passes anteriorly under cover of the oral mucosa, just inferior to the third molar tooth.

The **chorda tympani nerve,** a branch of CN VII (Fig. 8.25*B*), carries taste fibers from the anterior two thirds of the tongue and presynaptic parasympathetic secretomotor fibers for the submandibular and sublingual salivary glands. The chorda tympani joins the lingual nerve in the infratemporal fossa.

MANDIBULAR NERVE BLOCK

To produce a mandibular nerve block, an anesthetic agent is injected adjacent to the mandibular nerve where it enters the infratemporal fossa. This block usually anesthetizes the auriculotemporal, inferior alveolar, lingual, and buccal branches of the mandibular nerve.

Inferior Alveolar Nerve Block

An inferior alveolar nerve block—commonly used by dentists when repairing mandibular teeth—anesthetizes the inferior alveolar nerve, a branch of CN V_3. The anesthetic agent is injected around the **mandibular foramen,** the opening of the **mandibular canal** on the medial side of the ramus of the mandible, which gives passage to the inferior alveolar nerve, artery, and vein (Fig. 8.28). When this nerve block is successful, all mandibular teeth are anesthetized to the median plane. The skin and mucous membrane of the lower lip, the labial alveolar mucosa and gingiva, and the skin of the chin are also anesthetized because they are supplied by the mental branch of this nerve. Often there is some overlapping of the two mental nerves.

TEMPOROMANDIBULAR JOINT

The TMJ is a modified hinge type of synovial joint (Fig. 8.29, *A* and *B*) permitting movement in three planes. The articular surfaces involved are the **head of the mandible,** the **articular tubercle** of the temporal bone, and the **mandibular fossa.** The articular surfaces of the TMJ are covered by fibrocartilage rather than hyaline cartilage as in a typical synovial joint. An **articular disc** divides the joint cavity into two separate synovial compartments. The **fibrous capsule** attaches to the margins of the articular area on the temporal bone and around the neck of the mandible. The thick part of the articular capsule forms the intrinsic **lateral ligament** (temporomandibular ligament), which strengthens the TMJ laterally and, with the **postglenoid tubercle,** acts to prevent posterior dislocation of the joint (Fig. 8.29*C*).

Two extrinsic ligaments and the lateral ligament connect the mandible to the cra-

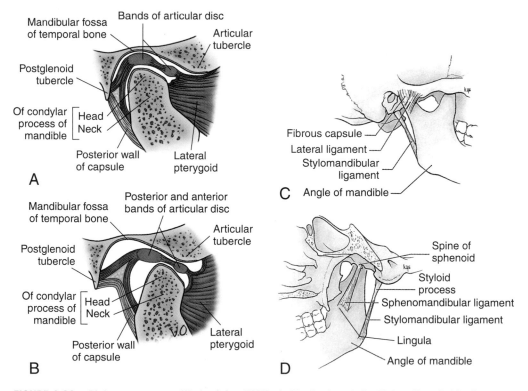

FIGURE 8.29   Right temporomandibular joint (TMJ). A. Mouth closed. Sagittal section. **B.** Mouth open. Sagittal section. **C.** Lateral view. **D.** Medial view.

nium. The **stylomandibular ligament**—actually a thickening in the fibrous capsule of the parotid gland—runs from the styloid process to the angle of the mandible (Fig. 8.29, *C* and *D*). It does not contribute significantly to the strength of the TMJ. The **sphenomandibular ligament** runs from the *spine of the sphenoid* to the *lingula of the mandible* (Fig. 8.29*D*).

Muscles (or forces) producing movements of the mandible at the TMJs are (Table 8.8):

- *Depression* (open mouth)
    Gravity (prime mover)
    Suprahyoid and infrahyoid muscles
    Note: Protrusion must occur for all but minimal depression.
- *Elevation* (close mouth—most powerful movement)
    Temporal
    Masseter
    Medial pterygoid
- *Protrusion* (protrude chin)
    Lateral pterygoid (prime mover)
    Masseter (oblique [superficial] fibers only—secondary synergist)
    Medial pterygoid (secondary synergist)
- *Retrusion* (retrude chin)
    Temporal (middle [oblique] and posterior [nearly horizontal] fibers only—prime mover)
    Masseter (vertical [deep] fibers only—secondary synergist)
- *Lateral movements* (side-to-side grinding and chewing)
    Retractors of same side (see above)
    Protruders of opposite side (see above)

To enable more than a small amount of depression of the mandible (Fig. 8.29*B*), that is, to open the mouth wider than just separating the upper and lower teeth, the head of the mandible and articular disc must move anteriorly on the articular surface until the head lies inferior to the articular tubercle (a movement referred to as "translation" by dentists). If this anterior gliding occurs unilaterally, the head of the mandible on the retracted side rotates (pivots) on the inferior surface of the articular disc, permitting simple side-to-side chewing or grinding movements over a small range. During protrusion and retrusion of the mandible, the head and articular disc slide anteriorly and posteriorly on the articular surface of the temporal bone, with both sides moving together. *TMJ movements are produced chiefly by the muscles of mastication.* The attachments, nerve supply, and actions of these muscles are described in Tables 8.7 and 8.8.

DISLOCATION OF TMJ

Sometimes during yawning or taking a very large bite, excessive contraction of the lateral pterygoids may cause the heads of the mandible to dislocate anteriorly (pass anterior to the articular tubercles). In this position, the mouth remains wide open and the person may not be able to close it. Most commonly, a sideways blow to the chin when the mouth is open dislocates the TMJ on the side that received the blow. *Fracture(s) of the mandible* may be accompanied by dislocation of the TMJ. Because of the close relationship of the facial and auriculotemporal nerves to the TMJ, care must be taken during surgical procedures to preserve both the branches of the facial nerve overlying it and the articular branches of the auriculotemporal nerve that enter the posterior part of the joint. Injury to articular branches of the auriculotemporal nerve supplying the TMJ—associated with traumatic dislocation and rupture of the articular capsule and lateral ligament—leads to laxity and instability of the TMJ.

TABLE 8.8. MOVEMENTS OF MANDIBLE AT TEMPOROMANDIBULAR JOINT

Elevation (Close Mouth)	Depression (Open Mouth)	Protrusion (Protrude Chin)	Retrusion (Retrude Chin)	Lateral Movements (Grinding and Chewing)
Temporal (vertical [anterior] part); masseter; medial pterygoid	Lateral pterygoid; suprahyoid and infrahyoid muscles[a]	Masseter; lateral pterygoid; medial pterygoid[b]	Temporal (horizontal [posterior] part); masseter	Temporal of same side Pterygoids of opposite side; masseter

[a]Prime mover normally is gravity—these muscles are mainly active against resistance.
[b]Lateral pterygoid is the prime mover.

ORAL REGION

The oral region includes the oral cavity (mouth), teeth, gingivae (gums), tongue, palate, and the region of the palatine tonsils. The oral cavity is where food is ingested and prepared for digestion. When food is chewed, the teeth and saliva from the salivary glands facilitate the formation of a manageable *food bolus* (L. lump).

ORAL CAVITY

The oral cavity consists of two parts: the *oral vestibule* and the *oral cavity proper* (Fig. 8.30). The **oral vestibule** is the slitlike space between the lips and cheeks superficially and the teeth and gingivae deeply. The oral vestibule communicates with the exterior through the **oral fissure** (orifice of mouth); the size of this opening is controlled by muscles such as the orbicularis oris. The **oral cavity proper** is the space posterior and medial to the upper and lower dental arches. It is limited laterally and anteri-

orly by the maxillary and mandibular alveolar arches housing the teeth and posteriorly by the terminal groove of the tongue (p. 560) and palatoglossal arches (p. 559). The *roof of the oral cavity* is formed by the **palate.** Posteriorly, the oral cavity communicates with the **oropharynx** (Fig. 8.33*B*). When the mouth is closed and at rest, the oral cavity is fully occupied by the tongue.

ORAL VESTIBULE

The **lips**—mobile, fleshy muscular folds surrounding the mouth—contain the orbicularis oris (Fig. 8.26) and superior and inferior labial muscles, vessels, and nerves. They are covered externally by skin and internally by mucous membrane. The upper lip has a vertical groove—the **philtrum** (Fig. 8.31*A*). As the

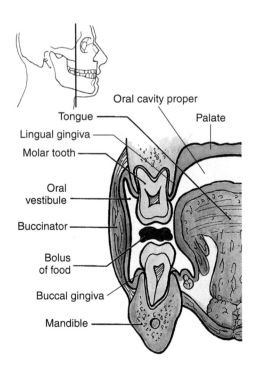

FIGURE 8.30 Oral cavity. Coronal section of the right side.

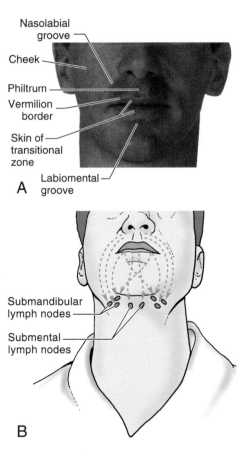

FIGURE 8.31 Cheeks, lips, and chin. Anterior view. **A.** Surface anatomy. **B.** Lymphatic drainage.

skin of the lips approaches the mouth, it changes color abruptly to red; this red margin of the lips is the **vermillion border,** a transitional zone between the skin and mucous membrane. The skin of the **transitional zone of the lips** is hairless and so thin that it appears red because of the underlying capillary bed. The upper lip is supplied by superior labial branches of the **facial** and **infraorbital arteries.** The lower lip is supplied by inferior labial branches of the **facial** and **mental arteries.** The upper lip is supplied by the superior labial branches of the **infraorbital nerves** (CN V_2), and the lower lip is supplied by the inferior labial branches of the mental nerves (CN V_3).

Lymph from the upper lip and lateral parts of the lower lip passes primarily to the **submandibular lymph nodes** (Fig. 8.31B), whereas lymph from the medial part of the lower lip passes initially to the **submental lymph nodes.**

The **cheeks** include the lateral distensible walls of the oral cavity and the facial prominences over the zygomatic bones. The cheeks have essentially the same structure as the lips, with which they are continuous. The principal muscle of the cheek is the **buccinator** (Fig. 8.30). The lips and cheeks function as an oral sphincter that pushes food from the oral vestibule into the oral cavity proper. The tongue and buccinator work together to keep the food between the occlusal surfaces of the molar teeth during chewing. The labial and **buccal glands** (Fig. 8.25A) are small mucous glands between the mucous membrane and the underlying orbicularis oris and buccinator muscles.

The **gingivae (gums)**—composed of fibrous tissue covered with mucous membrane—firmly attach to the alveolar processes of the jaws and the necks of the teeth. The **buccal gingivae** of the mandibular molar teeth are supplied by the **buccal nerve,** a branch of the mandibular nerve (Fig. 8.25B). The **lingual gingivae** of all mandibular teeth are supplied by the **lingual nerve** (Fig. 8.28). The **palatine gingivae** of the maxillary premolar and molar teeth are supplied by the **greater palatine nerve** and the palatine gingivae of the incisors by the **nasopalatine nerve** (see Fig. 8.35). The labial and buccal aspects of the maxillary gingivae are supplied by the anterior, middle, and posterior **superior alveolar nerves** (Fig. 8.28).

TEETH

Teeth are hard conical structures set in the alveoli of the upper and lower jaws that are used in mastication (chewing) and assisting in articulation. Children have *20 deciduous (primary) teeth.* The first tooth usually erupts at 6 to 8 months of age and the last tooth by 20 to 24 months of age. Eruption of the *permanent (secondary) teeth,* normally 16 in each jaw (three molars, two premolars, one canine, and two incisors on each side), usually is complete by the midteens (Fig. 8.32A), except for the third molars ("wisdom teeth"), which usually erupt during the late teens or early twenties. A tooth has a crown, neck, and root. Each type of tooth has a characteristic appearance (Fig. 8.32, B and C). The **crown** projects from the gingiva. The **neck** is the part of the tooth between the crown and root. The **root** is fixed in the alveolus (tooth socket) by a fibrous *periodontal membrane.* Most of the tooth is composed of **dentin** that is covered by **enamel** over the crown and **cement** (L. cementum) over the root. The **pulp cavity** contains connective tissue, blood vessels, and nerves. The **root canal** transmits the nerves and vessels to and from the pulp cavity.

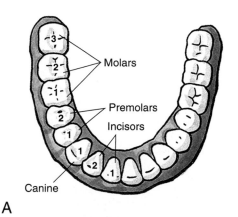

FIGURE 8.32   Teeth. A. Adult mandibular teeth. Inferior view.

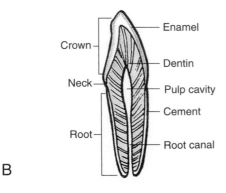

B

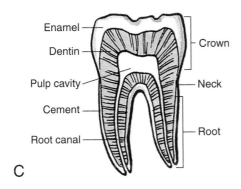

C

FIGURE 8.32 *Continued.* **B.** Incisor tooth. Sagittal section. **C.** Molar tooth. Sagittal section.

The **superior** and **inferior alveolar arteries,** branches of the **maxillary artery,** supply both the maxillary (upper) and mandibular (lower) teeth, respectively (Fig. 8.26). **Veins** with the same names and distribution accompany the arteries (Fig. 8.27). **Lymphatic vessels** from the teeth and gingivae pass mainly to the **submandibular lymph nodes** (Fig. 8.31*B*). The superior and inferior **alveolar nerves,** branches of CN V$_2$ and CN V$_3$, respectively, form superior and inferior dental plexuses that supply the maxillary and mandibular teeth (Fig. 8.28).

PULPITIS AND TOOTHACHE

Invasion of the pulp of the tooth by a carious lesion ("cavity") results in infection and irritation of the tissues in the pulp cavity. This condition causes an inflammatory process (*pulpitis*). Because the pulp cavity is a rigid space, the swollen pulpal tissues cause pain (*toothache*).

Gingivitis and Periodontitis

Improper oral hygiene results in food deposits in tooth and gingival crevices, which may cause inflammation of the gingivae (*gingivitis*). If untreated, the disease spreads to other supporting structures (including the alveolar bone), producing *periodontitis*. Periodontitis results in inflammation of the gingivae and may result in absorption of alveolar bone and gingival recession. Gingival recession exposes the sensitive cement of the teeth.

PALATE

The palate forms the arched roof of the oral cavity proper and the floor of the nasal cavities (Fig. 8.33*A*). The palate consists of hard and soft parts: the **hard palate** anteriorly and the **soft palate** posteriorly. The hard palate separates the anterior part of the oral cavity from the nasal cavities, and the soft palate separates the posterior part of the oral cavity from the nasopharynx superior to it (Fig. 8.33, *B* and *C*).

The **hard palate** is the anterior vaulted part; its cavity is filled with the tongue when it is at rest. The hard palate (covered by a mucous membrane) is formed by the palatine processes of the maxillae and the horizontal plates of the palatine bones (Fig. 8.34). Three foramina open on the oral aspect of the hard palate: the incisive fossa and the greater and lesser palatine foramina. The **incisive fossa** is a slight depression posterior to the central incisor teeth. The **nasopalatine nerves** pass from the nose through a variable number of incisive canals and foramina that open into the incisive fossa (Fig. 8.35). Medial to the 3rd molar tooth, the **greater palatine foramen** pierces the lateral border of the bony palate. The **greater palatine vessels and nerve** emerge from this foramen and run anteriorly on the palate. The **lesser palatine foramina** transmit the **lesser palatine nerves and vessels** to the soft palate and adjacent structures.

The **soft palate** is the posterior muscular part, which is suspended from the posterior border of the hard palate (Fig. 8.33). The soft palate extends posteroinferiorly as a curved free margin from which hangs a conical process, the **uvula** (Fig. 8.35). The soft palate is strengthened by the **palatine aponeurosis** formed by the expanded tendon of the **tensor veli palatini.** The aponeurosis, attached to the posterior margin of the hard palate, is thick anteriorly and thin posteriorly. The anterior part of the soft palate is formed mainly by the

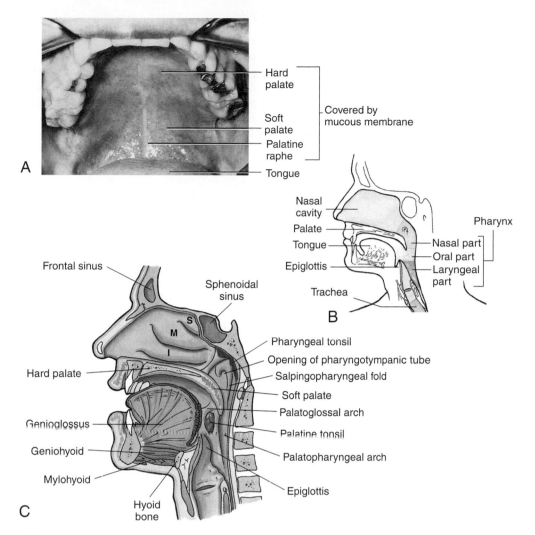

FIGURE 8.33 **Palate, teeth, nasal and oral cavities, and pharynx. A.** Anterior view of maxillary teeth and mucosa covering the bony palate in a living person. **B.** Parts of the pharynx. Medial view of the right half of the bisected head. **C.** Similar view showing the nose, mouth, and pharynx. The fauces (L. throat) is the passage from the oral cavity to the pharynx. *S,* superior concha; *M,* middle concha; *I,* inferior concha.

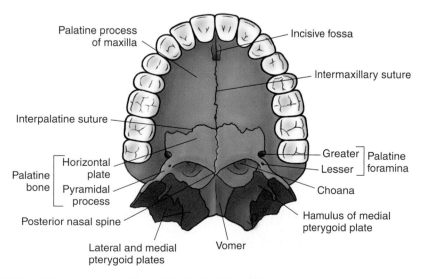

FIGURE 8.34 **Teeth and hard palate.** Inferior view of the bones forming the hard palate.

aponeurosis, whereas its posterior part is muscular. When a person swallows, the soft palate is initially tensed to allow the tongue to press against it, squeezing the bolus of food to the back of the oral cavity. The soft palate is then elevated posteriorly and superiorly against the wall of the pharynx, thereby preventing passage of food into the nasal cavity. Laterally the soft palate is continuous with the wall of the pharynx and is joined to the tongue and pharynx by the **palatoglossal** and **palatopharyngeal arches** (Figs. 8.33*C* and 8.35*A*), respectively. The **palatine tonsils,** often referred to as "the tonsils," are two masses of lymphoid tissue, one on each side of the oropharynx (Figs. 8.33*C* and 8.36*A*). Each tonsil lies in a *tonsillar sinus* (fossa), bounded by the palatoglossal and palatopharyngeal arches and the tongue. The **muscles of the soft palate** (Fig. 8.35) arise

from the cranial base and descend to the palate. The soft palate may be elevated so that it is in contact with the posterior wall of the pharynx, sealing off the oral passage from the nasopharynx (e.g., when swallowing or breathing through the mouth). The soft palate can also be drawn inferiorly so that it is in contact with the posterior part of the tongue, sealing off the oral cavity from the nasal passage (e.g., when breathing exclusively through the nose, even with the mouth open). For attachments, nerve supply, and actions of the five muscles of the soft palate, see Figure 8.35 and Table 8.9.

- The **levator veli palatini** (lifter of the soft palate) is a cylindrical muscle that runs inferoanteriorly, spreading out in the soft palate where it attaches to the superior surface of the palatine aponeurosis.

TABLE 8.9.   MUSCLES OF SOFT PALATE

Muscle	Superior Attachment	Inferior Attachment	Innervation	Main Action(s)
Tensor veli palatini	Scaphoid fossa of medial pterygoid plate, spine of sphenoid bone, and cartilage of pharyngotympanic tube	Palatine aponeurosis	Medial pterygoid nerve (a branch of mandibular nerve CN V_3) via otic ganglion	Tenses soft palate and opens mouth of pharyngotympanic tube during swallowing and yawning
Levator veli palatini	Cartilage of pharyngotympanic tube and petrous part of temporal bone			Elevates soft palate during swallowing and yawning
Palatoglossus	Palatine aponeurosis	Side of tongue	Cranial part of CN XI through pharyngeal branch of vagus nerve (CN X) via pharyngeal plexus	Elevates posterior part of tongue and draws soft palate onto tongue
Palatopharyngeus	Hard palate and palatine aponeurosis	Lateral wall of pharynx		Tenses soft palate and pulls walls of pharynx superiorly, anteriorly, and medially during swallowing
Uvular (L. musculus uvulae)	Posterior nasal spine and palatine aponeurosis	Mucosa of uvula		Shortens uvula and pulls it superiorly

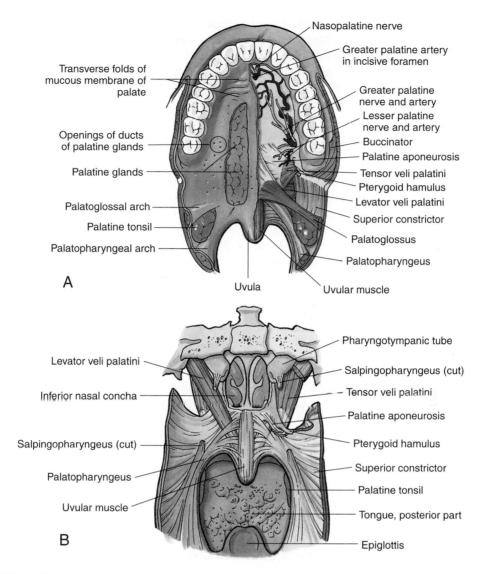

FIGURE 8.35 **Palate.** Inferior view. **A.** Part of the right side has been dissected to show the palatine glands. The left side has been dissected to show the muscles of the soft palate and palatine arteries and nerves. **B.** Posterior view of a dissection of the soft palate showing the muscles and their relationship to the posterior part of the tongue.

- The **tensor veli palatini** (tensor of the soft palate) is a muscle with a triangular belly that passes inferiorly; the tendon formed at its apex hooks around the **pterygoid hamulus**—the hook-shaped inferior extremity of the medial pterygoid plate—before spreading out as the palatine aponeurosis.

- The **palatoglossus** is a slender slip of muscle that is covered with a mucous membrane; it forms the **palatoglossal arch.**

Unlike the other muscles ending in "-glossus," the palatoglossus is a palatine muscle (in function and innervation) rather than a tongue muscle.

- The **palatopharyngeus** is a thin flat muscle also covered with a mucous membrane; it forms the **palatopharyngeal arch** and blends inferiorly with the longitudinal muscle of the pharynx.

- The **uvular muscle** (L. musculus uvulae) inserts into the mucosa of the uvula.

Vasculature and Innervation of Palate

The palate has a rich blood supply, chiefly from the **greater palatine artery** (Fig. 8.35A). The **lesser palatine artery**—a smaller branch of the descending palatine artery—enters the palate through the **lesser palatine foramen** and anastomoses with the ascending palatine artery, a branch of the facial artery. **Venous drainage of the palate,** corresponding and accompanying the branches of the maxillary artery, are tributaries of the **pterygoid venous plexus** (Fig. 8.27). The *sensory nerves of the palate* pass through the **pterygopalatine ganglion** and are considered branches of the maxillary nerve (see Fig. 8.41D). The **greater palatine nerve** supplies the gingivae, mucous membrane, and glands of most of the hard palate (Fig. 8.35A). The **nasopalatine nerve** supplies the mucous membrane of the anterior part of the hard palate. The **lesser palatine nerves** supply the soft palate. These nerves accompany the arteries through the greater and lesser palatine foramina, respectively. Except for the tensor veli palatini supplied by CN V_3, all muscles of the soft palate are supplied through the *pharyngeal plexus of nerves* (Chapter 9), derived from pharyngeal branches of the glossopharyngeal nerve (CN IX) and the vagus nerve (CN X).

TONGUE

The tongue is a mobile muscular organ that can assume a variety of shapes and positions. The tongue is partly in the oral cavity proper and partly in the pharynx (Fig. 8.33). At rest, it occupies essentially all the oral cavity proper. The tongue—mainly composed of muscles and covered by mucous membrane—assists with mastication (chewing), taste, deglutition (swallowing), articulation (speech), and oral cleansing. The tongue has a root, a body, an apex, a curved dorsal surface (dorsum), and an inferior surface. A V-shaped groove—the **terminal groove** (sulcus) of the tongue (Fig. 8.36)—marks the separation between the *anterior (presulcal) part* and the *posterior (postsulcal) part.*

The **root of the tongue** (base) is the posterior part. The anterior two-thirds of the tongue forms the **body of the tongue.** The pointed anterior part of the body is the **apex (tip) of the tongue.** The body and apex are extremely mobile. The **dorsum of the tongue** is the postero-

---

NASOPALATINE NERVE BLOCK

The nasopalatine nerves can be anesthetized by injecting anesthetic into the mouth of the *incisive fossa* in the hard palate. The needle is inserted posterior to the *incisive papilla,* a slight elevation of the mucosa that covers the incisive fossa. The affected tissues are the palatal mucosa, the lingual gingivae, and the alveolar bone of the six anterior maxillary teeth and the hard palate.

Greater Palatine Nerve Block

The greater palatine nerve can be anesthetized by injecting anesthetic into the greater palatine foramen. The nerve emerges between the 2nd and 3rd molar teeth. This nerve block anesthetizes, on the side concerned, all the palatal mucosa and lingual gingivae posterior to the maxillary canine teeth and the underlying bone of the palate.

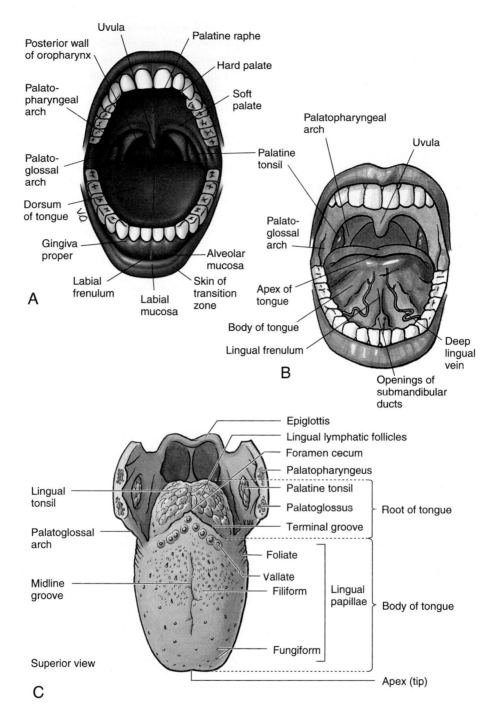

FIGURE 8.36 Tongue. A. Oral cavity and the dorsum of the tongue. **B.** Inferior surface of the tongue (dorsal surface) showing the veins. **C.** Features of the dorsum of the tongue.

superior surface of the tongue, which includes the **terminal groove.** At the apex of this groove is the **foramen cecum,** a small pit that is the nonfunctional remnant of the proximal part of the embryonic thyroglossal duct from which the thyroid gland developed. The mucous membrane on the anterior part of the tongue is rough because of the presence of numerous **lingual papillae** (Fig. 8.36*C*):

- **Vallate papillae** are large and flat-topped; they lie directly anterior to the terminal groove and are surrounded by deep moatlike trenches, the walls of which are studded by taste buds; the ducts of serous *lingual glands* (of von Ebner) open into these trenches.
- **Foliate papillae** are small lateral folds of lingual mucosa; they are poorly developed in humans.
- **Filiform papillae** are threadlike and scaly; they contain afferent nerve endings that are sensitive to touch.
- **Fungiform papillae** are mushroom-shaped and appear as pink or red spots; they are scattered among the filiform papillae but are most numerous at the apex and sides of the tongue.

The vallate, foliate, and most of the fungiform papillae contain taste receptors in the *taste buds.* A few taste buds are also in the epithelium covering the oral surface of the soft palate, the posterior wall of the oropharynx, and the epiglottis. The mucous membrane of the dorsum of the tongue is thin over the anterior part of the tongue and is closely attached to the underlying muscle. A depression on the dorsal surface, the **midline groove of the tongue** (median sulcus), divides the tongue into right and left halves (Fig. 8.36*C*); it also indicates the site of fusion of the embryonic distal tongue buds. Deep to the midline groove is a fibrous **lingual septum** that forms a vertical partition (Table 8.10).

The **posterior part of the tongue** lies within the oropharynx; it is located posterior to the **terminal groove** and the **palatoglossal arches** (Fig. 8.36). Its mucous membrane is thick and freely movable. It has no lingual papillae but the underlying nodules of **lingual lymphatic follicles** (lingual tonsil) give this part of the tongue its cobblestone appearance.

The **inferior surface of the tongue** (sublingual surface) is covered with a thin, transparent mucous membrane through which one can see the underlying **deep lingual veins.** With the tongue raised, observe the **lingual frenulum** (Fig. 8.36*B*)—a large midline fold of mucosa that passes from the gingiva covering the lingual aspect of the anterior alveolar ridge to the posteroinferior surface of the tongue. The frenulum connects the tongue to the floor of the mouth while allowing the anterior part of the tongue to move freely. At the base of the frenulum are the **openings of the submandibular ducts** from the submandibular salivary glands.

Muscles of Tongue

The tongue is essentially a mass of muscles that is mostly covered by mucous membrane (Fig. 8.37*A*). Although it is traditional to do so, providing descriptions of the actions of tongue muscles ascribing a single action to a specific muscle—or implying that a particular movement is the consequence of a single muscle—greatly oversimplifies the actions of the tongue and is misleading. The muscles of the tongue do not act in isolation, and some muscles perform multiple actions with parts of one muscle capable of acting independently, producing different—even antagonistic—actions. *In general, however, extrinsic muscles alter the position of the tongue and intrinsic muscles alter its shape.* The four intrinsic and four extrinsic muscles in each half of the tongue are separated by the fibrous lingual septum (Table 8.10). The **intrinsic muscles of the tongue** (superior and inferior longitudinal, transverse, and vertical) are confined to the tongue and are not attached to bone. The **extrinsic muscles of the tongue** (genioglossus, hyoglossus, styloglossus, and pala-toglossus) originate outside the tongue and attach to it. They mainly move the tongue but they can alter its shape as well. For attachments, nerve supply, and actions of the extrinsic and intrinsic muscles, see Table 8.10.

Innervation of Tongue

All the muscles of the tongue are supplied by the CN XII, the **hypoglossal nerve** (Fig. 8.37), except for the palatoglossus (actually a palatine muscle supplied by the *pharyngeal plexus*—formed by fibers from the cranial root of CN XI carried by CN X). For general sensation (touch and temperature), the mucosa of the anterior two thirds of the tongue is supplied by the **lingual nerve,** a branch of CN V₃. For special sensation (taste), this part of the tongue, except for the vallate papillae, is supplied through the **chorda tympani** nerve, a branch of CN VII. The chorda tympani joins the lingual nerve and runs anteriorly in its sheath (Fig. 8.37*A*). The mucous membrane of the posterior one third of the tongue and the vallate papillae are supplied by the lingual branch of the **glossopharyngeal nerve** (CN IX) for both general and special sensation (taste). Twigs of the **internal laryngeal nerve,** a branch of the vagus nerve (CN X), supply mostly general but some special sensation to a small area of the tongue just anterior to the epiglottis. These mostly sensory nerves also carry *parasympathetic secretomotor fibers* to serous glands in the tongue. These nerve fibers probably synapse in the **submandibular ganglion** suspended from the lingual nerve.

TABLE 8.10. MUSCLES OF TONGUE

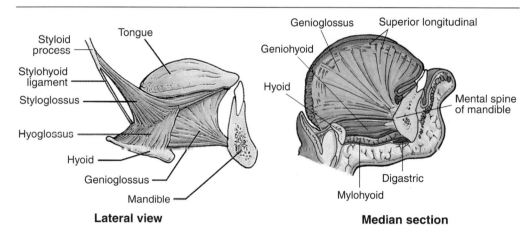

Lateral view   **Median section**

Extrinsic Muscles

Muscle	Origin	Insertion	Innervation	Action(s)
Genioglossus	Superior part of mental spine of mandible	Dorsum of tongue and body of hyoid		Depresses tongue; its posterior part protrudes tongue
Hyoglossus	Body and greater horn of hyoid	Side and inferior aspect of tongue	Hypoglossal nerve (CN XII)	Depresses and retracts tongue
Styloglossus	Styloid process and stylohyoid ligament			Retracts tongue and draws it up to create a trough for swallowing
Palatoglossus	Palatine aponeurosis of soft palate	Side of tongue	Cranial root of CN XI via pharyngeal branch of CN X and pharyngeal plexus	Elevates posterior part of tongue

Continued

TABLE 8.10. *CONTINUED*

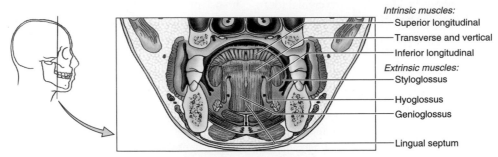

Frontal (coronal) section

Intrinsic muscles:
- Superior longitudinal
- Transverse and vertical
- Inferior longitudinal

Extrinsic muscles:
- Styloglossus
- Hyoglossus
- Genioglossus
- Lingual septum

Intrinsic Muscles

Muscle	Origin	Insertion	Innervation	Action(s)
Superior longitudinal	Submucous fibrous layer and median fibrous septum	Margins of tongue and mucous membrane	Hypoglossal nerve (CN XII)	Curls tip and sides of tongue superiorly and shortens tongue
Inferior longitudinal	Root of tongue and body of hyoid	Apex of tongue		Curls tip of tongue inferiorly and shortens tongue
Transverse	Median fibrous septum	Fibrous tissue at margins of tongue		Narrows and elongates the tongue[a]
Vertical	Superior surface of borders of tongue	Inferior surface of borders of tongue		Flattens and broadens tongue[a]

[a]Act simultaneously to protrude tongue.

Vasculature of Tongue

The **arteries of the tongue** derive from the **lingual artery,** which arises from the **external carotid artery** (Fig. 8.37C). On entering the tongue, the lingual artery passes deep to the hyoglossus muscle. *The main branches of the lingual artery are the:*

- **Dorsal lingual arteries,** which supply the posterior part the tongue and send a tonsillar branch to the palatine tonsil
- **Deep lingual artery,** which supplies the anterior part of the tongue; the dorsal and deep arteries communicate with each other near the apex of the tongue
- **Sublingual artery,** which supplies the sublingual gland and the floor of the mouth.

The **veins of the tongue** are the:

- *Dorsal lingual veins,* which accompany the lingual artery
- *Deep lingual veins* (Fig. 8.36B), which begin at the apex of the tongue and run posteriorly beside the lingual frenulum to join the *sublingual vein.* All lingual veins terminate, directly or indirectly, in the IJV.

Lymph from the tongue takes the following routes (Fig. 8.38):

- Lymph from the posterior third drains to the **superior deep cervical lymph nodes** on both sides

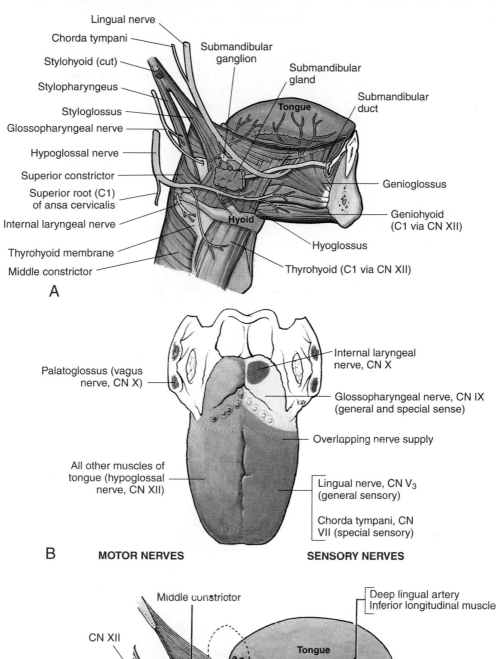

A

- Lingual nerve
- Chorda tympani
- Stylohyoid (cut)
- Stylopharyngeus
- Styloglossus
- Glossopharyngeal nerve
- Hypoglossal nerve
- Superior constrictor
- Superior root (C1) of ansa cervicalis
- Internal laryngeal nerve
- Thyrohyoid membrane
- Middle constrictor
- Submandibular ganglion
- Submandibular gland
- Tongue
- Submandibular duct
- Genioglossus
- Geniohyoid (C1 via CN XII)
- Hyoglossus
- Thyrohyoid (C1 via CN XII)
- Hyoid

B

MOTOR NERVES   SENSORY NERVES

- Palatoglossus (vagus nerve, CN X)
- All other muscles of tongue (hypoglossal nerve, CN XII)
- Internal laryngeal nerve, CN X
- Glossopharyngeal nerve, CN IX (general and special sense)
- Overlapping nerve supply
- Lingual nerve, CN V₃ (general sensory)
- Chorda tympani, CN VII (special sensory)

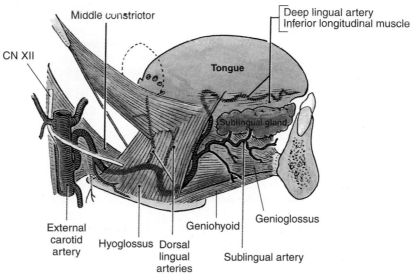

C

- Middle constrictor
- CN XII
- Deep lingual artery
- Inferior longitudinal muscle
- Tongue
- Sublingual gland
- External carotid artery
- Hyoglossus
- Dorsal lingual arteries
- Geniohyoid
- Sublingual artery
- Genioglossus

FIGURE 8.37 Muscles, nerves, and arteries of the tongue. A. Muscles and nerves. Right lateral view. The ansa cervicalis is a loop in the cervical plexus (see Chapter 9). **B.** Innervation. Superior view. **C.** Arteries. Right lateral view.

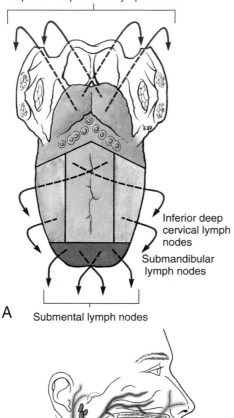

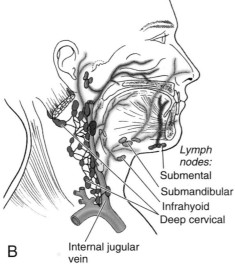

FIGURE 8.38   Lymphatic drainage of the tongue.
A. Superior view of the dorsum of the tongue.
B. Lateral view of the head and neck.

- Lymph from the *medial part of the anterior two thirds* drains to the **inferior deep cervical lymph nodes**
- Lymph from *lateral parts of the anterior two thirds* drains to the **submandibular lymph nodes**

- Lymph from the *apex of the tongue* drains to the **submental lymph nodes**
- Lymph from the *posterior third* and the area near the midline groove drain bilaterally.

GAG REFLEX
One may touch the anterior part of the tongue without feeling discomfort; however, when the pharyngeal part is touched, one usually gags. CN IX and CN X are responsible for the muscular contraction of each side of the pharynx. Glossopharyngeal branches (CN IX) provide the afferent limb of the gag reflex.

Paralysis of Genioglossus
When the genioglossus is paralyzed, the tongue mass has a tendency to shift posteriorly, obstructing the airway and presenting the risk of suffocation. Total relaxation of the genioglossus muscles occurs during general anesthesia; therefore, the tongue of an anesthetized patient must be prevented from relapsing by inserting an airway.

Injury to Hypoglossal Nerve
Trauma, such as a fractured mandible, may injure the hypoglossal nerve, resulting in paralysis and eventual atrophy of one side of the tongue. The tongue deviates to the paralyzed side during protrusion because of the "anchoring effect" of the inactive side.

Sublingual Absorption of Drugs
For quick transmucosal absorption of a drug—for instance, when nitroglycerin is used as a vasodilator in angina pectoris (chest pain)—the pill (or spray) is put under the tongue where the thin mucosa allows the absorbed drug to enter the deep lingual veins in less than a minute.

LINGUAL CARCINOMA
Malignant tumors in the posterior part of the tongue metastasize to the superior deep cervical lymph nodes on both sides. In contrast, tumors in the apex and anterolateral parts usually do not metastasize to the inferior deep cervical nodes until late in the disease. Because the deep nodes are closely related to the IJVs, carcinoma from the tongue may spread to the submental and submandibular regions and along the IJVs into the neck.

SALIVARY GLANDS

The **major salivary glands** include the parotid, submandibular, and sublingual glands (Fig. 8.39*A*). Saliva, the clear, tasteless, odorless viscid fluid secreted by these glands and the mucous glands of the oral cavity:

- Keeps the mucous membrane of the mouth moist
- Lubricates the food during mastication

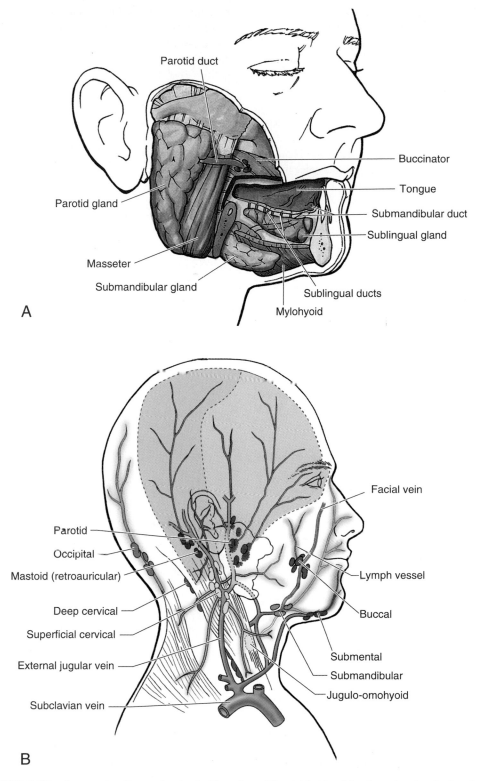

Parotid duct

Buccinator

Tongue

Submandibular duct

Sublingual gland

Parotid gland

Masseter

Submandibular gland

Sublingual ducts

Mylohyoid

A

Facial vein

Parotid

Occipital

Mastoid (retroauricular)

Lymph vessel

Deep cervical

Buccal

Superficial cervical

External jugular vein

Submental

Submandibular

Jugulo-omohyoid

Subclavian vein

B

FIGURE 8.39   Face and salivary glands. A. Dissection of the right side of the face showing the location of glands and ducts. Anterolateral view. **B.** Lymphatic drainage of the face and glands. Lateral view.

- Begins digestion of starches
- Serves as an intrinsic "mouthwash"
- Plays a significant role in the prevention of tooth decay and in the ability to taste.

In addition to the three major salivary glands there are small *minor salivary glands* in the palate, lips, cheeks, tonsils, and tongue.

The **parotid glands** are the largest of the major salivary glands. Each parotid gland has an irregular shape because it occupies the gap between the ramus of the mandible and the styloid and mastoid processes of the temporal bone. The purely serous secretion of the gland passes through the **parotid duct** and empties into the vestibule of the oral cavity opposite the second maxillary molar tooth (Fig. 8.39*A*). In addition to its digestive function, it washes food particles into the mouth proper. The **arterial supply** of the parotid gland and duct is from branches of the *external carotid* and *superficial temporal arteries*. The **veins** from the parotid gland drain into the *retromandibular veins* (p. 550). The **lymphatic vessels** from the parotid gland end in the **superficial and deep cervical lymph nodes** (Fig. 8.39*B*). For a discussion of the innervation of the parotid gland, see p. 513.

The **submandibular glands** (Fig. 8.39*A*) lie along the body of the mandible, partly superior and partly inferior to the posterior half of the mandible and partly superficial and partly deep to the mylohyoid muscle. The **submandibular duct** arises from the intra-oral part of the gland that lies between the mylohyoid and hyoglossus. Passing lateral to medial, the **lingual nerve** loops under the duct as it runs anteriorly to open by one to three orifices on a small, fleshy *sublingual caruncle* (papilla) on each side of the lingual frenulum (Figs. 8.36*B* and 8.37*A*). Its orifice is visible and saliva often sprays from it when the tongue is elevated and retracted (as when yawning). The **arterial supply** of the submandibular gland is from the **submental artery** (Fig. 8.26). The **veins** accompany the arteries. The submandibular gland is supplied by presynaptic parasympathetic secretomotor fibers conveyed from the facial nerve to the lingual nerve by the **chorda tympani** (Figs. 8.25*B* and 8.37*A*), which synapse with postsynaptic neu-

rons in the **submandibular ganglion.** The latter fibers accompany arteries to reach the gland, along with vasoconstrictive postsynaptic sympathetic fibers from the superior cervical ganglion. The **lymphatic vessels** of the submandibular gland drain into the **deep cervical lymph nodes,** particularly the **jugulo-omohyoid lymph nodes** (Fig. 8.39*B*).

The **sublingual glands** are the smallest and most deeply situated (Fig. 8.39*A*). Each almond-shaped gland lies in the floor of the mouth between the mandible and the genioglossus muscle. The glands from each side unite to form a horseshoe-shaped glandular mass around the lingual frenulum. Numerous small **sublingual ducts** open into the floor of the mouth. The **arterial supply** of the sublingual glands is from the **sublingual** and **submental arteries**—branches of the lingual and facial arteries (Figs. 8.26 and 8.37*C*). The **innervation** of the sublingual glands is the same as that described for the submandibular gland.

EXCISION OF SUBMANDIBULAR GLAND

Excision of a submandibular gland because of a *calculus* (stone) in its duct or a tumor in the gland is not uncommon. Risks to the mandibular branch of the facial nerve may be avoided by making the skin incision at least 2.5 cm inferior to the angle of the mandible.

Sialography

The parotid and submandibular salivary glands may be examined radiographically after the injection of a contrast medium into their ducts. This special type of radiograph (*sialogram*) demonstrates the salivary ducts and some secretory units. Because of the small size and number of sublingual ducts of the sublingual glands, one cannot usually inject contrast medium into them.

PTERYGOPALATINE FOSSA

The pterygopalatine fossa—*a small pyramidal space inferior to the apex of the orbit*—lies between the pterygoid process (consisting of medial and lateral **pterygoid plates**), the maxilla, and the palatine bone (Fig. 8.40*A*). The fragile vertical plate of the palatine bone forms its medial wall. The incomplete *roof of the pterygopalatine fossa* is formed by the **greater wing of the sphenoid** (Fig. 8.40*B*). The *floor of the pterygopalatine fossa* is formed by the **pyramidal**

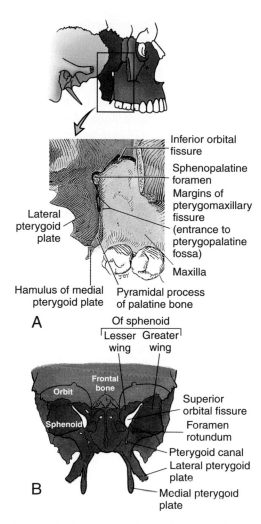

Inferior orbital fissure

Sphenopalatine foramen

Margins of pterygomaxillary fissure (entrance to pterygopalatine fossa)

Lateral pterygoid plate

Maxilla

Hamulus of medial pterygoid plate

Pyramidal process of palatine bone

A

Of sphenoid

Lesser wing — Greater wing

Frontal bone

Orbit

Sphenoid

Superior orbital fissure

Foramen rotundum

Pterygoid canal

Lateral pterygoid plate

B

Medial pterygoid plate

FIGURE 8.40   Pterygopalatine fossa and its communications. A. Right lateral view. **B.** Anterior view. Maxillae have been removed.

process of the palatine bone. Its superior, larger end opens into the **inferior orbital fissure;** its inferior end is closed except for the palatine canals. **The pterygopalatine fossa communicates:**

- Laterally with the *infratemporal fossa* through the *pterygomaxillary fissure* (Fig. 8.40*A*)
- Anterosuperiorly with the *orbit* through the *inferior orbital fissure*
- Posterosuperiorly with the *middle cranial fossa* through the *foramen rotundum* and *pterygoid canal* (Figs. 8.40*B* and 8.41, *A* and *B*)

- Medially with the *nasal cavity* through the *sphenopalatine foramen* (Figs. 8.40*A* and 8.41, *C* and *D*)
- Inferiorly with the *oral cavity* through the *palatine canals/foramina* (Fig. 8.41, *B* and *D*).

The **contents of the pterygopalatine fossa** (Figs. 8.41 and 8.42) are the:

- Third or pterygopalatine part of the maxillary artery and initial parts of its branches
- Maxillary nerve (CN V₂)
- Nerve of the pterygoid canal
- Pterygopalatine ganglion and the initial parts of its branches.

The **maxillary nerve** (CN V₂) enters the pterygopalatine fossa posterosuperiorly through the foramen rotundum and runs anterolaterally in the fossa (Fig. 8.41, *A* to *D*). Within the fossa, the maxillary nerve gives off the **zygomatic nerve,** which divides into **zygomaticofacial** and **zygomaticotemporal nerves.** These nerves emerge from the zygomatic bone through the cranial foramina of the same name and supply the lateral region of the cheek and the temple. The *zygomaticotemporal nerve* also gives rise to a **communicating branch** (Fig. 8.41*C*), which conveys parasympathetic secretomotor fibers to the lacrimal gland by way of the lacrimal nerve from CN V₁. While in the pterygopalatine fossa, the maxillary nerve also gives off the two **ganglionic branches** *(pterygopalatine nerves)* that suspend the parasympathetic **pterygopalatine ganglion** in the superior part of the pterygopalatine fossa (Fig. 8.41, *B* and *C*). The ganglionic branches convey general sensory fibers of the maxillary nerve, which pass through the pterygopalatine ganglion without synapsing and supply the nose, palate, tonsil, and gingivae. The maxillary nerve leaves the pterygopalatine fossa through the inferior orbital fissure, after which it is known as the **infraorbital nerve** (Fig. 8.41, *A* and *C*).

The *parasympathetic fibers to the pterygopalatine ganglion* come from the facial nerve by way of its first branch, the **greater**

petrosal nerve (Fig. 8.41*B*). This nerve joins the **deep petrosal nerve** as it passes through the cartilage occupying the foramen lacerum to form the **nerve of the pterygoid canal.** This nerve passes anteriorly through the pterygoid canal to the **pterygopalatine fossa** (Fig. 8.41, *B* and *C*). The presynaptic parasympathetic fibers of the greater petrosal nerve synapse in the pterygopalatine ganglion. The **deep petrosal nerve** is a sympathetic nerve from the internal carotid plexus. Its postsynaptic fibers are from nerve cell bodies in the superior cervical sympathetic ganglion. Thus, these fibers do not synapse in the pterygopalatine ganglion but pass directly to join the branches of the ganglion (maxillary nerve). The postsynaptic parasympathetic and sympathetic fibers pass to the lacrimal gland and the glands of the nasal cavity, palate, and upper pharynx (Fig. 8.41*D*).

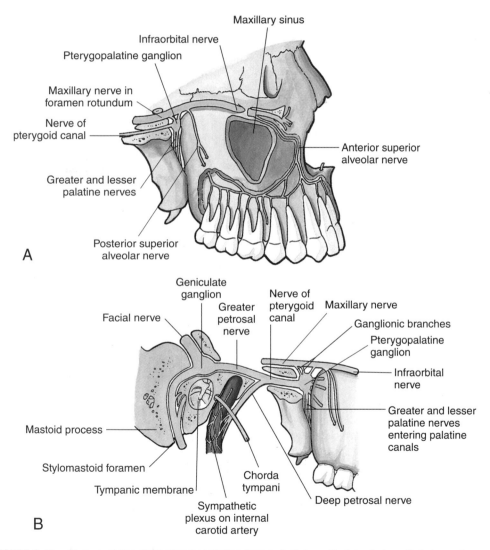

FIGURE 8.41   Nerves of the right pterygopalatine fossa. A. Schematic lateral view. **B.** Autonomic fibers to the pterygopalatine ganglion. Schematic lateral view.

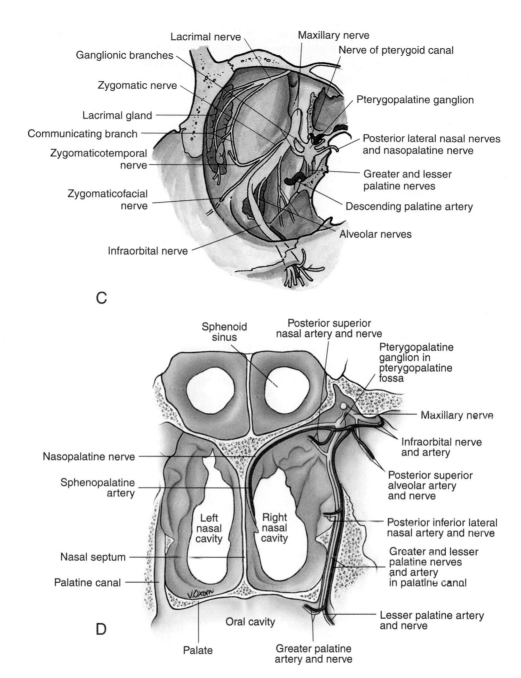

FIGURE 8.41 *Continued* **C.** Fossa viewed through the floor of the orbit showing the maxillary nerve (CN V₂) and its branches. **D.** Nasopalatine and greater and lesser palatine nerves. Posterior view of the cranium coronally sectioned through the nasal cavities and pterygopalatine fossa.

The **maxillary artery,** a terminal branch of the external carotid artery, passes anteriorly and traverses the infratemporal fossa. It passes over the lateral pterygoid muscle and enters the pterygopalatine fossa (Fig. 8.42). The *pterygopalatine part of the maxillary artery,* its third part, passes through the *pterygomaxillary fissure* and enters the pterygopalatine fossa, where it lies anterior to the **pterygopalatine ganglion.** The artery gives rise to branches that accompany all nerves in the fossa with the same names (Fig. 8.41). The **branches of the third or pterygopalatine part of the maxillary artery** are the:

- Posterior superior alveolar artery
- Descending palatine artery, which divides into greater and lesser palatine arteries
- Artery of the pterygoid canal
- Sphenopalatine artery, which divides into posterior lateral nasal branches to the lateral wall of the nasal cavity and its associated paranasal sinuses, and the posterior septal branches

- Infraorbital artery, which gives rise to the anterior superior alveolar artery and terminates as branches to the inferior eyelid, nose, and upper lip.

NOSE

The nose is the part of the respiratory tract superior to the hard palate and contains the peripheral organ of smell. It includes the external nose and nasal cavities, divided into right and left nasal cavities by the nasal septum. Each nasal cavity is divisible into an *olfactory area* and a *respiratory area*. **The functions of the nose and nasal cavities are:**

- Olfaction (smelling)
- Respiration (breathing)
- Filtration of dust
- Humidification of inspired air
- Reception of secretions from the nasal mucosa, paranasal sinuses, and nasolacrimal ducts.

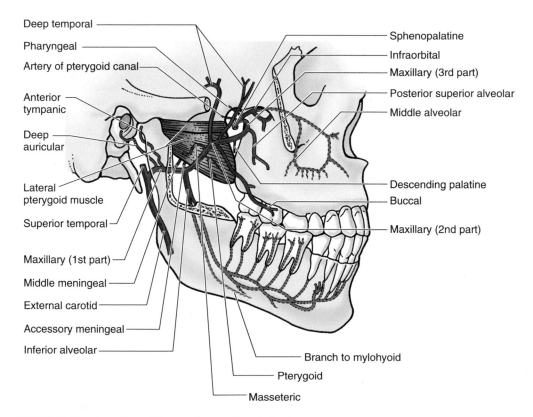

FIGURE 8.42   Branches of the maxillary artery. Lateral view.

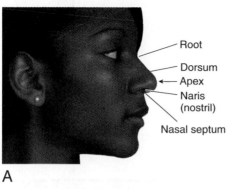

A

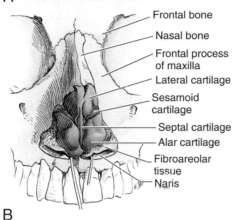

Root
Dorsum
Apex
Naris (nostril)
Nasal septum

Frontal bone
Nasal bone
Frontal process of maxilla
Lateral cartilage
Sesamoid cartilage
Septal cartilage
Alar cartilage
Fibroareolar tissue
Naris

B

FIGURE 8.43 External nose. A. Surface features. Lateral view. **B.** Nasal bones and cartilages (pulled inferiorly). Anterior view.

External Nose

External noses vary considerably in size and shape, mainly because of differences in the nasal cartilages. The **dorsum of the nose** extends from its superior angle—the **root** (Fig. 8.43A)—to the **apex** (tip) of the nose. The inferior surface of the nose is pierced by two piriform (pear-shaped) openings, the **nares** (nostrils), which are separated from each other by the **nasal septum.** The external nose consists of bony and cartilaginous parts (Fig. 8.43B). The **bony part of the nose** consists of the:

- Nasal bones
- Frontal processes of the maxillae
- Nasal part of the frontal bone and its nasal spine
- Bony nasal septum.

The **cartilaginous part of the nose** consists of five main cartilages: two **lateral cartilages,** two **alar cartilages,** and a **septal cartilage.** The septal cartilage has a tongue-and-groove articulation with the edges of the bony part of the septum (Fig. 8.44).

NASAL FRACTURES

Deformity of the external nose usually is present with a fracture, particularly when a lateral force is applied by someone's elbow, for example. When the injury results from a direct blow (e.g., from a hockey stick), the cribriform plate of the ethmoid bone may fracture, resulting in CSF rhinorrhea (p. 528).

NASAL CAVITIES

The nasal cavities, entered through the nares, open posteriorly into the nasopharynx through the **choanae** (p. 503). Mucosa lines the nasal cavities, except the *nasal vestibule,* which is lined with skin (Fig. 8.45A). The *nasal mucosa* is firmly bound to the periosteum and perichondrium of the supporting bones and cartilages of the nose. The mucosa is continuous with the lining of all the chambers with which the nasal cavities communicate: the nasopharynx posteriorly, the paranasal sinuses superiorly and laterally, and the lacrimal sac and conjunctiva superiorly. The inferior two thirds of the nasal mucosa is the *respiratory area,* and the superior one third is the *olfactory area.* Air passing over the respiratory area is warmed and moistened before it passes through the rest of the upper respiratory tract to the lungs. The **olfactory area** is specialized mucosa containing the peripheral organ of smell; sniffing draws air to the area. The central processes of the olfactory receptor neurons in the olfactory epithelium unite to form nerve bundles that pass through the cribriform plate and enter the **olfactory bulb** (see Fig. 8.45B and Chapter 10).

The boundaries of the nasal cavity are (Fig. 8.44):

- The *roof of the nasal cavity* is curved and narrow, except at the posterior end; the roof is divided into three parts (frontonasal, ethmoidal, and sphenoidal), which are named from the bones that form them.
- The *floor of the nasal cavity,* wider than the roof, is formed by the **palatine process of the maxilla** and the **horizontal plate of the palatine bone.**

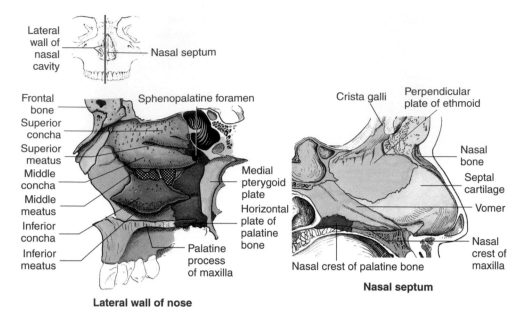

FIGURE 8.44 Lateral and medial (septal) walls of the right side of the nasal cavity.

- The *medial wall of the nasal cavity* is formed by the nasal septum. The main components of the nasal septum are the **perpendicular plate of the ethmoid, vomer, septal cartilage,** and the **nasal crests of the maxillary and palatine bones.**
- The *lateral wall of the nasal cavity* is uneven because of the **nasal conchae—superior, middle, and inferior**—three elevations that project inferiorly like scrolls.
- The conchae curve inferomedially, each forming a roof for a **meatus**—a passage in the nasal cavity.

The **nasal conchae** divide the nasal cavity into four passages (Figs. 8.44 and 8.46): sphenoethmoidal recess, superior meatus, middle meatus, and inferior meatus. The **sphenoethmoidal recess,** lying superoposterior to the superior concha, receives the *opening of the sphenoidal sinus.* The **superior meatus** is a narrow passage between the superior and middle nasal conchae (parts of the ethmoid bone) into which the posterior ethmoidal sinuses open by one or more orifices. The long **middle meatus** is wider than the superior one. The anterosuperior part of this passage communicates with the frontal sinus. The passage that leads inferiorly from each frontal sinus to the *ethmoidal infundibulum*—a funnel-shaped opening—is the *frontonasal duct.* The **semilunar hiatus** (L. hiatus semilunaris) is a semicircular groove into which the frontonasal duct opens. The **ethmoidal bulla** (L. swelling)—a rounded elevation located superior to the semilunar hiatus—is visible when the middle concha is removed. The bulla is formed by *middle ethmoidal cells* that constitute the **ethmoidal sinuses** (Fig. 8.46, *B* and *C*). The **maxillary sinus** also opens into the posterior end of the semilunar hiatus. The **inferior meatus** is a horizontal passage, inferolateral to the inferior nasal concha (an independent, paired bone). The **nasolacrimal duct** from the lacrimal sac (p. 534) opens into the anterior part of this meatus.

The arterial supply of the medial and lateral walls of the nasal cavity (Fig. 8.45*A*) is from branches of the **sphenopalatine artery, anterior and posterior ethmoidal arteries, greater palatine artery, superior labial artery,** and the **lateral nasal branches of the facial artery.** On the anterior part of the nasal septum is an area rich in capillaries (Kiesselbach area) where all

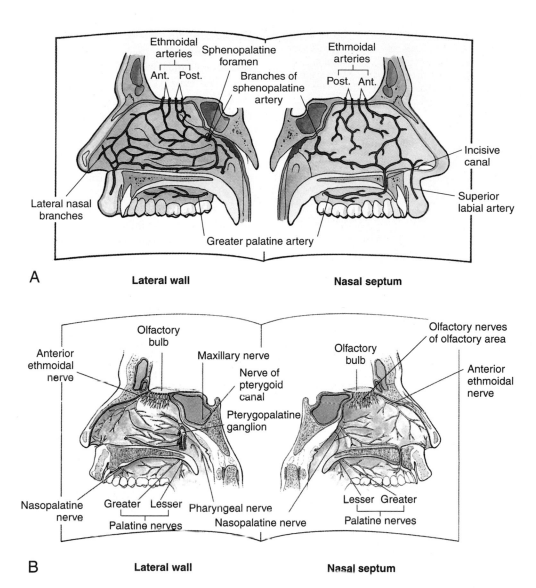

FIGURE 8.45   "Open book" view of the walls of the nasal cavity. **A.** Arterial supply. **B.** Innervation.

five arteries supplying the septum anastomose. Thus, this area is often where profuse bleeding from the nose occurs. A rich *plexus of veins* drains deep to the nasal mucosa into the sphenopalatine, facial, and ophthalmic veins. The *nerve supply of the posteroinferior half to two thirds of the nasal mucosa* is chiefly from the **maxillary nerve** (CN V$_2$) by way of the **nasopalatine nerve** to the nasal septum and posterior lateral nasal branches of the **greater palatine nerve** to the lateral wall (Fig. 8.45*B*). The anterosuperior part of the nasal mucosa

(both the septum and lateral wall) is supplied by the **anterior ethmoidal nerves,** branches of the nasociliary nerve CN V$_1$.

EPISTAXIS

Epistaxis (nose bleeding) is common because of the rich blood supply to the nasal mucosa. In most cases the cause is trauma and the bleeding is located in the anterior third of the nose (Kiesselbach's area). Recall that this area is supplied by the anastomosing of branches from five different arterial sources. Spurting of blood from the nose results from rupture of these arteries. Epistaxis is also associated with infections and hypertension.

CSF Rhinorrhea

Although nasal discharges are commonly associated with upper respiratory tract infections, a nasal discharge after a head injury may be CSF. CSF rhinorrhea results from fracture of the cribriform plate, tearing of the cranial meninges, and leakage of CSF from the nose (p. 528).

Rhinitis

The nasal mucosa becomes swollen and inflamed (*rhinitis*) during upper respiratory infections and allergic reactions (e.g., hayfever). Swelling of this mucous membrane occurs readily because of its vascularity and abundant mucosal glands. *Infections of the nasal cavities may spread to the:*

- Anterior cranial fossa through the cribriform plate
- Nasopharynx and retropharyngeal soft tissues
- Middle ear through the pharyngotympanic (auditory) tube
- Paranasal sinuses
- Lacrimal apparatus and conjunctiva.

PARANASAL SINUSES

The paranasal sinuses are air-filled extensions of the respiratory part of the nasal cavity into the following cranial bones: frontal, ethmoid, sphenoid, and maxilla (Fig. 8.46). They are named according to the bones in which they are located. The **frontal sinuses** are between the outer and inner tables of the frontal bone, posterior to the superciliary arches and the root of the nose. Each sinus drains through a **frontonasal duct** into the *infundibulum,* which opens into the **semilunar hiatus** of the middle meatus. The frontal sinuses are innervated by branches of the *supraorbital nerves* (CN V_1). The **ethmoidal sinuses** comprise several cavities—**ethmoidal cells**—that are located in the lateral mass of the ethmoid between the nasal cavity and orbit. The *anterior ethmoidal cells* drain directly or indirectly into the middle meatus through the infundibulum. The *middle ethmoidal cells* open directly into the middle meatus. The *posterior ethmoidal cells,* which form the **ethmoidal bulla,**

open directly into the superior meatus. The ethmoidal sinuses are supplied by the anterior and posterior ethmoidal branches (Fig. 8.45*B*) of the *nasociliary nerves* (CN V_1). The **sphenoidal sinuses,** unevenly divided and separated by a bony septum, occupy the body of the sphenoid bone; they may extend into the wings of this bone in the elderly. Because of these sinuses, the body of the sphenoid is fragile. Only thin plates of bone separate the sinuses from several important structures: the optic nerves and optic chiasm, the pituitary gland, the internal carotid arteries, and the cavernous sinuses. The *posterior ethmoidal artery* and *nerve* supply the sphenoidal sinuses (Fig. 8.46).

The **maxillary sinuses** are the largest of the paranasal sinuses (Fig. 8.46, *B* and *C*). These large pyramidal cavities occupy the entire bodies of the maxillae. The *apex of the maxillary sinus* extends toward and often into the zygomatic bone. The *base of the maxillary sinus* forms the inferior part of the lateral wall of the nasal cavity. The *roof of the maxillary sinus* is formed by the floor of the orbit. The *floor of the maxillary sinus* is formed by the alveolar part of the maxilla. The roots of the maxillary teeth, particularly the first two molars, often produce conical elevations in the floor of the maxillary sinus. Each sinus drains by an opening—the **maxillary ostium** (Fig. 8.46*A*)—into the middle meatus of the nasal cavity by way of the semilunar hiatus. Because of the superior location of this opening, it is impossible for the sinus to drain when the head is erect until the sinus is full. The **arterial supply of the maxillary sinus** is mainly from superior alveolar branches of the **maxillary artery;** however, branches of the **greater palatine artery** supply the floor of the sinus (Fig. 8.45*A*). **Innervation of the maxillary sinus** is from the anterior, middle, and posterior **superior alveolar nerves** (Fig. 8.28), branches of the maxillary nerve (CN V_2).

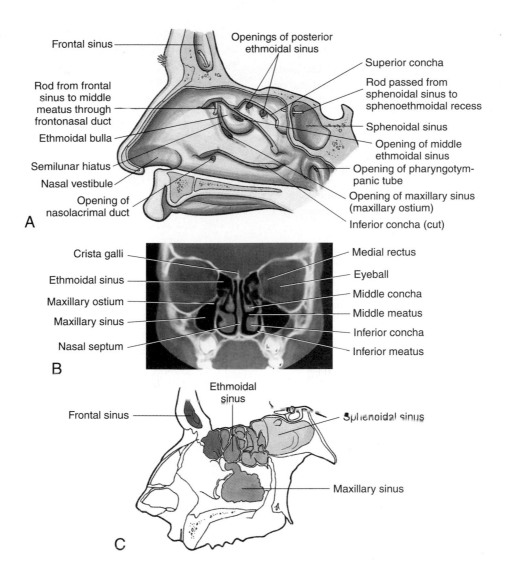

FIGURE 8.46 Paranasal sinuses. A. Lateral wall of the nasal cavity with parts of the conchae removed to show the openings of sinuses and other structures. Medial view. **B.** Coronal CT scan showing the paranasal sinuses. **C.** Right paranasal sinuses. Medial view.

INFECTION OF ETHMOIDAL CELLS

If nasal drainage is blocked, infections of the ethmoidal cells of the ethmoidal sinuses may break through the fragile medial wall of the orbit. Severe infections from this source may cause blindness because some posterior ethmoidal cells lie close to the optic canal, which gives passage to the optic nerve and ophthalmic artery. Spread of infection from these cells could also affect the dural sheath of the optic nerve, causing *optic neuritis.*

Infection of Maxillary Sinuses

The maxillary sinuses are the most commonly infected, probably because their ostia are located high on their su-

peromedial walls (Fig. 8.46B), a poor location for natural drainage of the sinus. When the mucous membrane of the sinus is congested, the maxillary ostia often are obstructed. The proximity of the molar teeth to the floor of the maxillary sinus poses potentially serious problems. During removal of a maxillary molar tooth, a fracture of a root may occur. If proper retrieval methods are not used, a piece of the root may be driven superiorly into the maxillary sinus. A communication (fistula) may be created between the oral cavity and the maxillary sinus. The maxillary sinus often can be cannulated and drained by passing a cannula through the nostril and into the maxillary ostium of the sinus.

EAR

The ear is divided into *external, middle,* and *internal parts* (Fig. 8.47). The external and middle parts are mainly concerned with the transference of sound to the internal ear, where the organ for equilibrium—the condition of being evenly balanced—and the organ for hearing are located. The **tympanic membrane** (eardrum) separates the external ear from the middle ear. The **pharyngotympanic (auditory) tube** joins the middle ear to the nasopharynx.

EXTERNAL EAR

The external ear comprises the **auricle** (pinna), which collects sound, and the **external acoustic meatus** (L. passage), which conducts sound to the tympanic membrane (Fig. 8.47*C*). The **auricle,** consisting of several parts, is composed of elastic cartilage covered with skin. The auricle has several depressions; the **concha**—the large hollow or floor of the auricle—is the deepest depression. The **lobule** (lobe) of the auricle—devoid of cartilage—consists of fibrous tissue, fat, and blood vessels. It is easily pierced for taking small blood samples and ornamentation. The **arterial supply** to the auricle is derived mainly from the *posterior auricular* and *superficial temporal arteries* (p. 548). The **nerves** to the auricle are mainly the great auricular, auriculotemporal, and lesser occipital nerves, with minor contributions from the facial (CN VII) and vagus (CN X) nerves.

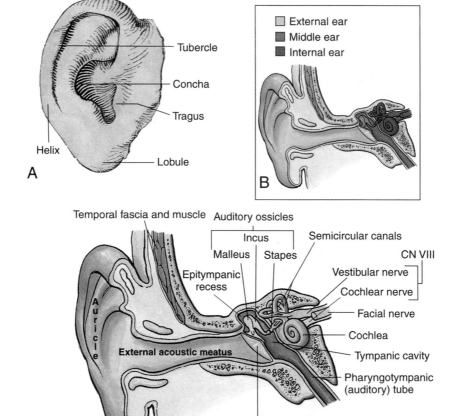

FIGURE 8.47   **Ear. A.** Auricle (pinna) of the right ear. Lateral view. **B.** External, middle, and internal ear. **C.** Schematic frontal (coronal) section.

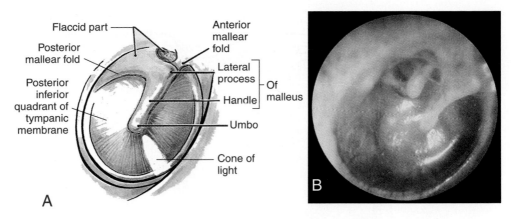

FIGURE 8.48 **Otoscopic views of the right tympanic membrane. A.** Schematic illustration. **B.** Normal otoscopic view, photograph.

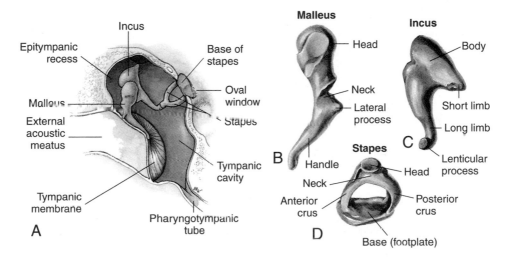

FIGURE 8.49 **Auditory ossicles. A.** Anterior view of the coronal section of the tympanic cavity showing ossicles in situ. **B.** Malleus. Posteromediul view. **C.** Incus. Posteromedial view. **D.** Stapes. Superolateral view.

Lymphatic drainage of the lateral surface of the superior half of the auricle is to the superficial **parotid lymph nodes.** Lymph from the medial surface of the superior half of the auricle drains to the **mastoid** and **deep cervical lymph nodes** (Fig. 8.39*B*). Lymph from the remainder of the auricle, including the lobule, drains to the **superficial cervical lymph nodes.**

The **external acoustic meatus** (Fig. 8.47*C*) leads inward from the concha through the tympanic part of the temporal bone (p. 546) to the tympanic membrane. The lateral third of the S-shaped meatus is cartilaginous and lined with skin, which is continuous with the skin of the au-

ricle. The medial two thirds of the meatus is bony and lined with thin skin that is continuous with the external layer of the tympanic membrane. The *ceruminous* and *sebaceous glands* produce *cerumen* (earwax). The **tympanic membrane** is a thin, oval, semitransparent membrane at the medial end of the external acoustic meatus. It forms a partition between the meatus and the **tympanic cavity** of the middle ear—an air chamber in the temporal bone containing small ear bones—the **auditory ossicles** (Fig. 8.47*C*). The tympanic membrane is covered with very thin skin externally and mucous membrane of the middle ear internally; it has a con-

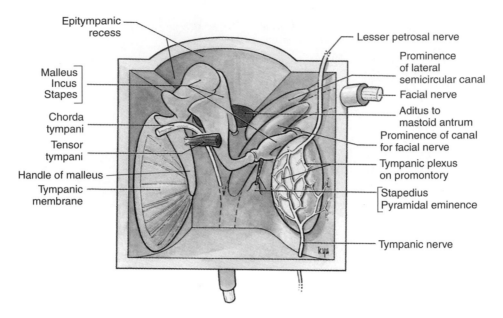

FIGURE 8.50   Walls of the tympanic cavity. Schematic drawing of the anterior view of the right middle ear.

cavity toward the external acoustic meatus with a shallow, conelike central depression, the **umbo** (Fig. 8.48). When observed with an *otoscope* (instrument for examining the tympanic membrane), a bright area—the **cone of light**—radiates anteroinferiorly from the umbo. Superior to the attachment of the malleus, the **flaccid part** (L. pars flaccida) of the tympanic membrane is thin and loose. It lacks the radial and circular fibers present in the remainder of the tympanic membrane—the **tense part** (L. pars tensa). The tympanic membrane moves in response to air vibrations that pass to it through the external acoustic meatus. Movements of the membrane are transmitted through the middle ear by the **auditory ossicles** (malleus, incus, and stapes) (Fig. 8.49). The external surface of the tympanic membrane is supplied mainly by the *auriculotemporal nerve,* a branch of CN V_3, although some innervation is supplied by a small auricular branch of the vagus nerve (CN X). The internal surface of the tympanic membrane is supplied by the *glossopharyngeal nerve* (CN IX).

MIDDLE EAR

The middle and internal parts of the ear are located in the petrous part of the temporal bone (Fig. 8.47C). The middle ear includes the **tym-** **panic cavity,** the space directly internal to the tympanic membrane, and the **epitympanic recess,** the space superior to the tympanic membrane (Figs. 8.50 and 8.51). The middle ear is connected anteromedially with the nasopharynx by the **pharyngotympanic (auditory) tube.** Posterosuperiorly, the tympanic cavity connects with the **mastoid cells** through the **aditus to the mastoid antrum.** The tympanic cavity is lined with mucous membrane that is continuous with the lining of the pharyngotympanic tube, mastoid antrum, and mastoid cells. *The contents of the middle ear are the:*

- Auditory ossicles—malleus, incus, and stapes
- Tendons of the stapedius and tensor tympani muscles
- Chorda tympani nerve—a branch of CN VII
- Tympanic plexus of nerves.

Walls of Tympanic Cavity
The middle ear, shaped like a narrow box with concave sides, has a roof, floor, and four walls (Figs. 8.50 and 8.51).

- The *tegmental wall* is formed by a thin plate of bone, the **tegmen tympani,** which separates the tympanic cavity from the dura on the floor of the middle cranial fossa.

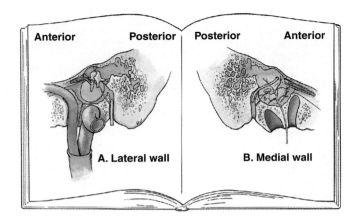

Anterior | Posterior | Posterior | Anterior

A. Lateral wall

B. Medial wall

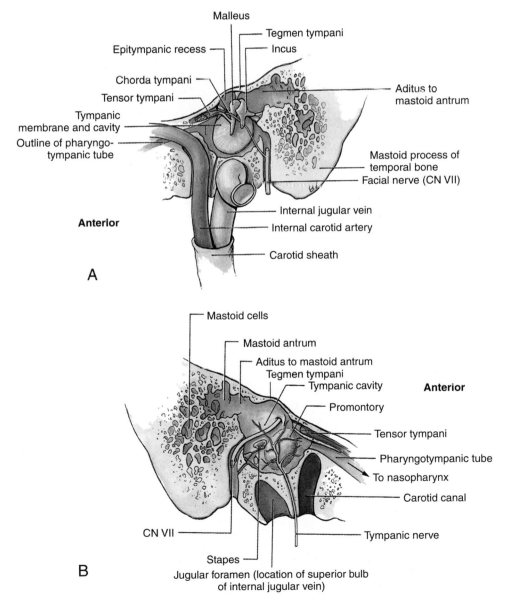

Malleus

Tegmen tympani

Epitympanic recess

Incus

Chorda tympani

Tensor tympani

Tympanic membrane and cavity

Outline of pharyngotympanic tube

Aditus to mastoid antrum

Mastoid process of temporal bone

Facial nerve (CN VII)

Anterior

Internal jugular vein

Internal carotid artery

Carotid sheath

A

Mastoid cells

Mastoid antrum

Aditus to mastoid antrum

Tegmen tympani

Tympanic cavity

Anterior

Promontory

Tensor tympani

Pharyngotympanic tube

To nasopharynx

Carotid canal

CN VII

Tympanic nerve

Stapes

Jugular foramen (location of superior bulb of internal jugular vein)

B

FIGURE 8.51 **Dissections of the right middle ear showing the contents and walls of the tympanic cavity. A.** Medial view of the lateral wall. **B.** Lateral view of the medial wall.

- The *jugular wall* (floor) is formed by a layer of bone that separates the tympanic cavity from the superior bulb of the IJV.
- The *membranous wall* (lateral wall) is formed almost entirely by the peaked convexity of the tympanic membrane; superiorly it is formed by the lateral bony wall of the **epitympanic recess.** The handle of the malleus is incorporated in the tympanic membrane and its head extends into the epitympanic recess.
- The *labyrinthine wall* (medial wall) separates the tympanic cavity from the internal ear and features the **promontory** of the initial part (basal turn) of the cochlea.
- The *carotid wall* (anterior wall) separates the tympanic cavity from the **carotid canal** (Fig. 8.51), which contains the *internal carotid artery;* superiorly the carotid wall has the opening of the pharyngotympanic tube and the canal for the **tensor tympani muscle.**
- The *mastoid wall* (posterior wall) features an opening in its superior part—the *aditus to the mastoid antrum*—connecting the tympanic cavity to the mastoid cells; the canal for the facial nerve descends between the mastoid wall and the antrum, medial to the aditus. The tendon of the **stapedius muscle** emerges from the apex of the **pyramidal eminence** (Fig. 8.50)—a hollow, bony cone enclosing the stapedius muscle (on the mastoid wall).

The **mastoid antrum** is a cavity in the mastoid process of the temporal bone (Fig. 8.50*B*). The mastoid antrum—like the tympanic cavity—is also separated from the middle cranial fossa by the thin, bony roof, the **tegmen tympani.** The floor of the antrum has several apertures through which it communicates with the mastoid cells. The antrum and mastoid cells are lined by mucous membrane that is continuous with the lining of the middle ear. Anteroinferiorly, the mastoid antrum is related to the canal for the facial nerve.

OTOSCOPY

Examination of the tympanic membrane begins by aligning the cartilaginous and bony parts of the meatus. In adults, the helix (margin) of the auricle is grasped and pulled posterosuperiorly (up, out, and

back). These movements straighten the meatus, facilitating use of the *otoscope.* The external acoustic meatus is relatively short (lacks a bony part) in infants; therefore, extra care must be taken to prevent damage to the tympanic membrane.

Otitis Media

A bulging red tympanic membrane may indicate pus or fluid in the middle ear, a sign of otitis media. Infection of the middle ear often is secondary to upper respiratory infections. Inflammation and swelling of the mucous membrane lining the tympanic cavity may cause partial or complete *blockage of the pharyngotympanic tube.* The tympanic membrane becomes red and bulges and the person may complain of "ear popping." If untreated, otitis media may produce impaired hearing as the result of scarring of the auditory ossicles, limiting the ability of these bones to move in response to sound.

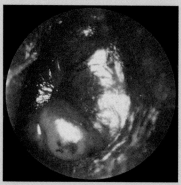

Otitis media

Perforation of Tympanic Membrane

Perforation of the tympanic membrane may result from *otitis media.* Perforation may also result from foreign bodies in the external acoustic meatus, trauma, or excessive pressure (e.g., during scuba diving). Because the superior half of the tympanic membrane is much more vascular than the inferior half, incisions (e.g., to release pus) are made posteroinferiorly through the membrane. This incision also avoids injury to the chorda tympani nerve and auditory ossicles. Severe bleeding through a ruptured tympanic membrane and the external acoustic meatus may occur after a severe blow to the head. Fractures of the floor of the middle cranial fossa may tear the meninges and result in loss of CSF through a ruptured tympanic membrane (*CSF otorrhea,* p. 528).

MASTOIDITIS

Infections of the mastoid antrum and mastoid cells (*mastoiditis*) result from middle ear infections (*otitis media*) that cause inflammation of the mastoid process. Infections may spread superiorly into the middle cranial fossa through the petrosquamous fissure (see Fig. 8.53*A*) in children or may cause *osteomyelitis* (bone infection) of the tegmen tympani. During operations for mastoiditis, surgeons are conscious of the course of the facial nerve so that it will not be injured.

One point of access to the tympanic cavity is through the mastoid antrum. In children, only a thin plate of bone must be removed from the lateral wall of the mastoid antrum to expose the tympanic cavity. In adults, bone must be penetrated for 15 mm or more. At present, most *mastoidectomies* are endaural (i.e., performed through the posterior wall of the external acoustic meatus).

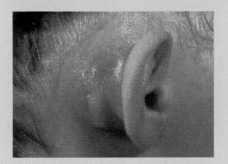

Mastoiditis (ruptured retroauricular abscess)

Auditory Ossicles

The auditory ossicles (malleus, incus, and stapes) form an articulating chain of small bones across the tympanic cavity from the tympanic membrane to the **oval window** (L. fenestra vestibuli) (Fig. 8.49*A*). The **malleus** is attached to the tympanic membrane, and the **stapes** occupies the oval window. The **incus** is located between these two bones and articulates with them. The ossicles are covered with the mucous membrane lining the tympanic cavity but, unlike other bones of the body, they are not directly covered with a layer of osteogenic periosteum. The rounded superior part, or **head of the malleus,** lies in the epitympanic recess. Its **neck** lies against the flaccid part of the tympanic membrane and its **handle** is embedded in the tympanic membrane (Fig. 8.48)—with its tip at the **umbo.** *The head of the malleus articulates with the incus;* the tendon of the *tensor tympani muscle* inserts into the handle of the malleus (Fig. 8.50). The **chorda tympani nerve** crosses the medial surface of the neck of the malleus.

The **body of the incus** lies in the epitympanic recess where it articulates with the head of the malleus. The **long limb of the incus** lies parallel to the handle of the malleus and its inferior end articulates with the stapes. The **short limb of the**

incus is connected by a ligament to the posterior wall of the tympanic cavity (Fig. 8.49*A*). The **base of the stapes** fits into the oval window on the medial wall of the tympanic cavity. Its head, directed laterally, articulates with the lenticular process of the incus. The base of the stapes is considerably smaller than the tympanic membrane; as a result, the vibratory force of the stapes is approximately 10 times over that of the tympanic membrane. Consequently, the auditory ossicles increase the force but decrease the amplitude of the vibrations transmitted from the tympanic membrane. Two muscles dampen or resist movements of the auditory ossicles; one also dampens movements (vibrations) of the tympanic membrane. The **tensor tympani** is a short muscle that arises from the superior surface of the cartilaginous part of the pharyngotympanic tube, the greater wing of the sphenoid, and the petrous part of temporal bone (Fig. 8.52). The tensor tympani inserts into the handle of the malleus. The tensor tympani—supplied by the mandibular nerve (CN V_3)—pulls the handle of the malleus medially, tensing the tympanic membrane and reducing the amplitude of its oscillations. This action tends to prevent damage to the internal ear when one is exposed to loud sounds. The **stapedius** is a tiny muscle inside the **pyramidal eminence** (Fig. 8.51), a hollow cone-shape prominence on the mastoid wall of the tympanic cavity. Its tendon enters the tympanic cavity by emerging from a pinpoint foramen in the apex of the pyramidal eminence and inserts on the neck of the stapes. The nerve to the stapedius arises from the facial nerve (CN VII). The stapedius pulls the stapes posteriorly and tilts its base in the oval window, thereby tightening the anular ligament and reducing the oscillatory range. It also prevents excessive movement of the stapes.

Pharyngotympanic Tube

The pharyngotympanic (auditory) tube connects the tympanic cavity to the nasopharynx (Fig. 8.52), where it opens posterior to the inferior meatus of the nasal cavity. The posterolateral third of the tube is bony and the remainder is cartilaginous. The pharyngotympanic tube is lined by mucous membrane that is continuous posteriorly with the lining of the tympanic cavity and anteriorly with the lining of the nasopharynx. *The function of the pharyngotympanic tube is to equalize pressure in the middle ear with the atmospheric pressure, thereby allowing free movement of the tympanic membrane.* By allowing air to enter and leave the tympanic cavity, this tube balances the pressure on both sides of the membrane. Because the walls of the cartilaginous part of the tube are normally in apposition, the tube must be actively opened. The tube is opened by the enlarged belly of the contracted **levator veli palatini** (Fig. 8.52) pushing against one wall while the **tensor veli palatini** pulls on the other. Because these are muscles of the soft palate, equalizing pressure ("popping the eardrums") is commonly associated with activities such as yawning and swallowing.

The **arteries of the pharyngotympanic tube** are derived from the *ascending pharyngeal artery,* a branch of the external carotid artery, the *middle meningeal artery,* and the *artery of the pterygoid canal*—branches of the maxillary artery (Fig. 8.42). The **veins of the pharyngotympanic tube** drain into the *pterygoid venous plexus* (p. 550). The **nerves of the pharyngotympanic tube** arise from the **tympanic plexus** (Fig. 8.51), which is formed by fibers of the facial and glossopharyngeal nerves. The anterior part of the tube also receives nerve fibers from the **pterygopalatine ganglion** (Fig. 8.46*B*).

PARALYSIS OF STAPEDIUS

The tympanic muscles have a protective action in that they dampen large vibrations of the tympanic membrane resulting from loud noises. Paralysis of the stapedius muscle (e.g., resulting from a lesion of the facial nerve) is associated with excessive acuteness of hearing—*hyperacusis* or hyperacusia. This condition results from uninhibited movements of the stapes.

BLOCKAGE OF PHARYNGOTYMPANIC TUBE

The pharyngotympanic tube forms a route for infections to pass from the nasopharynx to the tympanic cavity. This tube is blocked easily by swelling of its mucous membrane, even as a result of mild infections, because the walls of its cartilaginous part are normally already in apposition. When the pharyngotympanic tube is occluded, residual air in the tympanic cavity is usually absorbed into the mucosal blood vessels, resulting in lower pressure in the tympanic cavity, retraction of the tympanic membrane, and interference with its free movement. Finally, hearing is affected. The more sudden, usually temporary, pressure changes resulting from air flight can be equalized by swallowing (stimulated by gum chewing) or yawning; these movements open the pharyngotympanic tubes.

INTERNAL EAR

The internal ear contains the *vestibular* and *cochlear labyrinths* concerned with the reception of sound and the maintenance of balance, respectively. Buried in the petrous part of the temporal bone (Fig. 8.53*A*), the internal ear consists of the sacs and ducts of the **membranous labyrinth.** This labyrinth—containing *endolymph*—is suspended in the **bony labyrinth** by *perilymph;* both fluids carry sound waves to the end organs for hearing and balancing (Fig. 8.53, *B* and *C*).

Bony Labyrinth

The bony labyrinth of the internal ear is a series of cavities composed of three parts: cochlea, vestibule, and semicircular canals. It occupies

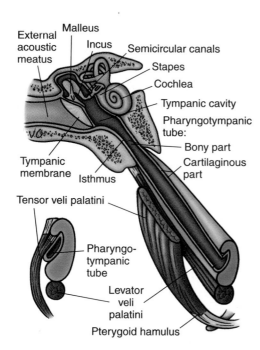

FIGURE 8.52   Right pharyngotympanic (auditory) tube. Anterior view. The tube is open throughout its length by removal of its membranous wall and the lateral part of its bony wall.

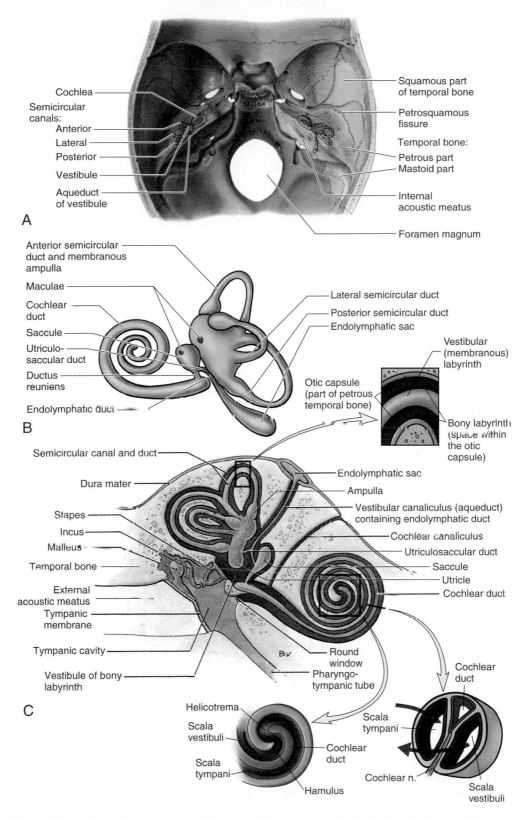

FIGURE 8.53 **Internal ear. A.** Parts of the temporal bone and bony labyrinth, in situ. Superior view. **B.** Left vestibular labyrinth. Anterolateral view. **C.** General scheme of the ear showing the relationship of the middle and internal parts. Superior view of a schematic transverse section of the right side. Observe that the membranous labyrinth is suspended in the bony labyrinth.

much of the lateral part of the petrous part of the temporal bone (Fig. 8.53). Its walls are made of bone that is denser than the remainder of the petrous temporal bone and constitutes the bony **otic capsule,** which can be isolated (carved) from the surrounding matrix of bone using a dental drill. The otic capsule is often illustrated and identified as being the **bony labyrinth;** however, the bony labyrinth is the *fluid-filled space,* which is surrounded by the otic capsule (Fig. 8.53C). The **cochlea** is the shell-shaped part of the bony labyrinth that contains the **cochlear duct**—the part of the membranous labyrinth that contains the organ of hearing. The *spiral canal of the cochlea* begins at the vestibule of the bony labyrinth and makes 2.5 turns around a bony core, the cone-shaped *modiolus,* in which there are canals for blood vessels and for distribution of the cochlear nerve (Fig. 8.54). The large basal turn of the cochlea produces the *promontory* on the medial wall of the tympanic cavity (Fig. 8.50).

The small oval chamber—the **vestibule of the bony labyrinth**—contains the **utricle** and **saccule**—parts of the balancing apparatus (membranous labyrinth). The vestibule features the **oval window** on its lateral wall, occupied by the base of the stapes (Fig. 8.49A). The vestibule is continuous with the bony cochlea anteriorly, the semicircular canals posteriorly, and the posterior cranial fossa by the **vestibular canaliculus** (aqueduct). The canaliculus extends to the posterior surface of the petrous part of the temporal bone, where it opens posterolateral to the *internal acoustic meatus.* The canaliculus transmits the **endolymphatic duct** and two small blood vessels. The **cochlear canaliculus** communicates with the subarachnoid space. The **semicircular canals** (anterior, posterior, and lateral) communicate with the vestibule of the bony labyrinth. The canals lie posterosuperior to the vestibule into which they open and are set at right angles to each other. They occupy three planes in space (Fig. 8.53B). Each semicircular canal forms about two thirds of a circle and is about 1.5 mm in diameter, except at one end where there is a swelling—the **ampulla.** The canals have only five openings into the vestibule because the anterior and posterior canals share a *common*

limb. Lodged within the canals are the **semicircular ducts** of the membranous labyrinth.

Membranous Labyrinth

The membranous labyrinth consists of a series of communicating sacs and ducts that are suspended in the bony labyrinth (Fig. 8.53). The membranous labyrinth contains *endolymph,* a watery fluid that differs in composition from the *perilymph* that fills the remainder of the bony labyrinth. *The membranous labyrinth consists of three parts:*

- Utricle and saccule, two small communicating sacs in the vestibule of the bony labyrinth
- Three semicircular ducts in the semicircular canals
- Cochlear duct in the cochlea.

The membranous labyrinth is suspended in the bony labyrinth; its chief divisions are the *cochlear labyrinth* and the *vestibular labyrinth.* The **spiral ligament** (Fig. 8.54), a spiral thickening of the periosteal lining of the cochlear canal, *secures the cochlear duct to the cochlear canal of the cochlea.* The various parts of the membranous labyrinth form a closed system of sacs and ducts that communicate with one another. The **semicircular ducts** open into the utricle through five openings, reflective of the way the surrounding semicircular canals open into the vestibule. The utricle communicates with the saccule through the **utriculosaccular duct** from which the **endolymphatic duct** arises (Fig. 8.53C). The saccule is continuous with the cochlear duct through a narrow communication—the **ductus reuniens** (Fig. 8.53B).

The utricle and saccule have specialized areas of sensory epithelium—the maculae. The **macula of the utricle** (L. macula utriculi) is in the floor of the utricle (Fig. 8.53B), whereas the **macula of the saccule** (L. macula sacculi) is vertically placed on the medial wall of the saccule. The *hair cells in the maculae* are innervated by fibers of the vestibular division of the *vestibulocochlear nerve* (CN VIII). The cell bodies of the sensory neurons are in the *vestibular ganglion,* which is in the **internal acoustic meatus** (Fig. 8.53A). The **endolymphatic duct** traverses the

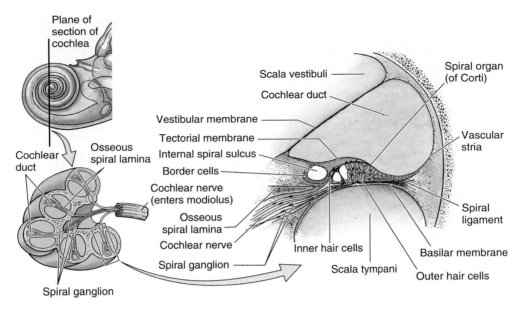

FIGURE 8.54 **Structure of the cochlea.** Section of the cochlea and spiral organ.

vestibular canaliculus (aqueduct) of the bony labyrinth and emerges through the bone of the posterior cranial fossa, where it expands into a blind pouch—the **endolymphatic sac.** It is located under the dura on the posterior surface of the petrous part of the temporal bone (Fig. 8.53, *A* and *C*). The endolymphatic sac is a storage reservoir for excess endolymph formed by the blood capillaries within the membranous labyrinth.

Each **semicircular duct** has an **ampulla** at one end containing a sensory area, the *ampullary crest* (L. crista ampullaris). The crests are sensors for recording movements of the endolymph in the ampulla resulting from rotation of the head in the plane of the duct. The hair cells of the crest, like those of the maculae, stimulate primary sensory neurons whose cell bodies are also in the *vestibular ganglia.*

The **cochlear duct** is a spiral, blind tube, triangular in cross-section (Fig. 8.53*C*), and firmly suspended across the cochlear canal between the **spiral ligament** on the external wall of the cochlear canal and the **osseous spiral lamina** of the modiolus (Fig. 8.54). Spanning the cochlear canal in this manner, the endolymph-filled cochlear duct divides the perilymph-filled spiral canal into two channels that

communicate at the apex of the cochlea at the **helicotrema** (Fig. 8.53*C*). Waves of hydraulic pressure created in the perilymph of the vestibule by the vibrations of the base of the stapes ascend to the apex of the cochlea by one channel, the **scala vestibuli;** then the pressure waves pass through the helicotrema and then descend back to the basal turn by the other channel, the **scala tympani.** There the pressure waves again become vibrations, this time of the *secondary tympanic membrane,* which occupies the **round window.** Here the energy initially received by the (primary) tympanic membrane is finally dissipated into the air of the tympanic cavity.

The roof of the cochlear duct is formed by the **vestibular membrane** (Fig. 8.54). The floor of the duct is formed by part of the duct, the **basilar membrane,** plus the outer edge of the **osseous spiral lamina.** The receptor of auditory stimuli is the **spiral organ** (of Corti), situated on the basilar membrane. It is overlaid by the gelatinous **tectorial membrane.** The spiral organ contains **hair cells,** the tips of which are embedded in the tectorial membrane. The spiral organ is stimulated to respond by deformation of the cochlear duct induced by hydraulic pressure waves in the perilymph, which ascend and descend in the surrounding scala vestibuli and tympani in the endolymph by sound waves.

Internal Acoustic Meatus

The internal acoustic meatus is a narrow canal that runs laterally for approximately 1 cm within the petrous part of the temporal bone (Fig. 8.53A). The opening of the meatus is in the posteromedial part of this bone, in line with the external acoustic meatus. The internal acoustic meatus is closed at its lateral end by a thin, perforated plate of bone that separates it from the internal ear. Through this plate pass the *facial nerve* (CN VII), branches of the *vestibulocochlear nerve* (CN VIII), and labyrinthine artery and vein. The vestibulocochlear nerve divides near the lateral end of the internal acoustic meatus into two parts, a *cochlear nerve* and a *vestibular nerve*.

MOTION SICKNESS

The maculae of the membranous labyrinth are primarily static organs, which have small dense particles—otoliths—embedded among the hair cells. Under the influence of gravity, the *otoliths* cause bending of the hair cells, which stimulate the vestibular nerve and provide awareness of the position of the head in space; the hairs also respond to quick tilting movements and to linear acceleration and deceleration. *Motion sickness* results mainly from fluctuating stimulation of the maculae.

High Tone Deafness

Persistent exposure to excessively loud sounds causes degenerative changes in the spiral organ, resulting in *high tone deafness*. This type of hearing loss commonly occurs in workers who are exposed to loud noises and do not wear protective earmuffs (e.g., persons working for long periods around jet engines). It has also been determined that individuals associated with chronic exposure to high volume stereo music via earphones exhibit high tone deafness.

Otic Barotrauma

Injury caused to the ear by an imbalance in pressure between ambient (surrounding) air and the air in the middle ear is called *otic barotrauma*. This type of injury occurs in fliers and divers.

MEDICAL IMAGING OF HEAD

Radiographs are a reliable method of detecting cranial fractures. Because crania vary considerably in shape, one must examine radiographs carefully for abnormalities (Fig. 8.55). **Computerized tomography** (CT) is a premier imaging method in neurodiagnosis (Fig. 8.56); it is quicker and less expensive than magnetic resonance imaging (MRI) and is more inform-

ative than plain cranial radiographs. The major advantages of CT are the speed and ease with which each image is obtained, thereby obviating problems of patient discomfort and motion. For reasons of cost, speed, and availability, CT is in wide use for evaluation of head injuries. It is especially useful for people who are neurologically or medically unstable, uncooperative, or claustrophobic, as well as for patients with pacemakers or other metallic implants.

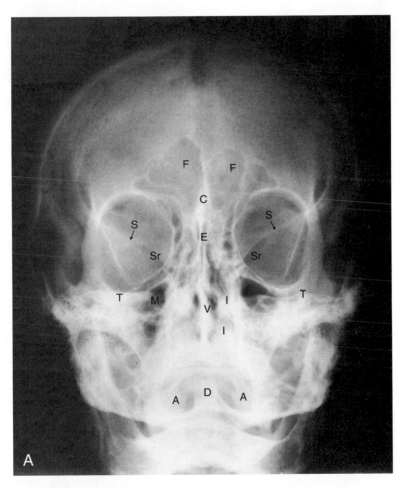

FIGURE 8.55   Radiographs of the cranium (skull). A. Anteroposterior view. Observe the superior orbital fissure (*Sr*), the lesser wings of the sphenoid (*S*), and the superior surface of the petrous part of the temporal bone (*T*). Also observe that the nasal septum is formed by the perpendicular plate of the ethmoid (*E*) and the vomer (*V*). Examine the inferior and middle conchae (*I*) of the lateral wall of the nose; the crista galli (*C*); the frontal sinus (*F*); and the maxillary sinus (*M*). Superimposed on the facial skeleton (viscerocranium or splanchnocranium) is the dens (*D*) and the lateral masses of the atlas (*A*).

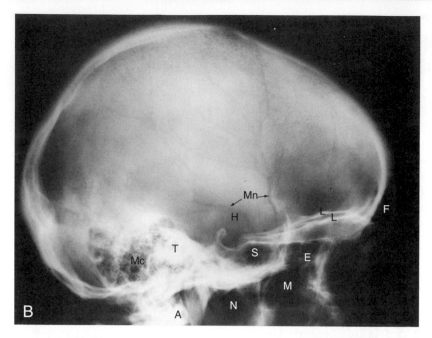

FIGURE 8.55 *Continued* **B.** Right lateral view of the cranium. Observe the paranasal sinuses: frontal (*F*), ethmoidal (*E*), sphenoidal (*S*), and maxillary (*M*). Also observe the hypophysial fossa (*H*) for the pituitary gland; the great density of the petrous part of the temporal bone (*T*); and the mastoid cells (*Mc*). Note that the right and left orbital parts of the frontal bone are not superimposed and, thus, the floor of the anterior cranial fossa appears as two lines (*L*). Observe the bony grooves for the branches of the middle meningeal vessels (*Mn*), the arch of the atlas (*A*), and the nasopharynx (*N*). (Courtesy of Dr. E. Becker, Associate Professor of Diagnostic Imaging, University of Toronto, Toronto, Ontario, Canada)

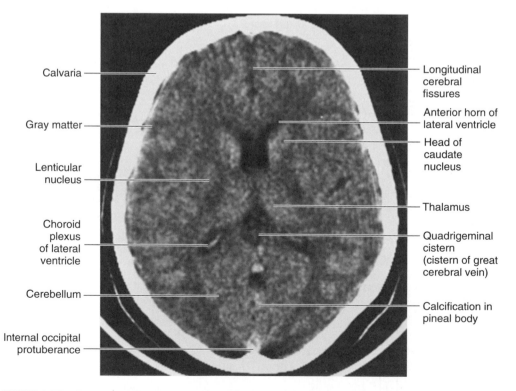

FIGURE 8.56 Transverse (axial) CT image of the brain. Observe the ventricles, various parts of the brain, and the choroid plexus of the lateral ventricle.

Magnetic resonance imaging (MRI) shows much more detail in the soft tissues than do CTs (Fig. 8.57). MRI is extremely good for detecting and delineating intracranial and spinal lesions. MRI provides good soft tissue contrast of normal and pathological struc- tures in the orbit, for example. It also per- mits multiplanar capability, which provides three-dimensional information and relation- ships that are not so readily available with CT. MRI can also demonstrate blood and CSF flow.

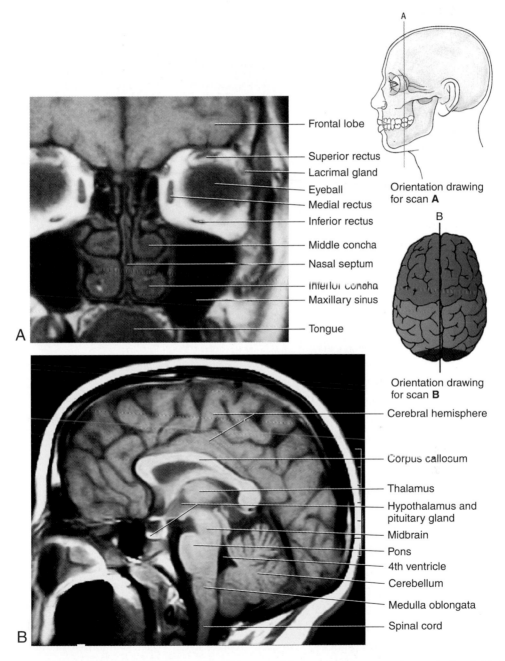

- Frontal lobe
- Superior rectus
- Lacrimal gland
- Eyeball
- Medial rectus
- Inferior rectus
- Middle concha
- Nasal septum
- Inferior concha
- Maxillary sinus
- Tongue

Orientation drawing for scan **A**

Orientation drawing for scan **B**

- Cerebral hemisphere
- Corpus callosum
- Thalamus
- Hypothalamus and pituitary gland
- Midbrain
- Pons
- 4th ventricle
- Cerebellum
- Medulla oblongata
- Spinal cord

FIGURE 8.57   **MRI images of head. A.** Frontal (coronal) MRI through the orbit and nose. **B.** Sagittal MRI of the brain.

9

Neck

*T*he neck is the major conduit between the head, trunk, and limbs. The neck (L. cervix) contains bones, muscles, vessels, nerves, and other structures connecting these areas. It also contains important endocrine glands such as the thyroid gland. The *skeleton of the neck* is formed by the seven cervical vertebrae, hyoid bone, manubrium of the sternum, and clavicles (Fig. 9.1*A*). See Chapter 5 for a description of the cervical vertebrae.

FASCIA OF NECK

Structures in the neck are compartmentalized by layers of cervical fascia. These fascial planes afford the slipperiness that allows structures in the neck to move and pass over one another without difficulty, as when swallowing and twisting the neck. The deep cervical fascial layers also determine the direction in which an infection in the neck may spread. The **subcutaneous tissue** (superficial cervical fascia) usually is a thin layer of connective tissue that lies between the dermis of the skin and the *investing layer of deep cervical fascia* (Fig. 9.1, *A* and *B*). It contains cutaneous nerves, blood and lymphatic vessels, and variable amounts of fat; anterolaterally it contains the platysma. The **muscular or deep cervical fascia** consists of three fascial layers (Fig. 9.1): **investing, pretracheal,** and **prevertebral.** These layers (sheaths) support the viscera (e.g., thyroid gland), muscles, vessels, and deep lymph nodes. *The fascial layers also form natural cleavage planes, allowing separation of tissues during surgery.* The fascial layers may deflect penetrating objects (such as knives) away from vital organs.

INVESTING LAYER OF DEEP CERVICAL FASCIA

The investing layer of deep cervical fascia—the most superficial deep fascial layer—surrounds the entire neck deep to the skin and subcutaneous tissue (Fig. 9.1, *A* and *B*). At the four "corners" of the neck, the investing layer splits into superficial and deep layers of fascia to enclose the sternocleidomastoid (SCM) and trapezius muscles. *Superiorly, the investing layer of fascia attaches to the:*

- Superior nuchal line of the occipital bone
- Mastoid processes of the temporal bones
- Zygomatic arches
- Inferior border of the mandible
- Hyoid bone
- Spinous processes of the cervical vertebrae.

Inferiorly, the investing layer of fascia attaches to the:

- Manubrium of the sternum
- Clavicles
- Acromions and spines of the scapulae.

Inferior to its attachment to the mandible, the investing layer of fascia splits to enclose the *submandibular gland;* posterior to the mandible, it splits to form the *fibrous capsule of the parotid gland.* Inferiorly, between the sternal heads of the SCM muscles and just superior to the manubrium of the sternum, the investing layer of fascia remains divided into the two layers that enclose the SCM, with one layer attaching to the anterior and the other to the posterior surface of the manubrium. A **suprasternal space** lies between these layers (Fig. 9.1*A*) and contains the inferior ends of the anterior jugular veins (AJVs), the jugular venous arch, fat, and a few deep lymph nodes.

PRETRACHEAL LAYER OF DEEP CERVICAL FASCIA

The pretracheal layer of deep cervical fascia is thin and limited to the anterior part of the neck (Fig. 9.1). This layer of fascia extends inferiorly from the **hyoid bone** into the thorax, where it blends with the fibrous pericardium covering the heart (see Chapter 2). It includes a thin *muscular layer,* which encloses the infrahyoid muscles (omohyoid, sternothyroid, sternohyoid, thyrohyoid), and a *visceral layer,* which encloses the thyroid gland, trachea, and esophagus (Fig. 9.1, *B* and *C*). The visceral layer is continuous posteriorly and superiorly with the **buccopharyngeal fascia** (Fig. 9.1*A* inset). The pretracheal layer of deep cervical fascia blends laterally with the carotid sheaths (Fig. 9.1, *B* and *C*). Each **carotid sheath** is a tubular, dense fibrous investment that extends from the base of the cranium to the root of the neck. This fascial sheath blends anteriorly with the investing and pretracheal layers of fascia and posteriorly with the prevertebral layer of deep cervical fascia.

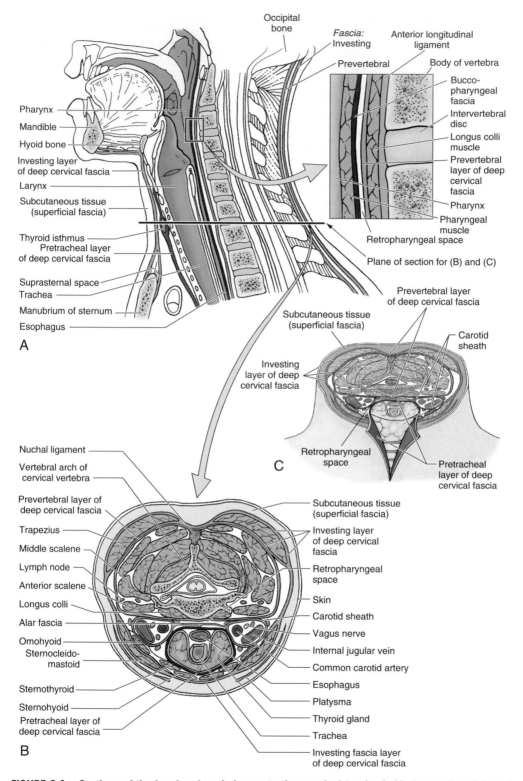

FIGURE 9.1 **Sections of the head and neck demonstrating cervical fascia. A.** Median section. Enlarged area on the right illustrates fascia in the retropharyngeal region. **B.** Superior view of the transverse section (at C7 vertebra). **C.** Anterosuperior view of **B.**

The carotid sheath contains the following major structures (Fig. 9.1*B*):

- Common (inferiorly) and internal (superiorly) carotid arteries
- Internal jugular vein (IJV)
- Vagus nerve (CN X).

Associated with these structures are the:

- Deep cervical lymph nodes
- Carotid sinus nerve
- Carotid periarterial branches of the sympathetic nerves.

PREVERTEBRAL LAYER OF DEEP CERVICAL FASCIA

The prevertebral layer of deep cervical fascia forms a tubular sheath for the vertebral column and muscles associated with it, such as the **longus colli** (Fig. 9.1). This layer of fascia extends from the base of the cranium to T3 vertebra, where it fuses with the **anterior longitudinal ligament.** It extends laterally as the axillary sheath, which surrounds the axillary vessels and brachial plexus. The **retropharyngeal space** *is a potential space consisting of loose connective tissue between the prevertebral layer of fascia and the buccopharyngeal fascia surrounding the pharynx superficially* (Fig. 9.1*A* inset). It is the largest and most important interfascial space in the neck because it is the major pathway for the spread of infection from the neck to the thorax. Inferiorly, the **buccopharyngeal fascia** is continuous with the pretracheal layer of cervical fascia. *The retropharyngeal space permits movement of the pharynx, esophagus, larynx, and trachea during swallowing.* This space is closed superiorly by the base of the cranium and on each side by the carotid sheath.

SPREAD OF INFECTION IN THE NECK
The investing layer of deep cervical fascia helps to prevent the spread of *abscesses*—circumscribed collections of pus caused by tissue destruction. If an infection occurs between the investing layer of fascia and that surrounding the infrahyoid muscles, the infection usually will not spread beyond the superior edge of the manubrium. If, however, the infection occurs between the investing and pretracheal layers of fascia, it can spread into the thoracic cavity anterior to the pericardium. Pus from an abscess posterior to the prevertebral layer of fascia may extend laterally in the neck and form a swelling posterior to the SCM. The pus may perforate the prevertebral layer of fascia and enter the *retropharyngeal space,* producing a bulge in the pharynx (*retropharyngeal abscess*). This swelling may cause difficulty in swallowing (dysphagia) and speaking (dysphonia).

SUPERFICIAL AND LATERAL NECK MUSCLES

There are three superficial muscles in the lateral aspect of the neck: platysma, SCM, and trapezius (Fig. 9.1*B*). The attachments, nerve supply, and main actions of these muscles are described in Table 9.1.

The **platysma**—*a broad, thin sheet of muscle in the subcutaneous tissue*—covers the anterolateral aspect of the neck. The superficial cervical veins and nerves are located deep to this muscle. Its fibers arise in fascia covering superior parts of the deltoid and pectoralis major muscles and sweep superomedially over the clavicle to the inferior border of the mandible. It is one of the muscles of facial expression (see Chapter 8) and is innervated by the cervical branch of the facial nerve (CN VII).

INJURY OF PLATYSMA
Paralysis of the platysma (e.g., resulting from injury to the cervical branch of the facial nerve) causes the skin to fall away from the neck in slack folds. Consequently, during surgical dissections of the neck, extra care is necessary to preserve this branch of the facial nerve. In incisions of the neck, it is imperative that the severed ends of the platysma be approximated to overcome unsightly postoperative skin defects.

The broad straplike **SCM** divides each side of the neck into anterior and posterior triangles (Fig. 9.2*A*). The SCM has two heads: the rounded tendon of the **sternal head of SCM** attaches to the manubrium of the sternum and the thick fleshy **clavicular head of SCM** attaches to the superior surface of the medial third of the clavicle. The two heads of the SCM join as they pass obliquely upward to the cranium posterior to the ear.

The **trapezius**—a large, flat, triangular muscle—covers the posterolateral aspect of the neck and thorax. It is a superficial muscle of the back, a muscle of the pectoral (shoulder) girdle, and a neck muscle. The trapezius attaches the pectoral girdle to the cranium and vertebral column and assists in suspending it.

INJURY OF SCM

Occasionally the SCM is injured when an infant's head is pulled excessively during a difficult birth, tearing its fibers. The lesion may include a branch of the accessory nerve, denervating part of the SCM. If untreated the lesion may result in *torticollis* (wry neck), a flexion deformity of the neck. There is a tilt and rotation of the head to one side and restricted rotation to the other side. Stiffness of the neck results from fibrosis and shortening of the SCM. Surgical release of a partially fibrotic SCM from its distal attachments to the manubrium and clavicle may be necessary to enable the person to tilt and rotate the head normally.

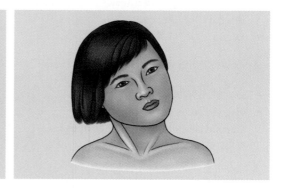

TABLE 9.1.   **SUPERFICIAL MUSCLES IN THE LATERAL ASPECT OF THE NECK**

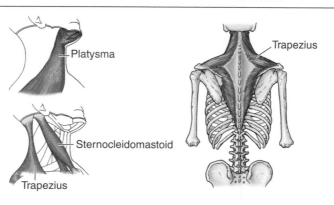

Muscle	Superior Attachment	Inferior Attachment	Innervation	Main Action(s)
Platysma	Inferior border of mandible, skin, and subcutaneous tissues of lower face	Fascia covering superior parts of pectoralis major and deltoid muscles	Cervical branch of facial nerve	Draws corners of mouth inferiorly and widens it as in expressions of sadness and fright; draws the skin of neck superiorly when teeth are "clenched"
Sternocleido-mastoid	Lateral surface of mastoid process of temporal bone and lateral half of superior nuchal line	Sternal head: anterior surface of manubrium of sternum Clavicular head: superior surface of medial third of clavicle	Spinal root of accessory nerve (motor) and C2 and C3 nerves (pain and proprioception)	Tilts head to one side, i.e., laterally; flexes neck and rotates it so face is turned superiorly toward opposite side; acting together, the two muscles flex the neck so chin is thrust forward
Trapezius	Medial third of superior nuchal line, external occipital protuberance, nuchal ligament, spinous processes of C7–T12 vertebrae, and lumbar and sacral spinous processes	Lateral third of clavicle, acromion, and spine of scapula	Spinal root of accessory nerve (motor) and C3 and C4 nerves (pain and proprioception)	Elevates, retracts, and rotates scapula; superior fibers elevate the scapula, middle fibers retract it, and inferior fibers depress it

Surface Anatomy of Neck

The skin of the neck is thin and pliable. The subcutaneous connective tissue contains the **platysma** (indicated by arrows). It can be observed by asking the person to contract it by pretending to ease a tight collar. The broad

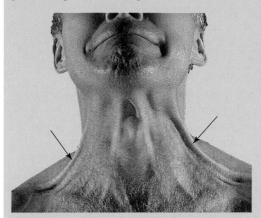

SCM—*the key landmark of the neck*—divides the neck into anterior and posterior triangles. It is easy to observe and palpate throughout its length as it passes superolaterally from the clavicle and manubrium to the mastoid process of the temporal bone. The SCM stands out when one moves the chin to the shoulder on the opposite side. The SCM is crossed by the platysma and EJV. This vein may be prominent, especially if the person is asked to take a breath and bear down (*Valsalva maneuver*). The **jugular notch** in the manubrium is easily palpated in the fossa between the sternal heads of the SCM. A slight triangular depression lies between the sternal and clavicular heads of the SCM. The inferior end of the IJV lies deep to this depression, where it can be entered by a needle or catheter. Deep to the superior half of the SCM lies the **cervical plexus**—a network of adjacent anterior primary rami of the first four cervical nerves (Fig. 9.4*B*). Deep to the inferior half of the SCM are the IJV, common carotid artery, and vagus nerve in the carotid sheath. Feel the narrow, tendinous sternal head of your left SCM. Move your finger laterally and palpate the broader clavicular head of the SCM. Lateral to this head is a large depression, the **supraclavicular fossa**. Another large muscle of importance in the neck is the **trapezius**. It can be observed and palpated by asking the person to shrug their shoulder against resistance.

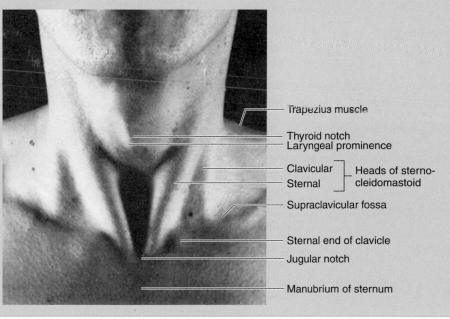

Trapezius muscle

Thyroid notch
Laryngeal prominence

Clavicular — Heads of sterno-
Sternal — cleidomastoid

Supraclavicular fossa

Sternal end of clavicle

Jugular notch

Manubrium of sternum

Essential Clinical Anatomy

TRIANGLES OF NECK

To facilitate description of cervical anatomy, each side of the neck is divided into anterior and posterior triangles by the obliquely placed SCM (Fig. 9.2).

The **posterior triangle of the neck has:**

- An *anterior boundary,* formed by the posterior border of the SCM
- A *posterior boundary,* formed by the anterior border of the trapezius
- An *inferior boundary,* formed by the middle third of the clavicle between the trapezius and SCM
- Its *apex,* where the SCM and trapezius meet on the superior nuchal line of the occipital bone
- A *roof,* formed by the investing layer of deep cervical fascia
- A *floor,* formed by muscles covered by the prevertebral layer of deep cervical fascia.

For more precise location of cervical structures, the posterior triangle is subdivided into supraclavicular and occipital triangles by the inferior belly of the omohyoid muscle (Fig. 9.2*B*).

The **anterior triangle of the neck has:**

- An *anterior boundary,* formed by the median line of the neck
- A *posterior boundary,* formed by the anterior border of the SCM
- A *superior boundary,* formed by the inferior border of the mandible
- An *apex* at the jugular notch in the manubrium of the sternum
- A *roof,* formed by subcutaneous tissue containing platysma
- A *floor,* formed by the pharynx, larynx, and thyroid gland covered by the pretracheal layer of deep cervical fascia.

The anterior triangle is subdivided into the unpaired **submental triangle** and three small paired triangles (**submandibular, carotid,** and **muscular**) by the digastric and omohyoid muscles (Fig. 9.2*B*). The contents of the triangles of the neck are listed in Table 9.2.

TABLE 9.2.   CONTENTS OF TRIANGLES OF NECK

Posterior Triangle	Main Contents
Occipital triangle	Part of external jugular vein, posterior branches of cervical plexus of nerves, accessory nerve, trunks of brachial plexus, transverse cervical artery, cervical lymph nodes
Supraclavicular (omoclavicular, subclavian) triangle	Subclavian artery (3rd part), part of subclavian vein (sometimes), supracapular artery, supraclavicular lymph nodes

Anterior Triangle	Main Contents
Submandibular (digastric) triangle	Submandibular gland almost fills triangle; submandibular lymph nodes, hypoglossal nerve, mylohyoid nerve, parts of facial artery and vein
Submental triangle	Submental lymph nodes, small veins that unite to form anterior jugular vein
Carotid triangle	Carotid sheath containing common carotid artery and its branches, internal jugular vein and its tributaries, and vagus nerve; external carotid artery and some of its branches; hypoglossal nerve and superior root of ansa cervicalis; accessory nerve; thyroid, larynx, and pharynx; deep cervical lymph nodes; branches of cervical plexus
Muscular (omotracheal) triangle	Sternothyroid and sternohyoid muscles, thyroid and parathyroid glands

598

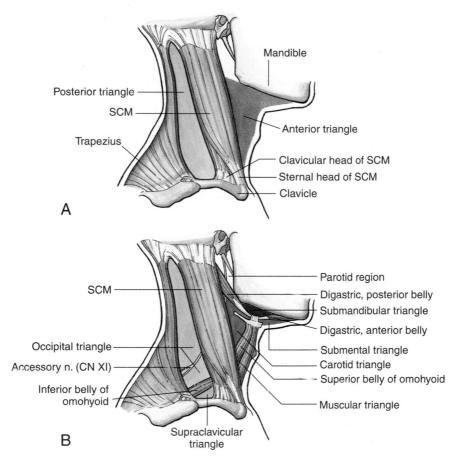

FIGURE 9.2 **Triangles of the neck.** Lateral views. **A.** Anterior and posterior triangles. **B.** Subdivisions of the anterior and posterior triangles.

POSTERIOR TRIANGLE

The posterior triangle is the region of the neck bounded by the SCM, trapezius, and clavicle (Figs. 9.2 and 9.3). The triangle wraps around the lateral surface of the neck like a spiral and is covered by skin and subcutaneous tissue containing the platysma. The **floor of the posterior triangle** is formed by the prevertebral layer of deep cervical fascia overlying four muscles (Table 9.3): splenius capitis, levator scapulae, middle scalene, and posterior scalene. Sometimes part of the anterior scalene muscle appears in the inferomedial angle of the triangle. Inferiorly, the posterior triangle is crossed by the **inferior belly of the omohyoid** (Fig. 9.2B). This muscle belly divides the pos-

terior triangle into the occipital and supraclavicular triangles. The important nerve crossing the **occipital triangle** is the **accessory nerve** (CN XI). The small **supraclavicular triangle** is bounded by the clavicle, the inferior belly of the omohyoid muscle, and the SCM. The external jugular vein (EJV) and **suprascapular artery** cross this triangle superficially, and the **subclavian artery** lies deep in it (Fig. 9.4B). The **EJV** begins near the angle of the mandible by the union of the posterior division of the **retromandibular vein** and the **posterior auricular vein** (Fig. 9.3). The EJV crosses the superficial surface of the SCM, deep to the platysma, and then pierces the investing layer of deep cervical fascia forming

TABLE 9.3.   MUSCLES OF POSTERIOR TRIANGLE (LATERAL PREVERTEBRAL MUSCLES)

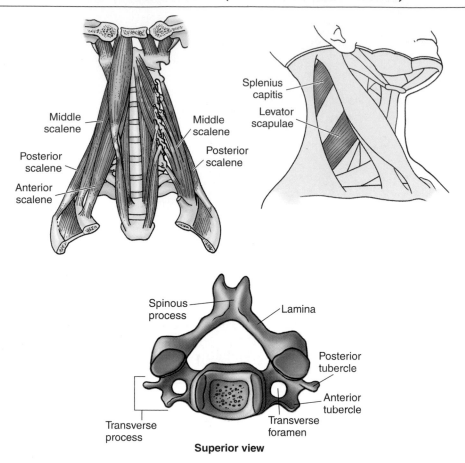

Superior view

Muscle	Superior Attachment	Inferior Attachment	Innervation	Main Action(s)
Splenius capitis	Inferior half of nuchal ligament and spinous processes of superior six thoracic vertebrae	Lateral aspect of mastoid process and lateral third of superior nuchal line	Posterior rami of middle cervical spinal nerves	Laterally flexes and rotates head and neck to same side; acting bilaterally, they extend head and neck[a]
Levator scapulae	Transverse process of C1–C2, posterior tubercles of transverse processes of C3–C4 vertebrae	Superior part of medial border of scapula	Dorsal scapular nerve (C5) and cervical spinal nerves (C3) and (C4)	Elevates scapula and tilts its glenoid cavity inferiorly by rotating scapula
Posterior scalene	Posterior tubercles of transverse processes of C4–C6 vertebrae	External border of 2nd rib	Anterior rami of cervical spinal nerves C7 and C8	Flexes neck laterally; elevates 2nd rib during forced inspiration
Middle scalene	Posterior tubercules of transverse processes of C3–C7 vertebrae	Superior surface of 1st rib, posterior groove for subclavian artery	Anterior rami of cervical spinal nerves	Flexes neck laterally; elevates 1st rib during forced inspiration
Anterior scalene	Anterior tubercules of transverse processes of C3–C7 vertebrae	1st rib	Cervical spine nerves C4, C5, and C6	Elevates 1st rib; laterally flexes and rotates neck

[a]Rotation of head occurs at atlantoaxial joints (p. 289).

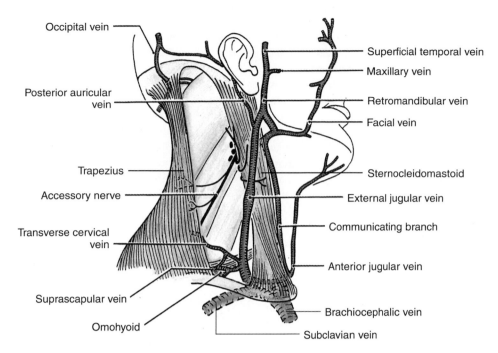

Occipital vein

Superficial temporal vein

Maxillary vein

Posterior auricular vein

Retromandibular vein

Facial vein

Trapezius

Accessory nerve

Sternocleidomastoid

External jugular vein

Transverse cervical vein

Communicating branch

Anterior jugular vein

Suprascapular vein

Brachiocephalic vein

Omohyoid

Subclavian vein

FIGURE 9.3 **Superficial veins of the right side of the neck.** Lateral view.

the roof of the posterior triangle at the posterior border of the SCM. The EJV descends to the inferior part of the triangle and terminates in the **subclavian vein.** Just superior to the clavicle, the EJV receives the **transverse cervical, suprascapular,** and **anterior jugular veins.** The major venous channel draining the upper limb, the **subclavian vein,** courses through the inferior part of the posterior triangle, passing anterior to the anterior scalene muscle and phrenic nerve (Fig. 9.4*B*). The subclavian vein joins the **IJV** to form the **brachiocephalic vein** posterior to the medial end of the clavicle (Figs. 9.3 and 9.4*B*).

SUBCLAVIAN VEIN PUNCTURE
The right subclavian vein often is the point of entry to the venous system for *central line placement.* This technique is used to administer parenteral fluids (nutritional fluid not introduced via the digestive system) and medications and to measure central venous pressure. The pleura and/or the subclavian artery are in danger of puncture during this procedure.

Prominence of External Jugular Vein
When venous pressure is within the normal range, the blood distending the EJV is either not apparent or observable for only a short distance at the base of the neck. However, when the pressure rises—as during *heart failure,* for example—the EJV becomes prominent throughout its course along the side of the neck. Consequently, routine observation for distention of the EJV during physical examinations may reveal diagnostic signs of *heart failure,* obstruction of the superior vena cava (e.g., by tumor cells), enlarged supraclavicular lymph nodes, or *increased intrathoracic pressure.*

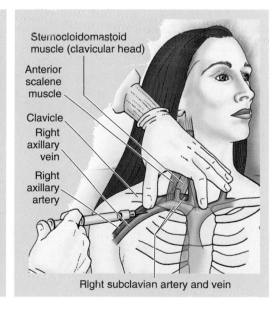

Sternocloidomastoid muscle (clavicular head)

Anterior scalene muscle

Clavicle

Right axillary vein

Right axillary artery

Right subclavian artery and vein

Arteries in Posterior Triangle

The arteries in the posterior triangle are the **transverse cervical** and **suprascapular arteries,** the third part of the **subclavian artery,** and part of the occipital artery (Fig. 9.4*B*). The **transverse cervical artery** originates from the **thyrocervical trunk,** a branch of the **subclavian artery.** The transverse cervical artery runs a primarily posteriorly directed course. Initially it runs superficially and laterally across the **phrenic nerve** and anterior scalene muscle, superior to the clavicle. The transverse cervical artery then crosses the **superior trunk of the brachial plexus** and passes beneath the trapezius, which it supplies. The superficial branch of the transverse cervical artery may arise independently from the thyrocervical trunk; in such cases it is known as the superficial cervical artery. The **suprascapular artery,** also a branch of the thyrocervical trunk, passes inferolaterally across the anterior scalene muscle and phrenic nerve. It then crosses the subclavian artery (third part) and brachial plexus and passes posterior to the scapula to supply muscles on the posterior aspect of this bone. The **occipital artery,** a branch of the external carotid artery (Figs. 9.5*A* and 9.6*B*), enters the posterior triangle at it superior angle and ascends on the back of the head to supply the posterior half of the scalp. The **third part of the subclavian artery,** supplying blood to the upper limb, lies posterosuperior to the subclavian vein in the inferior part of the posterior triangle (Fig. 9.4*B*). This is the most superficial part of the subclavian artery, and its pulsations can be felt on deep pressure in the supraclavicular triangle (Fig. 9.2*B*). Posteroinferiorly, the third part of the subclavian artery lies against the 1st rib; consequently, compression of it against the rib can control bleeding in the upper limb.

Nerves of Posterior Triangle

The **accessory nerve** (CN XI) has cranial and spinal roots (see Chapter 10). The *spinal root of the accessory nerve* separates immediately from the cranial root before exiting the jugular foramen of the cranium and enters the posterior triangle at or inferior to the junction of the superior and middle thirds of the posterior border of the SCM (Fig. 9.4*A*). It passes posteroinferiorly through the triangle, *superficial to the investing layer of deep cervical fascia.* CN XI then disappears deep to the anterior border of the trapezius at the junction of its superior two thirds with its inferior one third. The spinal root of CN XI passes deep to the SCM, supplying it before crossing the posterior triangle to supply the trapezius.

DISSECTIONS IN POSTERIOR TRIANGLE

Care is essential during surgical dissections in the posterior triangle inferior to the accessory nerve (CN XI) because of the presence of many vessels and nerves. To preserve the continuity of CN XI during dissections for removal of cancerous lymph nodes, for example, the nerve is isolated at the outset and separated from the nodes.

Lesions of Spinal Root of CN XI

Lesions of this root are uncommon; however, the nerve may be damaged by traumatic injury, neck lacerations, and surgical neck dissections. A unilateral lesion usually does not produce an abnormal position of the head; however, weakness can occur in turning the head to one side against resistance. *Drooping of the shoulder* is an obvious sign of injury to the spinal root of CN XI. *Unilateral paralysis of the trapezius* is evident by the patient's inability to elevate and retract the shoulder and by difficulty in elevating the arm superior to the horizontal level.

The **anterior rami of the spinal nerves** comprising the roots of the brachial plexus appear in the neck between the anterior and middle scalene muscles. Five rami (C5 through C8 and T1) unite to form the three **trunks of the brachial plexus** (Fig. 9.4*B*) that descend inferolaterally through the posterior triangle. The plexus then passes between the lst rib and clavicle (*cervicoaxillary canal*) and enters the axilla, providing innervation for most of the upper limb (see Chapter 7). The **cervical plexus** is located in the posterior triangle (Fig. 9.4*A*).

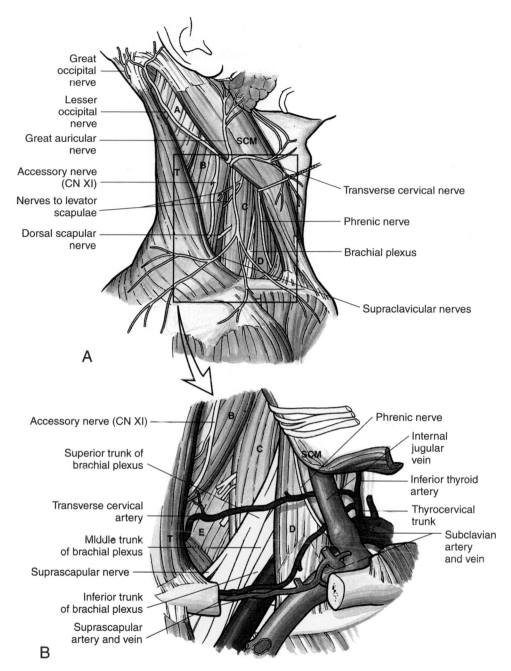

FIGURE 9.4   Dissections of the posterior triangle of the neck. Lateral views. **A.** Cervical plexus and muscles. **B.** Closer view of the brachial plexus, subclavian vessels, and muscles. *A,* splenius capitis; *B,* levator scapulae; *C,* middle scalene; *D,* anterior scalene; *E,* posterior scalene; *T,* trapezius; *SCM,* sternocleidomastoid.

This plexus, formed by union of the adjacent anterior rami of the first four cervical nerves, lies deep to the IJV and SCM. Cutaneous branches from the plexus emerge around the middle of the posterior border of the SCM and supply the skin of the neck and scalp. Close to their origin, the nerves of the cervical plexus receive communicating branches (L. rami communicantes), most of which descend from the *superior cervical ganglion* (cluster of postsynaptic neurons) in the superior part of the neck. The **branches of the cervical plexus** arising from the loop between C2 and C3 (Fig. 9.4*A*) are the:

- **Lesser occipital nerve** (C2), supplying the skin of the neck and scalp posterosuperior to the auricle
- **Great auricular nerve** (C2 and C3), ascending diagonally across the SCM onto the parotid gland, where it divides and supplies skin over the gland, posterior aspect of the auricle, and an area extending from the angle of the mandible to the mastoid process
- **Transverse cervical nerve** (C2 and C3), supplying the skin covering the anterior triangle; the nerve curves around the middle of the posterior border of the SCM and crosses it anteriorly and deep to the platysma.

Branches of the cervical plexus arising from the loop formed between the anterior rami of C3 and C4 are the **supraclavicular nerves,** which emerge as a common trunk under cover of the SCM and send small branches to the skin of the neck (Fig. 9.4*A*); they then cross the clavicle and supply skin over the shoulder. Branches of the anterior primary rami of cervical nerves supply the rhomboids (dorsal scapular nerve [C4 and C5], serratus anterior, long thoracic nerve [C5, **C6,** and C7]) and nearby prevertebral muscles. The **supra-scapular nerve,** which arises from the *superior trunk of the brachial plexus* (Fig. 9.4*B*), runs laterally across the posterior triangle to supply the supraspinatus and infraspinatus muscles; it also sends branches to the glenohumeral (shoulder) joint.

The **phrenic nerve** originates chiefly from the 4th cervical nerve (C4) but receives contributions from the 3rd and 5th cervical nerves (C3 and C5). *It contains motor, sensory, and sympathetic nerve fibers.* The pair of phrenic nerves provides the sole motor supply to the diaphragm as well as sensation to its central part. In the neck each phrenic nerve forms at the superior part of the lateral border of the anterior scalene muscle at the level of the superior border of the thyroid cartilage. Each nerve receives variable communicating fibers from the cervical sympathetic ganglia or their branches. Each phrenic nerve descends obliquely with the IJV across the anterior scalene muscle, deep to the prevertebral layer of the deep cervical fascia and the transverse cervical and suprascapular arteries. *On the left,* the phrenic nerve crosses the first part of the subclavian artery; *on the right,* it crosses anterior to the second part of this artery. On each side, the phrenic nerve runs posterior to the subclavian vein and anterior to the internal thoracic artery as it enters the thorax. The contribution from C5 to the phrenic nerve may derive from an *accessory phrenic nerve,* which is frequently a branch of the nerve to the subclavius. If present, the accessory phrenic nerve lies lateral to the main nerve and descends posterior and sometimes inferior to the subclavian vein. The accessory phrenic nerve joins the phrenic nerve either in the root of the neck or in the thorax.

SEVERANCE OF PHRENIC NERVE AND PHRENIC NERVE BLOCK

Severance of a phrenic nerve results in paralysis of the corresponding half of the diaphragm. A *phrenic nerve block* will produce a short period of paralysis of the diaphragm on one side (e.g., for a lung operation). The anesthetic agent is injected around the nerve where it lies on the anterior surface of the anterior scalene muscle.

Cervical and Brachial Plexus Blocks

Regional anesthesia often is used for surgical procedures in the neck region or upper limb. In a **cervical plexus block,** an anesthetic agent is injected at several points along the posterior border of the SCM, mainly at the junction of its superior and inferior thirds—the *nerve point of the neck.* For anesthesia of the upper limb, a **supraclavicular brachial plexus block** often is used where an anesthetic is injected into the axillary sheath around the supraclavicular part of the brachial plexus. The main injection site is superior to the midpoint of the clavicle.

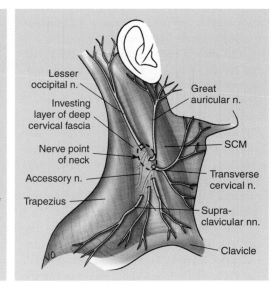

Lesser occipital n.
Great auricular n.
Investing layer of deep cervical fascia
Nerve point of neck
SCM
Accessory n.
Transverse cervical n.
Trapezius
Supra-clavicular nn.
Clavicle

ANTERIOR TRIANGLE

The anterior triangle of the neck is bounded by the anterior border of the SCM, the anterior midline of the neck, and the mandible. The anterior triangle is subdivided into four smaller triangles for descriptive purposes (Fig. 9.2, Table 9.2). The **submandibular triangle** is a glandular area between the inferior border of the mandible and the anterior and posterior bellies of the *digastric muscle* (Fig. 9.5). The **submandibular gland** nearly fills this triangle. The **submandibular duct** passes from the deep process of the submandibular gland, parallel to the tongue, to open by one to three orifices into the oral cavity. The *floor of the submandibular triangle* is formed by the mylohyoid muscle, hyoglossus muscle, and middle constrictor muscle of the pharynx (Fig. 9.5). **Submandibular lymph nodes** lie on each side of the submandibular gland and along the inferior border of the mandible. The **hypoglossal nerve** (CN XII), motor to the muscles of the tongue, passes into the submandibular triangle, as do the **nerve to the mylohyoid muscle,** parts of the **facial artery** and **vein,** and the **submental artery,** a branch of the facial artery (Fig. 9.5*B*).

The unpaired **submental triangle** is inferior to the chin. The *apex of the triangle* is at the mandibular symphysis and the *base of the triangle* is formed by the **hyoid bone.** Laterally it is bounded by the right and left anterior bellies of the *digastric muscles. The floor of the submental triangle* is formed by the two mylohyoid muscles, which meet in a median **fibrous raphe** (Fig. 9.5*C*). The submental triangle contains several small **submental lymph nodes.** The triangle also contains small veins that unite to form the **AJV.**

The **carotid triangle** is a vascular area bounded by the superior belly of the omohyoid, the posterior belly of the digastric, and the anterior border of the SCM (Fig. 9.5*A*). The **common carotid artery** ascends into the carotid triangle. At the level of the superior border of the thyroid cartilage (C4 vertebral level), the common carotid artery divides into the **internal** and **external carotid arteries** (Fig. 9.6*A*). At this bifurcation there is a slight dilation of the proximal part of the internal carotid artery—the **carotid sinus** (Fig. 9.6, *B* and *C*). Innervated principally by the glossopharyngeal nerve (CN IX) through the **carotid sinus nerve,** as well as the vagus nerve, *the carotid sinus is a* *baroreceptor (pressoreceptor) that is stimulated by changes in arterial blood pressure.*

The **carotid body,** an ovoid mass of tissue, lies on the medial (deep) side of the bifurcation of the common carotid artery in close relation to the carotid sinus (Fig. 9.6*C*). Supplied mainly by the carotid sinus nerve and CN X, *the carotid body is a chemoreceptor that monitors the level of oxygen and carbon dioxide in the blood.* It is stimulated by low levels of oxygen and initiates a reflex, which increases the rate and depth of respiration, cardiac rate, and blood pressure.

The **muscular triangle** is bounded by the superior belly of the omohyoid muscle, the anterior border of SCM, and the median plane of the neck (Fig. 9.5, *A* and *B*). *The muscular triangle contains the infrahyoid muscles and viscera of the neck,* such as the *thyroid* and *parathyroid glands.* In the anterolateral part of the neck, the **hyoid bone** provides attachments for the hyoid muscles (Figs. 9.5). The **hyoid muscles** steady or move the hyoid bone and larynx. For descriptive purposes, they are divided into suprahyoid and infrahyoid muscles whose attachments, innervation, and main actions are presented in Table 9.4.

The **suprahyoid muscles** are superior to the hyoid bone and connect it to the cranium. The suprahyoid muscle group includes the mylohyoid, geniohyoid, stylohyoid, and digastric.

- **Mylohyoid muscles** form the mobile but stable floor of the mouth and a muscular sling inferior to the tongue. These muscles support the tongue and elevate it and the hyoid bone when swallowing or protruding the tongue.
- **Geniohyoid muscles** are superior to the mylohyoid muscles, where they reinforce the floor of the mouth.
- **Stylohyoid muscles** form a slip on each side that is nearly parallel to the posterior belly of the digastric muscle.
- **Digastric muscles,** each of which has two bellies that descend toward the hyoid bone, are joined by an *intermediate tendon.* The **fibrous sling of digastric muscle**—connected to the body of the hyoid bone (Fig. 9.5*B*)—allows the tendon to slide anteriorly and posteriorly.

The **infrahyoid muscles** (strap muscles) are inferior to the hyoid bone. These four muscles anchor the hyoid bone, sternum, and clavicle and depress the hyoid bone and larynx during swallowing and speaking (Table 9.4). They also work with the suprahyoid muscles to steady the hyoid bone, providing a firm base for the tongue. The infrahyoid muscle group includes the sternohyoid, omohyoid, sternothyroid, and thyrohyoid, which are arranged in two planes: a *superficial plane* comprising the sternohyoid and omohyoid and a *deep plane* comprising the sternothyroid and thyrohyoid.

- The **sternohyoid,** a thin, narrow muscle, lies superficially, parallel and adjacent to the anterior median line.
- The **omohyoid,** lateral to the sternohyoid, has two bellies united by an intermediate tendon that connects to the clavicle by a fascial sling.
- The **sternothyroid** is wider than the sternohyoid, under which it lies. The sternothyroid covers the lateral lobe of the thyroid gland, attaching to the oblique line of the lamina of the thyroid cartilage immediately above it. This muscle limits upward expansion of the thyroid gland; thus, tumors or goiters resulting in enlargement cause the thyroid gland to expand anteriorly or inferiorly.
- The **thyrohyoid,** running superiorly from the oblique line of thyroid cartilage to the hyoid bone, appears to be a continuation of the sternothyroid muscle.

Arteries in Anterior Triangle

The **carotid system of arteries** lies in the anterior triangle (Figs. 9.5*B* and 9.6). It is formed by the common carotid artery and its terminal branches, the internal and external carotid arteries. The anterior triangle also contains the IJV and its tributaries and the AJVs. The **common carotid artery** and one of its terminal branches, the **external carotid artery,** are the main arterial vessels in the carotid triangle. Each common carotid artery ascends within the **carotid sheath** with and parallel to the descending IJV and vagus nerve to the level of the superior border of the thyroid cartilage. It terminates by dividing into the internal and

TABLE 9.4. SUPRAHYOID AND INFRAHYOID MUSCLES

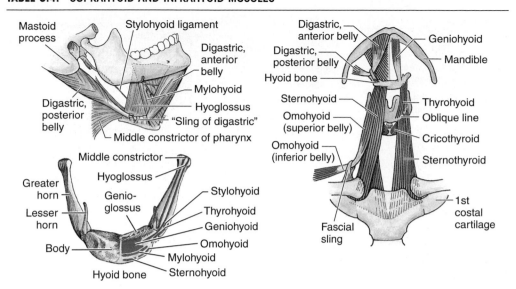

Muscle	Origin	Insertion	Innervation	Main Action(s)
Suprahyoid				
Mylohyoid	Mylohyoid line of mandible	Raphe and body of hyoid bone	Mylohyoid nerve, a branch of inferior alveolar nerve of CN V_3	Elevates hyoid bone, floor of mouth, and tongue during swallowing and speaking
Geniohyoid	Inferior mental spine of mandible	Body of hyoid bone	C1 via the hypoglossal nerve	Pulls hyoid bone anterosuperiorly, shortens floor of mouth, and widens pharynx
Stylohyoid	Styloid process of temporal bone	Body of hyoid bone	Cervical branch of facial nerve	Elevates and retracts hyoid bone, thereby elongating floor of mouth
Digastric	Anterior belly: digastric fossa of mandible. Posterior belly: mastoid notch of temporal bone	Intermediate tendon to body and greater horn of hyoid bone	Anterior belly: mylohyoid nerve, a branch of inferior alveolar nerve. Posterior belly: facial nerve	Depresses mandible; raises hyoid bone and steadies it during swallowing and speaking
Infrahyoid				
Sternohyoid	Manubrium of sternum and medial end of clavicle	Body of hyoid bone	C1–C3 by a branch of ansa cervicalis (Fig. 9.5B)	Depresses hyoid bone after it has been elevated during swallowing
Omohyoid	Superior border of scapula near suprascapular notch	Inferior border of hyoid bone	C1–C3 by a branch of ansa cervicalis (Fig. 9.5B)	Depresses, retracts, and steadies hyoid bone
Sternothyroid	Posterior surface of manubrium of sternum	Oblique line of thyroid cartilage	C2 and C3 by a branch of ansa cervicalis	Depresses hyoid bone and larynx
Thyrohyoid	Oblique line of thyroid cartilage	Inferior border of body and greater horn of hyoid bone	C1 via hypoglossal nerve	Depresses hyoid bone and elevates larynx

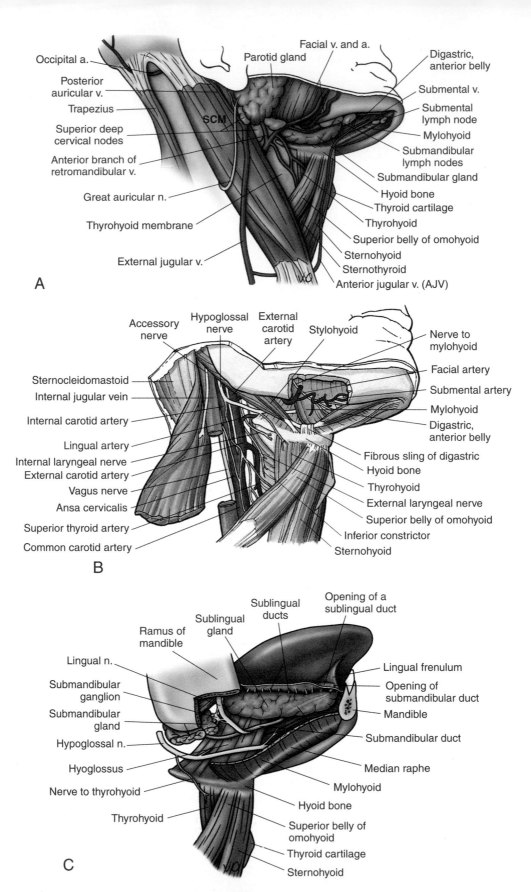

FIGURE 9.5 **Dissections of the anterior triangle of the neck and suprahyoid region. A.** Superficial dissection. Lateral view. **B.** Deep dissection. Lateral view. **C.** Suprahyoid region. Lateral view. The right half of the mandible and the superior half of the mylohyoid muscle have been removed.

external carotid arteries. The **right common carotid artery** begins at the bifurcation of the brachiocephalic trunk in the root of the neck. In contrast, the **left common carotid artery** arises from the arch of the aorta and ascends in the neck. Within the carotid sheath, each common carotid artery ascends parallel to the descending IJV and vagus nerve to the level of the superior border of the thyroid cartilage. The common carotid artery then terminates by dividing into the internal and external carotid arteries.

The **internal carotid arteries,** the direct continuation of the common carotid arteries, *have no branches in the neck.* They enter the cranium through the carotid canals and become the main arteries of the brain and structures in the orbits. *A sympathetic plexus of nerve fibers accompanies each artery* (see Fig. 9.10). During passage through the neck, the internal carotid artery lies anterior to the longus capitis muscle and the sympathetic trunk and posterolateral to the vagus nerve (CN X).

The **external carotid arteries** for the main part supply structures external to the cranium (Figs. 9.5*B* and 9.6). Each artery runs posterosuperiorly to the region between the neck of the mandible and the earlobe, where it is embedded in the parotid gland. Here it divides into two terminal branches, the **maxillary** and **superficial temporal arteries** (Fig. 9.6*B*). The 1st or 2nd branch of the external carotid artery, the **ascending pharyngeal artery,** arises medially and ascends on the pharynx and sends branches to the pharynx, prevertebral muscles, middle ear, and cranial meninges. The **superior thyroid artery,** the most inferior of the three anterior branches of the external carotid artery, runs anteroinferiorly deep to the infrahyoid muscles to reach the thyroid gland. In addition to supplying this gland, it gives off muscular branches to the infrahyoid muscles and SCM. It also gives rise to the *superior laryngeal artery,* which supplies the larynx. The **lingual artery** also arises from the external carotid artery where it lies on the middle constrictor muscle of the pharynx. It arches superoanteriorly and passes deep to the hypoglossal nerve (CN XII), stylohyoid muscle,

and posterior belly of the digastric muscle (Figs. 9.5*B* and 9.6*B*). It disappears deep to the hyoglossus muscle and turns superiorly at the anterior border of this muscle and becomes the *deep lingual and sublingual arteries.* The **facial artery** is the third anterior branch to arise from the external carotid artery, either in common with the lingual artery or immediately superior to it. The facial artery gives off a *tonsillar branch* and branches to the palate and submandibular gland. It then passes superiorly under cover of the digastric and stylohyoid muscles and the angle of the mandible. The facial artery loops anteriorly and enters a deep groove in the *submandibular gland.* It then hooks around the middle of the inferior border of the mandible and crosses the face (Fig. 9.6*C*). The **occipital artery** arises from the posterior aspect of the external carotid artery, superior to the origin of the facial artery (Fig. 9.5*A*). It passes posteriorly, parallel and deep to the posterior belly of the digastric muscle, and ends in the posterior part of the scalp. During its course, it passes superficial to the internal carotid artery and CN IX through CN XI. The **posterior auricular artery,** a small posterior branch of the external carotid artery, ascends posteriorly between the external acoustic meatus and mastoid process and contributes to the blood supply of adjacent muscles, parotid gland, facial nerve, structures in the temporal bone, auricle, and scalp.

LIGATION OF EXTERNAL CAROTID ARTERY

Sometimes ligation of an external carotid artery is necessary to control bleeding from one of its relatively inaccessible branches. This procedure decreases blood flow through the artery and its branches but does not eliminate it. Blood will flow retrogradely (pass backward) into the artery from the external carotid artery on the other side through communications between its branches (e.g., those in the face and scalp). When the external carotid or subclavian arteries are ligated, the descending branch of the occipital artery provides the main collateral circulation, anastomosing with the vertebral and deep cervical arteries.

Surgical Dissection of Carotid Triangle

The carotid triangle provides an important surgical approach to the carotid system of arteries, the IJV, the vagus and hypoglossal nerves, and the cervical sympathetic trunk. Damage or compression of the laryngeal branches of the vagus nerve during surgical dissection

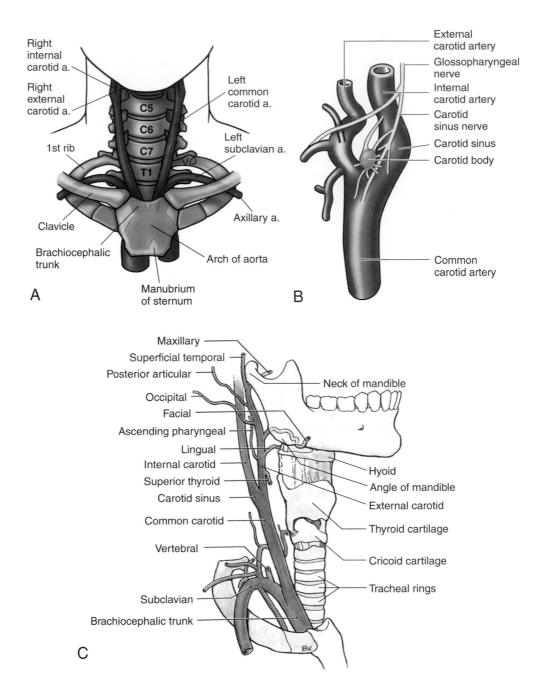

FIGURE 9.6   Arteries in the neck. A. Subclavian and carotid arteries in the anterior neck. Anterior view. **B.** Schematic illustration of the right carotid sinus and carotid body. Medial view. **C.** Branches of the subclavian and external carotid arteries. Lateral view.

Continued
of the triangle may produce an alteration in the voice because these nerves supply laryngeal muscles (p. 628).

Carotid Pulse

The carotid pulse (neck pulse) is easily felt by palpating the common carotid artery in the side of the neck, where it lies in a groove between the trachea and the infrahyoid muscles. It is usually easily palpated just deep to the anterior border of the SCM at the level of the superior border of the thyroid cartilage. It is routinely checked during cardiopulmonary resuscitation *(CPR)*. Absence of a carotid pulse indicates cardiac arrest.

Veins of Anterior Triangle

Most veins in the anterior triangle are tributaries of the **IJV,** usually the largest vein in the neck (Fig. 9.7). The *IJV* drains blood from the brain, anterior face, cervical viscera, and deep muscles of the neck. The IJV commences at the jugular foramen in the posterior cranial fossa as the direct continuation of the sigmoid sinus (see Chapter 8). From the dilation at its origin—the **superior bulb of IJV**—the vein runs inferiorly through the neck in the *carotid sheath* with the internal carotid artery and the common carotid artery and vagus nerve (CN X). The artery is medial and the vein lateral, and the nerve lies posteriorly between these vessels (Fig. 9.1*C*). The IJV leaves the anterior triangle by passing deep to the SCM. Posterior to the sternal end of the clavicle, the IJV unites with the subclavian vein to form the **brachiocephalic vein.** The inferior end of the IJV dilates to form the **inferior bulb of the IJV.** The *tributaries of the IJV* are the inferior petrosal sinus, facial, lingual, pharyngeal, and superior and middle thyroid veins. The **occipital vein** usually drains into the *suboc-*

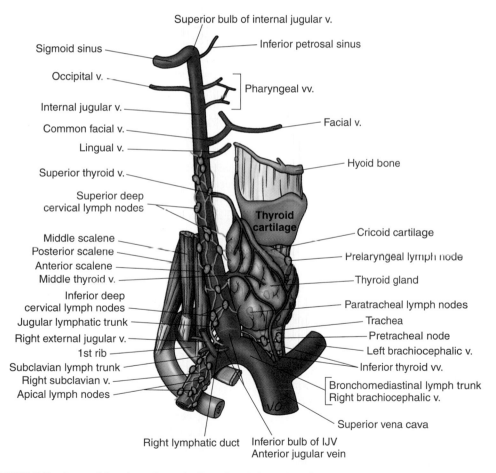

FIGURE 9.7   Internal jugular vein and tributaries. Lateral view. Deep cervical lymph nodes along the IJV are also shown.

cipital venous plexus, drained by the deep cervical vein and the vertebral vein.

Nerves of Anterior Triangle

The **transverse cervical nerve** (C2 and C3) supplies the skin covering the anterior triangle (see Fig. 9.4*A*). The **hypoglossal nerve** (CN XII), the motor nerve of the tongue, enters the submandibular triangle deep to the posterior belly of the digastric muscle to supply the tongue (Fig. 9.5*B*). Branches of CN IX and CN X are located in the digastric and carotid triangle.

DEEP STRUCTURES OF NECK

Notable deep structures of the neck are the brachial plexus, internal jugular and subclavian veins, muscles forming the floor of the posterior triangle, viscera of the neck (e.g., thyroid gland), and hyoid and prevertebral muscles (Fig. 9.8, Table 9.5). The **root of the neck** is the junctional area between the thorax and neck. It opens into the *superior thoracic aperture,* through which pass all structures going from the head to the thorax and vice versa (see Chapter 2). *The root of the neck is bounded:*

- *Laterally* by the 1st pair of ribs
- *Anteriorly* by the manubrium of the sternum and costal cartilages
- *Posteriorly* by the body of T1 vertebra.

ARTERIES IN ROOT OF NECK

The arteries in the root of the neck (Figs. 9.6*A* and 9.8), the large brachiocephalic trunk on the right side and the common carotid and subclavian arteries on the left side, originate from the *arch of the aorta.* The **brachiocephalic trunk,** covered anteriorly by the sternohyoid and sternothyroid muscles, is the largest branch of the aortic arch. It arises in the midline, posterior to the manubrium, passes superolaterally to the right, and *divides into the right common carotid and right subclavian arteries.* The **subclavian arteries** supply the upper limbs; they also send branches to the neck and to the brain. The **right subclavian artery** arises from the brachiocephalic trunk, posterior to the right sternoclavicular (SC) joint. The first part of the artery courses superolaterally, extending between its origin and the medial margin of the anterior scalene muscle. The cervical pleurae, apex of lung, and sympathetic trunk lie posterior to this part of the right subclavian artery (see Chapter 2). The **left subclavian artery** arises from the arch of the aorta and enters the root of the neck, posterior to the left SC joint. For purposes of description, *the anterior scalene muscle divides each subclavian artery into three parts:* the first part is medial to the muscle, the second is posterior to it, and the third is lateral to it (Fig. 9.8). *The branches of the subclavian arteries* (Figs. 9.8 and 9.9) *are the:*

- *Vertebral artery, internal thoracic artery, and thyrocervical trunk* from the first part of the subclavian artery
- *Costocervical trunk* from the second part of the subclavian artery
- *Dorsal scapular artery* (its origin is inconstant)—often arises as a branch of the transverse cervical artery but it may be a branch of the third or, less often, the second part of the subclavian artery.

The **cervical part of the vertebral artery** arises from the first part of the subclavian artery and ascends through the transverse foramina of C6 through C1 vertebrae; however, it may enter a foramen more superior than C6 vertebra. After passing through the

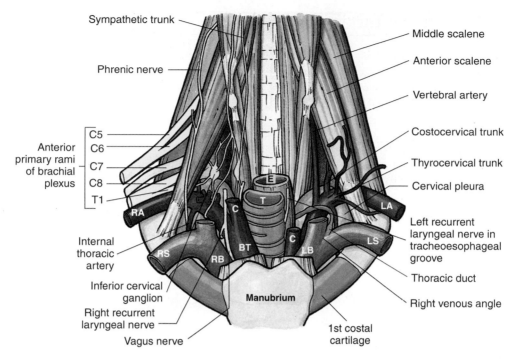

FIGURE 9.8 **Root of the neck and prevertebral region.** Anterior view. *E,* esophagus; *T,* trachea; *C,* left and right common carotid arteries; *RA,* right subclavian artery; *LA,* left subclavian artery; *RS,* right subclavian vein; *LS,* left subclavian vein; *RB,* right brachiocephalic vein; *LB,* left brachiocephalic vein; *BT,* brachiocephalic trunk.

C1 transverse foramen (placed more laterally than the others), the **suboccipital part of the vertebral artery** courses horizontally and medially in a groove on the posterior arch of the atlas before it enters the cranial cavity through the foramen magnum (p. 505). The **internal thoracic artery** arises from the anteroinferior aspect of the subclavian artery and descends inferomedially into the thorax (Figs. 9.8 and 9.9). *The internal thoracic artery has no branches in the neck;* its thoracic distribution is described in Chapter 2. The **thyrocervical trunk** arises from the anterosuperior aspect of the first part of the subclavian artery, near the

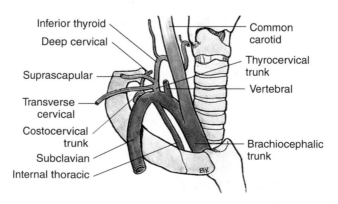

FIGURE 9.9 **Branches of the subclavian artery.** Lateral view.

TABLE 9.5.   ANTERIOR PREVERTEBRAL MUSCLES

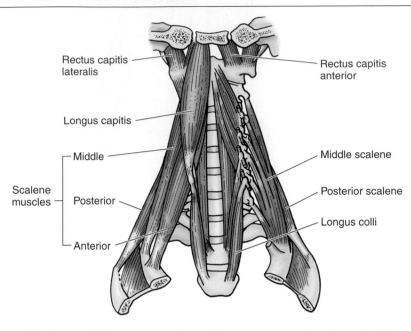

Muscle	Superior Attachment	Inferior Attachment	Innervation	Main Action(s)
Longus colli	Anterior tubercle of C1 vertebra (atlas); bodies of C1–C3 and transverse processes of C3–C6 vertebrae	Bodies of C5–T3 vertebrae, transverse processes of C3–C5 vertebrae	Anterior rami of C2–C6 spinal nerves	Flexes neck with rotation (torsion) to opposite side if acting unilaterally[a]
Longus capitis	Basilar part of occipital bone	Anterior tubercles of C3–C6 transverse processes	Anterior rami of C1–C3 spinal nerves	Flexes head[b]
Rectus capitis anterior	Base of skull, just anterior to occipital condyle	Anterior surface of lateral mass of C1 vertebra (atlas)	Branches from loop between C1 and C2 spinal nerves	Flexes head[b]
Rectus capitis lateralis	Jugular process of occipital bone	Transverse process of C1 vertebra (atlas)	Branches from loop between C1 and C2 spinal nerves	Flexes head and helps to stabilize it

[a]Flexion of neck = anterior (or lateral if so stated) bending of cervical vertebrae C2–C7.
[b]Flexion of head = anterior (or lateral if so stated) bending of head relative to vertebral column of atlanto-occipital joints.

medial border of the anterior scalene muscle. It has three branches, the largest and most important of which is the **inferior thyroid artery,** the primary visceral artery of the neck (Fig. 9.9). Other branches of the thyrocervical trunk are the **suprascapular artery,** supplying muscles on the posterior scapula, and the **transverse cervical artery,** sending branches to muscles in the posterior triangle, the trapezius, and the medial scapular muscles.

The **costocervical trunk** arises posteriorly from the second part of the subclavian artery—posterior to the anterior scalene muscle on the right side and usually just medial to it on the left side (Fig. 9.8). The trunk passes posterosuperiorly and divides into the superior intercostal and deep cervical arteries, which supply the first two intercostal spaces and the posterior deep cervical muscles, respectively.

VEINS IN ROOT OF NECK

Two large veins terminate in the root of the neck: the **EJV,** draining blood received mostly from the scalp and face (Figs. 9.3 and 9.7), and the **AJV.** The AJV typically arises near the hyoid bone from the confluence of superficial submandibular veins. At the root of the neck, the vein turns laterally, posterior to the SCM, and opens into the termination of the EJV or into the subclavian vein. Superior to the manubrium, the right and left AJVs commonly unite to form the *jugular venous arch.* There is considerable variation in the sizes of the jugular venous components (IJV, EJV, AJV, and communicating veins). The **subclavian vein**, the continuation of the axillary vein, begins at the lateral border of the 1st rib and ends when it unites with the **IJV,** posterior to the medial end of the clavicle, to form the **brachiocephalic vein** (Fig. 9.7). This union is commonly referred to as the "venous angle" and is the site where the **thoracic duct** (left side) and the **right lymphatic trunk** (right side) drain lymph collected throughout the body into the venous circulation (Fig. 9.8, see also Fig. 9.11*C*). Throughout its course, the IJV is enclosed by the carotid sheath.

NERVES IN ROOT OF NECK

Important nerves pass through the root of the neck (Figs. 9.8 and 9.10). Following their exit from the jugular foramen, each **vagus nerve** (CN X) passes inferiorly in the neck within the posterior part of the **carotid sheath** in the angle between and posterior to the IJV and common carotid artery (Fig. 9.1*C*). The **right vagus nerve** passes anterior to the first part of the subclavian artery and posterior to the brachiocephalic vein and SC joint to enter the thorax. The **left vagus nerve** descends between the left common carotid and left subclavian arteries and posterior to the SC joint to enter the

thorax. The nerves of the two sides have essentially the same distribution; however, they arise and recur (loop around) different structures and at different levels on the two sides. The **right recurrent laryngeal nerve** arises adjacent to and loops inferior to the right subclavian artery (Fig. 9.10), and the **left recurrent laryngeal nerve** (Fig. 9.8) arises adjacent to and loops inferior to the arch of the aorta (see Fig. 9.14). After looping, both recurrent nerves ascend to the posteromedial aspect of the thyroid gland, where they ascend in the **tracheoesophageal groove** (Fig. 9.8) to supply all the intrinsic muscles of the larynx except the cricothyroid. The cardiac branches of CN X originate in the neck as well as in the thorax and run along the arteries to the cardiac plexus of nerves (see Chapter 2).

The **phrenic nerves** are formed at the lateral borders of the anterior scalene muscles (Fig. 9.8)—mainly from C4 nerve with contributions from C3 and C5. The phrenic nerves descend anterior to the anterior scalene muscles under cover of the SCMs and IJVs. They pass under the prevertebral layer of deep cervical fascia between the subclavian arteries and veins and proceed through the thorax on each side of the mediastinum and supply the diaphragm (Chapter 2).

The **sympathetic trunks**, anterolateral to the vertebral column, begin at the level of C1 vertebra (Figs. 9.8 and 9.10). These trunks receive no white communicating branches (L. rami communicantes) in the neck; however, the three **cervical sympathetic ganglia**—superior, middle, and inferior—communicate with the anterior rami of the cervical spinal nerves by way of gray communicating branches. These ganglia receive presynaptic fibers from the superior thoracic spinal nerves and associated white communicating branches that convey them to the sympathetic trunk. After ascending in the trunk to the cervical sympathetic ganglia, postsynaptic fibers pass to the cervical spinal nerves via gray communicating branches, or leave as direct visceral branches (splanchnic nerves). Branches to the head and viscera of the neck pass via cephalic arterial branches to run with the arteries (periarterial plexus), especially the **vertebral** and **internal** and **external carotid arteries** (Fig. 9.10).

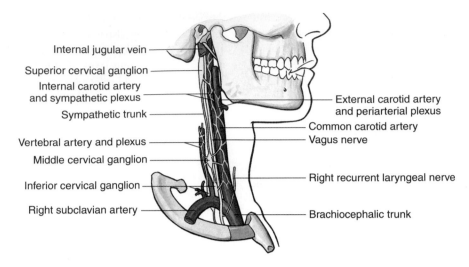

Internal jugular vein
Superior cervical ganglion
Internal carotid artery and sympathetic plexus
Sympathetic trunk
Vertebral artery and plexus
Middle cervical ganglion
Inferior cervical ganglion
Right subclavian artery

External carotid artery and periarterial plexus
Common carotid artery
Vagus nerve
Right recurrent laryngeal nerve
Brachiocephalic trunk

FIGURE 9.10   Vessels and nerves in the neck. Lateral view.

The **inferior cervical ganglion** usually fuses with the 1st thoracic ganglion to form the large *cervicothoracic* (stellate) *ganglion*. This star-shaped ganglion lies anterior to the transverse process of C7 vertebra, just superior to the neck of the 1st rib on each side and posterior to the origin of the vertebral artery. Some postsynaptic fibers from the ganglion pass via gray communicating branches to the anterior rami of C7 and C8 spinal nerves and others pass to the heart. The **middle cervical ganglion** (occasionally absent) lies on the anterior aspect of the inferior thyroid artery at the level of the cricoid cartilage and the transverse process of C6 vertebra, just anterior to the vertebral artery. Postsynaptic gray communicating branches (rami) pass from the ganglion to C5 and C6 spinal nerves and to the heart and thyroid gland. The **superior cervical ganglion** is at the level of C1 and C2 vertebrae. Because of its large size it forms a good landmark for locating the sympathetic trunk. Postsynaptic cephalic arterial branches pass from it to form the **internal carotid sympathetic plexus** and enter the cranial cavity (Fig. 9.10). This ganglion also sends arterial branches to the external carotid artery and gray communicating branches to the anterior rami of the superior four cervical spinal nerves. Other postsynaptic fibers pass from it to the *cardiac plexus of nerves* (see Chapter 2).

CERVICOTHORACIC GANGLION BLOCK
Anesthetic injected around the cervicothoracic (stellate) ganglion blocks transmission of stimuli through the cervical and superior thoracic ganglia. The cervicothoracic ganglion block may relieve vascular spasms involving the brain and upper limb. It is also useful when deciding if surgical resection of the ganglion would be beneficial to a person with excess vasoconstriction of the ipsilateral limb.

Lesion of Sympathetic Trunk
A lesion of a sympathetic trunk in the neck results in a sympathetic disturbance—*Horner syndrome*—characterized by:

* *Pupillary constriction*—resulting from paralysis of the dilator pupillae (p. 536)
* *Ptosis* (drooping of upper eyelid)—resulting from paralysis of smooth muscle intermingled with striated muscle of the levator palpebrae superioris (p. 532)
* Sinking in of the eye—possibly caused by paralysis of smooth muscle (orbitalis) in the floor of the orbit
* Vasodilation and absence of sweating on the face and neck—caused by a lack of sympathetic (vasoconstrictive) nerve supply to blood vessels and sweat glands.

LYMPHATICS OF NECK

Most superficial tissues of the neck are drained by lymphatic vessels that enter **superficial cervical lymph nodes** (Fig. 9.11*A*). These nodes are located along the course of the EJV. Lymph from these nodes drains into inferior **deep cervical lymph nodes** (Figs. 9.7 and 9.11*B*). The specific group of inferior deep cervical nodes involved descends across the posterior triangle with the accessory nerve. Most lymph from the six to eight nodes then drains into the *supraclavicular lymph nodes* that accompany the transverse cervical artery (see Fig. 9.4*B*). The main group of deep cervical nodes forms a chain along the IJV, mostly under cover of the SCM. Other deep cervical nodes include the prelaryngeal, pretracheal,

paratracheal, and retropharyngeal nodes (Fig. 9.7). Efferent lymphatic vessels from the deep cervical nodes join to form the **jugular lymphatic trunks** that, on the left side, usually join the thoracic duct and that, on the right side, enter the junction of the internal jugular and subclavian veins (*right venous angle*) directly (Fig. 9.11*C*) or via a short **right lymphatic duct.** A large lymphatic channel, the **thoracic**

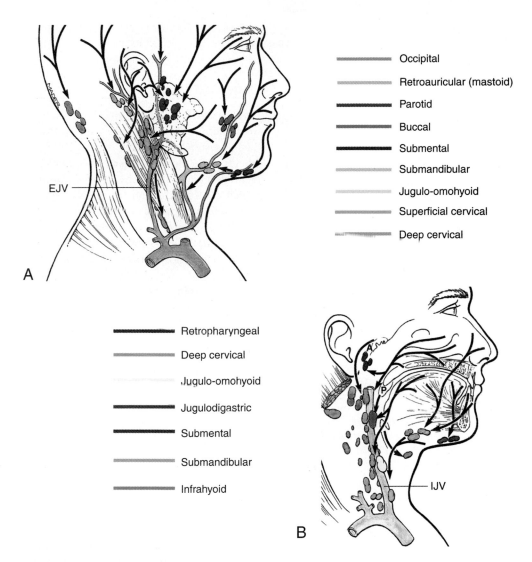

Occipital
Retroauricular (mastoid)
Parotid
Buccal
Submental
Submandibular
Jugulo-omohyoid
Superficial cervical
Deep cervical

EJV

A

Retropharyngeal
Deep cervical
Jugulo-omohyoid
Jugulodigastric
Submental
Submandibular
Infrahyoid

IJV

B

FIGURE 9.11 **Lymphatic drainage of the head and neck. A.** Superficial lymph nodes. Lateral view **B.** Deep lymph nodes. Lateral view.

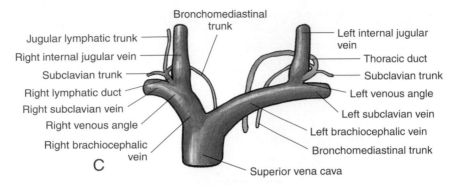

FIGURE 9.11 *Continued.* **C.** Termination of thoracic and right lymphatic ducts at venous angles.

duct, begins at the chyle cistern (L. cisterna chyli) in the abdomen (see Chapter 3) and passes superiorly through the posterior mediastinum (see Chapter 2) and superior thoracic aperture along the left border of the esophagus. It arches laterally in the root of the neck, posterior to the carotid sheath and anterior to the sympathetic trunk and vertebral and subclavian arteries (Fig. 9.8). The thoracic duct enters the left brachiocephalic vein at the junction of the subclavian and IJVs—**left venous angle** (Fig. 9.11C). The thoracic duct drains lymph from the entire body, except the right side of the head and neck, the right upper limb, and the right side of the thorax, which drain through the **right lymphatic duct.**

RADICAL NECK DISSECTIONS

In radical neck dissections performed when cancer invades the lymphatics, the deep cervical lymph nodes and the tissues around them are removed as completely as possible. While major arteries, the brachial plexus, CN X, and the phrenic nerve are preserved, most cutaneous branches of the cervical plexus are removed. The aim of the dissection is to remove all tissue that contains lymph nodes in one piece to try to prevent cancerous cells from escaping and circulating, thereby causing metastasis (spread) of the cancer.

VISCERA OF NECK

The cervical viscera are organized in three layers (Fig. 9.12). Superficial to deep, they are the *endocrine layer*—thyroid and parathyroid glands; the *respiratory layer*—pharynx, larynx, and trachea; and the *alimentary layer*—pharynx and esophagus. The names of the layers represent the functions of the viscera.

ENDOCRINE LAYER

The viscera in the endocrine layer—the **thyroid** and **parathyroid glands**—are part of the body's system of ductless, hormone-secreting glands. The **thyroid gland**—the largest endocrine gland—produces *thyroid hormone,* which controls the rate of metabolism, and *calcitonin,* a hormone controlling calcium metabolism. **Parathyroid glands** produce *parathormone* (PTH), which controls the metabolism of phosphorus and calcium in the blood.

The **thyroid gland** lies deep to the sternothyroid and sternohyoid muscles from the level of C5 to T1 vertebrae (Fig. 9.1A). It consists primarily of right and left lobes, anterolateral to the larynx and trachea. A relatively thin **isthmus** unites the lobes over the trachea, usually anterior to the 2nd and 3rd tracheal rings (Fig. 9.12). The thyroid gland is surrounded by a thin fibrous capsule, which sends septa deeply into the gland. Dense connective tissue attaches the fibrous capsule to the cricoid cartilage and superior tracheal rings. External to the capsule is a loose sheath formed by the visceral layer of the pretracheal deep cervical fascia (p. 593). The rich **blood supply of the thyroid gland** (essential to its endocrine function) is from the paired **superior** and **inferior thyroid arteries** (Fig. 9.13, *A* and *B*). Usually, the 1st branch of the external carotid artery, the **superior thyroid artery,** descends to the gland and divides into anterior and posterior branches. The **inferior thyroid artery,** the largest branch of the **thyrocervical trunk** (Fig. 9.13B), runs superomedially posterior to the carotid sheath to reach the posterior aspect of the thyroid gland. In approximately 10% of people, a **thyroid ima artery** (L. arteria thyroidea ima) arises from the brachiocephalic trunk or the arch of the aorta. This small artery ascends on the anterior surface of the trachea, which it supplies, and continues to the isthmus of the thyroid gland.

Three pairs of **thyroid veins** usually drain the thyroid plexus of veins on the anterior surface of the thyroid gland and trachea (Fig. 9.13, *A* and *C*). The **superior thyroid veins** drain the superior poles of the gland, the **middle thyroid veins** drain the middle of the lobes, and the **inferior thyroid veins** drain the inferior poles and/or isthmus. The superior and middle thyroid veins empty into the IJVs, and the inferior thyroid veins end in the brachiocephalic veins (most often, the left one).

The **lymphatic vessels of the thyroid gland** communicate with a capsular network of lymphatic vessels. From superior parts of the lobes and the isthmus of the gland, the lymphatic vessels pass to the **superior deep cervical lymph nodes** (Fig. 9.13*D*). Inferior to the thyroid gland, the lymphatic vessels pass to the **inferior deep cervical lymph nodes.** Some lymphatic vessels drain into brachiocephalic nodes or the thoracic duct. The **nerves of the thyroid gland** derive from the superior, middle, and inferior **cervical sympathetic ganglia** (Figs. 9.10 and 9.13*A*). They reach the gland through the cardiac and superior and inferior periarterial plexuses accompanying the thyroid arteries. These fibers are vasomotor, causing constriction of blood vessels.

The **parathyroid glands** lie external to the fibrous thyroid capsule but are embedded in the posterior surface of the thyroid gland (Figs. 9.12 and 9.14). There are usually two pea-sized **superior parathyroid glands** and two **inferior parathyroid glands.** Usually, the **inferior thyroid arteries** supply both the superior and inferior glands. The parathyroid veins drain into the **thyroid plexus of veins** (Fig. 9.13*C*). The

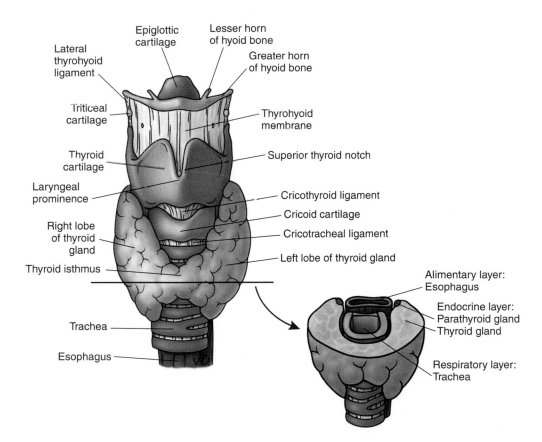

FIGURE 9.12   Relations of thyroid gland. Anterior view.

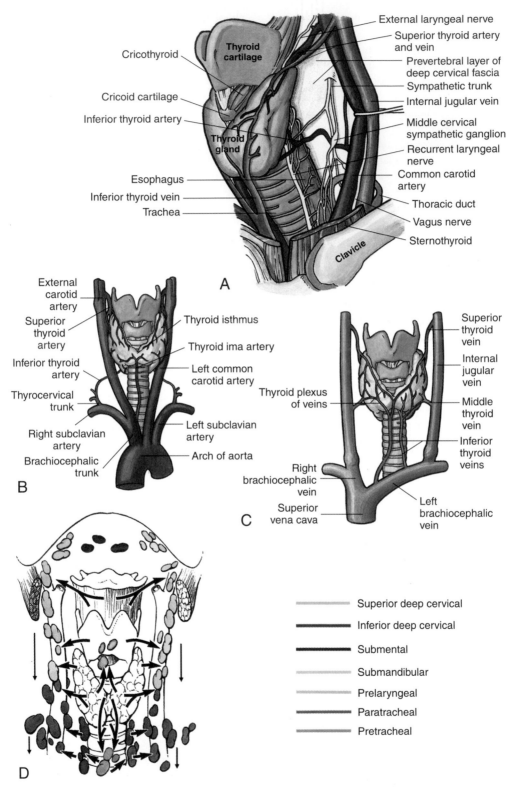

FIGURE 9.13 **Thyroid gland. A.** Root of the neck (anterolateral view of left side) showing vasculature and innervation. **B.** Arterial supply. Anterior view. **C.** Venous drainage. Anterior view. **D.** Lymphatic drainage. Anterior view.

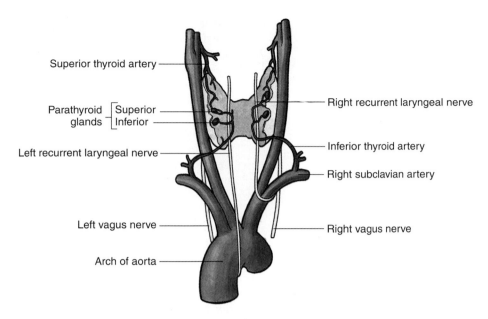

Superior thyroid artery

Parathyroid | Superior
glands | Inferior

Left recurrent laryngeal nerve

Left vagus nerve

Arch of aorta

Right recurrent laryngeal nerve

Inferior thyroid artery

Right subclavian artery

Right vagus nerve

FIGURE 9.14 **Parathyroid glands.** Posterior view. Dissection of the posterior surface of the thyroid gland showing the blood supply of the parathyroid glands. In this specimen the blood supply is from anastomoses between the superior and inferior thyroid arteries.

parathyroid lymphatic vessels drain with those of the thyroid gland into the **deep cervical** and **paratracheal lymph nodes** (Fig. 9.13D). The **nerves of the parathyroid glands** derive from thyroid branches of the superior or middle **cervical sympathetic ganglia** (Figs. 9.10 and 9.13A); the nerves are vasomotor but not secretomotor.

PYRAMIDAL LOBE OF THYROID GLAND

Approximately 50% of thyroid glands have a small prominence—the *pyramidal lobe*—on the superior surface of the isthmus of the thyroid gland, usually to the left of the median plane. A band of connective tissue containing muscle may continue from the pyramidal lobe to the hyoid bone.

Thyroidectomy and Inadvertent Removal of Parathyroid Glands

During a total thyroidectomy (excision of the thyroid gland), the parathyroid glands are in danger of being inadvertently damaged or removed; however, they are safe during *subtotal thyroidectomy* because the most posterior part of the thyroid gland usually is preserved. Variability in the position of the parathyroid glands, especially the inferior ones, puts them in danger of being removed during surgery on the thyroid gland. If the parathyroid glands are inadvertently removed during surgery, the patient suffers from *tetany*, a severe convulsive disorder. *The generalized convulsive muscle spasms result from a fall in blood calcium levels.*

Accessory Thyroid Gland

An accessory thyroid gland may develop in the neck lateral to the thyroid cartilage (*arrow*); usually it lies on the thyrohyoid muscle. Although functional, this tissue is often in-

sufficient to maintain normal function if the thyroid gland is removed. The pyramidal lobe and its connective tissue continuation may also contain thyroid tissue. Accessory thyroid tissue, like that of a pyramidal lobe, originates from remnants of the *thyroglossal duct*—a transitory endodermal tube extending from the posterior tongue region of the embryo carrying the thyroid-forming tissue at its descending distal end.

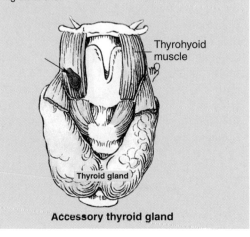

Thyrohyoid muscle

Thyroid gland

Accessory thyroid gland

RESPIRATORY LAYER

The viscera of the respiratory layer—**larynx, trachea,** and **pharynx**—contribute to the respiratory function of the body. *The main functions of viscera in the respiratory layer are:*

- Routing air and food into the respiratory tract and esophagus, respectively
- Providing a patent airway and a means of sealing it off temporarily
- Producing voice.

Larynx

The larynx lies in the anterior part of the neck at the level of the bodies of C3 through C6 vertebrae. *The larynx is the phonating mechanism designed for voice production,* connecting the inferior part of the pharynx (oropharynx) with the trachea. The larynx guards the air passages, especially during swallowing, and maintains a patent airway.

The **laryngeal skeleton** consists of nine cartilages joined by ligaments and membranes (Fig. 9.15). Three cartilages are single—thyroid, cricoid, and epiglottic—and three are paired—arytenoid, corniculate, and cuneiform. The **thyroid cartilage** is the largest of the cartilages. The inferior two thirds of its two plate-like **laminae** are fused anteriorly in the median plane to form the **laryngeal prominence.** Superior to this prominence, the laminae diverge to form a V-shaped **superior thyroid notch** (Fig. 9.12). The inferior thyroid notch is a shallow indentation in the middle of the inferior border of the cartilage. The posterior border of each lamina projects superiorly as the **superior horn** (L. cornu) and inferiorly as the **inferior horn** (Fig. 9.15*A*). The superior border and superior horns attach to the hyoid bone by the **thyrohyoid membrane.** The thick median part of this membrane is the median thyrohyoid ligament and its lateral parts (containing the triticeal cartilages) are the **lateral thyrohyoid ligaments.** The inferior horns of the thyroid cartilages articulate with the lateral surfaces of the cricoid cartilage at the **cricothyroid joints** (Fig. 9.15*B*). The main movements at these joints are rotation and gliding of the thyroid cartilage, which result in changes in the length of the vocal folds.

The **cricoid cartilage** forms a complete ring around the airway, the only laryngeal cartilage

Surface Anatomy of Larynx

The U-shaped **hyoid bone** (*H*) lies superior to the **thyroid cartilage** at the level of C4 and C5 vertebrae. The **laryngeal prominence** (*P*) is produced by the *laminae of the thyroid cartilage (T)* that meet in the median plane. The **cricoid cartilage** (*C*), another laryngeal cartilage, can be felt inferior to the laryngeal prominence. It lies at the level of C6 vertebra. The cartilaginous **tracheal rings** are palpable in the inferior part of the neck. The 2nd to 4th rings cannot be felt because the **isthmus** (*S*) of the thyroid, connecting its right (*RL*) and left (*LL*) lobes, covers them. The first tracheal ring (*1*) is just superior to the isthmus.

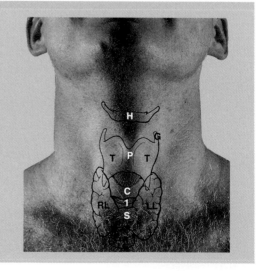

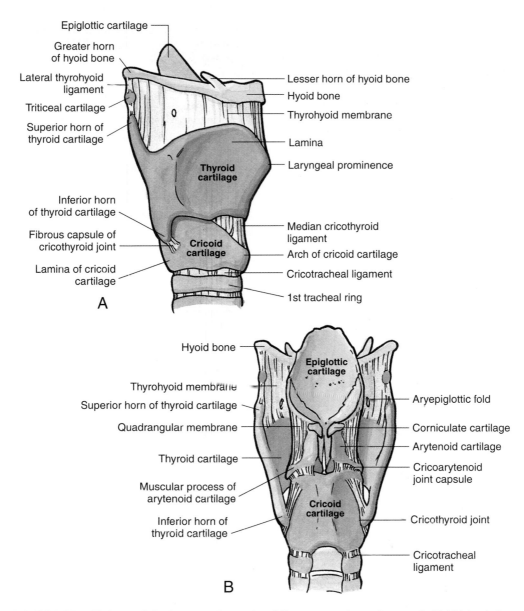

Epiglottic cartilage

Greater horn
of hyoid bone

Lateral thyrohyoid
ligament

Triticeal cartilage

Superior horn of
thyroid cartilage

Inferior horn
of thyroid cartilage

Fibrous capsule of
cricothyroid joint

Lamina of cricoid
cartilage

A

Lesser horn of hyoid bone

Hyoid bone

Thyrohyoid membrane

Lamina

Laryngeal prominence

Thyroid
cartilage

Median cricothyroid
ligament

Cricoid
cartilage

Arch of cricoid cartilage

Cricotracheal ligament

1st tracheal ring

Hyoid bone

Thyrohyoid membrane

Superior horn of thyroid cartilage

Quadrangular membrane

Thyroid cartilage

Muscular process of
arytenoid cartilage

Inferior horn of
thyroid cartilage

B

Epiglottic
cartilage

Aryepiglottic fold

Corniculate cartilage

Arytenoid cartilage

Cricoarytenoid
joint capsule

Cricoid
cartilage

Cricothyroid joint

Cricotracheal
ligament

FIGURE 9.15 **Skeleton of the larynx and associated ligaments and membranes. A.** Right lateral view.
B. Posterior view.

to do so. It is shaped like a signet ring with its
band facing anteriorly (Fig. 9.15). The opening
of the cartilage would fit on an average finger.
The posterior (signet) part of the cricoid cartilage is the **lamina,** and the anterior (band) part
is the **arch.** The cricoid cartilage is smaller but
thicker and stronger than the thyroid cartilage. The cricoid cartilage is attached to the inferior margin of the thyroid cartilage by the

median cricothyroid ligament and to the first
tracheal ring by the **cricotracheal ligament.**
Where the larynx is closest to the skin and
most accessible, the median cricothyroid ligament may be felt as a soft spot during palpation inferior to the thyroid cartilage.

The **arytenoid cartilages** are three-sided
pyramids that articulate with lateral parts of
the superior border of the cricoid cartilage

lamina. Each cartilage has an apex superiorly, a slender **vocal process** that extends anteriorly, and a large **muscular process** that projects laterally from the base (Figs. 9.15*B* and 9.16*C*). The *apex* of each arytenoid cartilage bears a **corniculate cartilage** and provides attachment for the **aryepiglottic fold.** The *vocal process of the arytenoid cartilage* provides the posterior attachment for the **vocal ligament** (Fig. 9.16, *B* and *C*), and the *muscular process of the arytenoid cartilage* serves as a lever to which the posterior and lateral cricoarytenoid muscles are attached.

The **cricoarytenoid joints**—between the bases of the arytenoid cartilages and the superolateral surfaces of the cricoid cartilage lamina (Figs. 9.15*B* and 9.16*C*)—permit the arytenoid cartilages to slide toward or away from one another, to tilt anteriorly and posteriorly, and to rotate. These movements are important in approximating, tensing, and relaxing the vocal folds. The elastic **vocal ligament** extends from the junction of the laminae of the thyroid cartilage anteriorly to the **vocal process** of the arytenoid cartilage posteriorly (Fig. 9.16, *B* and *C*). The vocal ligament forms the skeleton of the vocal fold; it is the thickened, free superior border of the lateral **cricothyroid ligament** (part of conus elasticus). This ligament blends anteriorly with the median cricothyroid ligament (also part of the **conus elasticus**).

The **epiglottic cartilage** gives flexibility to the **epiglottis** (Fig. 9.16, *A* and *B*). Situated posterior to the root of the tongue and hyoid bone and anterior to the laryngeal inlet (aditus), *the fibrocartilaginous epiglottic cartilage forms the superior part of the anterior wall and the superior margin of the laryngeal inlet—the aperture between the larynx and laryngopharynx.* The broad superior end of the epiglottic cartilage is free, and its tapered inferior end is attached to the angle formed by the thyroid laminae by the **thyroepiglottic ligament** (Fig. 9.16*C*). A thin submucosal sheet of connective tissue—the **quadrangular membrane**—extends between the lateral aspects of the arytenoid and epiglottic cartilages (Fig. 9.16*B*). Its free superior margin forms the core of the **aryepiglottic fold;** its

free inferior margin constitutes the **vestibular ligament,** which is covered loosely by the **vestibular fold** (Figs. 9.16*B* and 9.17). This fold lies superior to the vocal fold and extends from the thyroid cartilage to the arytenoid cartilage. The **corniculate and cuneiform cartilages** are small nodules in the posterior part of the aryepiglottic folds (Figs. 9.15 and 9.16, *B* and *C*). The corniculate cartilages attach to the apices of the arytenoid cartilages; the cuneiform cartilages do not directly attach to other cartilages.

The **laryngeal cavity** extends from the **laryngeal inlet** (L. aditus), through which it communicates with the laryngopharynx (Fig. 9.17), to the level of the inferior border of the cricoid cartilage. Here the laryngeal cavity is continuous with the lumen of the trachea. *The laryngeal cavity is divided into three parts* (Fig. 9.17):

- *Vestibule of the larynx*—superior to the vestibular folds
- *Ventricle of the larynx (*laryngeal sinus)— between the vestibular folds and superior to the vocal folds
- *Infraglottic cavity*—inferior cavity of the larynx extending from the vocal folds to the inferior border of the cricoid cartilage, where it is continuous with the lumen of the trachea.

The **vocal folds** (true vocal cords) control sound production (tone). The apex of each wedge-shaped fold projects medially into the laryngeal cavity (Figs. 9.16–9.18). **Each vocal fold includes:**

- A *vocal ligament* consisting of elastic tissue that is the thickened medial free edge of the lateral cricothyroid ligament (conus elasticus)
- A *vocalis muscle,* the fine fibers that form the most medial part of the thyroarytenoid muscle (Table 9.6).

The vocal folds are the source of sounds that come from the larynx (Fig. 9.18). The vocal folds produce audible vibrations when their free margins are closely—but not tightly—opposed during phonation (production of sounds) and air is forcibly expired in-

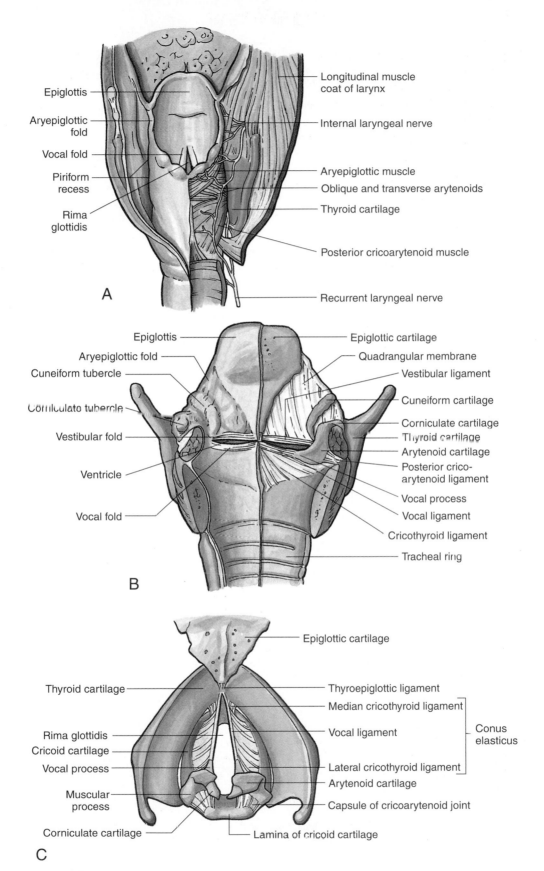

FIGURE 9.16 **A.** Muscles and nerves. Posterior view. *Pink,* mucosa. **B.** Interior of the larynx. Posterior view. **C.** Skeleton and ligaments of the larynx. Superior view.

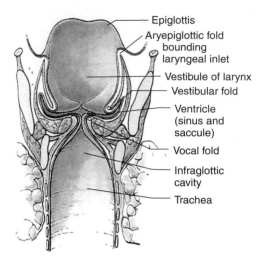

FIGURE 9.17   **Compartments of the larynx.**
Coronal section in the position of phonation.

termittently. The **vocal folds** also serve as the main sphincter of the respiratory tract when they are tightly closed. Complete adduction of the folds forms an effective sphincter that prevents entry or exit of air. The **glottis** (vocal apparatus of the larynx) comprises the vocal folds and processes, together with the **rima glottidis**—the aperture between the vocal folds (Fig. 9.18*A*). The shape of the rima (L. slit) varies according to the position of the vocal folds. During normal respiration, the rima is narrow and wedge-shaped; during forced respiration it is wide and kite-shaped. The rima glottidis is slitlike when the vocal folds are closely approximated during phonation

(Fig. 9.18*C*). Variation in the tension and length of the vocal folds at the level of the larynx (controlled by suprahyoid and infrahyoid muscles) and in the intensity of the expiratory effort produces changes in the pitch of the voice. The lower range of pitch of the male voice results from the greater length of the vocal folds due to the increased size of the thyroid cartilage. The **vestibular folds** (false vocal cords), extending between the thyroid and arytenoid cartilages (Figs. 9.16 and 9.17), play little or no part in voice production; they are protective in function. They consist of two thick folds of mucous membrane enclosing the **vestibular ligaments.**

Muscles of Larynx. The laryngeal muscles are divided into extrinsic and intrinsic groups:

* The **extrinsic laryngeal muscles** move the larynx as a whole (Table 9.4). The *infrahyoid muscles* are depressors of the hyoid bone and larynx, whereas the *suprahyoid* and *stylopharyngeus muscles* are elevators of the hyoid bone and larynx.

* The **intrinsic laryngeal muscles** move the laryngeal parts, making alterations in the length and tension of the vocal folds and in the size and shape of the rima glottidis. All but one of the intrinsic muscles of the larynx are supplied by the **recurrent laryngeal nerve** (Fig. 9.19), a branch of CN X; the cricothyroid muscle is supplied by the **external laryngeal nerve,** a branch of the **superior laryngeal nerve** (also derived from CN X). The actions of the intrinsic laryngeal muscles are described in Table 9.6.

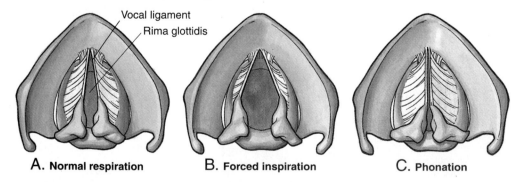

A. Normal respiration   **B. Forced inspiration**   **C. Phonation**

FIGURE 9.18   **Variations in the rima glottidis.** Superior views. Its shape varies according to the position of the vocal folds.

TABLE 9.6. MUSCLES OF LARYNX

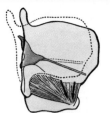

Lateral view
Cricothyroid

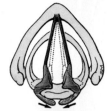

Superior view
Posterior cricoarytenoid

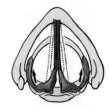

Superior view
Lateral cricoarytenoid

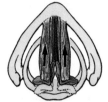

Superior view
Thyroarytenoid

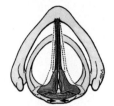

Superior view
Transverse arytenoid

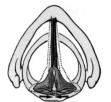

Superior view
Oblique arytenoid

Muscle	Origin	Insertion	Innervation	Main Action(s)
Cricothyroid	Anterolateral part of cricoid cartilage	Inferior margin and inferior horn of thyroid cartilage	External laryngeal nerve	Stretches and tenses vocal fold
Posterior cricoarytenoid	Posterior surface of laminae of cricoid cartilage	Muscular process of arytenoid cartilage	Recurrent laryngeal nerve	Abducts vocal fold (interligamentous part)
Lateral cricoarytenoid	Arch of cricoid cartilage	Muscular process of arytenoid cartilage	Recurrent laryngeal nerve	Adducts vocal fold
Thyroarytenoid[a]	Posterior surface of thyroid cartilage	Muscular process of arytenoid cartilage	Recurrent laryngeal nerve	Relaxes vocal fold
Transverse and oblique arytenoids[b]	One arytenoid cartilage	Opposite arytenoid cartilage	Recurrent laryngeal nerve	Closes intercartilaginous part of rima glottidis
Vocalis[c]	Depression between laminae of thyroid cartilage	Parts of vocal ligament and vocal process of arytenoid cartilage	Recurrent laryngeal nerve	Relaxes posterior vocal ligament while maintaining (or increasing) tension of anterior part

[a]Superior fibers of the thyroarytenoid muscle pass into the aryepiglottic fold, and some of them reach the epiglottic cartilage. These fibers constitute the thyroepiglottic muscle, which widens the inlet of larynx.
[b]Some fibers of oblique arytenoid muscle continue as the aryepiglottic muscle (Fig. 9.16A).
[c]This slender muscular slip is derived from inferior deeper and finer fibers of the thyroarytenoid muscle.

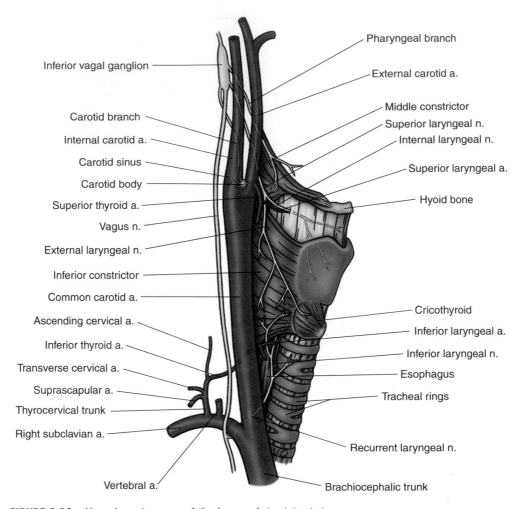

Inferior vagal ganglion

Carotid branch
Internal carotid a.
Carotid sinus
Carotid body
Superior thyroid a.
Vagus n.
External laryngeal n.
Inferior constrictor
Common carotid a.
Ascending cervical a.
Inferior thyroid a.
Transverse cervical a.
Suprascapular a.
Thyrocervical trunk
Right subclavian a.

Vertebral a.

Pharyngeal branch
External carotid a.
Middle constrictor
Superior laryngeal n.
Internal laryngeal n.
Superior laryngeal a.
Hyoid bone

Cricothyroid
Inferior laryngeal a.
Inferior laryngeal n.
Esophagus
Tracheal rings

Recurrent laryngeal n.
Brachiocephalic trunk

FIGURE 9.19   Vessels and nerves of the larynx. Anterolateral view.

Vessels of Larynx. The laryngeal arteries—branches of the superior and inferior thyroid arteries—supply the larynx (Fig. 9.19). The **superior laryngeal artery** accompanies the internal laryngeal nerve through the thyrohyoid membrane and branches to supply the internal surface of the larynx. The **inferior laryngeal artery** accompanies the inferior laryngeal nerve and supplies the mucous membrane and muscles in the inferior part of the larynx. Laryngeal veins accompany the laryngeal arteries. The **superior laryngeal vein** usually joins the superior thyroid vein and through it drains into the IJV. The **inferior laryngeal vein** joins the middle thyroid vein or the thyroid plexus of veins on the anterior aspect of the trachea.

The **lymphatics of the larynx** superior to the vocal folds accompany the superior laryngeal artery through the thyrohyoid membrane and drain into the **superior deep cervical lymph nodes** (Fig. 9.13D). The lymphatic vessels inferior to the vocal folds drain into the **pretracheal** or **paratracheal lymph nodes,** which drain into the **inferior deep cervical lymph nodes.**

Nerves of Larynx. The laryngeal nerves are superior and inferior branches of the **vagus nerve** (Fig. 9.19). The **superior laryngeal nerve** arises at the level of the **inferior vagal ganglion** and divides into two terminal branches: the internal laryngeal nerve (sensory and autonomic) and the external laryngeal nerve (motor). The **internal laryngeal nerve** pierces the thyrohyoid membrane with the superior laryngeal artery and supplies sensory fibers to the laryngeal mucous membrane superior to the vocal folds, including the superior surface of these folds. The **external laryngeal nerve** descends posterior to the sternothyroid muscle in company with the superior thyroid artery. At first the nerve lies on the inferior constrictor muscle of the pharynx, and then it pierces and supplies it and the cricothyroid muscle. The **recurrent laryngeal nerve** supplies all intrinsic muscles of the larynx except the cricothyroid, which is supplied by the external laryngeal nerve. It also supplies sensory fibers to the laryngeal mucous membrane inferior to the vocal folds. The continuation of the recurrent laryngeal nerve, the **inferior laryngeal nerve,** enters the larynx by passing deep to the inferior border of the inferior constrictor muscle of the pharynx. It divides into anterior and posterior branches that accompany the inferior laryngeal artery into the larynx.

INJURY TO LARYNGEAL NERVES

The recurrent laryngeal nerves are vulnerable to injury during thyroidectomy and other surgical operations in the anterior triangles of the neck. Because the inferior laryngeal nerve innervates the muscles moving the vocal fold, injury results in *paralysis of the vocal fold.* The voice is initially poor ("hoarse") because the paralyzed fold cannot meet the normal vocal fold. When paralysis of both vocal folds occurs, the voice is almost absent because the folds cannot be adducted sufficiently to produce tone. Further, patients suffer *dyspnea* (difficulty in breathing) during exertion because of the inability to abduct the vocal folds to permit increased respiration. The struggle to breath may result in stridor (high-pitched, noisy respiration) and panic. *Tracheostomy* (p. 630) may be required. *Hoarseness is the most common symptom of serious disorders of the larynx,* such as carcinoma of the vocal folds.

FRACTURES OF LARYNGEAL SKELETON

Laryngeal fractures result from blows received in sports such as kick boxing and hockey or from compression by a shoulder strap during an automobile accident. Laryngeal fractures produce submucous hemorrhage and edema, respiratory obstruction, hoarseness, and sometimes a temporary inability to speak. Calcification of the laryngeal cartilage occurs in elderly people. It is therefore more likely to fracture during compression (e.g., by a seatbelt).

Laryngoscopy

Laryngoscopy is any procedure used to examine the interior of the larynx. The larynx may be examined visually by *indirect laryngoscopy* using a laryngeal mirror or it may be viewed by *direct laryngoscopy* using an *endoscopic laryngoscope.* The vestibular folds normally appear pink and lie laterally, whereas the vocal folds are usually pearly white and appear medial to the vestibular folds.

Aspiration of Foreign Bodies

A foreign object, such as a piece of steak, may accidentally pass through the laryngeal inlet into the vestibule of the larynx, where it becomes trapped superior to the vestibular folds. When a foreign object enters the vestibule, the laryngeal muscles go into spasm, tensing the vocal folds. The rima glottidis closes and no air enters the trachea. *Emergency therapy must be given to open the airway.* The procedure used depends on the condition of the patient, the facilities available, and the experience of the person giving first aid. Because the lungs still contain air, sudden compression of the abdomen (*Heimlich maneuver*) causes the diaphragm to elevate and compress the lungs, expelling air from the trachea into the larynx. This maneuver usually dislodges the food or other material from the larynx.

Trachea

The trachea is an air tube composed of hyaline cartilaginous **tracheal rings** (Fig. 9.13*A*). These rings, which keep the trachea patent, are deficient posteriorly where the trachea is adjacent to the esophagus (Fig. 9.12). The posterior gap is spanned by the *trachealis muscle,* a band of smooth muscle in the fibrous membrane connecting the posterior ends of the tracheal rings. The trachea is surprisingly short (10–11 cm long). It extends from the inferior end of the larynx at the level of the 5th or 6th cervical vertebra. The trachea ends at the sternal angle or the T4/T5 IV disc, where *it divides into the right and left main bronchi* (see Chapter 2). Lateral to the trachea are the **common carotid arteries** and **thyroid lobes** (Fig. 9.19). Inferior to the thyroid gland, the **inferior thyroid veins** are anterior to the trachea. The **recurrent laryngeal nerves** ascend at the posterolateral borders of the trachea in the interval between the adjacent margins of the trachea and esophagus (see Fig. 9.8).

TRACHEOTOMY AND TRACHEOSTOMY

The trachea may be opened by making a median incision superior or inferior to the thyroid isthmus. An *emergency tracheotomy* (usually intended to be temporary) is more difficult inferior to the isthmus because the trachea recedes as it descends and it has hazardous anterior relations (discussed subsequently). A transverse incision through the skin of the neck and anterior wall of the trachea (*surgical tracheostomy*) establishes a long-term airway in persons with upper airway obstruction or respiratory failure. The sternohyoid and sternothyroid muscles are retracted laterally, and the isthmus of the thyroid gland is either divided or retracted superiorly. An opening is made in the trachea between the 1st and 2nd tracheal rings or through the 2nd through 4th rings. A *tracheostomy tube* is then inserted into the trachea and secured by neck straps. *To avoid complications during a tracheostomy, recall the following anatomical relationships:*

- The *inferior thyroid veins* arise from the thyroid plexus of veins and descend on the anterolateral surface of the trachea (Fig. 9.13, *A* and *C*).
- A small *thyroid ima artery* may be present and ascend to the isthmus of the thyroid gland (Fig. 9.13*B*).
- The *left brachiocephalic vein,* jugular venous arch, and pleurae may be encountered.
- The thymus covers the inferior part of the trachea in infants and children.
- The trachea is small, mobile, and soft in infants, making it easy to cut through its posterior wall and damage the esophagus.

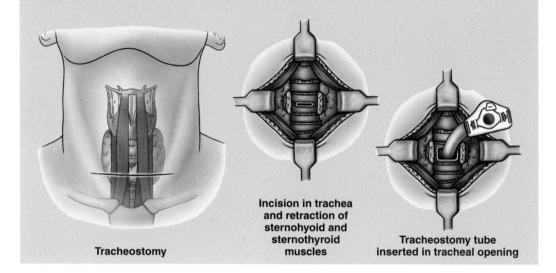

Tracheostomy

Incision in trachea and retraction of sternohyoid and sternothyroid muscles

Tracheostomy tube inserted in tracheal opening

ALIMENTARY LAYER

In the alimentary layer, cervical viscera take part in the digestive functions of the body. *The pharynx serves a role in both respiratory and alimentary activities.* Although the **pharynx** conducts air to the larynx, trachea, and lungs, its constrictor muscles direct—and the epiglottis deflects—food to the esophagus.

Pharynx

The **pharynx** is the part of the alimentary canal posterior to the nasal and oral cavities, extending inferiorly past the larynx (Fig. 9.20*A*). The pharynx extends from the base of the cranium to the inferior border of the cricoid cartilage anteriorly and the inferior border of C6 vertebra posteriorly. It is widest opposite the hyoid bone and narrowest at its inferior end, where it is continuous with the esophagus. The posterior wall of the pharynx lies against the prevertebral layer of deep cervical fascia (Fig. 9.1*A*). *The pharynx is divided into three parts:*

- *Nasopharynx*—posterior to the nose and superior to the soft palate
- *Oropharynx*—posterior to the oral cavity
- *Laryngopharynx*—posterior to the larynx.

Nasopharynx. The nasopharynx has a respiratory function. *It lies superior to the soft*

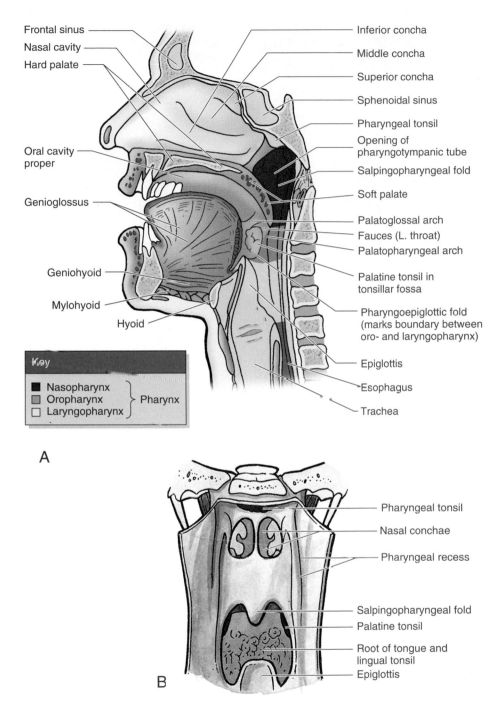

FIGURE 9.20 **Nasopharynx, oropharynx, and laryngopharynx. A.** Median section of the head and neck. **B.** Anterior wall of the nasopharynx and oropharynx, showing the anterior communications, pharyngeal recess, and palatine, pharyngeal, and lingual tonsils. Posterior view.

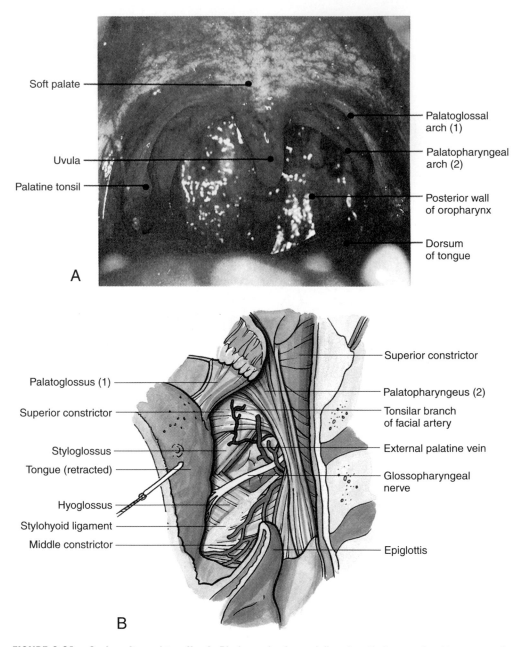

FIGURE 9.21   Oral cavity and tonsils. A. Photograph of an adult male with the mouth wide open and the tongue protruded. Anterior view. **B.** Deep dissection of the tonsillar bed. Medial view.

palate and is the posterior extension of the nasal cavities (Fig. 9.20A). The nose opens into the nasopharynx through two *choanae* (paired openings between the nasal cavities and naso-pharynx). A collection of lymphoid tissue, the **pharyngeal tonsil** ("adenoids"), is in the mucous membrane of the roof and posterior wall of the nasopharynx. Extending inferiorly from the medial end of the pharyngotympanic tube is a vertical fold of mucous membrane, the **salpingopharyngeal fold.** It covers the *salpingopharyngeus muscle* that

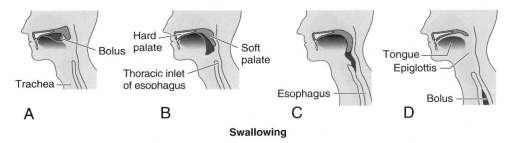

Swallowing

FIGURE 9.22 **Swallowing.** Lateral views. **A.** The bolus of food is pushed to the back of the oral cavity by pushing the tongue against the palate. **B.** The nasopharynx is sealed off and the larynx is elevated, enlarging the pharynx to receive food. **C.** The pharyngeal sphincters contract sequentially, squeezing food into the esophagus. The epiglottis closes the trachea. **D.** The bolus of food moves down the esophagus by peristaltic contractions.

participates in opening the pharyngeal orifice of the **pharyngotympanic tube** (auditory tube) during swallowing. The collection of lymphoid tissue in the submucosa of the pharynx near the pharyngeal orifice of the pharyngotympanic tube is the *tubal tonsil.* Posterior to the torus of the pharyngotympanic tube and the salpingopharyngeal fold is a slitlike lateral extension of the pharynx, the **pharyngeal recess** (Fig. 9.20*B*), which extends laterally and posteriorly.

Oropharynx. The oropharynx has a digestive function. Anteriorly, it is bounded by the soft palate superiorly, the base of the tongue interiorly, and the palatoglossal and palatopharyngeal arches laterally (Figs. 9.20 and 9.21). It extends from the level of the soft palate to that of the superior border of the epiglottis. **Deglutition** (act of swallowing) is the process whereby a bolus (masticated morsel of food) is transferred from the oral cavity through the pharynx and esophagus into the stomach (Fig. 9.22). Solid food is masticated and mixed with saliva to form a soft bolus during chewing. *Deglutition occurs in three stages:*

- The 1st stage is voluntary; the bolus is pushed from the oral cavity into the oropharynx, mainly by movements of the tongue and soft palate.
- The 2nd stage is automatic (reflex-driven) and rapid; the soft palate is elevated,

sealing off the nasopharynx from the oropharynx and laryngopharynx; the pharynx is now wide and short to receive the bolus of food as the suprahyoid muscles and longitudinal pharyngeal muscles contract, elevating the larynx.

- The 3rd stage is also automatic; sequential contraction of the three pharyngeal constrictor muscles forces food inferiorly into the esophagus.

The **palatine tonsils** are collections of lymphoid tissue on each side of the oropharynx in the interval between the **palatoglossal and palatopharyngeal arches** (Figs. 9.20 and 9.21*A*). The palatine tonsil lies in the **tonsillar bed,** between the palatoglossal and palatopharyngeal arches (Fig. 9.21*B*). The bed is formed by the superior constrictor of the pharynx and the thin sheet of **pharyngobasilar fascia** (Fig. 9.23). This fascia blends with the periosteum of the base of the cranium and defines the limits of the pharyngeal wall in its superior part.

Laryngopharynx. The laryngopharynx is the part of the pharynx posterior to the laryngeal inlet and the vestibule and ventricle of the larynx (Fig. 9.20). It extends from the superior border of the epiglottis to the esophagus at the level of the inferior border of the cricoid cartilage. Posteriorly, the laryngopharynx is related to the bodies of C4 through C6 vertebrae. The laryngopharynx communicates with the larynx through the *laryngeal inlet* (Fig. 9.17). The **pir-iform recess** is a small depression of the laryn-gopharyngeal cavity on each side of the inlet (Fig. 9.16*A*). This mucosa-lined recess is sepa-rated from the inlet by the **aryepiglottic fold.** Laterally, the piriform recess is bounded by the mucosa overlying the medial surfaces of the thyroid cartilage and the thyrohyoid mem-brane. Branches of the internal laryngeal and recurrent laryngeal nerves lie deep to the mu-cous membrane of the piriform recess.

The posterior and lateral **walls of the phar-ynx** are formed by the **constrictor muscles** (Fig. 9.23). Internally, the wall is formed by the **palatopharyngeus and stylopharyngeus mus-**

cles (Fig. 9.24). The walls of the pharynx are thus composed mainly of an external circular and an internal longitudinal layer of muscles, which is opposite to the muscular wall (muscu-laris externa) of the remainder of the alimen-tary canal. The external layer consists of three constrictor muscles—superior, middle, and in-ferior (Figs. 9.23 and 9.24, Table 9.7). The con-strictor muscles contract reflexively so that contraction takes place sequentially from the superior to the inferior end of the pharynx. This action propels food into the esophagus. All three constrictors are supplied by the **pha-ryngeal plexus of nerves** that lies on the lateral wall of the pharynx (Fig. 9.23, *B* and *C*), mainly

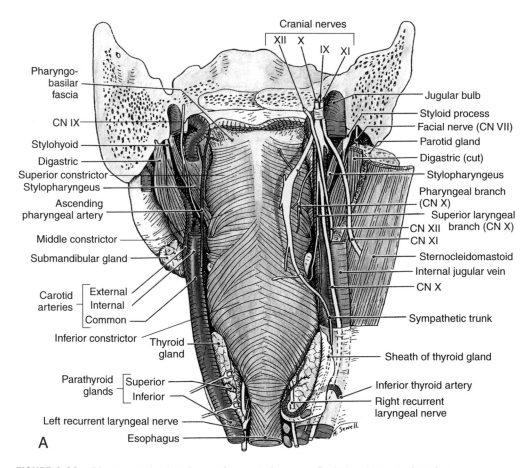

FIGURE 9.23   Pharynx and related vasculature and nerves. Posterior views. **A.** Overview.

TABLE 9.7. MUSCLES OF PHARYNX

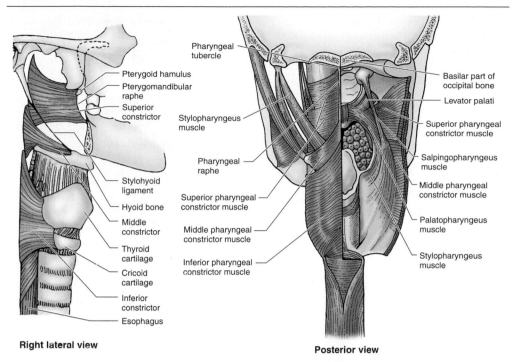

Right lateral view

Posterior view

Muscle	Origin	Insertion	Innervation	Main Action
External layer				
Superior-constrictor	Pterygoid hamulus, pterygomandibular raphe, posterior end of mylohyoid line of mandible, and side of tongue	Median raphe of pharynx and pharyngeal tubercle on basilar part of occipital bone	Cranial root of accessory nerve via pharyngeal branch of vagus and pharyngeal plexus	Constrict wall of pharynx during swallowing
Middle-constrictor	Stylohyoid ligament and superior (greater) and inferior (lesser) horns of hyoid bone	Median raphe of pharynx	Cranial root of accessory nerve as above, plus branches of external and recurrent laryngeal nerves of vagus	
Inferior-constrictor	Oblique line of thyroid cartilage and side of cricoid cartilage			
Internal layer				
Palato-pharyngeus	Hard palate and palatine aponeurosis	Posterior border of lamina of thyroid cartilage and side of pharynx and esophagus	Cranial root of accessory nerve via pharyngeal branch of vagus and pharyngeal plexus	Elevate (shorten and widen) pharynx and larynx during swallowing and speaking
Salpingo-pharyngeus	Cartilaginous part of pharyngotympanic tube	Blends with palatopharyngeus		
Stylo-pharyngeus	Styloid process of temporal bone	Posterior and superior borders of thyroid cartilage with palatopharyngeus	Glossopharyngeal nerve	

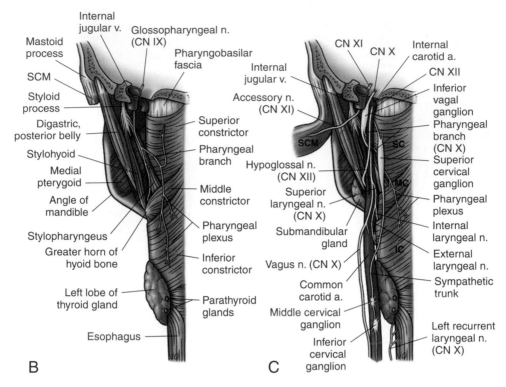

Internal jugular v.
Glossopharyngeal n. (CN IX)
Mastoid process
Pharyngobasilar fascia
SCM
Styloid process
Digastric, posterior belly
Stylohyoid
Medial pterygoid
Angle of mandible
Stylopharyngeus
Greater horn of hyoid bone
Left lobe of thyroid gland
Esophagus
Superior constrictor
Pharyngeal branch
Middle constrictor
Pharyngeal plexus
Inferior constrictor
Parathyroid glands
B

CN XI CN X
Internal carotid a.
Internal jugular v.
Accessory n. (CN XI)
SCM
CN XII
Inferior vagal ganglion
Pharyngeal branch (CN X)
Superior cervical ganglion
Hypoglossal n. (CN XII)
Superior laryngeal n. (CN X)
Submandibular gland
Vagus n. (CN X)
Common carotid a.
Middle cervical ganglion
Inferior cervical ganglion
SC
MC
Pharyngeal plexus
Internal laryngeal n.
IC
External laryngeal n.
Sympathetic trunk
Left recurrent laryngeal n. (CN X)
C

FIGURE 9.23   *Continued.* **B.** Muscles. **C.** Nerves and vessels. *SCM,* sternocleidomastoid.

on the middle constrictor. The overlapping of the constrictor muscles leaves the following four gaps in the musculature for structures to enter or leave the pharynx (Figs. 9.23 and 9.24):

- Superior to the superior constrictor, the levator veli palatini, pharyngotympanic tube, and ascending palatine artery pass through the gap between the superior constrictor and the cranium; it is here that the pharyngobasilar fascia blends with the buccopharyngeal fascia to form, with the mucous membrane, the thin wall of the **pharyngeal recess** (Fig. 9.20*B*).
- Between the superior and middle constrictors is a gap that forms the gateway to the oral cavity through which pass the stylopharyngeus, glossopharyngeal nerve (CN IX), and stylohyoid ligament.
- Between the middle and inferior constrictors is a gap for the internal laryngeal nerve and superior laryngeal artery and vein to pass to the larynx.

- Inferior to the inferior constrictor is a gap for the recurrent laryngeal nerve and inferior laryngeal artery to pass superiorly into the larynx.

The internal, mainly longitudinal, layer of pharyngeal muscles consists of the **palatopharyngeus, salpingopharyngeus,** and **stylopharyngeus.** These muscles shorten the pharynx and elevate the larynx during swallowing and speaking. The attachments, nerve supply, and actions of the pharyngeal muscles are described in Table 9.7.

The **nerve supply to the pharynx** (motor and most of sensory) derives from the **pharyngeal plexus of nerves** (Fig. 9.23, *B* and *C*), which is formed by pharyngeal branches of the vagus (CN X) and glossopharyngeal (CN IX) nerves and by sympathetic branches from the superior cervical ganglion. *Motor fibers in the pharyngeal plexus* derive from the cranial root of the *accessory nerve* and are carried by the vagus nerve (CN X)—via its pharyngeal branches—

to all muscles of the pharynx and soft palate, except the stylopharyngeus (supplied by CN IX) and the tensor veli palatini (supplied by CN V$_2$). *Sensory fibers in the pharyngeal plexus* derive from the glossopharyngeal nerve (CN IX). They supply most of the mucosa of all three parts of the pharynx. The sensory nerve supply of the mucous membrane of the nasopharynx is mainly from the maxillary nerve (CN V$_2$), a purely sensory nerve.

The **tonsillar branch of the facial artery** (Fig. 9.21*B*) passes through the superior constrictor muscle and enters the inferior pole of the tonsil. The tonsil also receives arterial twigs from the ascending palatine, lingual, descending palatine, and ascending pharyngeal arteries. The large **external palatine vein** descends from the soft palate and passes close to the lateral surface of the tonsil before it enters the pharyngeal venous plexus. The **tonsillar nerves** derive from the ton-sillar plexus of nerves formed by branches of the **glossopharyngeal** and **vagus nerves** and the pharyngeal plexus of nerves. The **tonsillar lymphatic vessels** pass laterally and inferiorly to the superior deep cervical lymph nodes near the angle of the mandible and the jugulodigastric node (Figs. 9.11*B* and 9.13*D*). The **jugulodigastric node** is referred to as the *tonsillar node* because of its frequent enlargement when the tonsil is inflamed *(tonsillitis)*. The palatine, lingual, and pharyngeal tonsils form the *pharyngeal lymphoid (tonsillar) ring,* an incomplete circular band of lymphoid tissue around the superior part of the pharynx. The anteroinferior part of the ring is formed by the **lingual tonsil,** a collection of lymphoid tissue in the posterior part of the tongue (Fig. 9.20*B*). Lateral parts of the ring are formed by the palatine and tubal tonsils, and posterior and superior parts are formed by the pharyngeal tonsil.

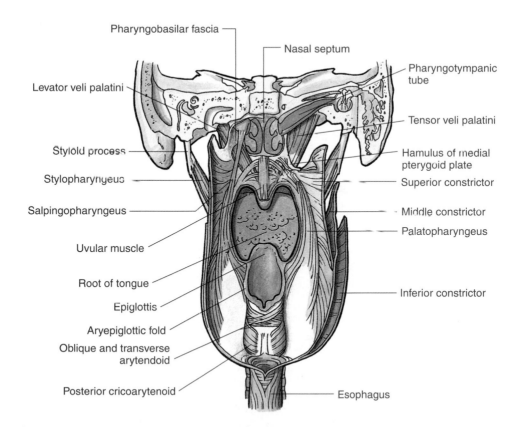

FIGURE 9.24 **Muscles of the soft palate and the interior of the pharynx.** Posterior view. The posterior wall of the pharynx has been cut in the midline and reflected laterally.

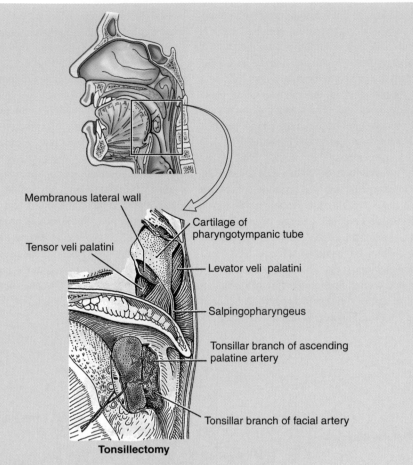

Membranous lateral wall

Cartilage of
pharyngotympanic tube

Tensor veli palatini

Levator veli palatini

Salpingopharyngeus

Tonsillar branch of ascending
palatine artery

Tonsillar branch of facial artery

Tonsillectomy

Tonsillitis and Tonsillectomy

Tonsillitis—inflammation of the tonsils, especially of the palatine tonsils—may result in a *tonsillectomy* being performed by dissecting the tonsil from the tonsillar bed. The operation involves removal of the tonsil and the fascial sheet covering the tonsillar bed. Because of the rich blood supply of the tonsil, bleeding may arise from the tonsillar artery or other arterial twigs; however, *bleeding commonly arises from the large external palatine vein* (Fig. 9.21*B*). The glossopharyngeal nerve (CN IX) accompanies the tonsillar artery on the lateral wall of the pharynx and is vulnerable to injury because this wall is thin. The majority of complications during tonsillectomy are vascular or septic (related to the presence of pus-forming and other pathogenic organisms, or their toxins, in the blood or tissues). The *internal carotid artery* is especially vulnerable when it is tortuous as it lies directly lateral to the tonsil.

Adenoiditis

Adenoiditis—inflammation of the pharyngeal tonsils (*adenoids*)—can obstruct passage of air from the nasal cavities through the choanae into the nasopharynx, making mouth breathing necessary. Infection from the enlarged pharyngeal tonsils may also spread to the tubal tonsils, causing swelling and closure of the pharyngotympanic tubes. Impairment of hearing may result from nasal obstruction and blockage of these tubes. Infection spreading from the nasopharynx to the middle ear causes *otitis media* (middle ear infection), which may produce temporary or permanent hearing loss.

FOREIGN BODIES IN LARYNGOPHARYNX

Foreign bodies entering the pharynx may become lodged in the *piriform recess*. If the object (e.g., a chicken bone) is sharp, it may pierce the mucous membrane and injure the superior laryngeal nerve and its internal laryngeal branch. Similarly, the nerves may be injured if the instrument used to remove the foreign body accidentally pierces the mucous membrane. Injury to these nerves may result in anesthesia of the laryngeal mucous membrane as far inferiorly as the vocal folds. Young children swallow various objects, most of which reach the stomach and subsequently pass through the gastrointestinal tract without difficulty. In some cases, the foreign body stops at the inferior end of the laryngopharynx, its narrowest part. A radiographic examination, CT scan, or MRI will reveal the presence of a radiopaque foreign body. Foreign bodies in the pharynx are often removed under direct vision through an *pharyngoscope*.

The **esophagus,** a highly muscular tube, extends from the pharynx to the stomach. It begins in the median plane at the inferior border of the cricoid cartilage, passes inferiorly, and enters the stomach at the cardial orifice (see Chapter 3). Its cervical part lies between the trachea and the cervical vertebral bodies (Fig. 9.20). On the right side, the esophagus is in contact with the cervical pleura at the root of the neck, whereas on the left side, posterior to the subclavian artery, the thoracic duct lies between the pleura and the esophagus. The **arteries to the cervical esophagus** are branches of the **inferior thyroid arteries** (Fig. 9.19). Each artery gives off ascending and descending branches that anastomose with each other and across the midline. The **veins of the cervical esophagus** are tributaries of the inferior thyroid veins. **Lymphatic vessels of the cervical esophagus** drain into the *paratracheal lymph nodes* and *inferior deep cervical lymph nodes* (Fig. 9.13*D*). The **nerve supply of the cervical esophagus** is somatic motor and sensory to the superior half and parasympathetic (vagal), sympathetic, and visceral sensory to the inferior half. The cervical esophagus receives the somatic fibers by way of branches from the **recurrent laryngeal nerves** and vasomotor fibers from the **cervical sympathetic trunks** (Fig. 9.13*A*) through the plexus around the inferior thyroid artery.

ZONES OF PENETRATING NECK TRAUMA

Three zones are common clinical guides to the seriousness of neck trauma. The zones provide an understanding of structures that are at risk when there are penetrating neck injuries.

- **Zone 1:** root of neck extending from the clavicles and manubrium to the cricoid cartilage. *Structures in jeopardy are:* cervical pleurae, apices of lungs, thyroid and parathyroid glands, trachea, esophagus, common carotid arteries, jugular veins, and cervical region of the vertebral column.

- **Zone II:** cricoid cartilage to the angles of the mandible. *Structures in jeopardy are:* apices of the thyroid gland, thyroid and cricoid cartilages, larynx, laryngopharynx, carotid arteries, jugular veins, esophagus, and cervical region of the vertebral column.

- **Zone III:** superior to the angles of the mandible. *Structures in jeopardy are:* salivary glands, facial nerve, oral and nasal cavities, oropharynx, and nasopharynx.

Injuries in Zones I and III obstruct the airway and have the greatest risk for morbidity (diseased state) *and mortality* (fatal outcome) *because injured structures are difficult to visualize and repair and because vascular damage is difficult to control.* **Injuries in Zone II are most common;** however, morbidity and mortality are lower because physicians can control vascular damage by direct pressure and surgeons can visualize and treat injured structures.

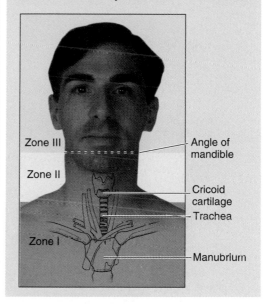

Zone III

Zone II

Zone I

Angle of mandible

Cricoid cartilage

Trachea

Manubrium

MEDICAL IMAGING OF NECK

Standard **radiographical examinations** of the neck include anteroposterior (AP), lateral, and oblique projections. Lateral projections are common for evaluating neck injuries. When taking a lateral projection, the person is usually sitting erect, with the neck slightly extended (Fig. 9.25). The central X-ray beam aims perpendicular to the X-ray film cassette at the level of the thyroid cartilage. When a fracture is suspected, the lateral projection is examined before the person is moved for other projections. Observe the anterior and posterior margins of the vertebral bodies. Any deviation from the smooth curvature of these margins suggests a fracture and tearing of associated ligaments. Observe that the IV disc spaces are wider anteriorly than posteriorly; this exists because the IV discs are wedge-shaped. As the discs degenerate, the vertical height of the disc spaces decreases.

Transverse computed tomography (CT) scans through the thyroid gland provide sections of the neck (Fig. 9.26). CTs are oriented to show how a horizontal section of the person's neck appears to the physician standing at the foot of the bed. The superior edge of the CT image represents the anterior surface of the neck, and the right lateral edge of the image represents the left lateral surface. CT scans are used mainly as a diagnostic adjunct to conventional radiography. They are superior to radiographs because they reveal radiodensity differences among and within soft tissues.

Magnetic resonance imaging (MRI) systems construct images of transverse, sagittal, and coronal sections of the neck and have the advantage of using no radiation (Fig. 9.27). MRIs of the neck are superior to CTs for showing detail in soft tissues.

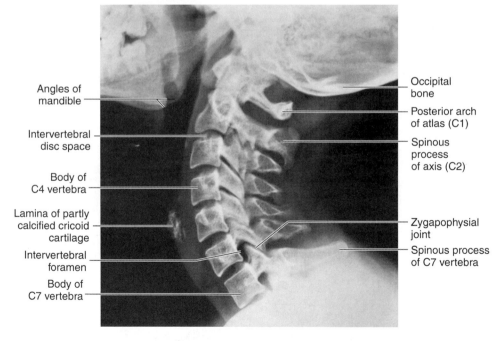

FIGURE 9.25   Radiograph of the cervical region of the vertebral column. Lateral projection.

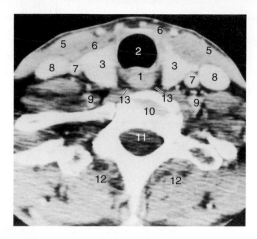

FIGURE 9.26 **Transverse CT scan of the neck through the thyroid gland.** *1,* esophagus; *2,* trachea; *3,* lobes of thyroid gland; *5,* SCM; *6,* sternohyoid muscles; *7,* common carotid artery; *8,* IJV; *9,* vertebral artery; *10,* vertebral body; *11,* spinal cord in cerebrospinal fluid; *12,* deep muscles of the back; *13,* retropharyngeal space. (Courtesy of Dr. M. Keller, Assistant Professor of Medical Imaging, University of Toronto, Toronto, Ontario, Canada.)

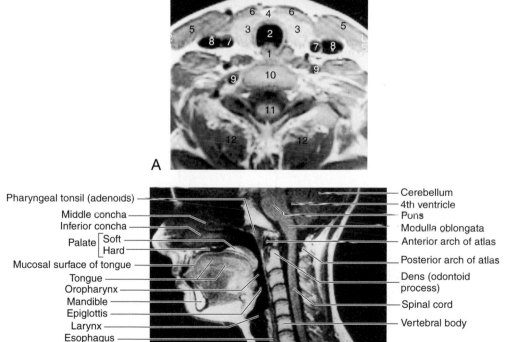

FIGURE 9.27 **MRI scans of the neck. A.** MRI through the thyroid gland. *1,* esophagus; *2,* trachea; *3,* lobes of thyroid gland; *4,* thyroid isthmus; *5,* SCM; *6,* sternohyoid muscles; *7,* common carotid artery; *8,* IJV; *9,* vertebral artery; *10,* vertebral body; *11,* spinal cord in cerebrospinal fluid; *12,* deep muscles of the back. **B.** Median MRI of the head and neck. Note that the air and food passages share the oropharynx. (Courtesy of Dr. W. Kucharczyk, Chair of Medical Imaging, and Clinical Director, Tri-Hospital Resonance Centre, Toronto, Ontario, Canada.)

Ultrasonography is also used for studying soft tissues of the neck. Ultrasound provides images of many abnormal conditions noninvasively, at relatively low cost, and with minimal discomfort. Ultrasound is useful for distinguishing solid from cystic masses, for example, which may be difficult to determine during physical examinations. **Vascular imaging of arteries and veins** of the neck is possible using *intravascular ultrasonography* (Fig. 9.28). The images are produced by placing the transducer within the blood vessel. *Doppler ultrasound techniques* help evaluate bloodflow through a vessel (e.g., for detecting stenosis [narrowing] of a carotid artery).

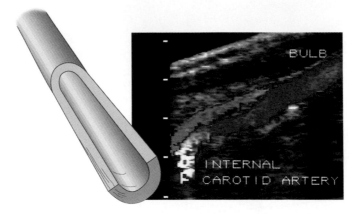

FIGURE 9.28   Normal Doppler color flow study of the internal carotid artery.

10 Review of Cranial Nerves

OVERVIEW OF CRANIAL NERVES

Cranial nerves, like spinal nerves, contain sensory or motor fibers or a combination of these fiber types (Fig. 10.1). Cranial nerves are bundles of processes from neurons that innervate muscles or glands or carry impulses from sensory areas. They were named cranial nerves because they emerge from foramina or fissures in the cranium and are covered by tubular sheaths derived from the cranial meninges.

The regional features of cranial nerves, especially those concerned with the head and neck, are described in preceding chapters. This chapter summarizes the cranial nerves and autonomic nervous system in schematic and tabular forms. Cranial nerve lesions, illustrating important clinical features, also are described.

The twelve pairs of cranial nerves are numbered I through XII, from anterior to posterior, according to their attachments to the brain (Fig. 10.2, Table 10.1). The fibers of cranial nerves connect centrally to *cranial nerve nuclei*—groups of neurons in which sensory or afferent fibers terminate and from which motor or efferent fibers originate. *Cranial nerves carry one or more of the following functional components:*

- *General sensory* (general somatic afferent): fibers transmit general sensation (e.g., touch) from the skin and mucous membranes mainly through the trigeminal nerve (CN V) but also through CNs VII, IX, and X; these sensations are usually (but not always) experienced consciously

- *Visceral sensory* (general visceral afferent): fibers convey visceral sensation from the parotid gland, carotid body, carotid sinus, middle ear, pharynx, larynx, trachea, bronchi, lungs, heart, esophagus, stomach, and intestines as far as the left colic flexure; this type of sensory information does not normally reach consciousness

- *Special sensory* (special visceral afferent): fibers transmit the sensation of taste and smell and serve the special senses of vision, hearing, and balance.

- *Somatic motor* (general somatic efferent): axons innervate striated muscles in the orbit and tongue, which are not derived from embryonic pharyngeal arches

- *Branchial motor* (special visceral efferent): axons innervate muscles, which are derived from embryonic pharyngeal (branchial) arches (face, larynx, and pharynx)

- *Visceral motor* (general visceral efferent): axons give rise to the cranial parasympathetic fibers that eventually innervate certain smooth muscles and glands; these presynaptic fibers are transmitted by CNs III, VII, IX, and X, but the postsynaptic fibers they contact are carried by branches of CN V

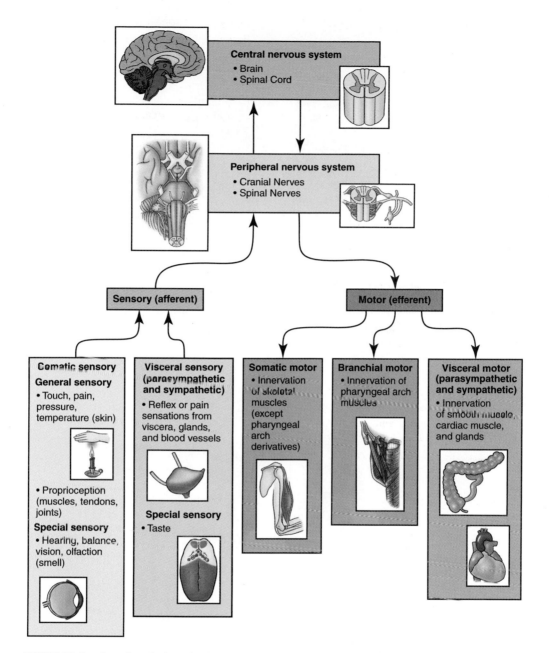

FIGURE 10.1 Overview (schema) of sensory and motor components of cranial and spinal nerves.

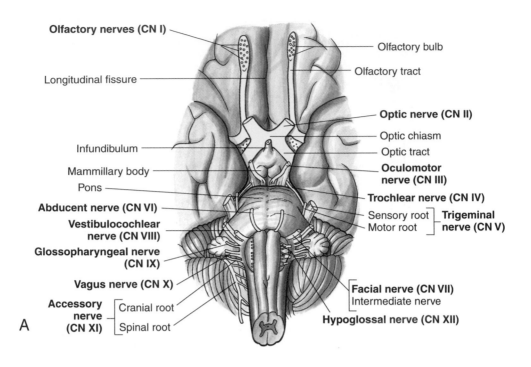

A. Olfactory nerves (CN I) — Olfactory bulb — Olfactory tract — Longitudinal fissure — **Optic nerve (CN II)** — Optic chiasm — Infundibulum — Optic tract — Mammillary body — **Oculomotor nerve (CN III)** — Pons — **Trochlear nerve (CN IV)** — **Abducent nerve (CN VI)** — Sensory root / Motor root / **Trigeminal nerve (CN V)** — **Vestibulocochlear nerve (CN VIII)** — **Glossopharyngeal nerve (CN IX)** — **Facial nerve (CN VII)** / Intermediate nerve — **Vagus nerve (CN X)** — **Accessory nerve (CN XI)** / Cranial root / Spinal root — **Hypoglossal nerve (CN XII)**

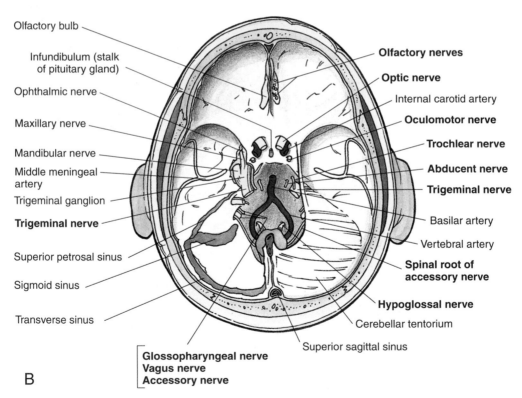

B. Olfactory bulb — Infundibulum (stalk of pituitary gland) — Ophthalmic nerve — Maxillary nerve — Mandibular nerve — Middle meningeal artery — Trigeminal ganglion — **Trigeminal nerve** — Superior petrosal sinus — Sigmoid sinus — Transverse sinus — **Olfactory nerves** — **Optic nerve** — Internal carotid artery — **Oculomotor nerve** — **Trochlear nerve** — **Abducent nerve** — **Trigeminal nerve** — Basilar artery — Vertebral artery — **Spinal root of accessory nerve** — **Hypoglossal nerve** — Cerebellar tentorium — Superior sagittal sinus — **Glossopharyngeal nerve / Vagus nerve / Accessory nerve**

FIGURE 10.2 Intracranial portions of cranial nerves. A. Inferior view of the brain showing the superficial origins of the cranial nerves. **B.** Interior of the cranial base showing the proximal parts of the cranial nerves, dura mater, and blood vessels.

TABLE 10.1. SUMMARY OF CRANIAL NERVES

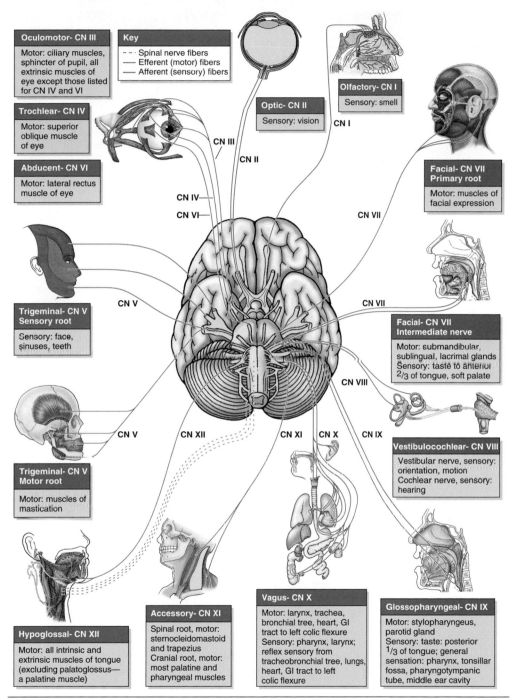

Oculomotor- CN III

Motor: ciliary muscles, sphincter of pupil, all extrinsic muscles of eye except those listed for CN IV and VI

Trochlear- CN IV

Motor: superior oblique muscle of eye

Abducent- CN VI

Motor: lateral rectus muscle of eye

Key
- - - Spinal nerve fibers
—— Efferent (motor) fibers
—— Afferent (sensory) fibers

Optic- CN II

Sensory: vision

Olfactory- CN I

Sensory: smell

Facial- CN VII Primary root

Motor: muscles of facial expression

Trigeminal- CN V Sensory root

Sensory: face, sinuses, teeth

Facial- CN VII Intermediate nerve

Motor: submandibular, sublingual, lacrimal glands
Sensory: taste to anterior 2/3 of tongue, soft palate

Trigeminal- CN V Motor root

Motor: muscles of mastication

Vestibulocochlear- CN VIII

Vestibular nerve, sensory: orientation, motion
Cochlear nerve, sensory: hearing

Hypoglossal- CN XII

Motor: all intrinsic and extrinsic muscles of tongue (excluding palatoglossus— a palatine muscle)

Accessory- CN XI

Spinal root, motor: sternocleidomastoid and trapezius
Cranial root, motor: most palatine and pharyngeal muscles

Vagus- CN X

Motor: larynx, trachea, bronchial tree, heart, GI tract to left colic flexure
Sensory: pharynx, larynx; reflex sensory from tracheobronchial tree, lungs, heart, GI tract to left colic flexure

Glossopharyngeal- CN IX

Motor: stylopharyngeus, parotid gland
Sensory: taste: posterior 1/3 of tongue; general sensation: pharynx, tonsillar fossa, pharyngotympanic tube, middle ear cavity

CN III
CN II
CN IV
CN VI
CN V
CN VII
CN VII
CN VIII
CN V
CN XII
CN XI
CN X
CN IX
CN I

continued

TABLE 10.1. *CONTINUED*

Nerve	Components	Location of Nerve Cell Bodies	Cranial Exit	Main Action(s)
Olfactory (CN I)	Special sensory	Olfactory epithelium (olfactory receptor neurons)	Foramina in cribriform plate of ethmoid bone	Smell from nasal mucosa of roof of each nasal cavity and superior sides of nasal septum and superior concha
Optic (CN II)	Special sensory	Retina (ganglion cells)	Optic canal	Vision from retina
Oculomotor (CN III)	Somatic motor	Midbrain		Motor to superior, inferior, and medial rectus, inferior oblique, and levator palpebrae superioris muscles; raises superior eyelid; turns eyeball superiorly, inferiorly, and medially
	Visceral motor	Presynaptic: midbrain; postsynaptic: ciliary ganglion	Superior orbital fissure	Parasympathetic innervation to sphincter pupillae and ciliary muscle; constricts pupil and accommodates lens of eye
Trochlear (CN IV)	Somatic motor	Midbrain		Motor to superior oblique that assists in turning eye inferolaterally
Trigeminal (CN V) Ophthalmic division (CN V$_1$)	General sensory	Trigeminal ganglion	Superior orbital fissure	Sensation from cornea, skin of forehead, scalp, eyelids, nose, and mucosa of nasal cavity and paranasal sinuses
Maxillary division (CN V$_2$)			Foramen rotundum	Sensation from skin of face over maxilla including upper lip, maxillary teeth, mucosa of nose, maxillary sinuses, and palate
Mandibular division (CN V$_3$)	Branchial motor	Pons	Foramen ovale	Motor to muscles of mastication, mylohyoid, anterior belly of digastric, tensor veli palatini, and tensor tympani
	General sensory	Trigeminal ganglion		Sensation from the skin over mandible, including lower lip and side of head, mandibular teeth, temporomandibular joint, and mucosa of mouth and anterior two-thirds of tongue
Abducent (CN VI)	Somatic motor	Pons	Superior orbital fissure	Motor to lateral rectus that turns eye laterally
Facial (CN VII)	Branchial motor	Pons	Internal acoustic meatus, facial canal, and stylomastoid foramen	Motor to muscles of facial expression and scalp; also supplies stapedius of middle ear, stylohyoid, and posterior belly of digastric
	Special sensory	Geniculate ganglion		Taste from anterior two-thirds of tongue, floor of mouth, and palate
	General sensory			Sensation from skin of external acoustic meatus
	Visceral motor	Presynaptic: pons; postsynaptic: pterygopalatine ganglion and submandibular ganglion		Parasympathetic innervation to submandibular and sublingual salivary glands, lacrimal glands, and glands of nose and palate

TABLE 10.1. *CONTINUED*

Nerve	Components	Location of Nerve Cell Bodies	Cranial Exit	Main Action(s)
Vestibulocochlear (CN VIII)				
Vestibular	Special sensory	Vestibular ganglion	Internal acoustic meatus	Vestibular sensation from semicircular ducts, utricle, and saccule related to position and movement of head
Cochlear		Spiral ganglion		Hearing from spiral organ
Glossopharyngeal (CN IX)	Branchial motor Visceral motor	Medulla Presynaptic: medulla Postsynaptic: otic ganglion		Motor to stylopharyngeus that assists with swallowing Parasympathetic innervation to parotid gland
	Visceral sensory	Superior ganglion of CN IX		Visceral sensation from parotid gland, carotid body and sinus, pharynx, and middle ear
	Special sensory	Inferior ganglion of CN IX		Taste from posterior third of tongue
	General sensory			Cutaneous sensation from external ear
Vagus (CN X)	Branchial motor	Medulla	Jugular foramen	Motor to constrictor muscles of pharynx, intrinsic muscles of larynx, and muscles of palate except tensor veli palatini, and striated muscle in superior two-thirds of esophagus
	Visceral motor	Presynaptic: medulla; postsynaptic: neurons in, on, or near viscera		Parasympathetic innervation to smooth muscle of trachea, bronchi, digestive tract, and cardiac muscle of heart
	Visceral sensory	Superior ganglion of CN X		Visceral sensation from base of tongue, pharynx, larynx, trachea, bronchi, heart, esophagus, stomach, and intestine
	Special sensory	Inferior ganglion of CN X		Taste from epiglottis and palate
	General sensory	Superior ganglion of CN X		Sensation from auricle, external acoustic meatus, and dura mater of posterior cranial fossa
Accessory (CN XI)				
Cranial root	Somatic motor	Medulla		Motor to striated muscles of soft palate, pharynx via fibers that join CN X; larynx
Spinal root	Branchial motor	Spinal cord		Motor to sternocleidomastoid and trapezius
Hypoglossal (CN XII)	Somatic motor	Medulla	Hypoglossal canal	Motor to muscles of tongue (except palatoglossus)

OLFACTORY NERVE (CN I)

The olfactory nerves convey the sense of smell. The cell bodies of the **olfactory receptor neurons** are in the **olfactory epithelium** in the roof of the nasal cavity (Fig. 10.3). The central processes of the bipolar olfactory neurons cells form approximately 20 bundles of **olfactory nerve fibers** on each side that collectively form the **olfactory nerves.** The olfactory receptor cells are true neurons, but they are unique in being the only neurons that undergo continuous turnover every 30 to 60 days (Sweazey, 2001). The fibers pass through foramina in the **cribriform plate** of the ethmoid bone, pierce the dura and arachnoid mater, and enter the **olfactory bulb** in the anterior cranial fossa (Fig. 10.3*B*). The olfactory nerve fibers synapse with **mitral cells** in the olfactory bulb. The axons of these cells form the **olfactory tract,** which conveys the impulses to the brain. An extension of the cranial meninges surrounds the bundles of olfactory nerves as they leave the cribriform plate. Hence, there are minute communications with the **subarachnoid space,** which contains cerebrospinal fluid (CSF).

LOSS OF SMELL

In severe head injuries, the olfactory bulbs may be torn away from the olfactory nerves, or some olfactory nerve fibers may be torn as they pass through a *fractured cribriform plate.* If all the nerve bundles on one side are torn, a complete loss of smell occurs on that side; consequently, *anosmia (loss of smell) may be a clue to a fracture in the base of the cranium, as may CSF rhinorrhea*—leakage of CSF through the nose. Viruses associated with nasal and paranasal diseases (rhinitis, sinusitis) may permanently damage the olfactory epithelium, preventing replacement of olfactory receptor neurons.

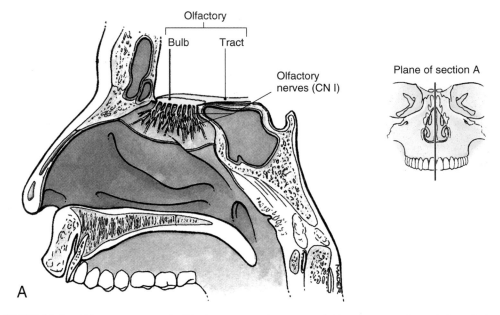

FIGURE 10.3   Olfactory system. A. Olfactory area and passage of olfactory nerves through the cribriform plate to end in the olfactory bulb.

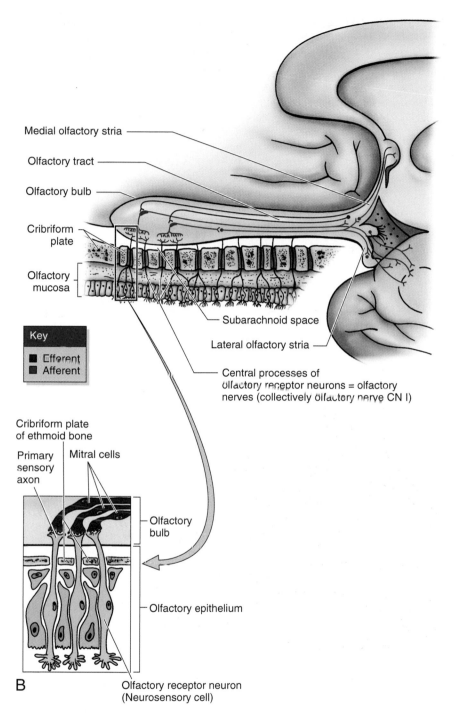

Medial olfactory stria

Olfactory tract

Olfactory bulb

Cribriform plate

Olfactory mucosa

Key
■ Efferent
■ Afferent

Subarachnoid space

Lateral olfactory stria

Central processes of olfactory receptor neurons = olfactory nerves (collectively olfactory nerve CN I)

Cribriform plate of ethmoid bone

Primary sensory axon

Mitral cells

Olfactory bulb

Olfactory epithelium

B

Olfactory receptor neuron (Neurosensory cell)

FIGURE 10.3 *Continued.* **B.** Medial view of the sagittal section through the cribriform plate of the ethmoid bone.

OPTIC NERVE (CN II)

The optic nerve conveys visual information. It is formed by axons of retinal ganglion cells. CN II is surrounded by extensions of the cranial meninges and subarachnoid space filled with CSF. CN II begins where the ax-

ons of the retinal ganglion cells pierce the sclera. The nerve passes posteromedially in the orbit and exits through the **optic canal** (Fig. 10.4*A*) and enters the middle cranial fossa where it forms the **optic chiasm** (G. chiasma). Here, fibers from the nasal or medial half of each retina decussate in the chiasm

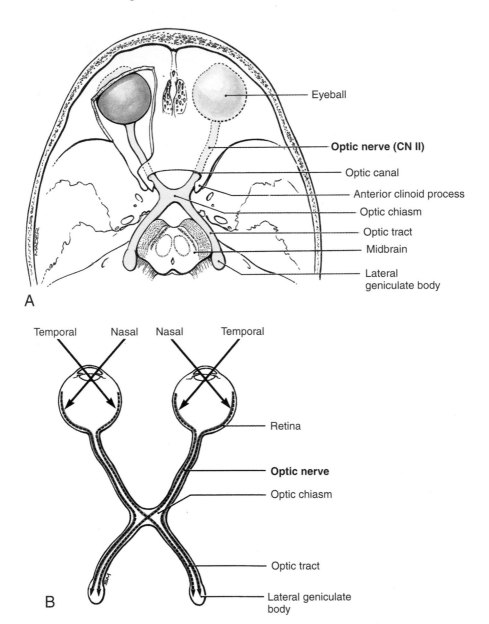

FIGURE 10.4   Visual system. A. Anterior half of the internal surface of the cranium showing the optic nerves, optic chiasm, optic tracts, and optic radiations. Superior view with the roof of the left orbit removed. **B.** Superior view of the schematically isolated visual apparatus. *Arrows,* rays of light from the nasal and temporal halves of a person's field of vision.

and join uncrossed fibers from the temporal or lateral half of the retina to form the **optic tract.** The partial crossing of optic nerve fibers in the chiasm is a requirement for binocular vision, allowing depth of field (three-dimensional vision). Fibers from the nasal half of each retina cross to the opposite side, whereas those from the temporal half of each retina are uncrossed (Fig. 10.4*B*). Thus, fibers from the right halves of both retinas form the right optic tract, and those from the left halves form the left optic tract. The decussation of nerve fibers in the chiasm results in the right optic tract conveying impulses from the left visual field and vice versa. The *visual field* is what is seen by a person with both eyes wide open and looking straight ahead. Most fibers in the optic tracts terminate in the **lateral geniculate bodies** of the thalamus. From these nuclei, axons are relayed to the *visual cortices* of the occipital lobes of the brain.

EDEMA OF RETINA

Because the optic nerves are surrounded by an extension of the cranial meninges, an increase in CSF pressure slows the return of venous blood, causing edema of the retina. This condition is apparent on ophthalmoscope examination as a swelling of the optic discs or papillae (*papilledema*). Swelling of the discs is an indication of increased intracranial pressure.

Visual Field Defects

Visual field defects result from lesions that affect different parts of the visual pathway; the type of defect depends on where the pathway is interrupted:

- *Section of right optic nerve* results in monocular blindness in temporal (*T*) and nasal (*N*) visual fields of the right eye (depicted in *black*)
- *Section of optic chiasm* reduces peripheral vision, resulting in *bitemporal hemianopsia*—loss of vision of one half of the visual field of both eyes
- *Section of right optic tract* eliminates vision from the left temporal and right nasal visual fields. A lesion of the right or left optic tract causes a contralateral *homonymous hemianopsia,* indicating that the visual loss is in similar fields. This defect is the most common form of visual field loss and is often observed in patients with strokes.

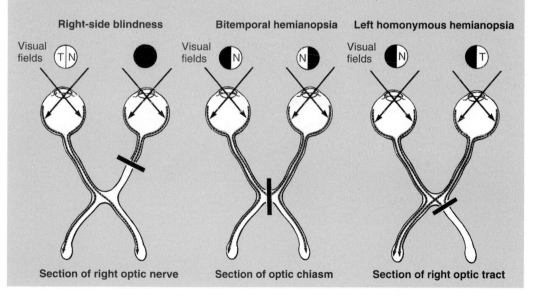

| Right-side blindness | Bitemporal hemianopsia | Left homonymous hemianopsia |

| Section of right optic nerve | Section of optic chiasm | Section of right optic tract |

OCULOMOTOR NERVE (CN III)

The oculomotor nerve is (Fig. 10.5):

- Motor to four of the six extraocular muscles (**superior, medial,** and **inferior rectus** and **inferior oblique**) and to the elevator of the upper eyelid (**levator palpebrae superioris**)
- Proprioceptive to the above muscles
- Parasympathetic—through the ciliary ganglion—to the sphincter of the pupil (sphincter pupillae), which causes constriction of the pupil, and to the ciliary muscle of the lens, which produces accommodation (thickening) of the lens for near vision.

CN III, the chief motor nerve to ocular and extraocular muscles, emerges from the midbrain, pierces the dura, and runs in the lateral wall of the *cavernous sinus* (Chapter 8). CN III leaves the cranial cavity and enters the orbit through the *superior orbital fissure.* Within this fissure, CN III divides into a *superior division* that supplies the superior rectus and levator palpebrae superioris and an *inferior division* that supplies the inferior and medial rectus and inferior oblique. The inferior division also carries presynaptic autonomic fibers to the **ciliary ganglion** where the parasympathetic fibers synapse. The postsynaptic fibers from this ganglion pass to the eyeball in the *short ciliary nerves* and supply the ciliary muscle (accommodation of the lens) and sphincter pupillae (constriction of the pupil). The *long ciliary nerves,* branches of the nasociliary nerve (CN V_1), transmit postsynaptic sympathetic fibers to the dilator pupillae and afferent fibers from the iris and cornea.

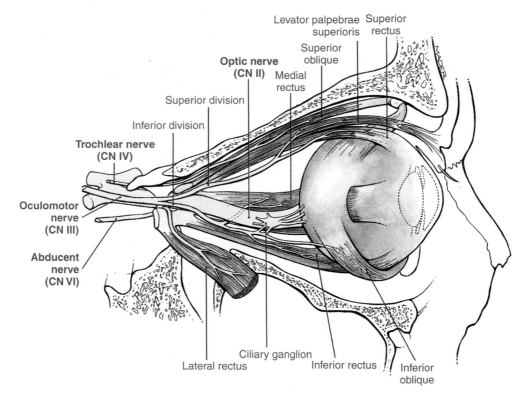

FIGURE 10.5   Innervation of the orbit. Distribution of oculomotor (CN III), trochlear (CN IV), and abducent (CN VI) nerves to extraocular muscles.

OCULOMOTOR NERVE PALSY

A lesion that interrupts CN III fibers causes paralysis of all extraocular muscles except the superior oblique and lateral rectus. The sphincter pupillae in the iris and the ciliary muscle in the ciliary body also are paralyzed. **Characteristic signs of a complete lesion of CN III are:**

- *Ptosis (drooping) of the upper eyelid,* caused by paralysis of the levator palpebrae superioris

- *Eyeball (pupil) abducted and directed slightly inferiorly* (down and out) because of unopposed actions of the lateral rectus and superior oblique

- *No pupillary (light) reflex* (constriction of the pupil in response to bright light) in the affected eye

- *Dilation of pupil,* resulting from the interruption of parasympathetic fibers to the sphincter of the iris, leaving the dilator pupillae unopposed

- *No accommodation of the lens* (adjustment to increase convexity for near vision) because of paralysis of the ciliary muscle.

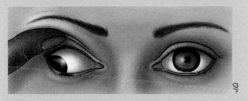

Right eye: Downward and outward gaze, dilated pupil, eyelid manually elevated due to ptosis   Left

Right oculomotor (CN III) nerve palsy

TROCHLEAR NERVE (CN IV)

The trochlear nerve provides motor and proprioceptive innervation to one extraocular muscle (**superior oblique**). *The trochlear nerve emerges from the dorsal surface of the midbrain,* winds around the brainstem (Fig. 10.2), pierces the dura, and passes anteriorly in the lateral wall of the cavernous sinus (Chapter 8). CN IV leaves the cranial cavity and passes through the superior orbital fissure into the orbit to supply the superior oblique (Fig. 10.5).

TROCHLEAR NERVE INJURY

CN IV may be torn in severe head injuries because of its long intracranial course; however, the superior oblique is rarely paralyzed in isolation. Damage to CN IV results in the person being unable to direct the affected eye inferolaterally. The characteristic sign of trochlear nerve injury is *diplopia* (double vision) when looking down (e.g., when going down stairs). Diplopia occurs because the inferior rectus normally assists the inferior oblique in depressing the pupil (directing the gaze downward), especially when it is adducted (in a medial position); thus, when the person tries to look in this direction, the gaze is directed differently in the affected and unaffected eye. The person can compensate for the diplopia by inclining the head anteriorly and to the side of the normal eye.

TRIGEMINAL NERVE (CN V)

The trigeminal nerve emerges from the pons by a *small motor root* and a *large sensory root* (Fig. 10.2A). CN V is the principal general sensory nerve for the head: face, teeth, mouth, nasal cavity, and dura (Fig. 10.6). Fibers in the sensory root are mainly central processes of neurons in the **trigeminal ganglion** (Fig. 10.2B). The peripheral processes of these neurons form the **ophthalmic nerve** (CN V_1), the **maxillary nerve** (CN V_2), and the sensory component of the **mandibular nerve** (CN V_3). For a summary of CN V, see Table 10.2. The fibers in the motor root of CN V are distributed through the mandibular nerve to the muscles of mastication, the mylohyoid, anterior belly of the digastric, tensor veli palatini, and tensor tympani.

TRIGEMINAL NERVE INJURY

CN V may be injured by trauma, tumors, aneurysms, or meningeal infections. **Injury to CN V causes:**

- Paralysis of the muscles of mastication with deviation of the mandible toward the side of the lesion

- Loss of the ability to appreciate soft tactile, thermal, or painful sensations in the face

- Loss of the corneal reflex (blinking in response to the cornea being touched) and the sneezing reflex.

Trigeminal neuralgia (tic douloureux), the principal condition affecting the sensory root of CN V, is characterized by attacks of excruciating pain in the area of distribution of the maxillary and/or mandibular divisions of CN V. The sudden attack is often set off by touching an especially sensitive facial area. Usually the cause of the *neuralgia*—pain of a severe, throbbing, or stabbing character—is undetectable.

ABDUCENT NERVE (CN VI)

The abducent (abducens) nerve provides motor and proprioceptive information to one ex-

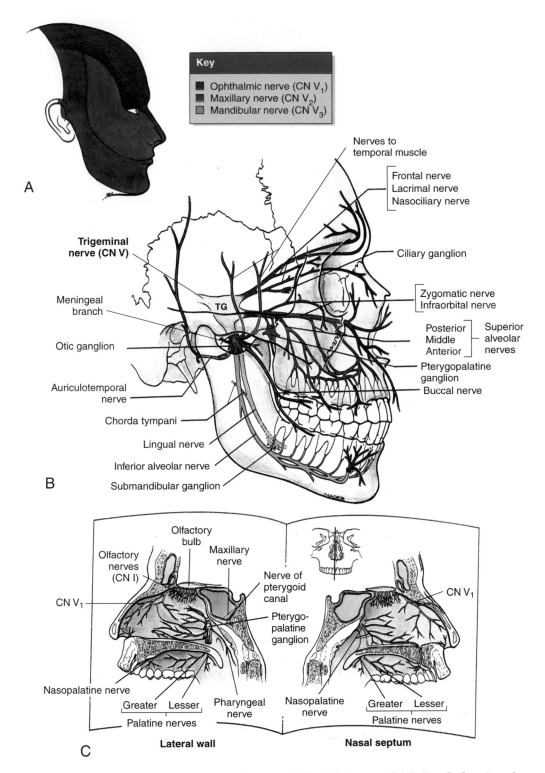

FIGURE 10.6 **Distribution of the trigeminal nerve (CN V). A.** Cutaneous distribution. **B.** Overview of branches. *TG,* trigeminal ganglion. **C.** Distribution of the maxillary nerve (CN V₂). The olfactory nerves (CN I) and a branch of the ophthalmic nerve (CN V₁) are shown also.

TABLE 10.2. SUMMARY OF TRIGEMINAL NERVE (CN V)

Divisions	Branches

Ophthalmic nerve (CN V₁), a sensory nerve, passes through the superior orbital fissure and supplies the eyeball, conjunctiva, lacrimal gland and sac, nasal mucosa, frontal sinus, external nose, superior eyelid, forehead, and scalp	Tentorial nerve
	Lacrimal nerve
	Frontal nerve
	   Supraorbital nerve
	   Supratrochlear nerve
	Nasociliary nerve
	   Short ciliary nerves
	   Long ciliary nerves
	   Infratrochlear nerve
	   Anterior and posterior ethmoidal nerves

Maxillary nerve (CN V₂), a sensory nerve, passes through the foramen rotundum	Meningeal branch
	Zygomatic nerve
	   Zygomaticofacial branch
	   Zygomaticotemporal branch
	Posterior superior alveolar branches
	Infraorbital nerve
	   Anterior and middle superior alveolar branches
	   Superior labial branches
	   Inferior palpebral branches
	   External nasal branches
	Greater palatine nerves
	   Posterior inferior lateral nasal nerves
	Lesser palatine nerves
	Posterior superior lateral nasal branches
	Nasopalatine nerve
	Pharyngeal nerve

Mandibular nerve (CN V₃), a motor and sensory nerve, passes through the foramen ovale
 	
General sensory branches
	Meningeal branch (nervus spinosum)
	Buccal nerve
	Auriculotemporal nerve
	Lingual nerve
	Inferior alveolar nerve
	   Nerve to mylohyoid
	   Inferior dental plexus
	   Mental nerve
	   Incisive nerve

Branchial branches to muscles	Masseter Temporal Medial and lateral pterygoids Tensor veli palatini Mylohyoid Anterior belly of digastric Tensor tympani

traocular muscle (**lateral rectus**). *The abducent nerve emerges from the brainstem between the pons and medulla* (Fig. 10.2) and enters the pontocerebellar (pontine) cistern (Chapter 8), where it runs along the basilar artery. It then pierces the dura and runs the longest course in the subarachnoid space of all the cranial nerves. It bends sharply over the crest of the petrous part of the temporal bone to enter the *cavernous sinus* (p. 521), coursing through it with the internal carotid artery. CN VI leaves this sinus to enter the orbit through the superior orbital fissure (Fig. 10.5) and runs anteriorly to supply the **lateral rectus,** which abducts the eye.

ABDUCENT NERVE INJURY

Because CN VI has a long intracranial course, often it is stretched when intracranial pressure rises, partly because of the sharp bend it makes over the crest of the petrous part of the temporal bone after entering the dura. A space-occupying lesion such as a brain tumor may compress CN VI, causing paralysis of the lateral rectus muscle. Thrombosis (clotting of blood in the veins) in the cavernous sinus may also compress CN VI. Complete paralysis of this muscle causes medial deviation of the affected eye; that is, it is fully adducted because of the unopposed action of the medial rectus, rendering the person unable to abduct the eye. *Diplopia* is present in all ranges of movement of the eyeball, except on gazing to the side opposite the lesion.

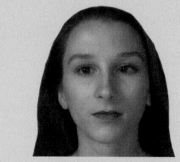

Abducent nerve injury

FACIAL NERVE (CN VII)

The facial nerve is:

- Sensory for taste from the anterior two thirds of the tongue and soft palate
- Sensory (general) from part of the external ear (concha of auricle)
- Motor to the muscles of facial expression, fauces (throat)—posterior belly of digastric, stylohyoid—and middle ear (stapedius)

- Proprioceptive to the above muscles
- Parasympathetic to the submandibular and sublingual salivary glands, lacrimal gland, and the glands of the nasal cavity and palate (Table 10.1).

The facial nerve emerges from the junction of the pons and medulla (Fig. 10.2*A*). CN VII has two divisions, the motor root (facial nerve proper) and the intermediate nerve (L. nervus intermedius). The larger *motor root* innervates the muscles of facial expression, and the smaller root (intermediate nerve) carries taste, parasympathetic, and somatic sensory fibers conveyed distally by the chorda tympani nerve (Fig. 10.7). During its course, CN VII traverses the posterior cranial fossa, internal acoustic meatus, facial canal in the temporal bone, stylomastoid foramen, and parotid gland. At the medial wall of the tympanic cavity, the facial canal bends posteroinferiorly where the **geniculate ganglion** (sensory ganglion of CN VII) is located. Within the facial canal, CN VII gives rise to the **greater petrosal nerve,** *the nerve to the stapedius*, and the **chorda tympani nerve.** After running the longest intraosseous course of any cranial nerve, CN VII then emerges from the cranium via the *stylomastoid foramen,* gives off branches to the auricular, facial, and occipitofrontal muscles, then enters the parotid gland, forming the *parotid plexus of nerves,* which gives rise to the following terminal branches: *posterior auricular, temporal, zygomatic, buccal, mandibular,* and *cervical.*

BRANCHIAL MOTOR

Terminal branches innervate the muscles of facial expression, the occipitalis, auricular muscles, posterior belly of digastric, stylohyoid, and stapedius muscles. These branches are all derivatives of the embryonic 2nd pharyngeal (branchial) arch.

GENERAL SENSORY

Some fibers from the **geniculate ganglion** (Fig. 10.7*A*) supply a small area of skin around the external acoustic meatus.

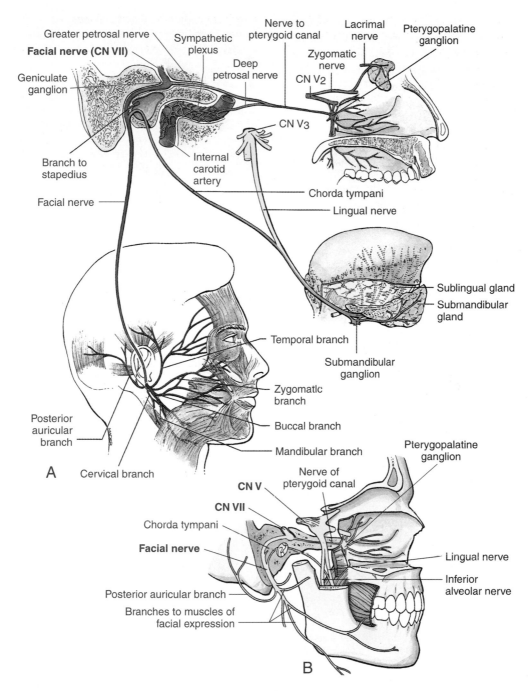

FIGURE 10.7 **Distribution of the facial nerve (CN VII). A.** Detailed regional distribution of facial nerve fibers. **B.** In situ relationships of branches of the facial nerve.

The parasympathetic distribution of the facial nerve is illustrated in Figure 10.8. Postsynaptic fibers from the **submandibular ganglion** (Fig. 10.7A) innervate the sublingual and submandibular salivary glands, while those from the **pterygopalatine ganglion** innervate lacrimal, nasal, pharyngeal, and palatine glands. The main features of parasympathetic ganglia associated with the facial nerve and other cranial nerves are illustrated in Table 10.3. Parasympathetic fibers synapse in these ganglia, whereas sympathetic and other fibers pass through them.

TASTE (SPECIAL SENSORY)

The chorda tympani receives fibers from the **lingual nerve** that convey taste sensation from the anterior two thirds of the tongue and soft palate to the geniculate ganglion.

FACIAL NERVE INJURY

Among motor nerves, *CN VII is the most frequently injured of all the cranial nerves.* Depending on the part of the nerve involved, injury to CN VII may cause paralysis of facial muscles without loss of taste on the anterior two thirds of the tongue or altered secretion of the lacrimal and salivary glands. A lesion of CN VII near its origin or near the geniculate ganglion is accompanied by loss of motor, gustatory (taste), and autonomic functions. The motor paralysis of facial muscles involves upper and lower parts of the face on the ipsilateral (same) side. Muscles in the lower quadrants of the face are influenced mainly from the contralateral cerebral hemisphere. A *cortical lesion of CN VII* results in paralysis of muscles in the lower face on the contralateral (opposite) side; however, forehead wrinkling on that side is not impaired. Lesions between the geniculate ganglion and the origin of the chorda tympani produce the same effects as that resulting from injury near the ganglion except that lacrimal secretion is not affected. Because it passes through the facial canal, CN VII is vulnerable to compression when a viral infection produces inflammation of the nerve (*viral neuritis*) with swelling of the nerve just before it emerges from the stylomastoid foramen. *Bell palsy,* the common disorder resulting from a lesion of CN VII, is described and illustrated on page 509. Because the branches of CN VII are superficial, they are also subject to injury from stab and gunshot wounds, cuts, and during birth.

A. Parasympathetic (visceral motor) to lacrimal gland

> Greater petrosal nerve arises from CN VII at the geniculate ganglion and emerges from the superior surface of the petrous part of the temporal bone to enter the middle cranial fossa.

> Greater petrosal nerve joins the deep petrosal nerve (sympathetic) at the foramen lacerum to form the nerve of the pterygoid canal.

> Nerve of pterygoid canal travels through the pterygoid canal and enters the pterygopalatine fossa.

> Parasympathetic fibers from the nerve of pterygoid canal in the pterygopalatine fossa synapse in the pterygopalatine ganglion.

> Postsynaptic parasympathetic fibers from this ganglion innervate the lacrimal gland via the zygomatic branch of CN V_2 and the lacrimal nerve (branch of CN V_1).

B. Parasympathetic (visceral motor) to submandibular and sublingual glands

> The chorda tympani branch arises from CN VII just superior to stylomastoid foramen.

> The chorda tympani crosses the tympanic cavity medial to handle of malleus.

> The chorda tympani passes through the petrotympanic fissure between the tympanic and petrous parts of the temporal bone to join the lingual nerve (CN V_3) in the infratemporal fossa; parasympathetic fibers of the chorda tympani synapse in the submandibular ganglion; postsynaptic fibers follow arteries to glands.

FIGURE 10.8   Flowchart showing the course of parasympathetic fibers in the facial nerve (CN VII). **A.** Parasympathetic (visceral motor) innervation of the lacrimal gland. **B.** Parasympathetic (visceral motor) innervation of the submandibular and sublingual glands.

VESTIBULOCOCHLEAR NERVE (CN VIII)

The 8th cranial nerve is the nerve of hearing and equilibrium (balance). *The vestibulocochlear nerve emerges from the junction of the pons and medulla* (Fig. 10.2*A*) and enters the *internal acoustic meatus* with the facial nerve. Here, CN VIII separates into the **vestibular** and **cochlear nerves** (Fig. 10.9).

- Vestibular fibers, concerned with equilibrium, are the central processes of neurons in the **vestibular ganglion;** peripheral processes of these neurons extend to the **maculae** of the utricle (utricular nerve) and saccule (saccular nerve) and the **ampullae of semicircular ducts** (anterior, lateral, and posterior ampullary nerves).
- Cochlear fibers, concerned with hearing, are the central processes of neurons in the **spiral ganglion;** the peripheral processes extend to the spiral organ (of Corti).

The **maculae** are primarily static organs that have small dense particles (otoliths) embedded among hair cells. Under the influence of gravity, the otoliths cause bending of the hair cells, which stimulates the vestibular nerve and provides awareness of the position of the head in space. The hairs also respond to quick tilting motion and to linear acceleration and deceleration.

The **ampulla** of each semicircular duct contains a sensory area. The hair cells of these areas are sensors for recording movements of the endolymph in the ampulla resulting from rotation of the head in the plane of the duct. The hair cells stimulate sensory neurons, the cell bodies of which are in the vestibular ganglia.

VESTIBULAR NERVE INJURIES
Although the vestibular and cochlear nerves are essentially independent, peripheral lesions often produce concurrent clinical effects because of their close relationship. Hence, lesions of CN VIII may cause *tinnitus* (ringing or buzzing of the ears), *vertigo* (dizziness, loss of balance), and impairment or loss of hearing. *There are two kinds of deafness:*

- *Conductive deafness,* involving the external or middle ear (e.g., otitis media, inflammation in the middle ear)
- *Sensorineural deafness,* the result of disease in the cochlea or in the pathway from the cochlea to the brain.

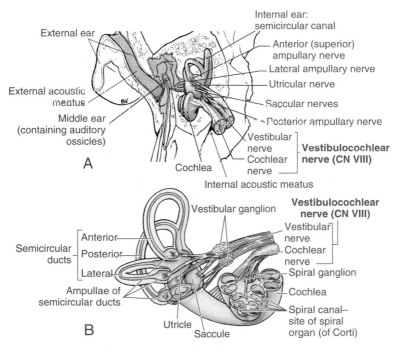

FIGURE 10.9 **Distribution of the vestibulocochlear nerve (CN VIII). A.** Parts of the ear. **B.** Schematic lateral view of the bony labyrinth showing innervation of the membranous labyrinth.

GLOSSOPHARYNGEAL NERVE (CN IX)

The glossopharyngeal nerve is:

- Sensory for taste from the posterior third of the tongue
- Sensory (general) from the mucosa of the pharynx, palatine tonsil, posterior third of the tongue, pharyngotympanic (auditory) tube, and middle ear
- Sensory for blood pressure and chemistry from the carotid sinus and carotid body
- Motor and proprioceptive to the stylopharyngeus
- Parasympathetic (secretomotor) to the parotid gland and glands in the posterior third of the tongue.

The glossopharyngeal nerve emerges from the medulla of the brain and passes anterolaterally to leave the cranium through the jugular foramen. At this foramen are the **superior** *and* **inferior ganglia of CN IX** *(Fig. 10.10), which contain the cell bodies for the afferent components of the nerve. CN IX follows the* **stylopharyngeus** *and passes between the superior and middle constrictor muscles of the pharynx to reach the oropharynx and tongue. It contributes to the pharyngeal plexus of nerves. The glossopharyngeal nerve is afferent from the tongue and pharynx (hence its name) and efferent to the stylopharyngeus and parotid gland.*

SENSORY (GENERAL VISCERAL)

The sensory branches of CN IX (Fig. 10.10) are the:

- Tympanic nerve
- Carotid branch to the carotid sinus and carotid body
- Nerves to the mucosa of the tongue and oropharynx, palatine tonsil, soft palate, and posterior third of the tongue.

TASTE (SPECIAL SENSORY)

Taste fibers pass from the posterior third of the tongue.

BRANCHIAL MOTOR

Motor fibers pass to the one muscle—the **stylopharyngeus**—derived from the 3rd pharyngeal (branchial) arch. The parasympathetic (visceral motor) distribution of CN IX is illustrated in Figure 10.11. **Parasympathetic ganglia** associated with CNs III, V, VII, and IX are illustrated in Table 10.3.

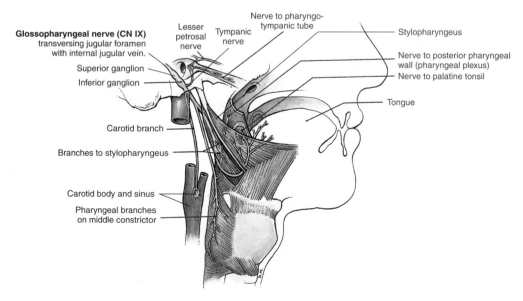

FIGURE 10.10   Distribution of the glossopharyngeal nerve (CN IX). Lateral view of the head and upper neck.

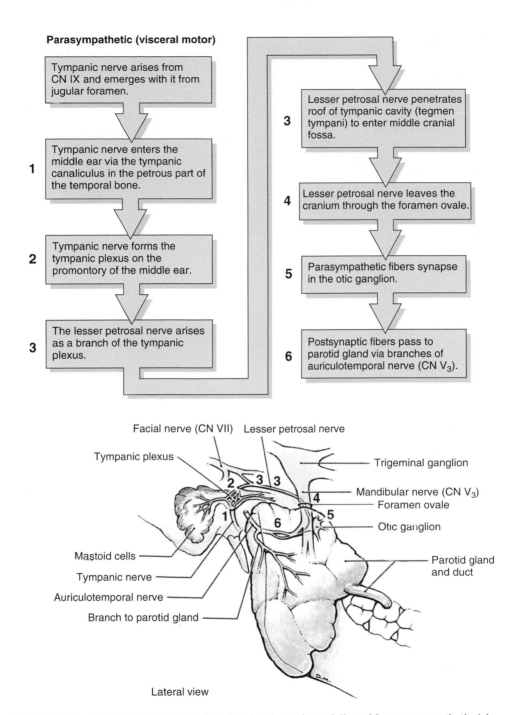

Parasympathetic (visceral motor)

1 Tympanic nerve arises from CN IX and emerges with it from jugular foramen.

Tympanic nerve enters the middle ear via the tympanic canaliculus in the petrous part of the temporal bone.

2 Tympanic nerve forms the tympanic plexus on the promontory of the middle ear.

3 The lesser petrosal nerve arises as a branch of the tympanic plexus.

3 Lesser petrosal nerve penetrates roof of tympanic cavity (tegmen tympani) to enter middle cranial fossa.

4 Lesser petrosal nerve leaves the cranium through the foramen ovale.

5 Parasympathetic fibers synapse in the otic ganglion.

6 Postsynaptic fibers pass to parotid gland via branches of auriculotemporal nerve (CN V₃).

Facial nerve (CN VII)   Lesser petrosal nerve
Tympanic plexus
Trigeminal ganglion
Mandibular nerve (CN V₃)
Foramen ovale
Otic ganglion
Mastoid cells
Tympanic nerve
Auriculotemporal nerve
Branch to parotid gland
Parotid gland and duct

Lateral view

FIGURE 10.11   Flowchart and illustration showing the pathway followed by parasympathetic (visceral motor) fibers of the glossopharyngeal nerve (CN IX) innervating the parotid gland.

LESIONS OF GLOSSOPHARYNGEAL NERVE
Isolated lesions of CN IX or its nuclei are uncommon and are not associated with perceptible disability. Taste is absent on the posterior third of the tongue, and the *gag reflex* is absent on the side of the lesion. Injuries of CN IX result- ing from infection or tumors usually are accompanied by signs of involvement of adjacent nerves. Because CNs IX, X, and XI pass through the jugular foramen, tumors in this region produce multiple cranial nerve palsies—*jugular foramen syndrome.*

VAGUS NERVE (CN X)

The vagus nerve is:

- Sensory from the inferior pharynx, larynx, and thoracic and abdominal organs
- Sensory for taste from the root of the tongue and the taste buds on the epiglottis
- Motor to the soft palate, pharynx, intrinsic laryngeal muscles (phonation), and a nominal extrinsic tongue muscle, the palatoglossus, which is actually a palatine muscle based on its derivation and innervation
- Proprioceptive to the above muscles
- Parasympathetic to thoracic and abdominal viscera.

The vagus nerve arises by a series of rootlets from the side of the medulla and leaves the cranium through the jugular foramen in company with CN IX and CN XI (Fig. 10.12). The **superior ganglion of CN X** is in this foramen and is mainly concerned with the general sensory component of the nerve. The **inferior ganglion of CN X** is inferior to the foramen and is concerned with the visceral sensory component of the nerve. In the region of the superior ganglion there are connections with CNs IX and XI (Fig. 10.12) and the superior cervical ganglion. CN X continues inferiorly in the carotid

TABLE 10.3. SUMMARY OF VAGUS NERVE

Divisions	Branches
Arises by a series of rootlets from medulla	
Leaves cranium through jugular foramen	Receives cranial root of accessory nerve (CN XI) Meningeal branch to dura mater Auricular nerve
Enters carotid sheath and continues to root of neck	Pharyngeal nerves Superior laryngeal nerves Right recurrent laryngeal nerve Cardiac nerves
Passes through superior thoracic aperture into thorax	Left recurrent laryngeal nerve Cardiac nerves Pulmonary branches to bronchi and lungs Esophageal nerves
Passes through esophageal hiatus in diaphragm and enters abdomen	Esophageal branches Gastric branches Pancreatic branches Branches to gallbladder Branches to intestine as far as left colic flexure

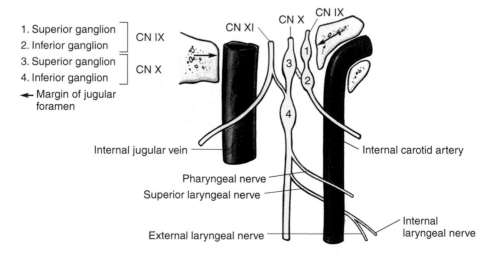

FIGURE 10.12   Relationship of CNs IX, X, and XI as they emerge from the jugular foramen. *Arrow,* margins of the foramen. Note the relationship of these nerves to the internal carotid artery and internal jugular vein.

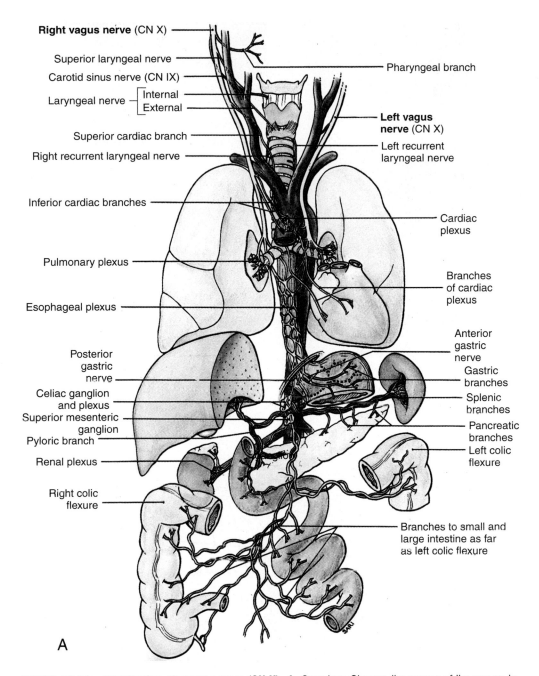

Right vagus nerve (CN X)

Superior laryngeal nerve

Carotid sinus nerve (CN IX)

Laryngeal nerve — Internal / External

Superior cardiac branch

Right recurrent laryngeal nerve

Inferior cardiac branches

Pulmonary plexus

Esophageal plexus

Posterior gastric nerve

Celiac ganglion and plexus

Superior mesenteric ganglion

Pyloric branch

Renal plexus

Right colic flexure

Pharyngeal branch

Left vagus nerve (CN X)

Left recurrent laryngeal nerve

Cardiac plexus

Branches of cardiac plexus

Anterior gastric nerve

Gastric branches

Splenic branches

Pancreatic branches

Left colic flexure

Branches to small and large intestine as far as left colic flexure

A

FIGURE 10.13 **Distribution of vagus nerves (CN X). A.** Overview. Observe the course of the nerves in the neck, thorax, and abdomen.

sheath to the root of the neck (Table 10.3). The course of the right and left vagi differs in the thorax (p. 107). In the neck and thorax the vagus supplies branches to the pharynx, larynx, trachea, lungs, heart, and esophagus (Fig. 10.13). The vagi join and contribute parasympathetic fibers to the **esophageal plexus** surrounding the esophagus; thus, this plexus is formed by intermingling branches of the bilateral sympathetic trunks. This plexus follows

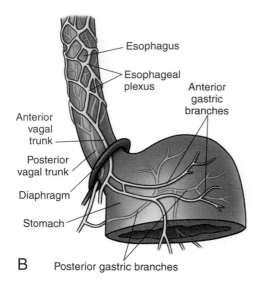

FIGURE 10.13 *Continued.* **B.** Anterior and posterior vagal trunks.

the esophagus through the diaphragm into the abdomen, where the **anterior** and **posterior vagal trunks** (Fig. 10.13*B*) break up into branches to innervate the esophagus, stomach, and intestinal tract as far as the left colic flexure.

LESIONS OF VAGUS NERVE

Isolated lesions of an entire vagus nerve are uncommon. *Injury to pharyngeal branches of CN X results in dysphagia* (difficulty in swallowing). *Lesions of the superior laryngeal nerve* produce anesthesia of the superior part of the larynx and paralysis of the cricothyroid muscle (see Chapter 9). The voice is weak and tires easily. Paralysis of the recurrent laryngeal nerves may result from cancer of the larynx and thyroid gland and from injury during surgery on the thyroid gland, neck, esophagus, heart, and lungs. Because of its longer course, lesions of the left recurrent laryngeal nerve are more common than those of the right. Proximal lesions of the vagus nerve affect the pharyngeal and superior laryngeal nerves, causing difficulty in swallowing and speaking.

ACCESSORY NERVE (CN XI)

The accessory nerve is motor to the soft palate and pharynx (*cranial root*—vagal part) and sternocleidomastoid (SCM) and trapezius (*spinal root*—spinal part). The accessory nerve has cranial and spinal roots, which are united for only a short distance (Fig. 10.14). (The cranial root of CN XI is often considered to be a part of CN X. Then, the spinal root is the accessory nerve.) The **cranial root** (vagal

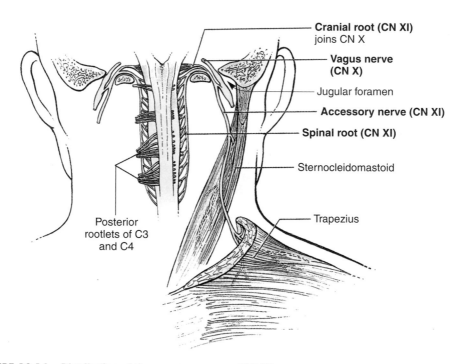

FIGURE 10.14 **Distribution of the accessory nerve (CN XI).**

part) of CN XI arises by a series of rootlets from the medulla and joins the vagus (CN X) intracranially. Its fibers are distributed by vagal branches to striated muscle of the soft palate, pharynx, larynx, and esophagus. The **spinal root** (spinal part) of CN XI emerges as a series of rootlets from the first five cervical segments of the spinal cord. It descends along the internal carotid artery, penetrates and innervates the SCM, and emerges from it at its posterior border near its middle. The nerve crosses the posterior triangle of the neck and innervates the trapezius. Branches of the cervical plexus conveying sensory fibers from spinal nerves C2 through C4 join the accessory nerve in the posterior triangle of the neck, providing these muscles with pain and proprioceptive fibers.

INJURY TO SPINAL ROOT OF CN XI

Because of its superficial passage through the posterior triangle of the neck, the spinal root of CN XI is susceptible to injury during surgical procedures such as lymph node biopsy and cannulation of the internal jugular vein. Lesions of CN XI produce weakness and atrophy of the trapezius and impairment of rotary movements of the neck and chin to the opposite side as a result of weakness of the SCM. Weakness of shrugging movements of the shoulder is the result of weakness of the trapezius. The SCM and trapezius muscles are influenced mainly by the ipsilateral cerebral hemisphere (Haines, 2002).

HYPOGLOSSAL NERVE (CN XII)

The hypoglossal nerve is motor to intrinsic and extrinsic muscles of the tongue (styloglossus, hyoglossus, genioglossus). It also conveys motor fibers from spinal nerves C1 and C2 to the hyoid muscles (thyrohyoid and geniohyoid), proprioceptive fibers to these muscles (Fig. 10.15), and general sensory to the dura of the posterior cranial fossa. *The hypoglossal nerve arises as a purely motor nerve by several rootlets from the medulla* (Fig. 10.2A) and leaves the cranium through the *hypoglossal canal*. After emerging from this canal, the nerve is joined by a branch of the cervical plexus (Fig. 10.15) conveying nerve fibers from C1 and C2 spinal nerves and by sensory fibers from the spinal ganglion of C2 spinal nerve. CN XII passes inferiorly, medial to the

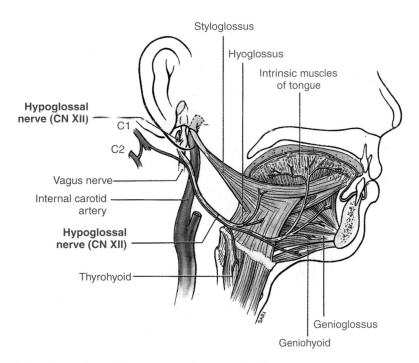

FIGURE 10.15 **Distribution of the hypoglossal nerve (CN XII).**

angle of the mandible, and then curves anteriorly to enter the tongue. CN XII ends in many branches that supply all the extrinsic muscles of the tongue, except the palatoglossus (which is actually a palatine muscle). The hypoglossal nerve is joined in the hypoglossal canal by the superior division of the C1 nerve. *CN XII has the following branches* (the list of branches includes both those of the hypoglossal nerve itself and those of cervical origin associated with it):

- Meningeal branch returns to the cranium through the hypoglossal canal and innervates dura on the floor and posterior wall of the posterior cranial fossa. The nerve fibers conveyed are from the sensory spinal ganglion of spinal nerve C2, not from CN XII.

- Descending branch joins *ansa cervicalis* (Chapter 9) to supply the infrahyoid muscles. This branch actually conveys fibers from the cervical plexus (loop between anterior rami of C1 and C2). The cervical spinal nerve fibers join the hypoglossal nerve proximally.

- Terminal branches are to the styloglossus, hyoglossus, genioglossus, and intrinsic muscles of the tongue.

INJURY TO HYPOGLOSSAL NERVE

The hypoglossal nerve accompanies the tonsillar artery on the lateral wall of the pharynx. Because this wall is thin, CN XII is vulnerable to injury during *tonsillectomy*. Injury to CN XII paralyses the ipsilateral half of the tongue. After some time the tongue atrophies, making it appear shrunken and wrinkled. When the tongue is protruded, its tip deviates toward the paralyzed side because of the unopposed action of the genioglossus in the normal side of the tongue.

TABLE 10.4.   PARASYMPATHETIC GANGLIA ASSOCIATED WITH CN III, V, VII, AND IX

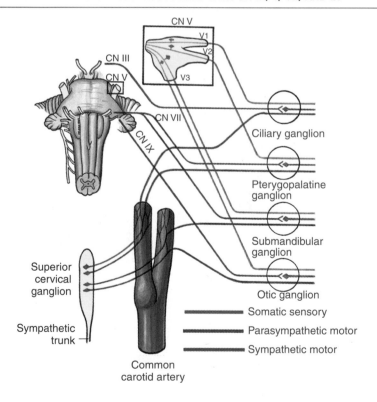

TABLE 10.4. *CONTINUED*

Ganglion	Location	Parasympathetic Root	Sympathetic Root	Main Distribution
Ciliary	Located between optic nerve and lateral rectus, close to apex of orbit	Inferior branch of oculomotor nerve (CN III)	Branch from internal carotid plexus in cavernous sinus	Parasympathetic postsynaptic fibers from ciliary ganglion pass to ciliary muscle and sphincter pupillae of iris; sympathetic postsynaptic fibers from superior cervical ganglion pass to dilator pupillae and blood vessels of eye
Pterygopalatine	Located in pterygopalatine fossa where it is suspended by pterygopalatine branches of maxillary nerve; located just anterior to opening of pterygoid canal and inferior to CN V_2	Greater petrosal nerve from facial nerve (CN VII)	Deep petrosal nerve, a branch of internal carotid plexus that is continuation of postsynaptic fibers of cervical sympathetic trunk; fibers from superior cervical ganglion pass through pterygopalatine ganglion and enter branches of CN V_2	Parasympathetic postsynaptic fibers from pterygopalatine ganglion innervate lacrimal gland via zygomatic branch of CN V_2; sympathetic postsynaptic fibers from superior cervical ganglion accompany those branches of pterygopalatine nerve that are distributed to blood vessels of the nasal cavity, palate, and superior part of the pharynx
Otic	Located between tensor veli palatini and mandibular nerve (CN V_3); lies inferior to foramen ovale	Tympanic nerve from glossopharyngeal nerve (CN IX); from tympanic plexus tympanic nerve continues as lesser petrosal nerve	Fibers from superior cervical ganglion come from plexus on middle meningeal artery	Parasympathetic postsynaptic fibers from otic ganglion are distributed to parotid gland via auriculotemporal nerve (branch of CN V_3); sympathetic postsynaptic fibers from superior cervical ganglion pass to parotid gland and supply its blood vessels
Submandibular	Suspended from lingual nerve by two short roots; lies on surface of hyoglossus muscle inferior to submandibular duct	Parasympathetic fibers join facial nerve (CN VII) and leave it in its chorda tympani branch, which unites with lingual nerve	Sympathetic fibers from superior cervical ganglion come from the plexus on facial artery	Parasympathetic postsynaptic fibers from submandibular ganglion are distributed to the sublingual and submandibular glands; sympathetic fibers supply sublingual and submandibular glands and appear to be secretomotor

References and Suggested Readings

Agur AMR, Lee M: *Grant's Atlas of Anatomy,* 10th ed. Baltimore: Lippincott Williams & Wilkins, 1999.

Amadio PC: Reaffirming the importance of dissection. *Clin Anat* 9:136, 1996.

Basmajian JV, DeLuca CJ: *Muscles Alive: Their Functions Revealed by Electromyography,* 5th ed. Baltimore: Williams & Wilkins, 1985.

Cahill DR, Leonard RJ: The role of computers and dissection in teaching anatomy: A comment. *Clin Anat* 10:140, 1997.

Callen PW: *Ultrasonography in Obstetrics and Gynecology,* 4th ed. Philadelphia: WB Saunders, 2000.

Cormack DH: *Essential Histology,* 2nd ed. Baltimore: Lippincott Williams & Wilkins, 2001.

Cotran RS, Kumar V, Collins T: *Robbin's Pathologic Basis of Disease,* 6th ed. Philadelphia: WB Saunders, 1998.

Federative Committee on Anatomical Terminology: *Terminologia Anatomica: International Anatomical Nomenclature.* Stuttgart: Thieme, 1998.

Gartner LP, Hiatt JL: *Color Textbook of Histology,* 2nd ed. Philadelphia: WB Saunders, 2001.

Ger R: Surgical anatomy of hepatic venous system. *Clin Anat* l:15, 1988.

Ger R, Abrahms, P, Olson TR: *Essentials of Clinical Anatomy,* 2nd ed. New York: The Parthenon Publishing Group, 1996.

Gross AE: Orthopedic surgery: Adult. *In* Gross A, Gross P, Langer B (eds): *A Complete Guide for Patients and Their Families.* Toronto: Harper & Collins, 1989.

Haines DE: *Neuroanatomy: An Atlas of Structures, Sections, and Systems,* 5th ed. Baltimore: Lippincott Williams & Wilkins, 1999.

Haines DE (ed): *Fundamental Neuroscience,* 2nd ed. New York: Churchill Livingstone, 2002.

Hutchins JB, Naftel JP, Ard MD: The cell biology of neurons and glia. *In* Haines DE (ed): *Fundamental Neuroscience,* 2nd ed. New York: Churchill Livingstone, 2002.

Kiernan JA: *Barr's The Human Nervous System: An Anatomical Viewpoint,* 7th ed. Baltimore: Lippincott, Williams & Wilkins, 1998.

Mihailoff GA, Haines DE: Motor system II: Corticofugal systems and the control of movement. *In* Haines DE (ed): *Fundamental Neuroscience,* 2nd ed. New York: Churchill Livingstone, 2002.

Moore KL: Anatomical terminology/clinical terminology. *Clin Anat* l:7, 1988.

Moore KL, Dalley AF: *Clinically Oriented Anatomy,* 4th ed. Baltimore: Lippincott Williams & Wilkins, 1999.

Moore KL, Persaud TVN: *The Developing Human: Clinically Oriented Embryology,* 6th ed. Philadelphia: WB Saunders, 1998.

Moore KL, Persaud TVN, Shiota K: *Color Atlas of Clinical Embryology,* 2nd ed. Philadelphia: WB Saunders, 2000.

Oelrich TM: The urethral sphincter in the male. *Am J Anat* 158:229, 1980.

Oelrich TM: The striated urogenital sphincter muscle in the female. *Anat Rec* 205:223, 1983.

Persaud TVN: *A History of Anatomy. The Post-Vesalian Era.* Springfield: Charles C Thomas, 1997.

Ross MH, Romrell LJ, Kaye G: *Histology. A Text and Atlas,* 3rd ed. Baltimore: Williams & Wilkins, 1994.

Rowland LP (ed): *Merritt's Textbook of Neurology,* 9th ed. Baltimore: Lippincott Williams & Wilkins, 1995.

Salter RB: *Textbook of Disorders and Injuries of the Musculoskeletal System,* 3rd ed. Baltimore: Lippincott Williams & Wilkins, 1998.

Skandalakis JE, Skandalakis PN, Skandalakis LJ: *Surgical Anatomy and Technique: A Pocket Manual.* New York: Springer-Verlag, 1995.

Swartz MH: *Textbook of Physical Diagnosis, History and Examination,* 4th ed. Philadelphia: WB Saunders, 2001.

Sweazy RD: Olfaction and taste. *In* Haines DE (ed): *Fundamental Neuroscience,* 2nd ed. New York: Churchill Livingstone, 2001.

Wendell-Smith C: Muscles and fasciae of the pelvis. *In* Williams PL, et al. (eds): *Gray's Anatomy. The Anatomical Basis of Medicine and Surgery,* 38th ed. New York: Churchill Livingstone, 1995.

Williams PL, Bannister LH, Berry MM, Collins P, Dussek JE, Ferguson MWJ (eds): *Gray's Anatomy. The Anatomical Basis of Medicine and Surgery,* 38th ed. New York: Churchill Livingstone, 1995.

Willis MC: *Medical Terminology: The Language of Health Care.* Baltimore: Lippincott, Williams & Wilkins, 1995.

Index